The Cystic Kidney

The Cystic Kidney

edited by

Kenneth D. Gardner, Jr.
Department of Medicine
University of New Mexico Hospital
Albuquerque
USA

Jay Bernstein
Department of Anatomic Pathology
William Beaumont Hospital
Royal Oak
USA

KLUWER ACADEMIC PUBLISHERS
DORDRECHT / BOSTON / LONDON

Distributors

for the United States and Canada: Kluwer Academic Publishers, PO Box
358, Accord Station, Hingham, MA 02018-0358, USA
for all other countries: Kluwer Academic Publishers Group, Distribution
Center, PO Box 322, 3300 AH Dordrecht, The Netherlands

Library of Congress Cataloging-in-Publication Data

The cystic kidney / edited by Kenneth D. Gardner, Jr., Jay Bernstein.
    p.   cm. – – (Developments in Nephrology : 27)
    Includes index.

    ISBN-13: 978-94-010-6690-7   e-ISBN-13: 978-94-009-0457-6
    DOI: 10.1007/978-94-009-0457-6

    1. Kidney, Cystic.   2. Polycystic kidney disease.   I. Gardner,
Kenneth D.   II. Bernstein, Jay.   III. Series.
[DNLM: 1. Kidney, Cystic.   W1 DE998EB v.27 / WJ 358 C9975]
RC918.6′1—dc20
DNLM/DLC
for Library of Congress   89-15555

Contents

Preface

This is a book about renal cysts and cystic kidneys. Its contributors have created a resource of current information in a field that once aroused only curiosity, but that now stands at the leading edge of molecular nephrology. Its authorship includes 'oldtimers', who bring the wisdom of experience, and 'newcomers', whose presence attests to the contributions made by the investigative and technological advances of the past decade.

Its text is organized to carry the reader from renal cyst to cystic renal disease. Each of its chapters defines or explores a challenge or an advance. Cells that line renal cysts are diverse in structure, type, and perhaps function. The cysts themselves lie within an interstitium that is not normal and may influence cyst development and growth. Experimental analogs of human disease offer increasing opportunities to basic researchers to examine, in sequence and under controlled circumstances, those events that favor nephron dilation, cyst growth and ultimate renal failure.

While models have provided clues important to pathogenesis, it is appropriate that the greatest advance has come from the application of human molecular genetics. Probes have identified the short arm of human chromosome 16 as the site of a mutant gene responsible for autosomal dominant polycystic kidney disease in 95% of affected families. This demonstration has, in turn, opened to debate such questions as the ethics of gene-linkage analysis for *in utero* diagnosis and preclinical detection, and the question of whether, in the affected population, gene modification or control of gene expression is the more practical therapeutic goal.

In the heart of the volume are chapters on classification, radiography, systemic manifestations and management. Their contents reflect the contributions made by intellectual dialog, technology, and experience to the detection and treatment of renal cysts and cystic disorders. Finally, there are chapters on the renal cystic diseases themselves, encompassing those disorders that have proven most challenging to clinician, diagnostician and therapeutician, with whom rests the ultimate responsibility for control of morbidity and mortality.

We, the editors, have made no attempt through censorship to conceal conflict of opinion, where it exists, among the contributors. We have, however striven to place on display the levels of sophistication that have been achieved in understanding the pathogenesis and in detecting and treating these disorders.

We thank our contributors. We acknowledge our failure to include all the researchers and clinicians who currently continue to make substantial contributions to the field. We hope that the essays that appear in this volume convey the excitement that now surrounds the renal cyst and the disorders with which it is associated.

Kenneth D. Gardner Jr.   *Jay Bernstein*
Albuquerque, New Mexico   *Royal Oak, Michigan*
December, 1989

List of Contributors

ED Avner
University of Washington School of
  Medicine
Children's Hospital and Medical Center
4800 Sand Point Way NE/PO Box C5371
Seattle, WA 98105
USA

JM Barry
Division of Nephrology
Oregon Health Sciences University
3181 S.W. Sam Jackson Park Road
Portland, OR 97201
USA

WM Bennett
Division of Nephrology
Oregon Health Sciences University
3181 S.W. Sam Jackson Park Road
Portland, OR 97201
USA

J Bernstein
Department of Anatomic Pathology
William Beaumont Hospital
Royal Oak, MI 48072
USA

BR Cole
Division of Nephrology
Washington University School of Medicine
400 South Kingshighway
St Louis, MO 63110
USA

LW Elzinga
Division of Nephrology
Oregon Health Sciences University
3181 S.W. Sam Jackson Park Road
Portland, OR 97201
USA

AP Evan
Department of Anatomy
Indiana University School of Medicine
635 Barnhill Drive
Indianapolis, IN 46223
USA

PA Gabow
Medical Service
Denver General Hospital
777 Bannock Street
Denver, CO 80204-4507
USA

KD Gardner Jr.
Division of Renal Diseases
Department of Medicine
University of New Mexico School of
  Medicine
Albuquerque, NM 87131
USA

JJ Grantham
Department of Medicine
University of Kansas Medical Center
Rainbow Blvd at 39th Stret
Kansas City, KS 66103
USA

I Ishikawa
Department of Internal Medicine
Kanazawa Medical University
Uchinada, Kahoku
Ishikawa 920-02
Japan

CJ Kelly
Renal Electrolyte Section
Hospital of University of Pennsylvania
3400 Spruce Street
Philadelphia, PA 19104
USA

JM Kissane
Department of Pathology
Washington University School of Medicine
Box 8118
St Louis, MO 63110
USA

E Levine
Department of Diagnostic Radiology
University of Kansas Medical Center
Rainbow Blvd at 39th Street
Kansas City, KS 66103
USA

JA McAteer
Department of Anatomy
Indiana University School of Medicine
635 Barnhill Drive
Indianapolis, IN 46223
USA

EG Neilson
Renal Electrolyte Section
Hospital of University of Pennsylvania
3400 Spruce Street
Philadelphia, PA 19104
USA

CF Piel
Department of Pediatrics
University of California, San Francisco
400 Parnassus Avenue, Rm A276
San Francisco, CA 94143-0314
USA

ST Reeders
Howard Hughes Medical Institute
Departments of Nephrology and Human
  Genetics
Yale University School of Medicine
New Haven, CT 16510
USA

VE Torres
Division of Nephrology and Internal
  Medicine
Mayo Clinic and Mayo Foundation
1734 7th Street S.W.
Rochester, MN 55905
USA

WB Weil
Department of Pediatrics and Human
  Development
B-240 Life Sciences Building
Michigan State University
East Lansing, MI 48824-1317
USA

LW Welling
Department of Pathology
University of Kansas Medical Center
4801 Linwood Boulevard
Kansas City, MO 64128
USA

E Yendt
Division of Endocrinology
Etherington Hall
Queen's University
Kingston
Ontario K7L 3N6
Canada

Developments in Nephrology

1. J.S. Cheigh, K.H. Stenzel and A.L. Rubin (eds.): *Manual of Clinical Nephrology of the Rogosin Kidney Center*. 1981   ISBN 90-247-2397-3
2. K.D. Nolph (ed.): *Peritoneal Dialysis*. 1981 ed.: out of print 3rd revised and enlarged ed. 1988 (not this series)   ISBN 0-89838-406-0
3. A.B. Gruskin and M.E. Norman (eds.): *Pediatric Nephrology*. 1981   ISBN 90-247-2514-3
4. O. Schück: *Examination of the Kidney Function*. 1981   ISBN 0-89838-565-2
5. J. Strauss (ed.): *Hypertension, Fluid-electrolytes and Tubulopathies in Pediatric Nephrology*. 1982   ISBN 90-247-2633-6
6. J. Strauss (ed.): *Neonatal Kidney and Fluid-electrolytes*. 1983   ISBN 0-89838-575-X
7. J. Strauss (ed.): *Acute Renal Disorders and Renal Emergencies*. 1984   ISBN 0-89838-663-2
8. L.J.A. Didio and P.M. Motta (eds.): *Basic, Clinical, and Surgical Nephrology*. 1985   ISBN 0-89838-698-5
9. E.A. Freidman and C.M. Peterson (eds.): *Diabetic Nephropathy*. Strategy for Therapy. 1985   ISBN 0-89838-735-3
10. R. Dzúrik, B. Lichardus and W. Guder: *Kidney Metabolism and Function. 1985*   ISBN 90-247-2749-3
11. J. Straus (ed.): *Homeostasis, Nephrotoxicity, and Renal Anomalies in the Newborn*. 1986   ISBN 0-89838-766-3
12. D.G. Oreopoulos (ed.): *Geriatric Nephrology*. 1986   ISBN 0-89838-781-7
13. E.P. Paganini (ed.): *Acute Continuous Renal Replacement Therapy*. 1986   ISBN 0-89838-793-0
14. J.S. Cheigh, K.H. Stenzel and A.L. Rubin (eds.): *Hypertension in Kidney Disease*. 1986   ISBN 0-89838-797-3
15. N. Deane, R.J. Wineman and G.A. Benis (eds.): *Guide to Reprocessing of Hemodialyzers*. 1986   ISBN 0-89838-798-1
16. C. Ponticelli, L. Minetti and G. D'Amico (eds): *Antiglobulins, Cryoglobulins and Glomerulonephritis*. 1986   ISBN 0-89838-810-4
17. J. Strauss (ed.): with the assistance of L. Strauss: *Persistent Renal Genitourinary Disorders*. 1987   ISBN 0-89838-845-7
18. V.E. Andreucci and A. Dal Canton (eds.): *Diuretics*. Basic, Pharmacological, and Clinical Aspects. 1987   ISBN 0-89838-885-6
19. P.H. Bach and E.H. Lock (eds): *Nephrotoxicity in the Experimantal and Clinical Situation*, Part 1. 1987   ISBN 0-89838-997-1
20. P.H. Bach and E.H. Lock (eds): *Nephrotoxicity in the Experimantal and Clinical Situation*, Part 2. 1987   ISBN 0-89838-980-2

21. S.M. Gore and B.A. Bradley (eds.): *Renal Transplantation*. Sense and Sensitization. 1988   ISBN 0-89838-370-6
22. L. Minetti, G. D'Amico and C. Ponticelli: *The Kidney in Plasma Cell Dyscrasias*. 1988   ISBN 0-89838-385-4
23. A.S. Lindblad, J.W. Novak and K.D. Nolph (eds.): *Continuous Ambulatory Peritoneal Dialysis in the USA*. Final Report of the National CAPD Registry 1981–1988. 1989   ISBN 0-7923-0179-X
24. V.E. Andreucci and A. Dal Canton (eds.): *Current Therapy in Nephrology*. 1989   ISBN 0-7923-0206-0
25. L. Kovàks and B. Lichardus: *Vasopressin*. Disturbed Secretion and its Effects. 1989   ISBN 0-7923-0249-4

Section 1

1
Cysts and Cystic Kidneys

K.D. Gardner, Jr

Abstract

Cysts are dilated nephrons or ducts. They are found in kidneys with disease that is acquired or inherited. They can be induced to form in normal kidneys. A mutant gene is not required for their development. Dilated or cystic nephrons give cystic kidneys their characteristic appearance and their name, and they provide the distinguishing feature that enables observers to differentiate cystic from non-cystic kidneys. Dilated tubules and ducts thus are the hallmark, the sine qua non, of every cystic kidney. This essay reviews evidence that renal cysts are individual and distinctive lesions, each perhaps unique unto itself. It proposes that greater recognition be given to the diverse nature of cysts and that cystic kidneys be regarded as mosaics, organs of heterogeneous rather than homogeneous structure and function.

Key words   Cyst;
Cystic disease;
Duct;
Nephron;
Pathogenesis;
Tubule.

1. Introduction

Cystic kidneys are remarkably disordered organs (Fig. 1.1)[25]. They differ from one another in appearance, function, symptomatology and situational occurrence. They may be large or small. They may contain few or many cysts. They may be discovered *in utero*. They may develop during life. They may appear after years of endstage renal disease. They may or may not cause pain, bleeding, or arterial hypertension. They do or do not retain the capacity to function normally.

Cystic kidneys provide unique opportunities to investigators. In no other renal lesion is it possible to obtain, in such large amounts fluid, cells and epithelial membrane for *in vitro* chemical analysis[24,37], culture[48], and functional evaluation[49]. Cystic kidneys provoke challenge and intrigue: How and why do cysts form within their parenchyma? How do cysts grow? Cystic kidneys tantalize, for hidden in the answers to these questions seemingly are keys to the prevention and arrest of cyst growth and the expression of hereditary cystic

4

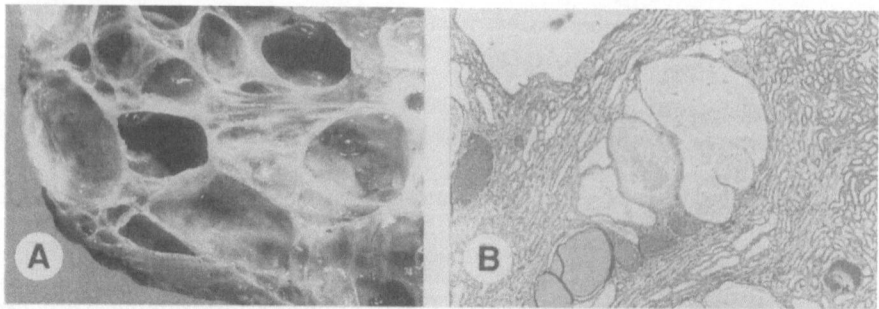

Figure 1.1 (A) Gross appearance of cut surface of kidney in late-stage autosomal polycystic kidney disease. Bulging, cavernous cysts chaotically distort renal architecture. (B) Microscopic appearance of cystic kidney from rat fed nordihydroguaiaretic acid to induce renal cystic disease (Gardner *et al.* 1986) (haematoxylin and eosin stain; approximately x 23). In this model, exposure to the cystogen is systemic. Cysts, however, develop along only some of the renal tubules and ducts. Note that cysts vary in size and content, with some containing proteinaceous and/or granular material, and that tubules adjacent to the larger cysts are compressed.

disease, and to potential savings to the endstage renal disease programme of hundreds of millions of dollars[31].

Research into the causes and candidate cures of renal cystic disease has intensified and diversified. While precise solutions have yet to be found, knowledge concerning the morphology of cysts and the circumstances under which they develop has expanded dramatically. Much new information has come from the study of models and has been interpreted (appropriately so, given prevalence and cost) in relation to its significance for human autosomal dominant polycystic kidney disease. To it is added the results of studies of the human genome.

Work to date identifies several alternative explanations for renal cyst formation: Epithelial cell hyperplasia, partial tubular obstruction, altered tubular basement membrane and net tubular secretion in place of reabsorption[19]. These choices are not mutually exclusive, but they sometimes prove difficult to reconcile with experience. Why, for example, should polycystic kidneys develop asynchronously[10,11,50] if all renal tubular basement membrane is excessively compliant[7,39,47]? Presumption that the product of a single mutant gene will prove to be responsible for one or more of the suspected pathogenetic mechanisms has been confounded by the identification of families with autosomal dominant polycystic disease in which the phenotype does not link to markers on chromosome 16[42,52].

This chapter provides an overview of cystic kidneys and the diseases they cause. It opens by focusing on the single characteristic that makes cystic kidneys recognizable and unique, namely the cysts themselves. It reviews evidence indicating that cysts in a cystic kidney, rather than being monotonously similar, are distinctive and perhaps even unique structures. Differences among cysts, among the cells that line their walls and the fluids that fill their lumens, dictate that cystic kidneys should be regarded as mosaics, composed of varying numbers of dissimilar cysts, really enormously dilated nephrons, interspersed among relatively normal tubules and ducts (Fig. 1.1A).

2. Cysts and cystic nephrons

In most organs, cysts develop as blind, fluid-filled sacs. In the kidney some cysts are of this type[30]. Other renal cysts, however, communicate with the lumens of the tubules or ducts from which they arise. Cysts with this configuration appear as dilated segments of nephrons (Fig. 1.2). Both types have been identified in kidneys of autosomal dominant polycystic disease; both occur in the same polycystic kidney[30].

Within any given kidney, cysts differ in lining and content. Cyst wall epithelium is cuboidal or columnar, may or may not be hyperplastic, and sometimes forms small polypoid structures[14,15,32]. Differences in cell type exist not only among cysts but also among sites on the wall of a single cyst[4,15,32]. Cysts, at least those in polycystic and medullary cystic kidneys, contain fluids of differing appearance, chemical composition[24,37], cellular contents[14,35] and cytokine-like activity[23]. Hydrostatic pressures are elevated in the cysts of some polycystic kidneys[6,12] and in some models[25]. These findings seemingly make it difficult to challenge the statement that cysts are individual structures. Nonetheless, the literature continues to contain allusions to two types of cyst fluids in polycystic kidney disease[24,37], and to imply that epithelium from polycystic kidneys is a single type when, at least on morphological grounds, it is not[15,45,55].

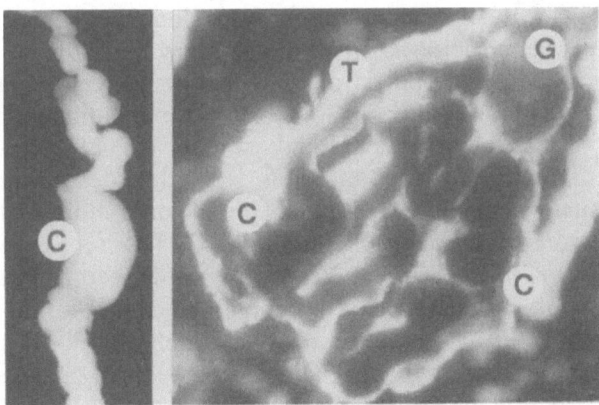

Figure 1.2 Latex castings of cystic nephrons in experimental cystic disease. (*Left*) A single area of focal dilation (C) along a collecting duct. (*Right*) Multiple dilated segments (C) along a proximal tube (T) of otherwise normal diameter. Latex also has filled Bowman's space (G). (Each approximately x38).

6

In the past no definitive criteria were used to distinguish *cystic* from merely *dilated* nephrons or ducts. The choice of designation was left to the opinion of the moment, and observers were inconsistent in their choice of terms. The results were a lack of uniformity in the naming of identical lesions and the appearance in the literature of such imaginative, but non-specific, terms as *cystoid* and *thyroidization* [33], terms that beg the issue of whether cysts are present and whether a given kidney is or should be considered cystic. To avoid further confusion the suggestion was made recently that the term *cyst* be used to designate tubules or ducts that have dilated to diameters greater that four times normal, that is, to diameters of 200 microns or more[25].

In themselves dilated nephrons and ducts are common pathological findings and are not unique to cystic kidneys. They occur in many renal disorders, including the interstitial nephritides and some of the glomerulonephritides. They are remarkable in cystic kidneys because of their size. Why ducts and tubules in cystic kidneys grow to such enormous proportions is not clear. The nature, duration, or intensity of the etiopathologic insult might govern final size. For example, a severe, acute process might favor dilation, while a milder and more chronic one might favor peritubular fibrosis, shrinkage, and tubular collapse and atrophy instead. Whether the pathogenesis of cyst expansion is the same as that responsible for the dilation seen in kidneys with chronic interstitial nephritis and other non-cystic, chronic nephropathies is not known. Suspicions are aroused[8,41].

Dilation, when it is present, usually is segmental. That is to say, it involves portions rather than entire lengths of affected, cystic structures[1,25,43].

Multiple influences evidently interact to cause nephrons to dilate. Some of these influences are general. For example, in some diseases, such as in multiple myeloma with amyloidosis or in diabetes mellitus, a systemic insult is held responsible for the development of renal lesions in which tubular dilation is striking in degree and extent[33]. In other disorders, heritable influences seem to predispose kidneys to nephron dilation and cyst development. Two outstanding examples of these diseases are the autosomal dominant and recessive forms of polycystic kidney disease. Medullary cystic disease–nephronophthisis is a third, but unlike the former conditions, it is a disorder in which renal cyst formation is inconstant[26]. Heredity also predisposes animals to renal cyst development, as exemplified by CFWwd[54] and CPK[17,27] mice.

While systemic influences can readily be implicated as predisposing or conditioning factors in renal cyst development, the configuration and distribution of cystic nephrons within a cystic kidney imply that local, not systemic, conditions determine whether a given duct or tubule will dilate sufficiently to become cystic. Several experimental examples are available of a more generalized insult leading to localized cyst formation. In rodents, the feeding of certain drugs and chemicals results in cyst formation along only some of the nephrons and ducts in the animals' kidneys[25]. In the fetal rabbit, ligation of the ureter, a lesion that obstructs outflow from the entire kidney, results in seg-

segmental dilations (cyst development) along a fraction of the tubules in the obstructed organ[16]. Papillectomy in rabbits is followed by cyst development along the course of a few of the interrupted tubules[9]. In each of these examples, cyst development involves only a fraction of the nephrons that are present, even though the insult that provokes it is generalized and sometimes even extrarenal.

Cystic ducts and tubules also can be induced to form after the insults that are reasonably well localized. "Figure 8" ties around the kidney and searing of the renal surface are two experimental approaches that lead to the subsequent development of dilated, cystic tubules that are restricted in their distribution to areas adjacent to the sites of trauma[25].

Nephrons can be made cystic at will. This fact indicates that heritable factors are not solely responsible for cyst development and, perhaps, that they need not be involved. The diverse observations that systemic or generalized insults lead to the segmental dilation of some but not other nephrons in a kidney, in my judgement, strongly implicate local factors in the pathogenesis of cysts. This impression is reinforced by the singular phenomenon of asynchronicity in autosomal dominant polycystic kidney disease. Cyst development can be far more dramatic in one kidney than the other as the lesion evolves and before endstage is reached[11,50].

3. Cystic kidneys

A *cystic kidney* is a kidney with 3–5 or more cystic (enormously dilated) nephrons or ducts[25].

Cystic kidneys have disordered rather than ordered structure and function. They contain a variable number of tubules and ducts, usually a small fraction of the total, that are massively dilated. The rest appear normal in their structure and function[5,30]. To the extent that generalizations can be made, it is the dilated nephrons and ducts (Fig. 1.2) that selectively exhibit proliferating epithelial cells and altered tubular basement membrane, are surrounded by an interstitium that is infiltrated by inflammatory and round cells, and possess disparate glomerular filtration rates and intranephron hydrostatic pressures.

As frivolous as the points may seem, both the number of cystic nephrons that must be present in order to characterize a kidney as cystic and the apportionment of cystic nephrons between the two kidneys in order to define the disease as bilateral have emerged as issues relevant to clinical diagnosis. For example, a single cyst in the kidney of a chronic dialysis patient may represent acquired renal cystic disease. It may be, on the other hand, a simple renal cyst and little worthy of further clinical consideration. Cyst *number* is invoked in order that kidneys with simple cysts can be distinguished from those with acquired renal cystic disease. The greater the number of cysts, the more likely the possibility that they represent disease. Therefore, some minimum number greater than one or two seems to be the reasonable criterion to apply when designating a kidney as cystic. We have suggested the number three or more[25]; others have suggested five, leaving little room for doubt[18,36].

Bilaterality is a useful criterion in the diagnosis of autosomal dominant polycystic kidney and acquired renal cystic diseases[10,11,18,36,47]. However, both dominant polycystic disease and acquired renal cystic disease may develop asynchronously, more and larger cysts in one kidney than the other, and therefore, may present at a stage when only one kidney is detectably cystic[25,50]. In this situation, the criterion of a minimum number of cysts necessary to designate a kidney as cystic needs to be modified. When other circumstances give reason to suspect autosomal dominant polycystic kidney disease, for example a family history that is positive for the disorder, the finding of but one cyst in each kidney or one cyst in one kidney and one or more liver cysts is adequate grounds for clinical diagnosis[18]. A history of long-standing renal failure, dialysis, or renal transplantation is helpful in establishing the probability of acquired disease in the presence of one or two cysts in each kidney. In brief, the plausibility of a diagnosis of cystic kidney disease is strengthened when renal cysts are multiple and/or bilateral.

4. Models of renal cyst development

A variety of animal models that are suitable for the laboratory study of renal cyst development are available. Those in which hereditary factors participate include CPK mice[17,27], CFWwd mice[54], the springbok[38] and rat[53]. In all, disease occurs as a recessive trait. There is no good animal model of dominantly inherited cyst development available at present.

Models provide numerous advantages for the study of cyst development. They can be created and manipulated at the convenience of the investigator. They mimic human disease. In most, the lesion which develops does so in the same way that it appears to develop in man–progressively in kidneys whose previous morphology was normal. The study of models has disclosed or confirmed at least three major abnormalities of function and structure in cystic kidneys: elevated hydrostatic pressures in cystic nephrons (Figs. 1.3A and 1.3B); widely disparate single nephron glomerular filtration rates (Fig. 1.3C); and new cell growth[25]. Elevated pressures and altered cell growth occur in human disease; single nephron filtration rates have not been measured. Observations in models have been responsible for the rediscovery of the epithelial proliferation that exists in so many different kinds of cystic kidneys[25].

Drugs and chemicals that are known to induce cyst development include antioxidants, such as diphenylamine, diphenylthiazole and nordihydroguaiaretic acid; streptozotocin; and *cis*-platinum and lithium chloride, two agents that cause cyst development in the kidneys of animals and humans[13,34]. In general terms, dietary exposure to, or parenteral administration of one of these substances on a chronic basis leads to slowly evolving renal disease.

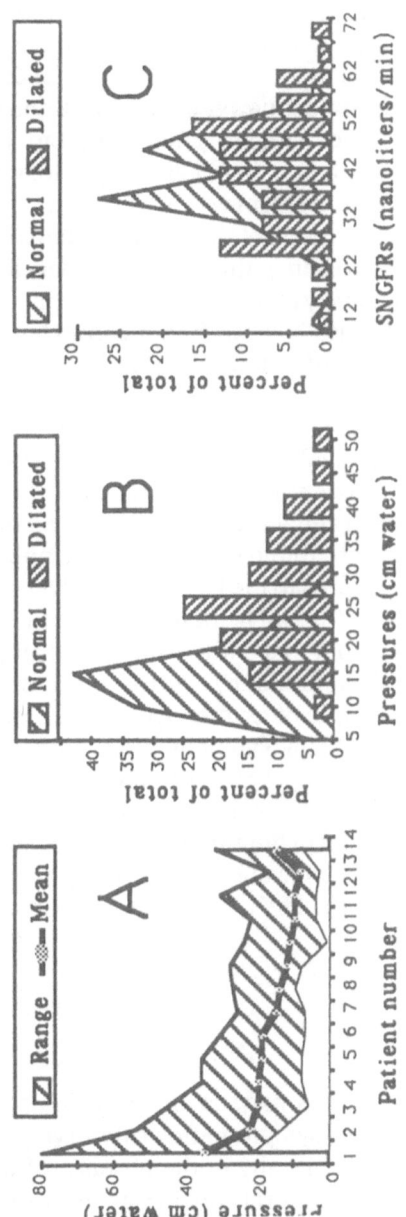

Figure 1.3 Functional heterogeneity in cystic human and experimental kidneys. (A) Intracystic hydrostatic pressures in human polycystic kidneys. Means and ranges of pressure are shown for each of 14 subjects in whom intracystic pressures were measured *in vivo* by direct manometry. Means and ranges vary among subjects; the overall pattern of pressures (hatched area) is highly variable (adapted from data in Bjerle *et al.* 1971). (B) Histogram of intraluminal pressure readings. Pressures were measured directly using a servo-nulling device in 41 dilated (cystic) and 27 normal surface proximal tubules of rats with induced renal cystic disease (personal observation). Approximately 50% of pressures in dilated tubules are similar to those measured in normal tubules; the remaining 50% (and the overall mean) are higher. (C) Histogram of single nephron glomerular filtration rates (SNGFRs) in dilated (cystic) and normal tubules. SNGFRs were measured in 61 dilated cortical nephrons of 21 kidneys from rats with chemically induced renal cystic disease, and are contrasted here with SNGFRs measured in 41 nephrons of 10 normal rat kidneys. Means are similar in the two types (dilated: 40.3 ± 1.9 nl/min; normal: 40.4 ± 1.7 nl/min). However, SNGFRs vary to a significantly greater degree among the dilated tubules (*P*

Clearly, heredity alone is not the ultimate determinant for the formation of renal cysts.

Manipulation of the ambient environment can determine not only whether cysts form, but also the rate at which cysts develop. Germ-free rats that are fed nordihydroguaiaretic acid in a sterile environment develop renal cysts when they are exposed to lipopolysaccharide, either by feeding them endo-toxin-containing bacteria or by injecting them intraperitoneally with endo-toxin[20,22]. Rats maintained under similar conditions, but not exposed to endotoxin, develop little or no change in renal morphology after the same interval of dietary exposure to the cystogen.

This observation underscores the fact that host and environment interact in the expression of nephrotoxity, seen in this case as the development of renal cysts. The behavior of this model may contain lessons relevant to the pathogen-esis of acquired renal cystic disease in man. Endotoxin exposure, as a conse-quence of either urinary tract infection or dialysis, might provoke cyst development in this entity.

Cyst development in models does not resemble human disease in every respect. One major difference involves the symmetry of cyst formation. In virtually all models, cyst development is bilateral. The exceptions are models in which surgical manipulation or renal trauma has occurred unilaterally[25]. In these models, dilated nephrons are found only in the manipulated kidney.

There is no evidence that trauma to the kidney is involved in the formation of cysts in man. Ureteral obstruction can be demonstrated in many congenital multiplastic (dysplastic) kidneys, but that entity is the sole example of complete obstruction among humans with cystic kidneys. Autosomal dominant polycystic kidney disease is the classic example of asymmetric cyst development in man. Some 25–50% of cases present with involvement in one kidney that is far more advanced than in the other[10,11,50]. There is no predilection as to side. Some as yet unidentified factor(s) operating within the kidneys of these individuals must determine not whether cysts will form but the rates at which they will develop. Partial obstruction of individual nephrons has been implicated as one local condition favoring cyst development[4,15]. The microenvironment of dilating nephrons is a second[23,25].

5. Renal cysts in man

Cyst development in human kidneys may be single or multiple; regional or diffuse; acquired or inherited; and symptomatic or non-symptomatic. One or two cysts, found unilaterally or bilaterally in the absence of familial disease, usually represent simple cysts. Unilateral renal cysts most often represent a congenital multicystic (dysplastic) kidney. Cysts that are diffuse and bilateral, especially if present in enlarged kidneys, most likely represent the expression of autosomal dominant or recessive polycystic kidney disease. Cysts that are multiple and bilateral but present in endstage (small) kidneys are most likely indicative of acquired renal cystic disease. The possibility of medullary cystic disease should be considered when cyst development dominates at the corticomedullary junction and where the family history is positive.

Autosomal dominant polycystic kidney disease is the most prevalent of the human renal cystic diseases. The responsible mutation may occupy either of at least two different chromosomal sites. One site, accounting for the disorder in over 95% of affected families, is located on the short arm of chromosome 16[51]. The site of the second remains unidentified[42,52].

Gene expression appears to be virtually 100% by the age of 80 years, but renal failure is not inevitable[10]. Roughly 50% of affected individuals achieve that age without manifesting renal failure[2]. Uncontrollable pain and infection currently are considered indications for cyst puncture or deroofing by experienced physicians under carefully monitored circumstances[3]. The medical treatment of hypertension and urinary tract infection appears to offer the best means available to control morbidity and perhaps delay endstage disease.

A progressive decline in renal function characterizes the clinical course of one half of affected individuals. Intraluminal hydrostatic pressures are variably elevated, both within and among cysts in autosomal dominant polycystic kidneys (Fig. 1.3A), lending credence to the hypothesis that cyst expansion, with compression of adjacent normal nephrons, is the cause of progressing azotemia. In this disorder, at least, progressive nephron dilation, therefore, becomes the critical determinant in targeting any therapeutic strategy that is intended to slow or stop the development of endstage disease.

Cellular hyperplasia and micropolyp formation also occur in autosomal dominant polycystic kidney disease. Deaths from metastatic adenocarcinoma of the kidney are infrequent.

Acquired renal cystic disease is a term denoting the appearance of bilateral multiple cysts in the previously non-cystic kidneys of chronic dialysis patients. The entity is well established, affecting approximately 40% of patients on chronic dialytic therapy. Acquired renal cystic disease has proven to be a significant cause of morbidity in this population. Cyst rupture and the development of adenomas and renal adenocarcinomas occur with increased frequencies. The factor(s) responsible for acquired renal cystic disease have not been identified. Exposure to dialysis membranes has been considered, but can be ruled out by the fact that the lesion occurs in patients who have never received hemodialysis[40]. Factors related to senescence seem more likely candidates. The occurrence of acquired renal cystic disease in individuals whose chronic renal failure has never been treated by dialysis suggests that the characteristics of the lesion reflect kidneys that have lived beyond their time.

The occurrence of renal adenocarcinoma among dialysis patients with acquired renal cystic disease approximates 45 times that of the general population[21] (Fig. 1.4). Given this astounding figure, it is curious that more individuals with the lesion do not die of metastatic adenocarcinoma. Together,

12

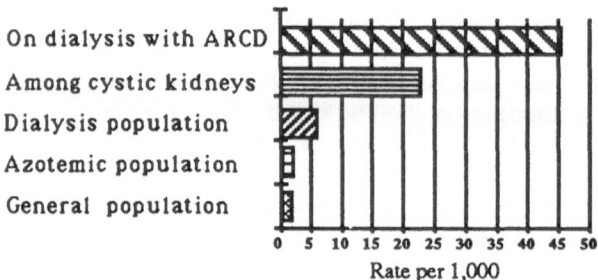

Figure 1.4 Prevalence of renal adenocarcinoma in various sub-groups of the population (adapted from Gardner and Evan 1984). The frequency of reported malignancy is significantly greater ($P < 0.05$) among cystic kidneys and among subjects who develop acquired renal cystic disease while on dialysis.

autosomal dominant polycystic kidney disease and acquired renal cystic disease account for more than 95% of all renal cystic disease in humans.

6. Pathogenesis

The pathogenesis of cyst development in these and other renal cystic disorders remains poorly understood, in spite of intensified investigative efforts over the past decade. Proliferation and fluid accumulation are involved. It is not established, however, whether either of these events are primary or are secondary to other abnormalities in the kidney. Any theory of pathogenesis must consider the heterogeneous nature of the cystic kidney, the disparate hydrostatic pressures that are found among the tubular structures, the fact that dilating nephrons need not be totally obstructed, and the focal and local patterns of epithelial hyperplasia that occur.

In the past, increased compliance of tubular basement membrane was an attractive theoretical possibility to explain cyst development, in autosomal dominant polycystic disease at least. Basement membrane is abnormal in its appearance and structure around most cystic nephrons. The change in appearance, however, is more often thickening rather than thinning, and *in vitro* studies fail to demonstrate an increase in the degree of its elasticity[29]. Intracystic pressures that vary among cysts in the same polycystic kidney (Figs. 1.3A and 1.3B) offer what is perhaps the strongest argument against a causative role for altered compliance of basement membrane in the development of cysts. One would expect intracystic pressures to be similar, were intervening membrane and interstitium to offer no significant barrier to the equalization of pressures throughout a cystic kidney.

Net secretion into rather than reabsorption from cystic nephrons is a second theoretical consideration. It is strengthened by *in vitro* observations that MDCK cells form fluid-filled cysts when grown under carefully controlled conditions in the laboratory[28,45,46,55], and that cyst development in kidneys from CPK mice involves the presence of increased amounts of Na–K ATPase[1]. In the intact kidney, however, active solute secretion into a cystic lumen has not been demonstrated and *in vitro* cyst walls, if they transport at all, do so in an outward direction[49].

Elevated pressures in dilated nephrons (Figs. 1.3A and 1.3B) suggest that resistance to their outflow is increased, offering a third conceptual suggestion as to how dilation might occur. The idea is reinforced by the finding that some dilating nephrons may be partially occluded at their distal outlets by the tiny micropolyps that develop in these kidneys[4,15]. However, polyps are not invariably found at these critical locations, indicating that this alternative may not be universally applicable.

Advances in molecular biology promise to change current concepts regarding cyst development. For example, studies in SV40 transgenic mice, in which renal cyst formation is dramatic, demonstrate a high degree of gene expression in the abnormal kidney[44]. Abnormal proteins can be demonstrated in western blots of cellular material from kidneys in autosomal dominant polycystic kidney disease[28,55]. Both reflect the possibility that abnormal genetic material is preferentially expressed in the affected organ. In addition to variability in the chemical composition of their contents, cysts in autosomal dominant polycystic kidney disease also contain a variety of monokines and lymphokines[23], raising the possibility that epithelial hyperplasia, fluid accumulation and altered collagen are secondary rather than primary manifestations of the phenotype.

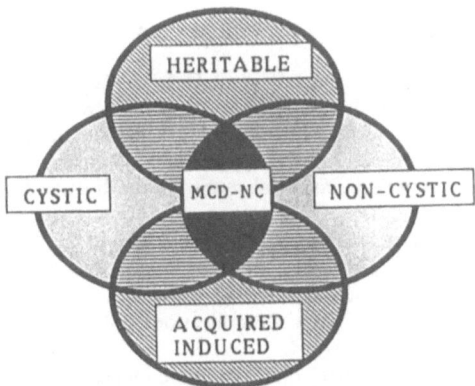

Figure 1.5 Cartoon of the universe of renal disease. Cystic disease is inherited, acquired or induced. The medullary cystic disease–nephronophthisis complex (MCD–NC) occupies an intermediate position in that it may be inherited or acquired and may be cystic or non-cystic in character. The extent to which heritable factors influence the acquisition of renal cysts in man may be considerable (Gardner 1988), but is not established and thus no overlap is shown. (Not drawn to scale.)

7. Final comments

As a group, cystic diseases of the kidney comprise a fraction, perhaps 12–14%[31], of all renal disease (Fig. 1.5). Among all cystic diseases, morphologic, genetic and clinical criteria distinguish individual entities. An entity, once segregated and identified, usually has been regarded *in toto* [1,8,10,11,15,26,29,31,39,41,43,47,50], with its manifestations considered to be similar among all affected subjects. The tendency to "group" extends to organ pathology, which is often thought of as being relatively constant from kidney to kidney. This approach is misleading to the extent that it glosses over the differences in appearance, configuration, lining, content and function that distinguish cysts from one another, even in the same kidney. It is not surprising, then, that different approaches to the study of pathogenesis have led to several concepts rather than to a single unifying explanation of why cysts form and how they grow[19]. Individual investigators tend to pursue their own individual interests and often interpret the results of successful studies as "representative" of all cystic kidneys or of all kidneys in a particular disease. The art of grouping may be justified only when it can be shown that the heterogeneity of structure and function that exists in the cystic kidney is irrelevant to pathogenesis and failure. No such demonstration has been forthcoming to date. For the future, it seems wise to ask: "Why does a cyst form?" "How does a cyst grow?". And to seek an answer to a third question: "What accounts for the differences that are observed among cysts in almost every cystic kidney?".

References

1. Avner ED. Renal cystic disease: Insights from recent experimental investigations. Nephron 1988, 48, 89–93.
2. Bear JC, McManamon P, Morgan J, Payne RH, Lewis H, Gault MH and Churchill ON. Age at clinical onset and at ultrasonic detection of adult polycystic kidney disease: Data for genetic counselling. American Journal of Medical Genetics 1984, 18, 45–53.
3. Bennett W, Elzinga L, Golper T and Barry J. Reduction of cyst volume for symptomatic management of autosomal dominant polycystic kidney disease. Journal of Urology 1987, 137, 620–622.
4. Bernstein J, Evan AP and Gardner KD. Human cystic kidney diseases: Epithelial hyperplasia in the pathogenesis of cysts and tumors. Pediatric Nephrology 1987, 1, 393–396.
5. Bernstein J. Morphology of human renal cystic disease. In: Cummings NB and Klahr S, eds., Chronic Renal Disease: Causes, Complications, and Treatment. New York: Plenum Medical Book Company 1985, 47–54.
6. Bjerle P, Lindqvist B and Michaelson G. Pressure measurements in renal cysts. Scandinavian Journal of Laboratory and Clinical Medicine 1971, 27, 135–138.
7. Butkowski RJ, Carone FA, Granthan JJ and Hudson BG. Tubular basement membrane changes in 2-amino-4,5-diphenylthiazole-induced polycystic disease. Kidney International 1985, 28, 744–751.
8. Carone FA. Functional changes in polycystic kidney disease are tubulo-interstitial in origin. Seminars in Nephrology 1988, 8, 89–93.

9. Cuttino JT, Herman PG and Mellins HZ. The renal collecting system after medullary damage. Investigative Radiology 1977, 12, 241–245.
10. Dalgaard OA. Bilateral polycystic disease of the kidneys. A follow-up of two hundred and eighty four patients and their families. Acta Medica Scandinavica 1957, 158 (Suppl 328), 1–255.
11. Delaney VB, Adler S, Bruns FJ, Licinia M, Segal DP and Fraley DS. Autosomal dominant polycystic kidney disease: Presentation, complications, and prognosis. American Journal of Kidney Disease 1985, 5, 104–111.
12. Derezuc D and Cecuk L. Possible role for enzyme inhibition in controlling kidney cysts (Letter). Lancet 1978, 1, 217.
13. Dobyan DC, Hill D, Lewis T and Bulger RE. Cyst formation in rat kidney induced by cis-platinum administration. Laboratory Investigation 1981, 45, 260–268.
14. Duncan KA, Cuppage FE and Grantham JJ. Urinary lipid bodies in polycystic kidney disease. American Journal of Kidney Disease 1985, 5, 49–53.
15. Evan AP, Gardner KD and Berstein J. Polypoid and papillary epithelial hyperplasia: A potential cause of ductal obstruction in adult polycystic disease. Kidney International 1979, 16, 743–750.
16. Fetterman GH, Ravitch MM and Sherman FE. Cystic changes in fetal kidneys following ureteral ligation: Studies by microdissection. Kidney International 1974, 5, 111–121.
17. Fry JL, Koch WE, Jennette JC, McFarland E, Fried FA and Mandell J. A genetically determined murine model of infantile polycystic kidney disease. Journal of Urology 1985, 134, 828–833.
18. Gabow PA, Inklerman DW and Holmes JH. Polycystic kidney disease: Prospective analysis of nonazotemic patients and family members. Annals of Internal Medicine 1984, 101, 238–247.
19. Gardner KD Jr. Pathogenesis of human renal cystic disease. Annual Review of Medicine 1988, 39, 185–191.
20. Gardner KD, Evan AP and Reed WP. Accelerated renal cyst development in deconditioned germ-free rats. Kidney International 1986, 29, 1116–1123.
21. Gardner KD and Evan AP. Cystic kidneys: An enigma evolves. American Journal of Kidney Diseases 1984, 3, 403–413.
22. Gardner KD, Reed WP, Evan AP, Zedalis J, Hylarides MD and Leon AA. Endotoxin provocation of experimental renal cystic disease. Kidney International 1987, 32, 329–334.
23. Gardner KD, Sadick MD, Elzinga LW, Bennett WM and Locksley RM. Evidence of cytokine-like substances and inhibitor(s) in human renal cyst fluid (Abstract). Kidney International 1989, 35, 369.
24. Gardner KD. Composition of fluid in twelve cysts of a polycystic kidney. New England Journal of Medicine 1969, 281, 985–988.
25. Gardner KD. Cystic kidneys. Kidney International 1988, 33, 610–621.
26. Gardner KD. Juvenile nephronophthisis and renal medullary cystic disease. In: Gardner KD, ed., Cystic Diseases of the Kidney. New York: John Wiley & Sons, 1976, 173–185.
27. Gattone VH, Calvet JP, Cowley BD Jr, Evan AP, Shaver TS, Helmstadter K and Grantham JJ. Autosomal recessive polycystic kidney disease in a murine model: A gross and microscopic description. Laboratory Investigation 1988, 59, 231–238.
28. Granot Y, Van Putten V, Summer S, Granot H, Gabow P and Schrier R. The biosynthesis of intra- and extracellular proteins by cultured human polycystic kidney (HPKD) cells (Abstract). Clinical Research 1988, 135A.
29. Grantham JJ, Donoso VS, Evan AP, Carone FA and Gardner KD. Intrinsic viscoelastic properties of tubule basement membranes in experimental renal cystic disease. Kidney International 1987, 32, 187–197.
30. Grantham JJ, Geiser JL and Evan AP. Cyst formation and growth in autosomal dominant polycystic kidney disease. Kidney International 1987, 31, 1145–1152.
31. Grantham JJ. Polycystic kidney disease – an old problem in a new context. New England Journal of Medicine 1988, 319, 944–946.

32. Gregiore JR, Torres VE, Holley KE and Farrow GM. Renal epithelial hyperplastic and neoplastic proliferation in autosomal dominant polycystic kidney disease. American Journal of Kidney Diseases 1987, 9, 29–38.

33. Heptinstall RH. Pathology of the Kidney, 3rd Edition. Boston: Little, Brown and Company, 1983, 1024.

34. Hestbech J, Hansen HE, Amdisen A and Olsen S. Chronic renal lesions following long-term treatment with lithium. Kidney International 1977, 12, 205–213.

35. Hilpert PL, Friedman AC, Radecki PD, Caroline DF, Fishman EK, Meziane MA, Mitchell DG and Kressel HY. MRI of hemorrhagic renal cysts in polycystic kidney disease. American Journal of Roentgenology 1986, 146, 1167–1172.

36. Hossack KF, Leddy CL, Johnson AM, Schrier RW and Gabow PA. Echocardiographic findings in autosomal dominant polycystic kidney disease. New England Journal of Medicine 1988, 319, 907–912.

37. Huseman R, Grady A, Welling D and Grantham J. Macropuncture study of polycystic disease in adult human kidneys. Kidney International 1980, 118, 375–385.

38. Iverson WO, Fetterman GH, Jacobson ER, Olsen JH, Senior DF and Schobert EE. Polycystic kidney and liver disease in springbok: I. Morphology of the lesions. Kidney International 1982, 22, 146–155.

39. Kanwar JS and Carone FA. Reversible changes of tubular cell and basement membrane in drug-induced cystic disease. Kidney International 1984, 26, 35-43.

40. Katz A, Sombolos K and Oreopoulos DG. Acquired cystic disease of the kidney in association with chronic ambulatory peritoneal dialysis. American Journal of Kidney Diseases 1987, 9, 426–429.

41. Kelly CJ and Neilson EG. Medullary cystic disease: An inherited form of autoimmune interstitial nephritis? American Journal of Kidney Diseases 1987, 10, 389–395.

42. Kimberling WJ, Fain PR, Kenyon JB, Goldgar D, Sujansky E and Gabow PA. Linkage heterogeneity of autosomal dominant polycystic kidney disease. New England Journal of Medicine 1988, 319, 913–918.

43. Lambert PP. Polycystic disease of the kidney: A review. Archives of Pathology 1947, 44, 34–58.

44. MacKay K, Striker LJ, Pinkert CA, Brinster RL and Striker GE. Glomerulosclerosis and renal cysts in mice transgenic for the early region of SV40. Kidney International 1987, 32, 827–837.

45. McAteer JA, Carone FA, Grantham JJ, Kempson SA, Gardner KD Jr and Evan AP. Explant culture of human polycystic kidney. Laboratory Investigation 1988, 59, 126–128.

46. McAteer JA, Dougherty GS, Gardner KD Jr and Evan AP. Polarized epithelial cysts in vitro: A review of cell and explant culture systems that exhibit epithelial cyst formation. Scanning Microscopy 1988, 1739–1763.

47. Milutinovic J and Agodoa LY. Potential causes and pathogenesis in autosomal dominant polycystic kidney disease. Nephron 1983, 33, 139–144.

48. Muther RS and Bennett WM. Cyst fluid antibiotic concentration in polycystic kidney disease: Differences between proximal and distal cysts. Kidney International 1981, 20, 519–522.

49. Perrone RD. In vitro function of cyst epithelium from human polycystic kidney disease. Journal of Clinical Investigation 1985, 76, 1688–1691.

50. Porch P, Noe HN and Stapleton FB. Unilateral presentation of adult-type polycystic kidney disease in children. Journal of Urology 1986, 135, 744–746.

51. Reeders ST, Breuning MH, Davies KE, Nicholls RD, Jarman AP, Higgs DR, Pearson PL and Weatherall DJ. A highly polymorphic DNA marker linked to adult polycystic kidney disease on chromosome 16. Nature 1985, 317, 542–543.

52. Romeo G, Devoto M, Costa G, Roncuzzi L, Catizone L, Zuchelli P, Germino GG, Keith T, Weatherall DJ and Reeders ST. A second genetic locus for autosomal dominant polycystic kidney disease. Lancet 1988, 2, 8–11.

53. Solomon S. Inherited renal cysts in rats. Science 1973, 181, 451–452.

54. Werder AA, Amos MA, Nielsen AH and Wolfe GH. Comparative effects of germ-free and ambient environments on the development of cystic kidney disease in CFWwd mice. Journal of Laboratory and Clinical Medicine 1984, 103, 399–407.

55. Wilson P, Schrier RW, Breckon RD and Gabow PA. A new method for studying human polycystic kidney disease epithelia in culture. Kidney International 1986, 30, 381–378.

Section 2

2
Cyst Cells and Cyst Walls

A.P. Evan and J.A. McAteer

Abstract

Tubular dilatation to the point of cyst formation is found in a number of disease entities. It involves epithelial hyperplasia and fluid accumulation, preceded by cell injury. Hyperplasia in the cyst wall takes many forms and is commonly accompanied by inflammatory cell infiltration and tubular atrophy. Cells of the cyst wall include not only the lining epithelium, but also migratory cells of the immune system that may be promoters of cell proliferation and altered epithelial function. Renal cysts arise as focal sites of tubular dilatation and communicate with the nephron or collecting tubule. Cells of newly formed cysts exhibit morphologic features that are typical of their tubular segments of origin. As cysts enlarge, most lose connection with renal tubules and come to be lined by an unidentifiable cell type. The early-stage cystic kidney has not been studied in detail. Understanding of the progression of the cystic lesion is limited.

Key words   Cyst;
                 Epithelium;
                 Histopathology;
                 Hyperplasia;
                 Ultrastructure.

1. Introduction

The morphology of cyst cells and cyst walls has been defined in kidneys from animals and humans with heritable, induced, and acquired renal cystic diseases. The bulk of information comes from observations on the kidneys of human autosomal dominant polycystic kidney disease (ADPKD)[32]. ADPKD is a common progressive form of renal cystic disease[2,3,4,13], but understanding of its ontogeny is limited. There is evidence that tubular and glomerular dilatation occurs in the fetus. It is unknown whether fetal onset is typical of ADPKD, and one does not know when cysts begin. Most of what is known about cyst cells and cyst walls comes from studies of advanced disease. Greater understanding is needed of the earliest stages of renal cyst development.

2. The early-stage cystic kidney

2.1. Acquisition of material

Because the early stages of renal cyst development are asymptomatic, it is not possible to define the exact moment at which cyst formation begins. The investigator is handicapped by at least three circumstances. First, taking ADPKD as the example, in cases without a positive family history and no symptoms or signs of cyst development, it is unlikely that a search for renal cysts will be made. As a consequence, early cystic kidneys go undetected, and the opportunity to examine their structure is missed. Second, even in the presence of positive family history and positive gene-linkage analysis, small cysts may escape clinical detection. Present-day diagnostic imaging techniques are not sensitive enough to resolve the "precystic" dilated tubule that can easily be recognized by histological examination[29,41,42]. Third, kidneys in the early stages of cyst formation tend to be fully functional and do little, therefore, to call attention to themselves. They are recognized only when hematuria, pain, or hypertension ultimately focuses attention upon them[2,21,29,42]. Thus, opportunities to examine early cystic lesions are limited.

ADPKD has been diagnosed on the basis of positive family history and gene-linkage analysis in a nine-week fetus[39]. Kidneys from this case showed tubular dilatations that were multiple and measured up to $200\,\mu$m in diameter; multiple glomerular cysts of diameters as great as $300\,\mu$m also were present. Other, earlier reports describe cystic tubules in a set of 14-week post-conception twins and in stillborn fetuses of 27 and 29 weeks gestation, respectively[8,15]. These reports are important because they clearly demonstrate that renal cyst development can begin during the fetal period.

2.2. General features

General features of the early cystic lesion in ADPKD include dilatation at any site along the nephron, hyperplasia of the epithelium that lines cysts, tubular cell injury and atrophy, hypertrophy of proximal tubular cells, glomerular sclerosis, glomerular and basement membrane thickening, interstitial fibrosis and scarring, and inflammatory cell infiltration (Fig. 2.1). These changes occur against a background of normal renal structure.

2.3. Cyst distribution and occurrence

Cysts in early ADPKD are scattered from cortex to inner medulla. Most appear as focal, spherical tubular dilatations (Fig. 2.2). Their appearance is unlike that in autosomal recessive polycystic kidney disease (ARPKD), in which lengthy

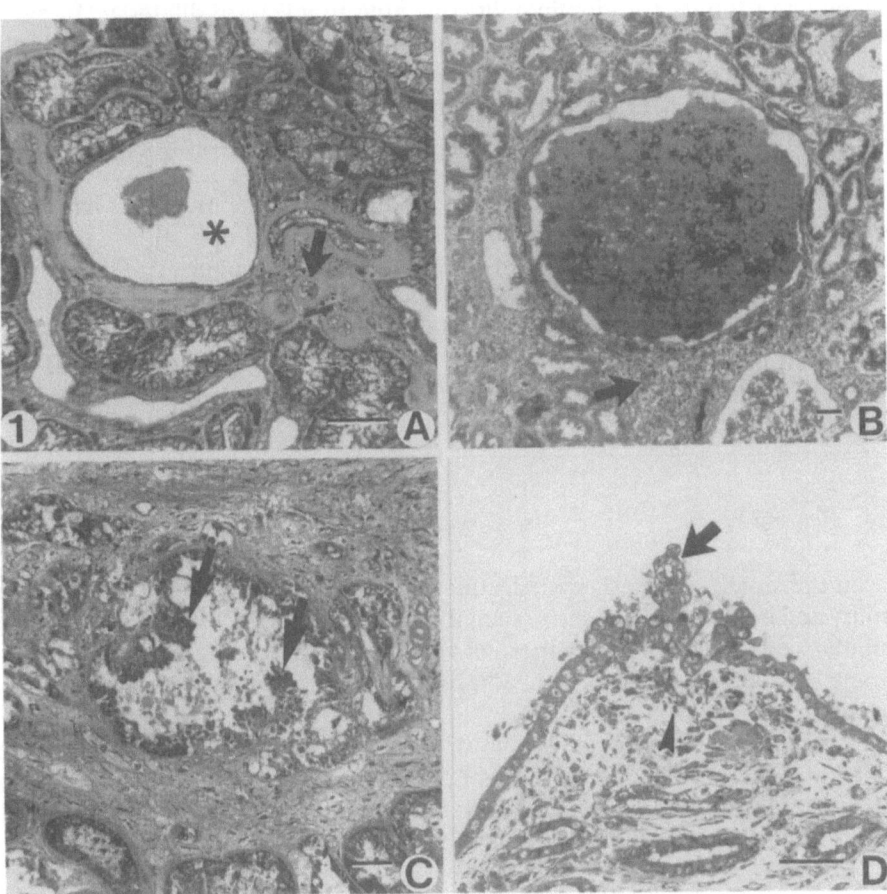

Figure 2.1 A–D. General features of the early-stage ADPKD kidney. (A) Low magnification light micrograph showing a small cortical cyst (asterisk). Adjacent to the cyst is a region showing tubular atrophy (arrow) and tubular basement membrane thickening. (Bar = 50 micrometres). (B) Low magnification light micrograph demonstrating a cyst that possesses a cast of PMNs. The interstitium adjacent to this cyst contains numerous inflammatory cells (arrow). Normal tubular segments are also seen. (Bar = 50 micrometres). (C) Epithelial hyperplasia is commonly seen in cysts of the early-stage ADPKD kidney. The cyst seen in this light micrograph possesses several micropolyps (arrows). The surrounding interstitium is fibrotic and contains a number of atrophic tubules. (Bar = 50 micrometres). (D) Micropolyps often appear as single, focal structures along the cyst wall. In this field, numerous inflammatory cells (arrowhead) are seen to fill the interstitium beneath a micropolyp (arrow). (Bar = 50 micrometres).

segments of tubule (predominately collecting tubule) are dilated[37]. In early ADPKD affected tubules can contain multiple dilatations that are completely or incompletely separated by narrow segments of epithelial wall (Figs. 2.2A–C). These give the cysts a septated or corkscrew appearance[1]. Glomerular cysts are relatively common in infants with both symptomatic and asymptomatic ADPKD.

Most early cysts average 300–500 μm, although some may be as large as 2 cm in diameter. They are lined with a simple polarized epithelium, in which the cell types of particular tubular segments can be recognized. Thus, at the earliest stages of their development, cysts appear to form along identifiable segments of the nephron and to incorporate phenotypically normal, differentiated cell populations. Cells that line early cysts, i.e. cysts detectable in the fetus[8,39], evidently undergo normal differentiation in spite of their incorporation into developing cysts.

2.4. Cell injury

Even the smallest of early cysts frequently display distinct regions of cellular injury and necrosis; cells may be shed into dilated lumens (Fig. 2.2F). Proximal tubular cells may contain numerous vacuoles. Surrounding basement membrane may be thickened, with adjacent fibrotic interstitium. Tubules may become atrophic (Figs. 2.1A–D).

Evidence of injury in the kidney of early ADPKD is of great interest, since cell injury and necrosis are early, if not the first, discernible morphologic events in the evolution of induced renal cystic disease in animal models[17,21]. Cell injury is followed by a burst of cell proliferation; thereafter, the number of cells

Figure 2.2 A–F. Cyst morphology in the early-stage ADPKD kidney. (A) Low magnification scanning electron micrograph showing the corkscrew appearance characteristic of some cystic nephrons of the early-stage kidney. This nephron shows several areas of focal dilatation separated by narrow septa (arrows). (Bar = 150 micrometres). (B) Many cysts possess narrow segments of epithelial wall that project into the cyst lumen. Such septa (arrow) usually divide the cyst (incompletely) into multiple chambers. A micropolyp (arrowhead) is noted in this cyst. (Bar = 150 micrometres). (C) Scanning electron micrograph of a small cortical cyst from an early-stage ADPKD kidney showing a patent connection (arrow) with a nephron. Approximately 50% of cysts 1 mm or less in diameter have one or more connections to a nephron. The patency of this connection is easily seen in the enlarged inset. (Bar = 50 micrometres). (D) Light micrograph showing a cyst (C) of the cortical collecting tubule. This cyst has at least one patent connection with a normal tubule (arrow). (Bar = 50 micrometres). (E) Scanning electron micrograph of the epithelium of a medullary cyst. The apical morphology of these cyst lining cells resembles that of the loop of Henle. (Bar = 1.25 micrometres). (F) Light micrograph showing a field of proximal tubules that are undergoing cell injury and necrosis (asterisk). The interstitium adjacent to these damaged tubular segments shows an increased number of interstitial cells embedded in regions of fibrosis and inflammatory cell infiltration. An adjacent renal corpuscle possesses a thickened basement membrane of the parietal layer of Bowman's capsule (arrowhead). (Bar = 50 micrometres).

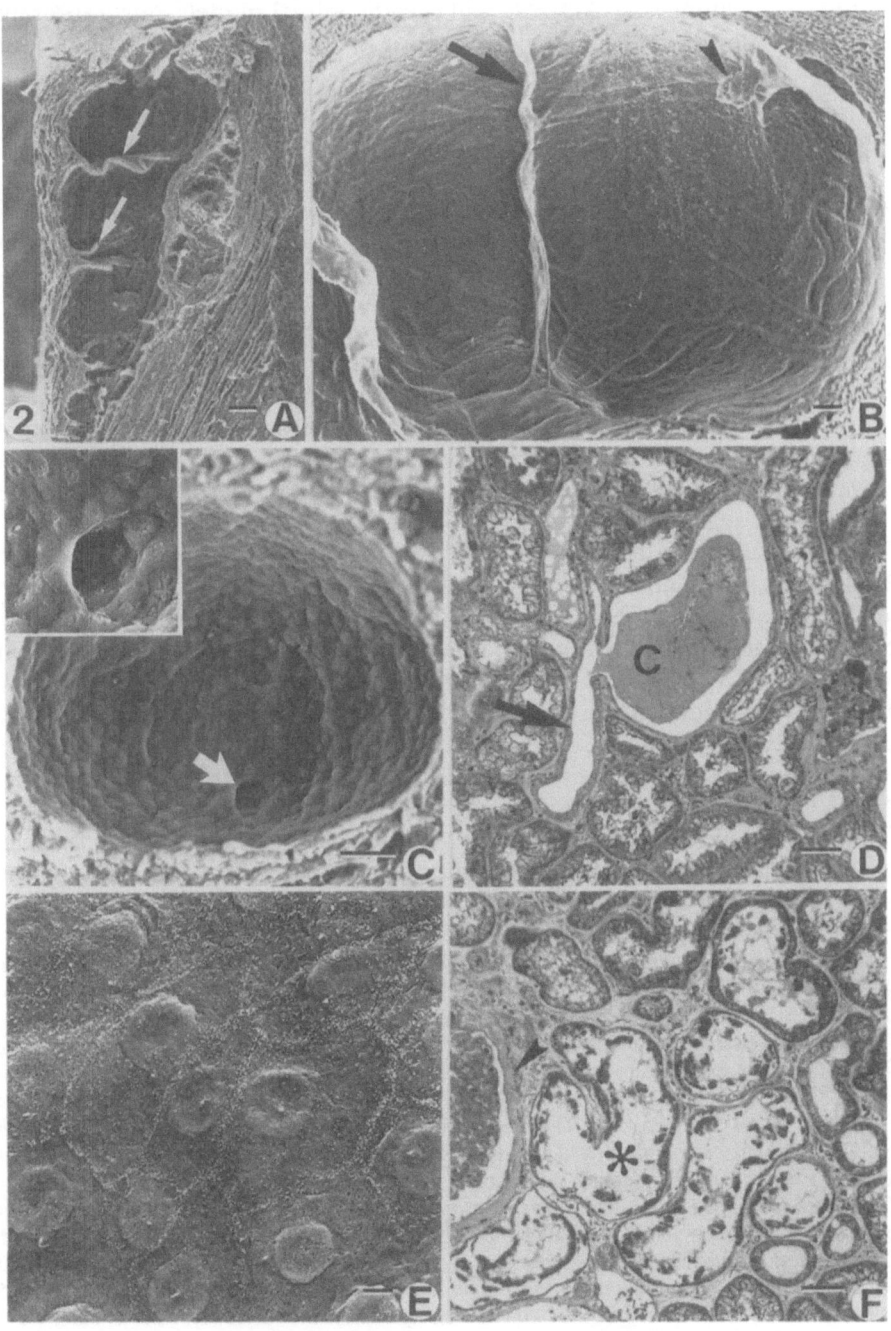

lining tubules is increased and tubules dilate[21]. Focal cell injury, seemingly shared by the kidneys of ADPKD and several animal models, may represent an important event in the early pathogenesis of cyst development.

2.5. Hyperplasia

Cellular hyperplasia is an important feature of early cysts in ADPKD and experimental models. It was first recognized in cystic kidneys over a century ago[9,40] and occurs in three recognizable forms[27]: (1) *regular hyperplasia* in which the cells of the cyst or dilated tubule appear normal or are only moderately attenuated; (2) *irregular hyperplasia* in which cells are tall cuboidal to columnar and form papillae or micropolyps that project from the cyst wall; and (3) *neoplastic proliferation* in the form of solid epithelial tumors.

Regular hyperplasia is seen in all cysts regardless of size, since the dilated segments are lined with an increased number of cells. This appears to involve elevated mitotic activity, and the cells may or may not be recognizable as to their tubular segments of origin (Figs. 2.1A, 2.2A–D).

Irregular hyperplasia is also identifiable in the early cysts of ADPKD (Figs. 2.1C–D, 2.3A–F) and occurs as regions of dense, tall columnar cells that are not identifiable as to their segment(s) of origin. Irregular hyperplasia is associated with micropolyp formation. Micropolyps are minute focal lesions that usually measure less than 0.1 mm, although some may be as large as 0.25 mm. They may be pedunculated and may possess vascularized connective tissue cores. They commonly stud cyst walls, and in one study were found at the outflow ends of 74% of cysts in early ADPKD kidneys[27]. In developing ADPKD, irregular hyperplasia is associated with interstitial infiltrates of inflammatory cells (neutrophils and lymphocytes) (Fig. 2.1D). The significance of this relationship is conjectural; it may or may not reflect the local release

Figure 2.3A–F. Epithelial hyperplasia in the early-stage ADPKD kidney. (A) Low magnification scanning electron micrograph showing a cyst that is lined by cord-like folds of epithelium characteristic of one form of irregular hyperplasia. (Bar = 50 micrometres). (B) This micrograph shows the same cyst seen in Fig. 1A, but at a higher magnification. The numerous cord-like folds are lined by cells that are fusiform in shape. These cells do not resemble any normal tubular cell type. (Bar = 1.25 micrometres). (C) Areas of irregular hyperplasia are commonly seen in cysts from the early-stage ADPKD kidney. Micropolyps (arrow) are usually associated with regions of irregular hyperplasia and are found along the walls of both minimally dilated tubules as well as larger cysts. Frequently, micropolyps are found at the outflow end of a cyst. (Bar = 50 micrometres). (D) This higher magnification scanning electron micrograph shows a cluster of micropolyps (arrow) along a cyst wall. Clearly the cells of micropolyps are continuous with the cyst lining epithelium. (Bar = 50 micrometres). (E) As seen is this micrograph, the cells that form micropolyps commonly do not resemble identifiable renal tubular cell types. (Bar = 5 micrometres). (F) This scanning electron micrograph shows the surface features of one type of micropolyp in which epithelial cells rest atop a central core of connective tissue. Usually a capillary is found traversing this connective tissue core. (Bar = 50 micrometres).

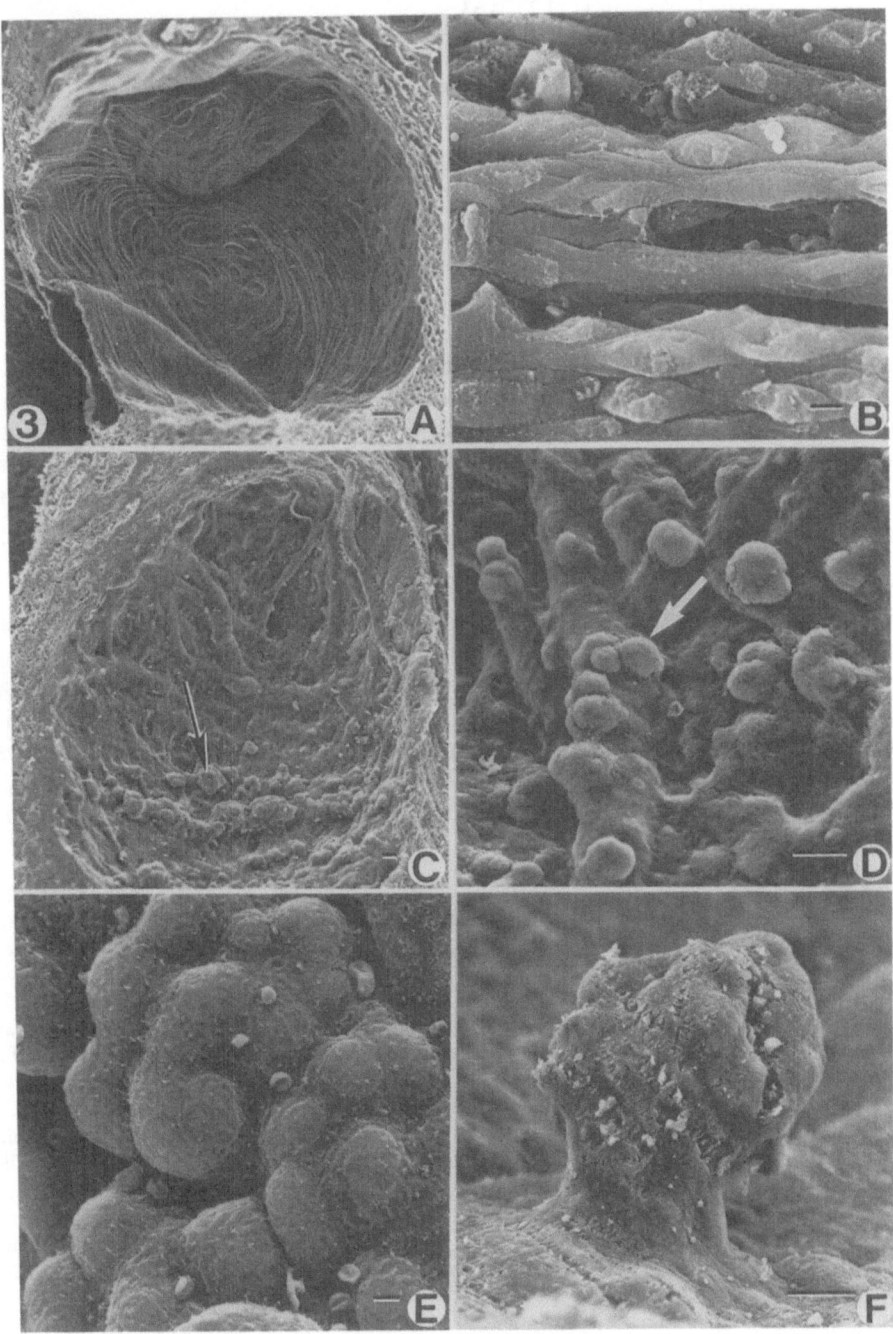

and subsequent impact of cytokines, superoxides, or other cell products on nearby cyst cells and walls[11,21,23,24,33].

3. The Late (Endstage) Cystic Kidney

3.1 General features

Several morphologic changes occur in ADPKD as the disease progresses (Fig. 2.4A–F). Renal architecture becomes highly disordered[3,31.35]. Glomeruli and the angle of the loop of Henle are common sites of cyst development[1,28], although cysts persist in their distribution along the entire nephron and collecting duct[28,32,35,36]. The endstage kidney commonly contains some voluminous cysts, separated by regions of condensed to morphologically normal interstitium in which dilated, normal, and atrophic nephrons are found (Fig. 2.4A). Cysts alter relationships among nephrons, collecting ducts and blood vessels. Connections with nephrons are often lost, and a majority of cysts become isolated as blind sacs[26].

3.2 Gross cyst morphology

The stage at which cysts lose connections with their nephrons is not known. A relationship seems to exist, however, between cyst size and patency. Approximately 50% of 1 mm cysts of early-stage kidneys have at least one tubular connection (Fig. 2.1C), while only 27% of 2 mm cysts of late-stage kidneys communicate with tubules or ducts[26]. Older, larger cysts appear to lose connection with their nephrons.

Figure 2.4 A–F. General morphological features of the endstage ADPKD kidney. (A) Light micrograph showing an island of dilated tubules (arrows) bordered by the walls of three individual cysts. Note the extensive amount of interstitial fibrosis. Similar regions of parenchyma may be occupied by normal nephrons. (Bar = 50 micrometres). (B) Many cysts of the endstage ADPKD kidney have an irregular contour. These irregularities can appear as trabecular projections (arrows) lined by a continuous layer of epithelium. The tissue trapped between the two epithelial layers of these septa includes fibroblastic cells, inflammatory cells, vessels, tubular segments and varying amounts of extracellular matrix material. (Bar = 50 micrometres). (C) Some cysts contain cystalline inclusions (asterisk) within the lumen. In this light micrograph, cysts also form the core of a large micropolyp lined at its surface by hyperplastic epithelial cells (arrow). (Bar = 50 micrometres). (D) Occasionally, cystalline inclusions (arrow) form the core of small irregularities in the cyst wall. (Bar = 25 micrometres). (E) Epithelial microcysts (arrow) represent another form of irregular morphology associated with epithelial hyperplasia of the endstage ADPKD kidney. These fluid-filled microcysts are part of the cyst wall and may be enclosed by as few as two to several epithelial cells. (Bar = 50 micrometres). (F) A relatively common feature noted in the cyst lining epithelium is the presence of pigmented deposits (arrow) in the cytoplasm. Some of these inclusions may represent hemosiderin-like material. (Bar = 25 micrometres).

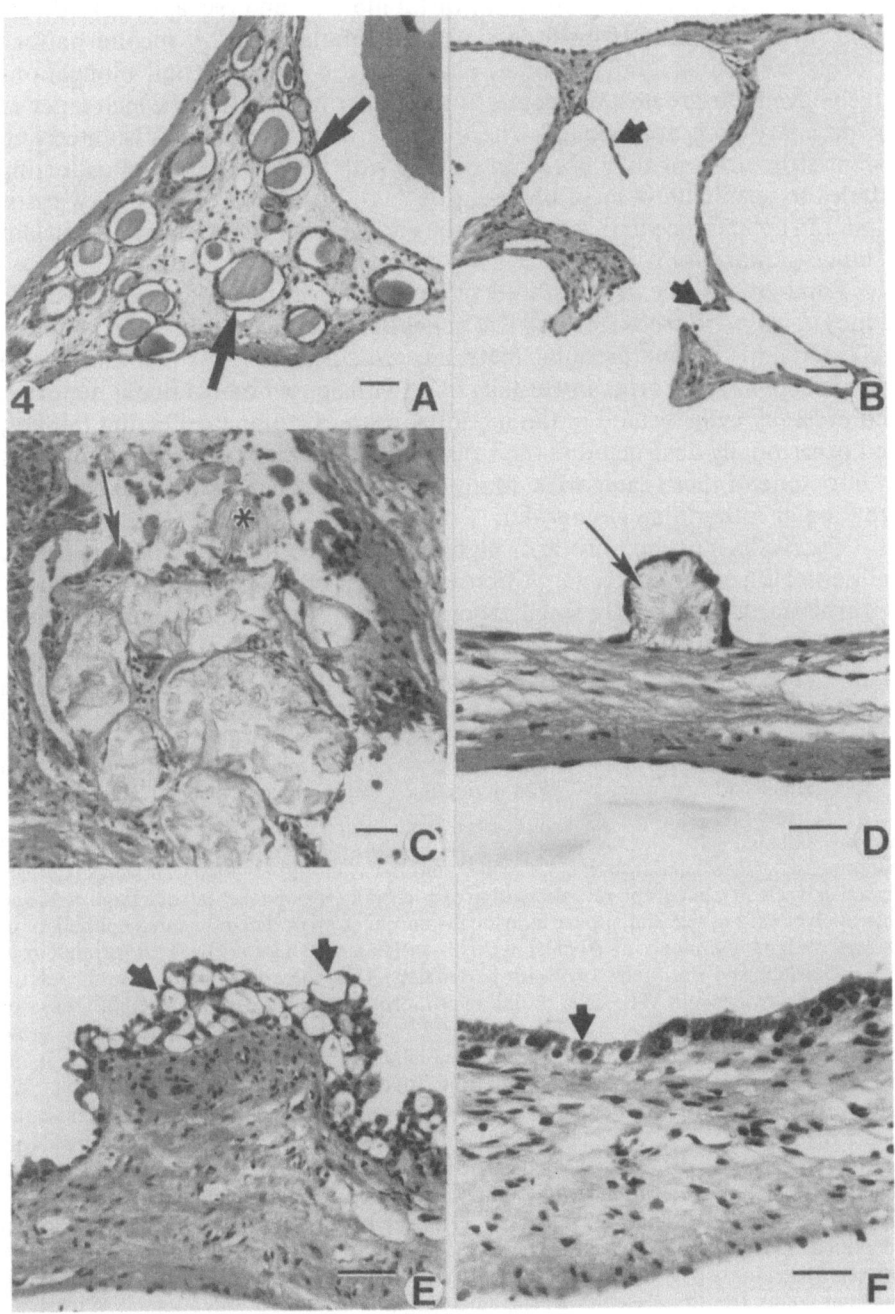

Cysts come to assume one of several predictable forms. They are commonly spherical, whether glomerular or tubular. Often cysts appear as diverticula or outpouchings from one side of a tubular wall. A second pattern involves collecting tubules, and is characterized by segmental elongations which have their greatest diameters at their proximal ends and which taper as the papillary tip is approached. These structures may remain as isolated and patent structures, or they may join distally with adjacent tapering collecting tubules to terminate in large blind cul-de-sacs. Loculated or corkscrew cysts, similar in appearance to those seen in the early lesion, persist as a third variant in late cyst morphology.

Lambert also described three types of cysts in the endstage polycystic kidney[32]: *glomerular cysts* located just beneath the renal capsule and containing small amounts of fine granular material; *tubular cysts* (proximal and distal) found deeper in the cortex and usually filled with dense homogeneous material; and *excretory cysts* located in the medulla, primarily along collecting tubules, and occasionally obstructed at their distal ends. In our experience many cysts fit into none of these categories. Many cysts at the renal surface, for example, are tubular rather than glomerular.

Cyst walls must be fibrotic or highly cellular and may contain fibroblastic cells and infiltrating leukocytes. Microcysts form, typically in areas of irregular hyperplasia. Microcysts are small spheres, usually less than $20\,\mu$m in diameter,

Figure 2.5A–F. Epithelial hyperplasia in the endstage ADPKD kidney. (A) Light micrograph showing a series of micropolyps (arrow) along the wall of a cyst from an end-stage ADPKD kidney. The cells of the cyst that are adjacent to and continuous with the epithelium of the micropolyp are also hyperplastic in appearance. (Bar = 50 micrometres). (Reprinted from Evan, Gardner and Bernstein, 1979 with permission). (B) At a higher magnification it can be noted that some polyps possess a central vascularized core surrounded by numerous densely packed epithelial cells. These cells do not resemble any identifiable tubular cell. (Bar = 50 micrometres). (Reprinted from Evan, Gardner and Bernstein, 1979 with permission). (C) This scanning electron micrograph reveals a group of micropolyps along the wall of a large cyst. The micropolyps vary in size and appear individually and in clusters. The remaining epithelium of the cyst wall shows evidence of irregular hyperplasia. (Bar = 50 micrometres). (Reprinted from Evan, Gardner and Bernstein, 1979 with permission). (D) The epithelium that forms micropolyps is heterogeneous. The cells of one micropolyp do not necessarily resemble those of another, even within the same cyst. Note the irregular shape of the cells of this micropolyp. Some cells bear a few short microvilli and a prominent cilium (arrow) while other cells are bulbous and rather smooth. (Bar = 5 micrometres). (Reprinted from Evan, Gardner and Bernstein, 1979 with permission). (E) This scanning electron micrograph shows a large cyst oriented from the upper right to lower left. At the upper right of the micrograph a cluster of small micropolyps (arrow) are identifiable. At the lower left where the cyst narrows, a larger micropolyp (P) is seen. Micropolyps is commonly seen at the outflow ends of cysts. (Bar = 100 micrometres). (Reprinted from Evan, Gardner and Bernstein, 1979 with permission). (F) The same micropolyp identified in Figure 2.4E is seen at a much higher magnification in this micrograph. The micropolyp is lined by a layer of columnar shaped cells while the central core of the polyp contains connective tissue elements. This micropolyp is associated with a region of irregular hyperplasia in which columnar cells line the cyst wall. (Bar = 25 micrometres). (Reprinted from Evan, Gardner and Bernstein, 1979 with permission).

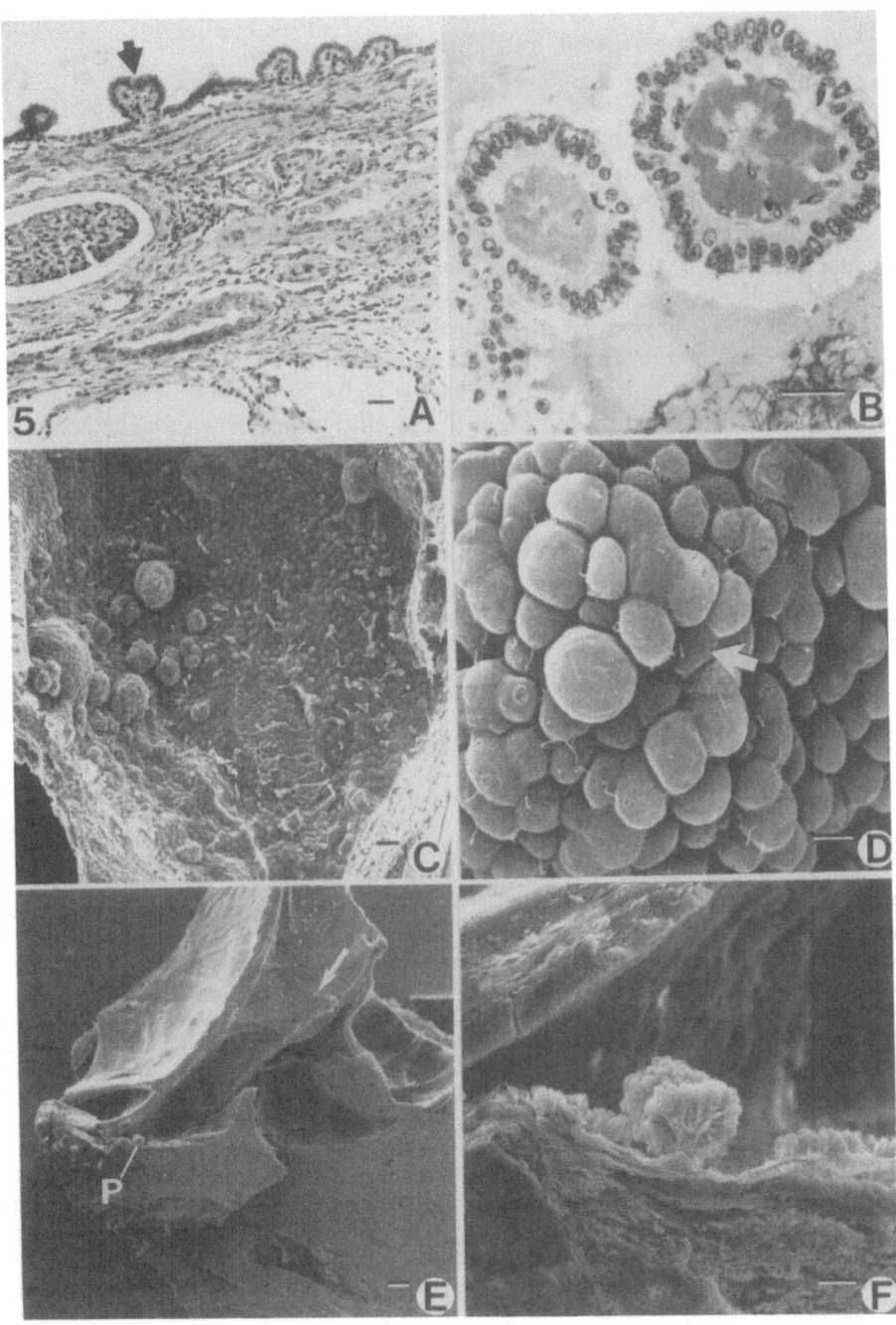

and may be enclosed by only a few epithelial cells (Fig. 2.4E). Arterioles occasionally project into cyst lumens[5]. Cysts may contain calcium oxalate crystals, which are also found in the interstitium (Fig. 2.4C–D).

3.3. Interstitium

The regions of interstitium that separate adjacent cysts are fibrotic to highly cellular and sparsely to plentifully vascular, and may be populated by various circulating cell types. Fibroblastic cells are commonly the predominant cell type, although bundles of hypertrophic spindle cells (smooth muscle) may form the major tissue component. Smooth muscle in the cyst wall may be a metaplastic response to increased cyst wall tension[5]. Diffuse lymphocytic infiltration is common within the interstitium and cyst walls. Interstitial neutrophils are also common immediately subjacent to the epithelium or within the cores of micropolyps. Neutrophils and lymphocytes may be observed within cyst lumens and within the epithelium.

Although some regions of apparently normal renal parenchyma may be found in highly cystic kidneys, the interstitium around cysts rarely contains more than a scattering of normal tubules. Tubules adjacent to cysts tend to be dilated, to exhibit mild to profound cellular injury, and to be atrophic. In fortuitous sections, dilated tubules in longitudinal profile continue to show the characteristic corkscrew pattern seen in the earlier lesions.

Figure 2.6A–F. Other forms of renal cystic disease that show epithelial hyperplasia. *A and B: Acquired renal cystic disease* – (A) Scanning electron micrograph of a cyst from an endstage kidney in acquired renal cystic disease. Cysts are commonly lined by a hyperplastic epithelium that forms micropapillae and small intraluminal tumours. (Bar = 25 micrometres). (B) Acquired renal cystic disease is characterized by numerous cysts of the proximal tubule. The epithelium lining these cysts still possess a distinct brush border (arrow) suggesting that these cells have retained some degree of differentiation. (Bar = 5 micrometres). *C and D: Tuberous sclerosis* – (C) Tuberous sclerosis, a dominantly inherited disorder, is sometimes characterized by numerous renal cysts. The cells lining both non-cystic and cystic nephrons in this disease present a unique form of hyperplasia. By routine light microscopy these cells would be identified by their intense eosinophilia. (Bar = 1.25 micrometres). (D) Large glomerular cysts are found in the kidney of patients with tuberous sclerosis. Note the distortion of the glomerular tuft (arrow) in this glomerular cyst. (Bar = 100 micrometres). *E and F: Autosomal recessive PKD* – (E) The recessive form of polycystic kidney disease is characterized by numerous elongated cysts of the cortical and medullary collecting tubules (arrow). These cysts show evidence of regular hyperplasia, but lack the irregular and neoplastic forms that are seen in ADPKD. (Bar = 150 micrometres). (F) Proximal tubular cysts can be identified in the recessive form of PKD. However, unlike the dominant form the cells that line proximal tubular cysts may retain a brush border (arrow). It should be noted that cysts of the proximal tubule are uncommon in autosomal recessive polycystic kidney disease. (Bar = 2.5 micrometres).

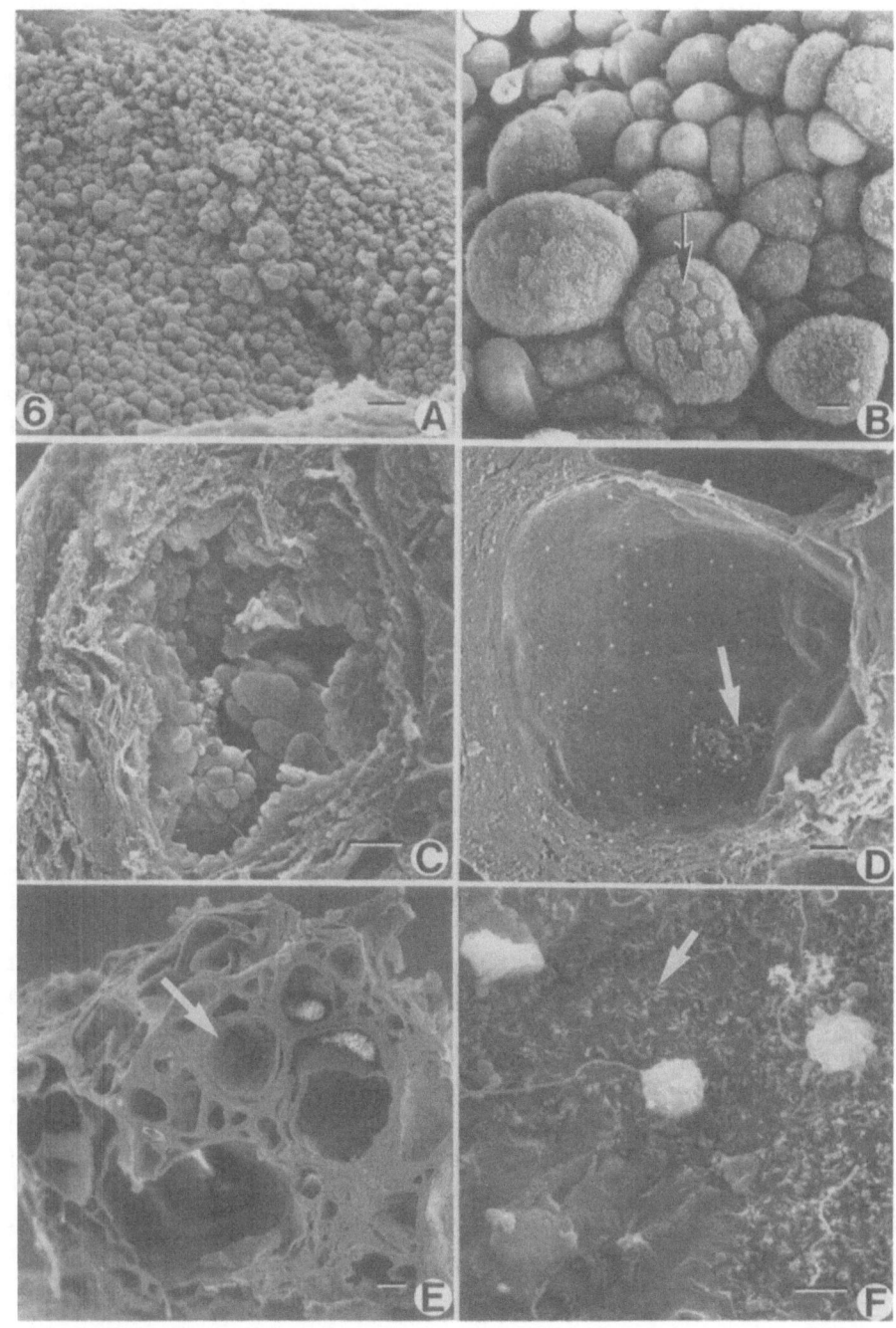

3.4. Cyst lining

Morphological studies have yet to identify ultrastructural features of cell types that are uniquely characteristic of renal cyst walls in ADPKD. The lining epithelium of renal cysts may be either characteristic of the renal tubule or identifiable as a specific segment of the nephron. Renal cysts are believed to be derived from all nephron segments, and a cyst wall may possess the differentiated epithelium of its tubular or glomerular segment of origin. So, a cyst wall may possess the differentiated epithelium of its tubular segment of origin, or of the glomerulus. Alternatively, the epithelium may be unidentifiable. That is, the cell types may not be characteristic of any tubule segment. Cysts that bear an unidentifiable or undifferentiated epithelium have been termed *undefined* cysts[26]. In a study of 387 cysts collected from 10 patients, scanning electron microscopy showed that 84% of cysts were of the undefined type, while 11% had an epithelium typical of a nephron segment[26]. The remaining 5% of cysts showed hyperplastic epithelial patterns.

3.5. Hyperplasia

Epithelial hyperplasia is a characteristic of cysts in several different forms of cystic disease, including ADPKD. However, not all cysts exhibit the same type of cellular hyperplasia. Cysts may possess broad areas or discrete foci of irregular to bulbous cuboidal cells. Cord-like epithelial bundles may be tightly organized in parallel array[26]. Hyperplastic cells of the cyst wall frequently form micropolyps projecting into the lumen[18]. The cells of micropolyps tend to be undifferentiated, irregular and cuboidal or short columnar. Two forms of polyps have been described, one in which cells form random aggregates and one in which the cells are polarized against a central core (Fig. 2.5A–F)[5,6,7,16,17,18,26,27]. Identifiable renal cell types may also be present in any cyst (Fig. 2.5B, D).

Hyperplasia in ADPKD can be distinguished from the hyperplasia that occurs in other forms of renal cystic disease (Fig. 2.6A–F). Cysts in von Hippel–Lindau disease are usually lined with irregular hyperplastic cells and with mural nodules of clear cell carcinoma[6]. Histopathological studies of the renal cysts in acquired renal cystic disease[25] show hyperplastic and atypical or dysplastic lining cells (Fig. 2.6A–B). Micropapillae and small intraluminal tumors are common. Renal cysts in tuberous sclerosis have a unique form of hyperplasia characterized by large eosinophilic epithelial cells (Fig. 2.6C–D)[6]. Finally, the recessive form of polycystic kidney disease shows regular hyperplasia while irregular and neoplastic forms are only rarely observed (Fig. 2.6E–F)[22].

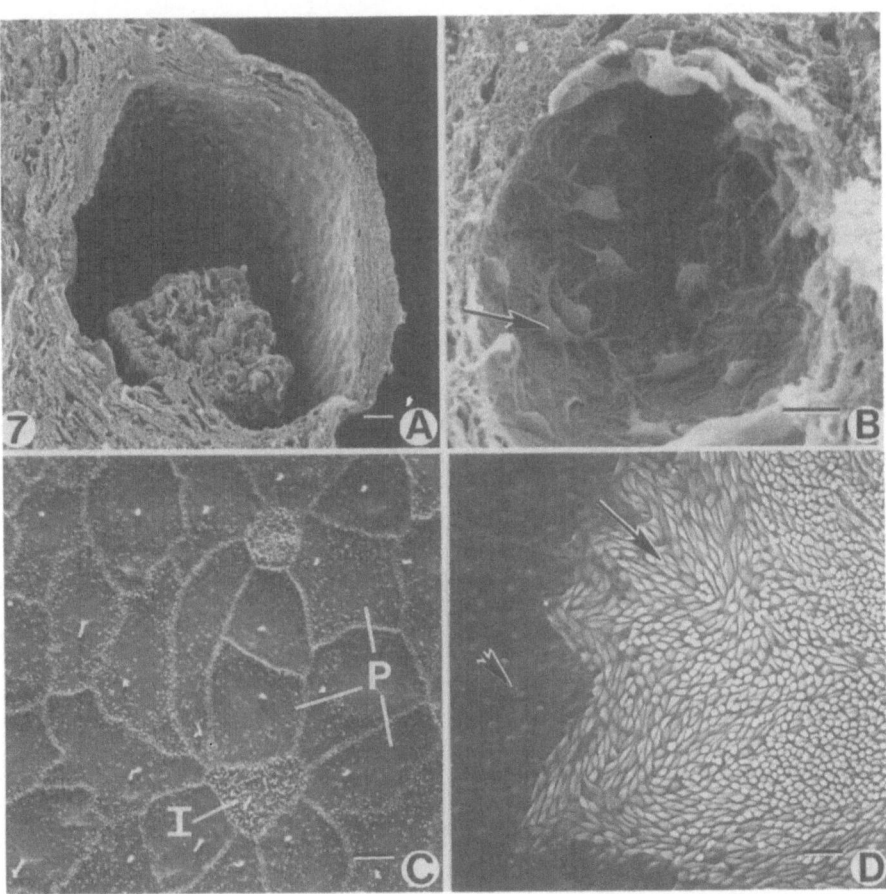

Figure 2.7 A–D. Morphology of cyst lining cells in ADPKD. (A) Glomerular cysts are common in the endstage ADPKD kidney. Usually these cysts are lined by an attenuated cell type that is characteristic of the normal glomerular parietal epithelium. (Bar = 50 micrometres). (B) Occasionally the parietal layer possesses cells that resemble those of the visceral layer of Bowman's capsule. These podocyte-like cells (arrow) possess numerous interdigitating foot processes. (Bar = 50 micrometres). (C) Some cortical and medullary cysts are lined by cells that closely resemble those of the normal collecting tubule. This scanning electron micrograph shows cells that have apical surface features characteristic of the principal cell (P) and the intercalated cell I. (Bar = 2.5 micrometres). (D) Most cysts of the ADPKD kidney are lined by an unidentifiable epithelium. These cells appear to be either undifferentiated (arrowhead) or hyperplastic (arrow). (Bar = 25 micrometres).

3.6. Micropolyps

The occurrence of micropolyps along renal cyst wall in ADPKD has been used in support of the hypothesis that partial tubular obstruction plays a role in cyst formation[5,6,7,16,17,18,21,23]. Micropolyps are frequently observed within small diameter cysts or at the narrow outflow port of large cysts. It is reasoned that occlusion or restriction of the tubule lumen may impede outflow and lead to increased fluid retention within the lumen. This may be a critical stimulus to the events that result in cyst enlargement.

3.7. Epithelium

It has not been determined if the nature of the epithelium is related to the size of the cyst. Both small and large cysts may possess homogeneous cell populations that are either identifiable or undifferentiated. Alternatively, small and large cysts occur in which differentiated and undifferentiated cells are present together. In ADPKD, cells of one type tend to occupy large portions of a cyst surface and to remain segregated. Thus, the transition between epithelial types is discrete.

3.8. Epithelium and type of cyst

Epithelial morphology along the wall of a cyst bearing a differentiated epithelium may closely resemble that of the nephron segment from which the cyst derived. It is not uncommon, for example, to observe a large diameter (> 1 cm) cyst in which the lining cells resemble the collecting duct, with intercalated cells

Figure 2.8 A–F. Ultrastructural features of the cyst lining cells in ADPKD. (A) Scanning electron microscopy shows the cells of this cyst to be squamous in shape. The central region of the cell is enlarged (arrow) and represents the position of the nucleus. The rest of the cell is extremely attenuated with pronounced cell boundaries. (Bar = 2.5 micrometres). (B) The same cyst wall seen in Fig. 2.8A is now viewed by transmission electron microscopy. The lining cells have a highly attenuated cytoplasm (arrow). A thickened and multilayered basal lamina is seen beneath the epithelium. (Bar = 2.5 micrometres). (C) Some cysts are lined by irregularly shaped cells, as seen in this scanning electron micrograph. The cells are pleiomorphic with no particular alignment. Also, the apical surface features of these cells is not uniform. Some regions bear short microvilli (arrow) while other areas are smooth. (Bar = 5 micrometres). (D) The same cyst seen in Fig. 2.8C is now viewed by transmission electron microscopy. The cells are irregular in shape and some have narrow processes (arrow). (Bar = 2.5 micrometres). (E) This scanning electron micrograph shows a cyst lined by a homogeneous epithelium. The apical cell surface is studded by numerous short microvilli. Intercellular margins (arrow) are distinct. (Bar = 2.5 micrometres). (F) The same cyst seen in Fig. 2.8E is now viewed by transmission electron microscopy. These cells possess a cuboidal shape. The apical surface is lined by short microvilli while the basal surface possesses numerous basal infoldings (arrow). These features are characteristic of the principal cell of the collecting tubule. (Bar = 2.5 micrometres).

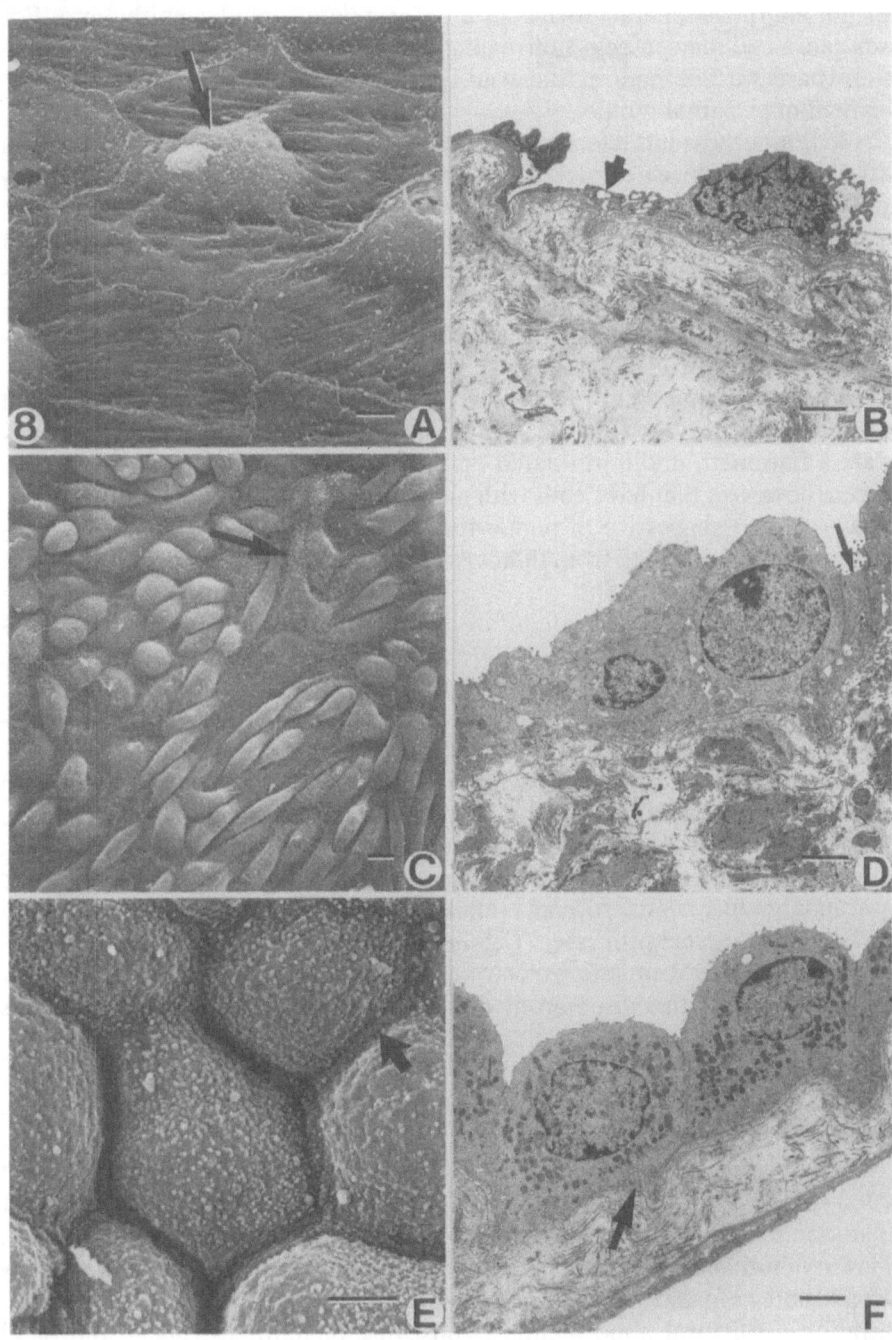

interspersed among principal cells (Fig. 2.7C). Some cysts may possess some, but not all, of the characteristics of a differentiated tubular epithelium. For example, a cell may possess an irregular brush border, but with indeterminate lateral basal surface features that would positively identify its origin as a specific segment of proximal tubule.

In both early- and late-stage ADPKD, cysts rarely possess an epithelium with a prominent brush border. Cysts in acquired renal cystic disease frequently have cells with a brush border that is typical of the normal proximal tubule[14]. In ADPKD, cysts must often be identified as proximal tubule on the basis of intercellular junction morphology. Faraggiana *et al.* [19] have found that, although cysts in ADPKD may lose their brush border, the epithelium still retains positive staining for the proximal tubule-specific marker lectin *Lotus tetrago-nolobus* agglutinin.

The glomerular cyst often retains the tuft, commonly with its atypical but identifiable podocytes (Fig. 2.7A–B). The wall of a glomerular cyst usually bears a flattened, undifferentiated epithelium. Glomerular cysts can be observed, however, that have cells with unusual characteristics, including elongated processes suggestive of podocytes[16,26]. In such cases normal podocytes may have been displaced from their visceral origins to parietal positions by the process of cyst enlargement.

Undefined cysts possess undifferentiated cells. Undifferentiated cell types are atypical of the normal renal tubule and may show several phenotypes (Fig. 2.7D). The cells that occupy hyperplastic foci are usually irregular cuboidal to bulbous in form, and may have a polarized distribution of cytoplasmic organelles. These cells are most commonly not identifiable as to type.

Broad "non-hyperplastic" regions of the cyst wall are frequently lined with cells that are somewhat flattened and irregular rather than polygonal in form. These cells commonly possess a scant and irregularly distributed population of short apical microvilli (Fig. 2.8A–B). Their intercellular boundaries, observed by scanning electron microscopy, tend to be distinct and highlighted by short interdigitating apical processes (Fig. 2.8A). These cells usually possess a solitary cilium. By transmission electron microscopy they have an apparently unpolarized and otherwise unremarkable component of typical membranous organelles (Fig. 2.8B).

3.9. Basement membrane

One hypothesis proposed to explain cyst formation in ADPKD is that tubular dilatation occurs because basement membranes have increased compliance[10]. It is thought that a weakened, excessively compliant basement membrane may stretch and deform under the continual pressure generated by glomerular filtration. Structural abnormalities, consisting of multilayering of the basal lamina in tubular and glomerular basement membranes, have been observed in early and late-stage ADPKD kidneys[34]. It does not follow, however, that structural abnormality supports the compliant basement membrane hypothesis. A morphologic correlate of a basement membrane with increased compliance has not been determined. It is neither known nor is it predictable from available information what structural characteristics a weakened basement membrane should possess.

3.10. Structure in relation to function

Little is known about the function of the renal cyst wall. An important question is whether cysts actively function to modify their fluid content and thereby influence fluid accumulation and cyst growth. Analyses of cyst fluid suggests that some walls possess ion transport activity and retain functional attributes reflecting their tubular origin. Proximal cysts have higher Na^+ and Cl^- and lower creatinine, K^+, and H^+ concentrations than do distal cysts, whereas distal cysts maintain steep concentration gradients for K^+, Cl^-, and creatinine[12,20,30].

Ultrastructural study of functionally distinct cyst walls suggests that differences in cyst content may be reflected by differences in morphology[12]. When intercellular junctions were examined, distal cysts were observed to possess lanthanum-impermeable, tight (occluding) apical junctions and to have dilated intercellular spaces. The majority of proximal cysts were lined by a so-called "leaky" epithelium in which the junctions were intermediate (adherens) type and intercellular spaces were narrow. Cysts in this study apparently were representative of the *undefined* type and did not possess differentiated cells typical of normal nephron segments. The only other published study that attempted to characterize the function of human renal cyst wall did not correlate function with morphology[38].

4. Summary

Studies of human renal cystic disease have been largely descriptive in nature and limited primarily to characterization of the endstage kidney. Such data as are available indicate that cyst formation may begin *in utero*, is progressive, and is associated with changes in the character of cyst linings, the size and number of visible cysts, and the prevalence of altered patterns of epithelial growth.

References

1. Baert L. Hereditary polycystic kidney disease (adult form): A microdissection study of two cases at an early stage of the disease. Kidney International 1978, 13, 519–525.
2. Bear JC, McManamon P, Morgan J, Payne RH, Lewis H, Gault MH and Churchill ON.

Age at clinical onset and at ultrasonic detection of adult polycystic kidney disease: Data for genetic counselling. American Journal of Medical Genetics 1984, 18, 45–53.

3. Bernstein J. The classification of renal cysts. Nephron 1973, 11, 91–100.

4. Bernstein J. Hereditary renal diseases. In: Churg B, Spargo H, Mostofi FK and Abell MR, eds, Kidney Disease: Present Status. Baltimore: Williams & Wilkins, 1979, 295–326.

5. Bernstein J. Morphology of renal cystic disease. In: Cummings NB and Klahr S, eds, Chronic Renal Disease. New York: Plenum Medical Book Company, 1985, 47–68.

6. Bernstein J, Evan AP and Gardner KD. Epithelial hyperplasia in human polycystic kidney disease: Its role in pathogenesis and risk of neoplasia. American Journal of Pathology 1987, 129, 92–101.

7. Bernstein J, Evan AP and Gardner KD. Human cystic kidney diseases: Epithelial hyperplasia in the pathogenesis of cysts and tumors. Pediatric Nephrology 1987, 1, 393–396.

8. Blyth H and Ockenden BG. Polycystic disease of the kidneys and liver presenting in childhood. Journal of Medical Genetics 1971, 8, 257–284.

9. Brigidi DV and Severi A. Contributo alla patogenesi: Delle cisti renal. Sperimentale 1880, 46, 1–25.

10. Carone FA, Rowland RG, Perlman SG and Ganote CE. The pathogenesis of drug-induced renal cystic disease. Kidney International 1974, 5, 411–421.

11. Caverzasio J, Rizzoli R, Dayer JM and Bonjour JP. Interleukin-1 decreases renal sodium reabsorption: Possible mechanisms of endotoxin-induced natriuresis. American Journal of Physiology 1986, 252, F943–F946.

12. Cuppage FE, Huseman RA, Chapman A and Grantham JJ. Ultrastructure and function of cysts from human adult polycystic kidneys. Kidney International 1980, 17, 372–381.

13. Dalgaard OZ. Bilateral polycystic disease of the kidney: A followup of two hundred eighty-four patients and their families. Acta Medica Scandinavica (Suppl) 1957, 328, 1–233.

14. Dunnill MS, Millard PR and Oliver D. Acquired cystic disease of the kidneys: A hazard of long-term intermittent maintenance haemodialysis. Journal of Clinical Pathology 1977, 30, 868–877.

15. Eulderink P and Hogewind BL. Renal cysts in premature children. Archives of Pathology and Laboratory Medicine 1978, 102, 592–595.

16. Evan AP and Gardner KD. Comparison of human polycystic and medullary cystic kidney disease with diphenylamine-induced cystic disease. Laboratory Investigation 1976, 35, 93–101.

17. Evan AP and Gardner KD. Morphology of polycystic kidney disease in man and experimental models. In: Cummings NB and Klahr S, eds, Chronic Renal Disease. New York: Plenum Medical Book Company, 1985, 55–68.

18. Evan AP, Gardner KD and Bernstein J. Polypoid and papillary epithelial hyperplasia: A potential cause of ductal obstruction in adult polycystic disease. Kidney International 1979, 16, 743–750.

19. Faraggiana T, Bernstein J, Strauss L and Churg J. Use of lectins in the study of histogenesis of renal cysts. Laboratory Investigation 1985, 53, 575–579.

20. Gardner KD. Composition of fluid in twelve cysts of a polycystic kidney. New England Journal of Medicine 1969, 281, 985–988.

21. Gardner KD. Cystic Kidneys. Kidney International 1988, 33, 610–621.

22. Gardner KD and Evan AP. Cystic diseases of the kidney. In: Gonick HC, ed, Current Nephrology. Chicago: Year Book Medical Publishers, Inc., 1987, 37–65.

23. Gardner KD and Evan AP. Cystic kidneys: An enigma evolves. American Journal of Kidney Disease 1984, 3, 403–413.

24. Gardner KD, Reed WP, Evan AP, Zedalis J, Hylarides MD and Leon OA. Endotoxin provocation of experimental renal cystic disease. Kidney International 1987, 32, 329–334.

25. Graham PC and Lindop GBM. The anatomy of the renin-containing cell in adult polycystic kidney disease. Kidney International 1988, 33, 1084–1090.

26. Grantham JJ, Geiser JL and Evan AP. Cyst formation and growth in autosomal dominant polycystic kidney disease. Kidney International 1987, 31, 1145–1152.
27. Gregoire JR, Torres VE, Holley KE and Farrow GM. Renal epithelial hyperplastic and neoplastic proliferation in autosomal dominant polycystic kidney disease. American Journal of Kidney Disease 1987, 9, 27–38.
28. Heggo O. A microdissection study of cystic disease of the kidneys in adults. Journal of Pathology and Bacteriology 1966, 91, 311–315.
29. Holmes JH and Gabow P. Early polycystic kidney disease. In: Cummings NB and Klahr S, eds, Chronic Renal Disease. New York: Plenum Medical Book Company, 1985, 105–112.
30. Huseman RA, Grady A, Welling D and Grantham JJ. Micropuncture study of polycystic disease in adult human kidneys. Kidney International 1980, 18, 375–385.
31. Kissane JM. The morphology of renal cystic disease. In: Gardner KD, ed, Cystic Diseases of the Kidney. New York: John Wiley and Sons, 1976, 31–63.
32. Lambert PP. Polycystic diseases of the kidney. Archives of Pathology 1947, 44, 34–58.
33. Le J and Vilcek J. Biology of disease: Tumor necrosis factor and interleukin 1: Cytokines with multiple overlapping biological activities. Laboratory Investigation 1987, 56, 234–248.
34. Milutinivic J and Agodoa LY. Potential causes and pathogenesis in autosomal dominant polycystic kidney disease. Nephron 1983, 33, 139–144.
35. Norris RF and Herman L. The pathogenesis of polycystic kidneys: Reconstruction of cystic elements in four cases. Journal of Urology 1941, 46, 147–176.
36. Osathanondh V and Potter EL. Pathogenesis of polycystic kidneys: Type 3 due to multiple abnormalities of development. Archives of Pathology 1964, 77, 485–501.
37. Osathanondh V and Potter EL. Pathogenesis of polycystic kidneys: Type 1 due to hyperplasia of interstitial portions of collecting tubules. Archives of Pathology 1964, 77, 466–473.
38. Perrone RD. In vitro function of cyst epithelium from human polycystic kidney. Journal of Clinical Investigation 1985, 76, 1688–1691.
39. Reeders ST, Gol A, Propping P, Waldherr R, Davis KE, Zerres K, Hogenkamp T, Schmidt W, Dolata MM and Weatherall DJ. Prenatal diagnosis of autosomal dominant polycystic kidney disease with a DNA probe. Lancet 1986, 2, 6–8.
40. Strum P. Über das Adenom der Niere und über die Beziehung desselben zu einigen anderen Neubildungen der Niere. Arch Heilk 1975, 16, 193–237.
41. Zerres K. Genetics of cystic kidney diseases: Criteria for classification and genetic counselling. Pediatric Nephrology 1987, 1, 397–404.
42. Zerres K, Volpel MC and Weiss H. Cystic kidneys: Genetics, pathologic anatomy, clinical picture, and prenatal diagnosis. Human Genetics 1984, 60, 104–135.

3
The Interstitium of the Cystic Kidney

C.J. Kelly and E.G. Neilson

Abstract

Two differing lines of research indicate that interstitial leukocytes link to renal cyst development. The degree of cystic change provoked by endotoxin in the kidneys of germfree rats fed nordihydroguaiaretic acid correlates directly with the degree of interstitial inflammatory cell infiltration. Microcysts develop in association with interstitial infiltrates in the hereditary T cell mediated autoimmune nephritis of kdkd mice. Details of these experimental observations, reviewed here, indicate that interstitial inflammatory cells may be either etiopathogenic or permissive for the expression of some forms of injury in cystic kidneys.

Abbreviations TBM, tubular basement membrane;
NDGA, nordihydroguaiaretic acid;
TGF, transforming growth factor-beta.

Key words   Autoimmunity;
Cystogenesis;
Immune cells;
Interstitium;
Lymphokines;
Tubular basement membrane.

1. Introduction

The most striking changes in the histology of polycystic and medullary cystic disease occur within the tubulointerstitial compartment of the kidney[34]. It is appropriate, therefore, given recent advances in cell biology, to review the current state of knowledge regarding cells both native and foreign to the tubulointerstitium and the functional mechanisms that may influence the expression of cystic kidney disease. The significance of changes within the tubulointerstitium have become better appreciated in recent years[48]. While it has long been clear in primary tubulointerstitial disease that the degree of renal functional impairment correlates well with evidence of chronically progressive interstitial fibrosis and tubular atrophy, such correlations in primary glomerular diseases have been more controversial. There is growing evidence, however, that even in primary glomerular diseases the degree of interstitial damage may not only be related to the degree of functional impairment, but may, in fact, be a more important factor than the degree of glomerular involvement[5,46,48]. In this chapter we will review the described pathologic abnormalities of the interstitium in polycystic and medullary cystic disease, and then consider how native and infiltrating interstitial cells may influence cyst development.

2. Pathologic alterations of the tubulointerstitium and tubular basement membrane in human and experimental cystic kidney disease

In most cases the appearance of polycystic kidneys and medullary cystic disease by light and electron microscopy has been detailed at rather advanced stages of injury[34]. Whether, in fact, such alterations are representative of those present in the early stages of cystogenesis is uncertain. Careful analyses of tubulointerstitial pathology at multiple time points throughout the course of disease can, from a practical standpoint, only be performed in a reproducible experimental model[29]. Findings in experimental models, however, are always vulnerable to the criticism that they do not faithfully represent the human disease. With these caveats in mind, there are some generalities that can be applied to the pathologic abnormalities of the tubulointerstitium observed in human and experimental cystic disease.

In autosomal dominant polycystic kidney disease, the cysts appear to be quite heterogeneous in the nature of their lining cells. There is morpho-logic[13,23] as well as functional[45] evidence that they are derived from proximal and distal tubules and perhaps Bowman's capsule. One possible implication of such diffuse cell proliferation, which is a requirement for this type of cysto-genesis[23], is that if abnormalities in growth factors or cell surface receptors for such factors play a role in cystogenesis, the abnormal growth mechanism is not specific for a discrete region of the nephron.

Cultured epithelia from human polycystic kidneys demonstrate markedly abnormal proliferation as compared to cultured normal proximal straight tubules and cortical collecting tubules[56]. Polycystic epithelial cells in culture synthesize morphologically bizarre basement membranes, consisting of banded collagen and proteoglycan[56]. Other studies of human polycystic tissue have, by immunofluorescence techniques, demonstrated alterations in the extracellular matrix. Employing antibodies with specificity for laminin, type IV collagen, basement membrane heparan sulphate–proteoglycan and fibro-nectin, Carone and co-workers[8] stained renal tissues from five patients with endstage polycystic kidney disease. They found focal diminution of fluor-escence with antiheparan sulphate–proteoglycan antibodies, probable normal reactivity with antilaminin and antitype IV collagen antibodies, and markedly increased staining of the peritubular interstitium for fibronectin.

It is not yet clear which component(s) of the complex heparan sulphate–proteoglycans were diminished in these studies, although the antibody used in this report was directed against the 18,000 Mr core protein[8]. Since these studies were performed on endstage polycystic kidneys which have likely endured multiple renal infections as well as the cystogenic stimuli of maintenance hemodialysis[19], the relevance of these findings to the primary disease is still uncertain. Arguing against the idea that such findings are epiphenomena related to infection or hemodialysis is the fact that similar alterations in heparan sulphate proteoglycans and fibronectin are found by immunofluorescence techniques in 2-amino-4,5-diphenylthiazole-induced cystic disease in rats[8]. Carone et al [7] have also found in this experimental model that de novo synthesis of sulphated proteoglycans is reduced to less than 50% of normal values, and that suppressed biosynthesis is reversible. It should be noted, however, that these investigators have not been able to demonstrate an alteration in basement compliance secondary to these changes in basement membrane composition[22].

Basement membrane alterations have also been described in the medullary cystic disease–nephronophthisis complex. Most studies demonstrate thickened basement membrane at advanced histologic and clinical stages of disease[4,51,59]. A more recent ultrastructural evaluation of the TBM in nephronophthisis with relatively well-preserved renal function[11] supported a previous one[59] and showed extreme variability in basement membrane thickness throughout an affected kidney. The thickness of the TBM ranged from 36 nm to 2,000 nm. The same study also showed abrupt transitions from very thick TBM to markedly attenuated TBM. Both laminin and type IV collagen appear to be normal by immunofluorescence. Staining with antiTBM antisera with specificity for the 3M-1 glycoprotein[9,10] was reduced in some areas. With these findings, the authors suggested that nephronophthisis may represent a primary tubular basement membrane defect with absence of some normal antigenic components[11].

Inflammatory cells within the tubulointerstitium have been noted in both polycystic kidney disease and medullary cystic disease, although they are more impressive in the latter. In fact, in early stages of medullary cystic disease, the interstitium may be heavily infiltrated with mononuclear cells. Some patients who clinically have this disease never really develop many corticomedullary cysts[4,51]. The kidneys in these cases display all the features of chronic interstitial nephritis with eventual tubular atrophy and fibrosis. The function of these infiltrating mononuclear cells has not been well studied. While it is possible that they represent a non-specific inflammatory response in the setting of damaged tissue and, perhaps, the exposure of normally hidden antigenic sites, it is also possible that they have a more primary role in the pathogenesis of cystic kidney disease.

3. Interstitial nephritis and cystogenesis

In considering a role for interstitial infiltrates in the process of cystogenesis, we will consider evidence that such cells may be either etiopathogenic or permissive for the expression of some forms of cystic kidney injury. The first model in which the issue has been explored is that of renal cystic disease induced by chemical cystogens. The antioxidant nordihydroguaiaretic acid (NDGA) is known to produce progressive renal cyst formation in experimental animals[15]. Gardner and co-workers[20,21] have shown that the natural history of this induced cystic disease can be dramatically altered by environmental manipulation. If, for example, this agent is fed to germfree rats kept in a sterile environment, cysts do not develop. When these NDGA-fed, germfree rats are either moved to an ambient environment or injected with endotoxin, however, renal cysts predictably develop[20,21]. In the studies performed with endotoxin, the authors were able to correlate the severity of tubular dilatation with elevated circulating polymorphonuclear leukocyte (PMN) and lymphocyte counts, as well as more pronounced interstitial infiltrates containing PMNs and lymphocytes. Based on these studies in NDGA-induced renal cystic disease, Gardner and co-workers[21] have hypothesized that following tubular damage by agents such as NDGA, leukocytes may accumulate in previously damaged tubulointerstitial areas where they potentially contribute to a cystic nephropathy through the release of cytotoxic oxygen radicals and other less well-defined mediators.

We have arrived at similar conclusions regarding the potential importance of inflammatory cells within the tubulointerstitium in the process of cystogenesis[32]. One of our major research interests has been studying T cell mediated immune responses targeted to native tubulointerstitial antigens. In these studies, which have been largely performed in two distinct models of autoimmune interstitial nephritis[40,43], we have frequently seen microcysts in kidneys displaying severe interstitial nephritis. This finding led us to question whether there were recognized mediators through which inflammatory cells, in particular lymphocytes and macrophages, could be mechanistically linked to cystogenesis[32].

There are currently several major theories as to the mechanism of cyst formation, and they are by no means mutually exclusive[1]. In a model of cortisone-induced proximal tubular cyst formation, Na^+–K^+ATPase activity is critical, leading Avner et al. to propose that cystogenesis relates to a sodium-dependent increase in organic anion uptake with obligate intratubular fluid accumulation[1-3]. Another proposed mechanism is that of partial or complete tubular obstruction by hyperplastic or polypoid foci of tubular epithelial cells[15,16]. In this scenario, continued accumulation of tubular fluid would potentially lead to tubular dilation and cyst formation proximal to the obstruction. Other investigators have favored the hypothesis that the tubular basement membrane may be intrinsically abnormal in certain types of cystic kidney disease[6,8,14,26,29], leading to diminished radial tensile strength of the TBM.

Lastly, there is recent evidence that abnormal tubular cell proliferation may be a primary phenomenon in cystogenesis. Increased expression of the c-mycon-cogene is seen both in settings of tubular cell proliferation and in genetically determined murine cystic disease[12]. Inhibition of c-myc expression inhibits cycling cell entry into S phase[27]. Moreover, transgenic mice carrying a c-myc construct driven by an SV-40 viral enhancer and human β-globin promoter, develop polycystic kidney disease and progressive renal failure[52]. This should prove to be a fruitful area for continued research. Arguments for and against these mechanisms are reviewed in more detail elsewhere in this volume. We will simply use these hypotheses as a framework to discuss mechanisms where-by autoimmune interstitial nephritis could represent a potential cystogenic process.

In 1971, Lyon and Hulse[35] described an inherited kidney disease that arose spontaneously in an inbred strain of CBA/Ca mice. Lyon developed an inbred strain of these affected mice which she named "kdkd" (kidney disease). The kidneys of kdkd mice are normal at birth. At approximately 10 weeks of age the earliest histologic changes appear, consisting of focal, peritubular accumu-lation of mononuclear cells. Over the next several weeks tubular dilatation occurs focally in both the medulla and cortex, primarily in areas of mononuclear cell infiltration. Both the inflammatory cell infiltrates and tubular dilatation become more widespread with time, eventually occurring throughout the cortex and medulla[35,40]. By 24–28 weeks of age, the tubulointerstitium has become fibrotic and the glomeruli, which remain remarkably normal in ap-pearance up until this time, become sclerotic. By this time the mononuclear cell infiltrates are much less extensive. There is a good correlation between these changes and renal functional abnormalities: at 8–10 weeks there is a concentrating defect, by 16 weeks azotemia, and from then on, a progressive decline in GFR with uremia. Because of the striking tubular dilatation and microcyst formation in the setting of progressive renal failure, Lyon and Hulse[35] proposed that kdkd mice might serve as a useful model of medullary cystic disease.

The spontaneous interstitial nephritis of kdkd mice, like nephronoph-thisis, is inherited as an autosomal recessive trait[35,40]. In early studies Fernan-dez et al [17] demonstrated this experimental disease, like autoimmune glomerulonephritis in NZB/W mice, could be markedly inhibited by caloric (although not protein) restriction. Their findings suggested that autosomal recessive disease in kdkd mice, characterized by tubulointerstitial nephritis and microcysts, might also be mediated by the immune system.

Studies performed in our laboratory over the last several years support the hypothesis that kdkd mice inherit an autoimmune disease[31,33,40]. Susceptibility to develop this disease can be transferred with kdkd bone marrow cells into CBA/Ca or kdkd mice via radiation bone marrow chimeras. Thymectomy at 4 weeks of age inhibits disease development, implying that thymic processing of the T cell repertoire is critical for disease expression[40]. The disease can also be transferred by kdkd spleen and/or lymph node cells into CBA/Ca recipients[31]. As opposed to many other models of autoimmune renal disease, there does not appear to be an important humoral component to this immune response.

We have not identified an antibody with renal specificity from either renal eluates of diseased kidneys or serum from immune mice. A more detailed evaluation of the effector T cells responsible for disease transfer has shown that they fall into the CD8+, CD4- T cell subpopulation, and like most CD8+ cells, recognize their target antigen in association with class I major histocompatibility complex antigens[31]. These CD8+ T cells recognize a tubulointerstitial protein antigen that retains its antigenicity following purification and collagenase solubilization of renal tubules[31]. We have not yet completed purification studies of this antigen. However, it is clearly a distinct protein by Mr and immunogenicity from the 48,000 Mr 3M-1 glycoprotein which is the target antigen of human and experimental antitubular basement membrane disease[9,10].

Having established that kdkd mice inherit a T cell mediated autoimmune disease, which has histologic features of both interstitial nephritis and microcyst formation, we need to understand how antigen-specific and non-specific immune cells and their products might contribute to cystogenesis. In a broad sense one can envisage immune cells and cytokines as either having a primary role or as secondarily acting to create an environment permissive for continued cyst development. Clearly these are not mutually exclusive roles.

There are now adequate phenotypic characterizations of interstitial inflammatory cell infiltrates in several clinical and experimental renal diseases. For example, phenotypic analyses of the interstitial cells in interstitial injury associated with transplant rejection[24] and drug hypersensitivity have consistently demonstrated the presence of both CD4+ and CD8+ T cells, as well as B cells, macrophages and natural killer cells. Likewise, in both experimental antiTBM disease and the spontaneous interstitial nephritis of kdkd mice, the interstitial infiltrates are composed of a variety of inflammatory cells[36,40,58]. Although the hallmark of a targeted immune response is the differentiation and directed trafficking of antigen-specific T and B cells, antigen non-specific immune cells arrive at these sites as well. Ultimately, these non-specific cell types may be equally, if not more, important in altering the structural integrity of the tubulointerstitium. For example, although macrophages are traditionally regarded primarily as phagocytic or antigen-presenting cells, they also produce a variety of secreted enzymes that may be potentially damaging to parenchymal structures[39]. Macrophage products include interleukin-I (IL-1), collagenases and elastases[54]. The latter two products could theoretically diminish the structural integrity of TBM and thus facilitate cyst formation under conditions of increased tubular pressure or altered solute transport.

Although it is not yet clear whether IL-1, IL-4, and IL-6 can primarily increase TBM degradation, at least IL-1 has been shown to stimulate collagenase production, by other parenchymal cells[37]. The number of properties ascribed to IL-1, tumor necrosis factor, and lymphotoxin, including those not traditionally regarded as immunological, is growing rapidly. Our traditional notion that production of these "lymphokines" is largely restricted to immune cells is also becoming outdated. There is abundant evidence that IL-1 is made by many different types of cells.. Most relevant to the kidney is that IL-1 has been shown to be produced by mesangial cells[55] and cultured proximal tubular epithelial cells[28]. Presumably IL-1 production and release by these cells is regulated and occurs in response to specific stimuli. These stimuli, however, are not yet well-characterized for any renal cell. Thus, native renal cells have the capacity to produce cytokines that may become a pathogenic liability in the setting of unregulated production or underlying structural predisposition to cyst formation.

Our knowledge regarding the interactions of T and B cells with their target antigens and how T and B cell products may lead to tubular dilatation is also evolving. Studies from our laboratory have shown that renal proximal tubular cells can function as antigen-presenting cells for a glycoprotein they normally synthesize, 3M-1, the target antigen of antitubular basement membrane disease[28]. Through their capacity to express this self-antigen, and class II MHC antigens and to secrete a cytokine(s) with IL-1 bioactivity, they can support the growth of CD4 +, class II-restricted, 3M-1-specific helper T cells[28]. The cellular effector limb of the autoimmune response in experimental antiTBM disease, as well as in kdkd mice, is mediated by CD8 + class I-restricted T cells[41]. The CD8 + T cell population in these systems is both reactive in mediating DTH responses as well as in mediating directed cytotoxicity[31,41,43].

There may be several discrete mechanisms by which cytotoxic T cells injure their targets. Current evidence shows an important one is directed exocytosis of cytoplasmic granules containing serine proteases or pore-forming proteins[44,57] which are structurally and mechanistically similar to activated proteins in the complement cascade[53]. Clearly with cytotoxicity of tubular cells, the circumferential integrity of the tubule could be compromised. Even sublethal tubular cell damage by serine proteases might critically alter synthesis of structurally important tubular basement membrane components. Either way, T cell-mediated tubular cell damage with a secondary change in TBM structure may be one important mechanistic link between the immune system and cystogenesis.

Autoimmune antibodies directed against tubular cell antigens could elicit tubular damage by a similar mechanism using antibody-dependent cell-mediated cytotoxicity reactions[42]. Antibodies directed against cell surface antigens may also alter TBM and matrix synthesis via complex pathways. For example, antibodies to the 3M-1 antigen on proximal tubular cells can downregulate class II MHC antigen expression[25]. Lastly, although in studies of autoimmune disease we think of cell-surface glycoproteins as target antigens, these proteins must subserve some cell function. If a tubular cell glycoprotein which functions in ion transport is bound by an antibody, this transport function may be altered leading to diminished solute and water transport, a possible cystogenic mechanism[1].

Epithelial cell hyperplasia is another possible cystogenic mechanism, either alone or in consort with other factors altering TBM integrity. T cells, particularly activated T cells, synthesize and secrete transforming growth factor beta (TGF), a peptide that appears to play a major role in cell proliferation and differentiation[49,50]. TGF has been described as having a multiplicity of functions, but it clearly stimulates fibroblast proliferation and can affect tubular cell hypertrophy[18,47]. By the latter mechanism it may be another cytokine linking T cells to cystogenesis.

This discussion has explored a number of mechanisms whereby immune and inflammatory cells may be involved in the process of cystogenesis. We have, out of necessity, reviewed experimental work performed in many different systems and have made analogies to situations which might exist in the kidney under defined circumstances. Many of these mechanisms are largely untested in experimental cystic disease. With the growing availability of well-characterized renal cells in culture, recombinant cytokines, and molecular probes for gene expression, the hypotheses discussed above can be more directly addressed by experimental analysis.

References

1. Avner ED. Renal cystic disease. Insights from recent experimental investigations. Nephron 1988, 48, 86–88.
2. Avner ED, Sweeney WE and Finegold DW. Sodium–potassium ATPase activity mediates cyst formation in metanephric organ culture. Kidney International 1985, 28, 447–455.
3. Avner ED, Sweeney WE, Piesco MP and Ellis D. Triniodothyronine-induced cyst formation in metanephric organ culture; the role of increased Na$^+$–K$^+$ ATPase activity. Journal of Laboratory and Clinical Medicine 1987, 109, 441–448.
4. Bernstein J and Gardner KD. Hereditary tubulointerstitial nephropathies. In: Cotran R, Brenner B and Stein J, eds, Tubulointerstitial Nephropathies. New York: Churchill Livingston, 1983, 335–357.
5. Bohle A, Mackensen-Haen S and Gise HV. Significance of tubulointerstitial changes in the renal cortex for the excretory function and concentration ability of the kidney: A morphometric contribution. American Journal of Nephrology 1987, 7, 421–433.
6. Butkowski RJ, Carone FA, Grantham JJ and Hudson BG. Tubular basement membrane changes in 2-amino-4,5-diphenylthiazole-induced polycystic disease. Kidney International 1985, 28, 744–751.
7. Carone FA. Functional changes in polycystic kidney disease are tubulointerstitial in origin. Seminars in Nephrology 1988, 8, 89–93.
8. Carone FA, Makino H and Kanwar YS. Basement membrane antigens in real polycystic kidney disease. American Journal of Pathology 1988, 130, 466–471.
9. Clayman MD, Martinez-Hernandez A, Michaud L, Alper R, Mann R, Kefalides MA and Neilson EG. Isolation and characterization of the nephritogenic antigen producing antitubular basement membrane disease. Journal of Experimental Medicine 1985, 161, 290–305.
10. Clayman MD, Michaud L, Brentjens J, Andres GA, Kefalides NA and Neilson EG.

Isolation of the target antigen of human anti-tubular basement membrane antibody-associated interstitial nephritis. Journal of Clinical Investigation 1986, 77, 1143–1147.

11. Cohen AH and Hoyer JR. Nephronophthisis. A primary tubular basement membrane defect. Laboratory Investigation 1986, 55, 564–572.

12. Cowley BD, Smardo FL, Grantham JJ and Calvet JP. Elevated c-myc expression in mouse polycystic kidney disease. Kidney International 1987, 31, 163.

13. Cuppage RE, Huseman RA, Chapman A, et al. Ultrastructure and function of cysts from human adult polycystic kidneys. Kidney International 1980, 17, 372–381.

14. Ebihara I, Killen PD, Laurie GW, Huang T, Yamada Y, Martin GR and Brown KS. Altered mRNA expression of basement membrane components in a murine model of polycystic kidney disease. Laboratory Investigation 1988, 58, 262–272.

15. Evan AP and Gardner KD. Nephron obstruction in norhydroguaiaretic acid-induced renal cystic disease. Kidney International 1979, 15, 7–19.

16. Evan AP, Gardner KD and Bernstein J. Polypoid and papillary epithelial hyperplasia: a potential cause of ductal obstruction in adult polycystic disease. Kidney International 1979, 16, 743–750.

17. Fernandez G, Yunis EJ, Miranda M, Smith J and Good RA. Nutritional inhibition of genetically determined renal disease and autoimmunity with prolongation of life in kdkd mice. Proceedings of the National Academy of Sciences (USA) 1978, 75, 2888–2892.

18. Fine LG, Holley RW, Nasri H et al.BSC-1 growth inhibitor transforms a mitogenic stimulus into a hypertrophic stimulus for renal proximal tubular cells: relationship to Na^+/H^+ antiport activity. Proceedings of the National Academy of Sciences (USA) 1985, 82, 6163–6166.

19. Gardner KD. Cystic kidneys. Kidney International 1988, 33, 610–621.

20. Gardner KD, Evan AP and Reed WP. Accelerated renal cyst development in deconditioned germ-free rats. Kidney International 1986, 29, 1116–1123.

21. Gardner KD, Reed WP, Evan AP, Zedalis J, Hylarides MD and Leon AA. Endotoxin provocation of experimental renal cystic disease. Kidney International 1987, 32, 329–334.

22. Grantham JJ, Donosos VS, Evan AP, Carone FA and Gardner KD. Viscoelastic properties of tubular basement membranes in experimental renal cystic disease. Kidney International 1987, 32, 187–197.

23. Grantham JJ, Geiser JL and Evan AP. Cyst formation and growth in autosomal dominant polycystic kidney disease. Kidney International 1987, 31, 1145–1152.

24. Hancock WW, Thomson NM and Atkins RC. Composition of intersititial cellular infiltrate identified by monoclonal antibodies in renal biopsies of rejecting human renal allografts. Transplantation 1983, 35, 458–463.

25. Haverty T, Kelly CJ, Watanabe M and Neilson EG. Immunoregulation of class II MHC gene expression by tubular epithelium influences susceptibility to murine interstitial nephritis. Kidney International 1988, 33, 158.

26. Haverty T and Neilson EG. Basement membrane gene expression in polycystic kidney disease. Laboratory Investigation 1988, 58, 245–248.

27. Heikkala R, Schwab G, Wickstrom E, Loke SL, Pluznik DH, Watt R and Neckers LM. A c-myc antisense oligodeoxynucleotide inhibits entry into S phase but not progress from G_0 to G_1. Nature 1987, 328, 445–449.

28. Hines WH, Kelly CJ, Haverty T and Neilson EG. Recognition of antigen-secreting renal epithelial cells by antigen specific helper T cells. Kidney International 1988, 33, 317.

29. Kanwar YS and Carone FA. Reversible changes of tubular cell and basement membrane in drug-induced renal cystic disease. Kidney International 1984, 26, 35–43.

30. Kehrl JH, Wakefield LM and Roberts AB. Production of transforming growth factor β by tumor T lymphocytes and its potential role in the regulation of a T cell growth. Journal of Experimental Medicine 1986, 163, 1037–1050.

31. Kelly CJ, Korngold R, Mann R, Clayman M, Haverty T and Neilson EG. Spontaneous interstitial nephritis in kdkd mice. II. Characterization of a tubular antigen-specific,

H-2K-restricted Lyt-2$^+$ effector T cell that mediates destructive tubulointerstitial injury. Journal of Immunology 1986, 136, 526–531.

32. Kelly CJ and Neilson EG. Medullary cystic disease: an inherited form of autoimmune interstitial nephritis? American Journal of Kidney Disease 1987, 10, 389–395.

33. Kelly CJ and Neilson EG. Contrasuppression in autoimmunity. Journal of Experimental Medicine 1987, 165, 107–123.

34. Kissane JM. Congenital malformations. In: Heptinstall RH ed, Pathology of the Kidney. Boston: Little Brown, 1983, 83–140.

35. Lyon MF and Hulse EV. An inherited kidney disease of mice resembling human nephronophthisis. Journal of Medical Genetics 1971, 8, 41–48.

36. Mampaso FM and Wilson CB. Characterisation of inflammatory cells in autoimmune tubulointerstitial nephritis in rats. Kidney International 1983, 23, 448–457.

37. Mizel SB, Dayer JM, Krane SM et al. Stimulation of rheumatoid synovial cell collagenase and prostaglandin production by partially purified lymphocyte activating factor (interleukin-1). Proceedings of the National Academy of Sciences (USA) 1981, 78, 2474–2477.

38. Naparstek Y, Cohen IR, Fuks Z, et al. Activated T lymphocytes produce a matrix degrading heparan sulphate endoglycosidase. Nature 1984, 310, 241–244.

39. Nathan C. Secretory products of macrophages. Journal of Clinical Investigation 1987, 79, 319–326.

40. Neilson EG, McCafferty E, Feldman A, Clayman MD, Zakheim B and Korngold R. Spontaneous interstitial nephritis in kdkd mice. I. An experimental model of autoimmune renal disease. Journal of Immunology 1984, 133, 2560–2565.

41. Neilson EG, McCafferty E, Mann R, Michaud L and Clayman M. Murine interstitial nephritis. III. The selection of phenotypic and idiotypic T cell preferences by genes in Igh-1 and H-2K characterizes the cell-mediated potential for disease expression: susceptible mice provide a unique effector T cell repertoire in response to tubular antigen. Journal of Immunology 1985, 134, 2375–2382.

42. Neilson EG and Phillips SM. Cell-mediated immunity in interstitial nephritis. IV. Antitubular basement membrane antibodies can function in antibody-dependent cellular cytotoxity reactions: observations on a nephritogenic effector mechanism acting as an information bridge between the humoral and cellular immune response. Journal of Immunology 1981, 126, 1990–1994.

43. Neilson EG and Phillips SM. Murine interstitial nephritis. I. Analysis of disease susceptibility and its relationship to pleiomorphic gene products defining both immune-response genes and a restrictive requirement for cytotoxic T cells at H-2K. Journal of Experimental Medicine 1982, 155, 1075–1085.

44. Pasternack MS, Verret CR, Liu MA and Eisen HN. Serine esterase in cytolytic T lymphocytes. Nature 1986, 322, 740–743.

45. Perrone RD. In vitro function of cyst epithelium from human polycystic kidney disease. Journal of Clinical Investigation 1985, 76, 1688–1691.

46. Risdon RA, Sloper JC and de Wardener HE. Relationship between renal function and histological changes found in renal-biopsy patients with persistent glomerular nephritis. Lancet 1968, 2, 363–366.

47. Roberts AB, Sporn MB, Assoian RK, et al. Transforming growth factor–β: rapid induction of fibrosis and angiogenesis in vivo and stimulation of collagen formation in vitro. Proceedings of the National Academy of Sciences (USA) 1986, 83, 4167–4171.

48. Sloper JC, de Wardener H and Woodrow DF. Relationship between renal structure and function deduced from renal biopsies. In: Leaf A, Giebisch G, Bolis L and Gorini S, eds, Renal Pathophysiology – Recent Advances. New York: Raven Press, 1980, 109–120.

49. Sporn MB and Roberts AB. Peptide growth factors are multifunctional. Nature 1988, 332, 216–219.

50. Sporn MB, Roberts AB and Wakefield LM. Transforming growth factor–β : Biological function and chemical structure. Science 1986, 233, 532–534.

51. Steele BT, Lirenman DS and Beattie CW. Nephronophthisis. American Journal of Medicine 1980, 68, 531–538.
52. Trudel M, D'Agati V and Costantini F. The c-myc oncogene induces kidney cysts in transgenic mice. Kidney International 1989 (in press).
53. Tschopp J, Masson D and Stanley KK. Structural/functional similarity between proteins involved in complement- and cytotoxic T-lymphocyte-mediated cytolysis. Nature 1986, 322, 831–834.
54. Werb Z, Banda MJ and Jones PA. Degradation of connective tissues matrices by macrophages. I. Proteolysis of elastin, glycoproteins, and collagen by proteinases isolated from macrophages. Journal of Experimental Medicine 1980, 152, 1340–1357.
55. Werber HI, Emancipator SN, Tykocinski MI and Sedor JR. The interleukin 1 gene is expressed by rat glomerular mesangial cells and is augmented in immune complex glomerulonephritis. Journal of Immunology 1987, 138, 3207–3212.
56. Wilson PD, Schrier RW, Breckon RD and Gabow PA. A new method for studying human polycystic kidney disease epithelia in culture. Kidney International 1986, 30, 371–378.
57. Young JD-E, Leong LG, Liu CC, et al. Isolation and characterization of a serine esterase from cytolytic T cell granules. Cell 1986, 47, 183–194.
58. Zakheim B, McCafferty E, Phillips SM and Neilson EG. Murine interstitial nephritis. II. The adoptive transfer of disease with immune T lymphocytes produces a phenotypically complex interstitial lesion. Journal of Immunology 1984, 133, 234–239.
59. Zollinger HU, Mihatsch MJ, Edefonti A, Gaboardi F, Imbascrati E and Lennert T. Nephronophthisis (medullary cystic disease of the kidney): A study using electron microscopy, immunofluorescence, and a review of the morphological findings. Helvetica Pediatrica Acta 1980, 35, 509–517.

4
Models of Cysts and Cystic Kidneys

E.D. Avner, J.A. McAteer and A.P. Evan

Abstract

The mechanisms of cyst formation and progressive enlargement have been the subject of intense experimental investigation in both in vivo and in vitro model systems. Animal studies have focused on induction of cystic disease in various species by cystogenic chemicals, by surgical induction of renal cysts, and by genetic analysis. In vitro studies have focused on the production and modulation of renal cysts in murine metanephric organ culture, the study of epithelial cell culture from natural and experimental cystic renal tissue, and the culture of established cell lines. Studies in models have identified hyperplasia, obstruction, basement membrane abnormalities and fluid transport as potential pathogenic factors. It is suggested that similar factors operate in human renal cystic diseases. Theories generated from experimental models can be synthesized into a working hypothesis of the pathogenesis of renal cyst formation.

Key words   Cyst;
Experimental models.

Abbreviations ADH, Antidiuretic hormone;
ADPKD, Autosomal dominant polycystic kidney disease;
AH 2835, 5, 6, 7, 8, Tetrahydrocarbazole-3-acetic acid;
cAMP, Cyclic adenosine monophosphate;
CPK, C57BL/6J-CPK mouse;
DOCA, 11-Deoxycorticosterone acetate;
DPA, Diphenylamine;
DPT, Diphenylthiazole;
MDCK, Madin–Darby canine kidney cell line;
Na–K ATPase, Sodium–potassium activated adenosine triphosphatase;
NDGA, Nordihydroguaiaretic acid;
TF/P, Tubular fluid to plasma.

1. Introduction

Renal cysts are central pathologic features in several human disease states. Mechanisms of their formation and progressive enlargement have been subjects of significant experimental investigation over the past three decades.

In this chapter we review the variety of experimental models that have been developed to study the pathogenesis of renal cystic disease. Since a number of excellent reviews have previously been published[51,160], we will focus on recent developments.

Table 4.1. Chemically-induced experimental renal cystic disease

I. Well-characterized models

Agent	Species[a]	References
Diphenylamine/Biphenyl	Rat (f,nb,y,a)	1,30,50,58,64,68,85,114, 171,180,182,185,206
	Chicken (nb)	59,125
Nordihydroguaiaretic acid	Rat (y,a)	65,82–84,90,94,97
Diphenylthiazole	Rat (y,a)	38–43,62,81,94,102,108,109,188
Corticosteroids	Rabbit (nb,y)	21,78,144–147,152,166,167,193
	Rat (nb,y)	52,54,140,197
	Hamster (nb)	71
	Dog (y)	140

a (f = fetal, nb = newborn, y = young, a = adult)

II. Incompletely characterized models

Alloxan	Rat	192
Bacitracin	Rat	34
Cis-platinum	Rat	60,61
Arabinoside	Rat/Mouse	151
5-Idododeoxyuridine	Rat/Mouse	151
Lead acetate	Rat	31
Lithium	Dog	157
	Rat	45
Santoquin	Rat	205
Sedormid®	Rat	31
Stilbestrol	Pig	44
Streptozotocin	Rat	115
2,4,5-Trichlorophenoxyacetic acid	Mouse	46
Di (2-ethylhexyl) phthalate	Rat	53

The pathogenesis of renal cyst formation and of subsequent enlargement has been studied in both *in vivo* and *in vitro* model systems. Animal studies *in vivo* have focused on the induction of cystic disease in several species by cystogenetic chemicals or surgical manipulation, and on the analysis of genetically transmitted cystic diseases in certain animal species. *In vitro* studies have focused on the production and modulation of renal cysts in murine renal organ culture, on primary cell culture of epithelia from animal and human cystic diseases, and on the culture of established renal cell lines.

2. In vivo models: Chemically-induced experimental renal cystic disease

Several different chemical agents produce renal cysts in experimental animals (Table 4.1). In all such models, kidneys are normal prior to treatment, and the cysts produced by drug administration progressively increase in size and number over time. These models provide important insights into the mechanisms of acquisition and growth of cysts in previously normal renal tissue. The chemical induction of cysts has permitted characterization of the structure and function of the cystic nephron, and demonstrated that environmental factors can modulate cyst formation and growth. The best characterized chemical cystogens include potent antioxidants, diphenylamine, diphenylthiazole, and nordihydroguaiaretic acid; corticosteroids; and 5, 6, 7, 8 tetrahydrocarbazole-3-acetic acid.

2.1. Diphenylamine (Figure 4.1A–F)

DPA was the first chemical cystogen to be extensively studied. Thomas et al. [185] showed that long-term feeding of 1.5% diphenylamine (DPA) produced renal cysts primarily at the corticomedullary junction. It was later shown that the severity of the cystic lesion was dose-dependent and that the lesion could be induced in kidneys of both young and mature rats[50,114,185,186].

Kime et al. [114] correlated functional changes of the kidney in response to DPA with a more detailed morphologic examination of the cystic lesion. Epithelial damage (cell injury) was identified in the proximal tubule, while cyst formation was localized to the distal and collecting tubules. These morphologic changes were accompanied by a decrease in creatinine clearance and a diminished concentrating ability. The DPA-cystic kidney was more susceptible to pyelonephritis. Kime et al. emphasized the similarities of the DPA-induced cystic lesion to human autosomal dominant polycystic kidney disease (ADPKD) by noting that in both conditions: (1) there is a loss of concentrating ability; (2) cysts develop in otherwise normal nephron segments; (3) the lesion is heterogeneous; and (4) cysts are focal in distribution and are surrounded by structurally normal tubules. Subsequent data showed that cell injury is involved in cyst formation in the collecting tubule, and confirmed that the first detectable change in renal function is a decreased maximal concentrating capacity[171,206]. Cyst formation is closely associated with interstitial inflammation and scarring. Thickened tubular basal laminae encase cystic and injured tubules.

Darmady et al. [58] found ultrastructural changes in the cyst-lining cells suggesting that an injury repair process may be involved in cyst formation. Cell repair followed cell injury after administration of DPA, and the newly proliferative epithelium was irregularly hyperplastic with thickened basal laminae. Darmady et al. hypothesized that cyst formation was a response of tubular cells

58

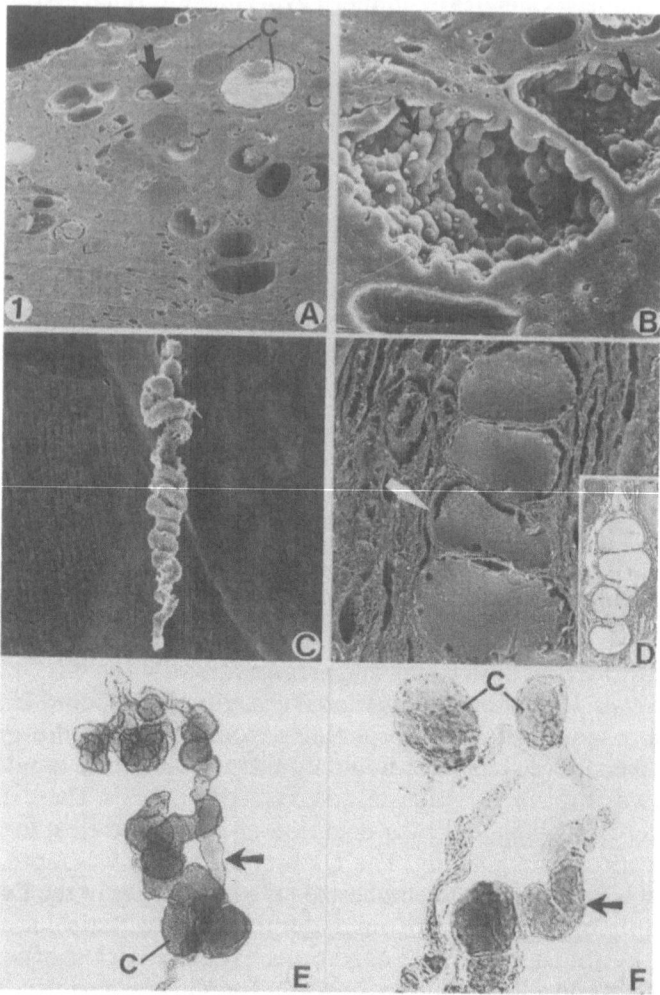

Figure 4.1. (A–F). The DPA model of renal cystic disease. (A) Low magnification scanning electron micrograph showing the renal cortex of an animal treated with DPA for 1 year. Numerous cysts of the renal corpuscle (arrow) and different segments of the nephron (C) are seen. (B) Higher magnification of two cortical cysts along a collecting tubule from the same kidney as Fig. 4.1A. The epithelium lining the cyst wall is characterised by irregular hyperplasia with micropolyp formation (arrows). (C) Scanning electron micrograph of an isolated medullary collecting tubule from an animal treated with DPA for 6 months. The corkscrew appearance of nephrons early in the development of the lesion is a consequence of epithelial hyperplasia. (D) This scanning electron micrograph shows a longitudinal fracture through a dilated medullary collecting tubule. The corkscrew pattern (arrow) of the lesion is clearly evident here and in tissue section (inset). (E) Microdissected cortical collecting tubule from an animal treated with DPA for 1 year. Cysts can appear as regions of dilation (tubular enlargement) (arrow) or focal sac-like structures (C). (F) This light micrograph also shows a microdissected cortical collecting tubule as in Figure 4.1E. A region of dilation (arrow) is seen, as well as two cystic diverticuli (C).

to prolonged exposure to a toxic substance. He suggested that human PKD may be linked to a long-acting genetically determined toxic metabolite.

In 1976, Gardner *et al.* [85] suggested that the pathogenesis of cyst formation in DPA-exposed kidneys may involve tubular obstruction. They found that dilated tubules exhibited elevated intraluminal pressures and that microperfused cystic nephrons had prolonged elimination of [^{3}H]inulin. Both findings suggested partial tubular obstruction, and morphologic examination showed dilated collecting tubules to contain debris and focal sites of narrowing. Evan *et al.* [64] further observed that epithelial hyperplasia was a consistent feature of affected tubules. They found that some cells of collecting tubule cysts were large and irregularly shaped, and frequently formed polyp-like structures projecting into the tubular lumens. The dilated tubules possessed an increased number of cells, further evidence of cellular hyperplasia. These findings led to the hypothesis that cellular hyperplasia was a primary event by which tubules undergo dilatation and cyst formation.

Despite the similarities of the DPA-induced model to ADPKD and despite its value in elucidating potential roles of cellular hyperplasia and tubular obstruction in cyst formation, interest in the model has waned in recent years. This situation may be due, in part, to the finding by Crocker *et al.* [50] that an unidentified contaminant of DPA, not DPA itself, is responsible for the cystic abnormality.

2.2. Diphenylthiazole (DPT) (Figure 4.2A–F)

Carone *et al.* [42,43] showed that a new cystogenic agent, DPT, produced functional and structural kidney changes during an 11-week period in which adult rats were fed a diet containing 1.0% DPT. By one week, treated animals demonstrated a marked impairment of maximal urine concentrating ability that was not corrected by exogenous antidiuretic hormone. After 1–2 weeks, cells of the medullary collecting ducts were focally degenerated and necrotic, with subsequent regeneration. The first morphologic evidence of cystic change was noted as dilatation of the outer medullary collecting tubules between 1 and 3 weeks. By 4–5 weeks all outer medullary collecting tubules were cystic, and the abnormality progressed to involve most inner medullary collecting ducts, distal tubules and loops of Henle. The proximal tubule and papillary collecting ducts were unaffected, and interstitial fibrosis and tubular obstruction were not noted. Electron microscopy showed normal epithelia in early cysts, with later loss of morphologic phenotype, cytoplasmic organelles, and basolateral membrane complexity. Functional analysis by micropuncture of cystic nephrons revealed normal GFR, normal intraluminal pressures in 95% of tubules, and preservation of normal tubular transport function (characterized by normal TF/P inulin ratios and osmolal gradients of proximal and distal tubular fluids).

60

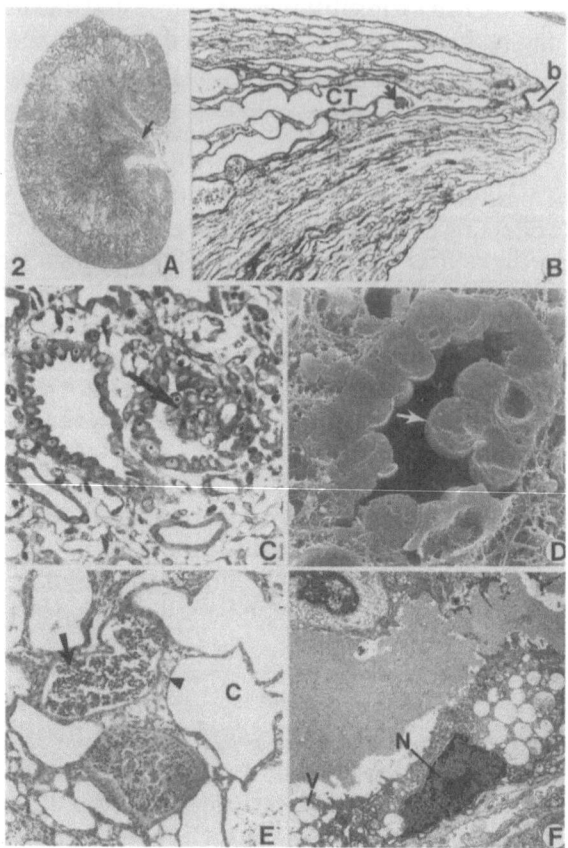

Figure 4.2A–F. Morphology of DPT-induced renal cystic disease. (A) Light micrograph of a kidney from an animal that was exposed to DPT for 4 months. The arrow marks a group of dilated medullary collecting tubules that are seen at a higher magnification in Fig. 4.2B. Cysts have a diffuse distribution throughout the entire kidney. (Reprinted from *Kidney International* [81] with permission). (B) Light micrograph of an enlargement of the papilla illustrated in Figure 4.2A. A large polyp (arrow) is located at a branching point of a duct of Bellini (B). The inner medullary collecting tubule (CT) proximal to the polyp are dilated. (Reprinted from *Kidney International* [81] with permission). (C) Cross-section of the inner medulla from an animal treated with DPT for 3 weeks. Two dilated collecting tubules with hyperplastic walls are seen. The tubule on the right bears a micropolyp (arrow) that has obstructed approximately 80% of the lumen. (D) Scanning electron micrograph showing a micropolyp (arrow) originating from the wall of a dilated collecting tubule, from an animal treated with DPT for 3 weeks. (E) Light micrograph of the renal cortex of an animal treated with DPT for 7 weeks. Numerous cysts (C) are seen. Two cysts are filled with polymorphonuclear leukocytes (arrow). Inflammatory cells are also noted in the adjacent interstitium (arrowhead). (F) Transmission electron micrograph of an outer medullary collecting tubule from an animal treated with DPT for 7 weeks. This model is characterized by extensive cell injury and necrosis. Several cells in this micrograph show evidence of degeneration noted by numerous large vacuoles (V) and electron dense nuclei (N). Basement membrane thickening at cystic sites is common for the DPT-induced model of renal cystic disease. (Reprinted from *Kidney International* [81] with permission).

Dousa et al. [62] demonstrated a reduced response of renal medullary adenylate cyclase to ADH, suggesting a diminished formation of cAMP in this model.

On the basis of their findings, Carone et al. [42] hypothesized the primary cause of tubular cystic change to be a defect in the elastic characteristics of the tubular basement membrane. They suggested that DPT alters the molecular structure of the collagen-like components of the tubular basement membrane, resulting in diminished elasticity and reduced tensile strength and allowing progressive tubular distention under conditions of normal intratubular pressure.

Kanwar and Carone[108] found progressive thickening and an abnormal, laminated fine structure of the basal lamina of DPT-induced cystic tubules. Concomitant with basal lamina thickening was a loss of alcian blue and ruthenium red staining, suggesting a change in the sulphated proteoglycan or anionic glycoprotein components. Structural changes in the cyst-lining cells prior to alterations of the tubular basal lamina suggested that cellular metabolic mechanisms had been affected. Butkowski et al. [38] found significant changes in the content of specific basal lamina components during the development of DPT-induced renal cysts: a four- to five-fold increase in fibronectin, a three-fold increase in type I collagen, and a decrease in both Mr 55,000 polypeptide and a sulphated proteoglycan. The concentrations of laminin, entactin and type IV collagen did not change. The content of defined extracellular matrix components (except type I collagen) in the tubular basal lamina returned to normal values within a four-week recovery period, a change paralleled by a return to normal in basal lamina morphology[38]. Immunofluorescent staining of cyst walls with antiheparan sulphate proteoglycan was reduced, while staining with anti-fibronectin, antilaminin and antitype IV collagen was increased[40], but changes were not in full agreement with the previously noted biochemical findings. These alterations in matrix may modulate epithelial behavior and direct cyst growth.

These studies on the DPT-induced model of PKD demonstrate changes in the tubular basal lamina of cystic nephrons. It is still not known, however, if these alterations represent primary events in the disease process or are secondary to other pathophysiologic mechanisms. To quantitate the mechanical properties of the supporting walls of normal and cystic nephrons, both deformability and viscoelastic creep were determined for individual microdissected nephrons from four models of cystic disease (two chemical, DPT and NDGA; and two genetic, CPK and CFW$_{wd}$) and controls[94]. The analyses showed no difference in the values obtained for the cystic nephrons of all models versus control nephrons, and do not support the idea that a change in basal lamina compliance is the primary mechanism of DPT-induced cyst formation.

Additional studies by Gardner and Evan on the DPT model[81] demonstrated that epithelial hyperplasia preceded fluid accumulation, cyst formation and other morphologic changes. Thymidine labelling increased within one week, and dilated collecting tubules radiated from the inner medulla to the cortex within two weeks. Micropolyps appeared to obstruct lumens in medullary collecting ducts, primarily in the inner medulla. Given the pattern of the dichotomous branching of the renal collecting ducts, a single polyp in this position could theoretically interfere with flow from several hundred nephrons. Other morphologic features of this model included extensive cellular injury and necrosis, interstitial fibroplasia and infiltration by neutrophils and lymphocytes. Functional studies showed mean basal hydrostatic pressures between normal and cystic nephrons not to be different. However, intratubular pressures were significantly elevated in cystic nephrons when they were challenged by microperfusion with a known volume of fluid. The structural and functional data suggest the presence of partial collecting duct obstruction in the DPT-induced cyst model.

Torres et al. [188] showed that the development of DPT-induced cysts can be influenced by experimental manipulation of the renin–angiotensin system. Sodium restriction, renovascular hypertension and furosemide administration enhanced cyst formation, wheras sodium-loading, DOCA-salt hypertension and enalapril administration decreased cyst growth. Angiotensin II may, therefore, regulate cyst growth by affecting cell proliferation, interstitial pressure, or tubular compliance.

While the acute changes in nephron structure and function following DPT-treatment have been well characterized, little attention has been given to chronic changes in the model. Carone et al. [41] found a gradual loss in renal function over 30 weeks. An early and persistent impairment of concentrating ability was followed by a progressive drop in glomerular filtration and by moderate proteinuria. Epithelial hyperplasia was superseded by tubular atrophy, with basal lamina thickening and interstitial fibrosis.

Thus, like ADPKD and the DPA-induced model, the DPT-induced model of renal cystic disease comprises a concentrating defect, a gradual decline in GFR, basal lamina changes, epithelial hyperplasia and fluid accumulation. Unlike ADPKD, however, the DPT model has fusiform cysts located primarily along collecting ducts. The cystic lesion is diffuse in that all collecting ducts appear to be involved, and rampant cell injury and necrosis eventually result in decreased cyst size.

2.3. Nordihydroguaiaretic Acid (NDGA) (Figure 4.3A–G)

NDGA is an antioxidant that has been used as both a food preservative and an anticancer agent[37,194]. NDGA is known as an extremely potent inhibitor of anaerobic and aerobic glycolysis[37] and of intracellular lipoxygenase activity[101]. Goodman et al. [90] were the first to identify the cystic nephropathy induced by NDGA. In adult rats fed a diet containing 2% NDGA, cysts progressively developed along the entire nephron following initial proximal tubular involvement. Cysts were lined with nondescript flattened or cuboidal cells and con-

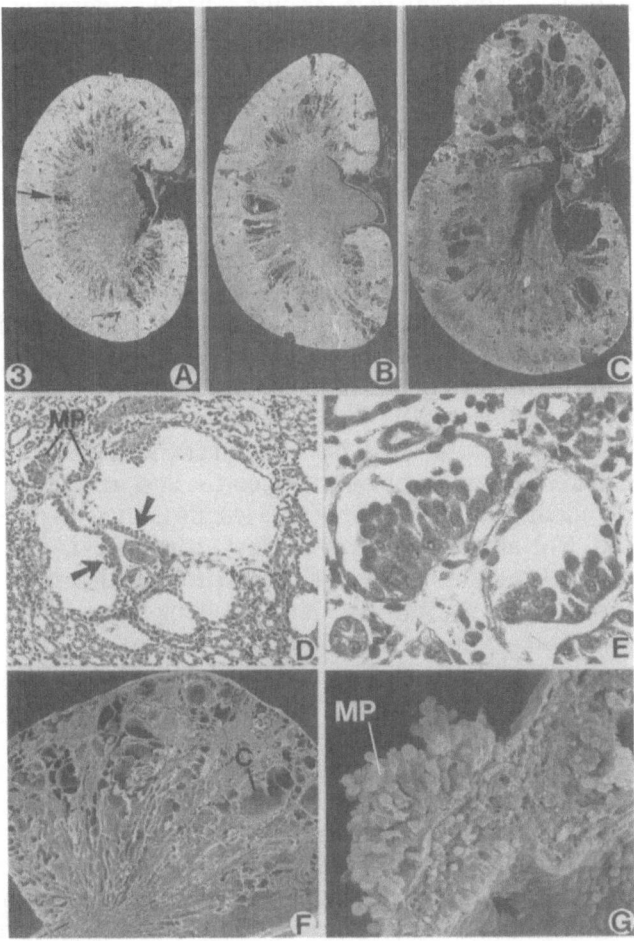

Figure 4.3A–G. Structure of the NDGA-treated rat model of renal cystic disease. Figs. 4.3A, B and C show a series of light micrographs from animals treated with NDGA. There is a progression in the severity of the cystic lesion with time, (4.3A) one week, (4.3B) one month, (4.3C) six months. At one week (4.3A), the only change noted is the appearance of small dilated collecting tubules in the inner cortex and outer medullar (arrow). By six months (4.3C) numerous cysts (arrow) of varying sizes are found throughout the kidney. (Reprinted from Kidney International [65] with permission). (D) Light micrograph showing a series of dilated inner medullary collecting tubules in cross section. Areas of irregular hyperplasia (arrows) are seen in several dilated tubules. In addition, micropolys (MP) are noted projecting into the tubular lumen of two dilated collecting tubules. (Reprinted from Kidney International [65] with permission). (E) Higher magnification field demonstrating a pair of dilated collecting tubules shown in Fig. 4.3D. Both tubules possesses micropolyps. The cells of the micropolyps are not characteristic of normal inner medullary collecting tubular cells. (Reprinted from Kidney International [65] with permission). (F) Scanning electron micrograph showing cystic nature of a kidney from an animal treated with NDGA for 6 months. Cysts (C) are seen throughout the kidney. (G) Scanning electron micrograph showing a micropolyp (MP) and an area of irregular hyperplasia (arrow) in two adjacent cysts.

tained foci of degenerating and regenerating cells. Degenerating tubules were seen adjacent to cystic nephrons. A marked interstitial reaction included fibroplasia and infiltration by lymphocytes and histiocytes. Cyst formation was thought to result from epithelial cell desquamation, producing tubular obstruction and cysts. Large cysts were thought to form by the coalescence of adjacent affected tubules.

Evan and Gardner[65] identified focal epithelial proliferation in a population of outer medullary collecting ducts as the first morphologic event in cyst formation. Many collecting ducts appeared unchanged. The initial burst of mitotic activity was followed by dilatation in some of the collecting ducts. Epithelial hyperplasia included a proliferation of the original differentiated cell type and focal collections of densely packed, undifferentiated, columnar cells. Micropolyps projected into the lumens, and some polyps were of a sufficient size to occlude 80% of the ductal lumen. Microdissection revealed that additional segments of the nephron dilated and formed fusiform to saccular cysts. Cysts were found throughout the cortex and medulla by six months, and the corticomedullary junctions became less distinct, with distortion of the inner medulla. Not all nephrons were affected in the NDGA model. This pattern of cyst progression is strikingly similar to that described in ADPKD (see Chapter 2). Tubular atrophy also occurred with progression of the disease. Dilated tubules were commonly surrounded by clusters of atrophic tubules as well as islands of apparently normal nephrons. Interstitial changes included fibrosis, interstitial cell proliferation, and infiltration by small lymphocytes, neutrophils and numerous macrophages.

Microperfusion of 50 nl of fluid into cysts over a two-minute interval caused the intraluminal pressure to rise significantly. Microinjection of [³H] inulin into individual nephrons demonstrated reduced fluid excretion in cystic compared to unaffected tubules. Thus, partial obstruction of ducts by hyperplastic polyps reduced urine outflow and contributed to cyst formation.

The expression of NDGA-induced renal cystic disease is influenced by environmental factors (Fig. 4.4A–D). Germ-free animals showed no cyst formation, but animals deconditioned after three weeks showed an accelerated rate of cyst formation and growth when compared to all previously published NDGA studies[82]. Deconditioning was accompanied by cellular injury, epithelial proliferation and tubular dilatation in the outer medullary collecting ducts. Several morphologic features were unique to NDGA-treated, deconditioned animal model. First, cell injury was clearly the first morphologically detectable alteration to occur, followed by epithelial proliferation. Second, hyperplastic micropolyps, often occurring in clusters, were common in affected segments throughout the nephron, and were larger and more numerous than those of conventional animals. Third, neutrophils and, to a lesser degree, lymphocytes, plasma cells and macrophages were prevalent within the interstitium and microvessels immediately subjacent to the cyst epithelium, particularly at regions of epithelial hyperplasia.

Secondary infection of cystic kidneys and colonization by specific micro-organisms were excluded as possible provocateurs of accelerated nephropathy in the deconditioned animals[82]. Cyst formation was enhanced, however, by treatment of germfree NDGA-exposed animals with endotoxin or by exposure to endotoxin-producing bacteria[84]. There was a high correlation between the degree of cystic change and the number of neutrophils and lymphocytes in the

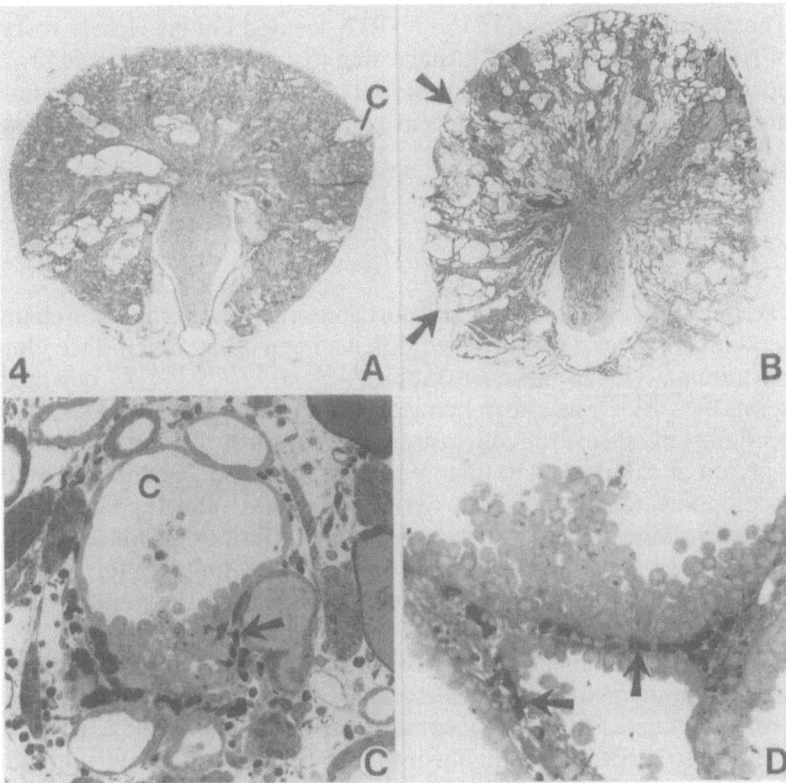

Figure 4.4A–D. Environmental modulation of the NDGA cystic lesion. These micrographs demonstrate acceleration of the cystic lesion by bacterial contamination. (A) Ligh micrograph showing a cross section of a kidney from a conventional Sprague–Dawley rat treated with NDGA for 42 days. Cysts (C) of various sizes are present, but they are fewer in number and smaller in size than cysts in an animal challenged by microbial contamination (Fig. 4.4B). (Reprinted from Kidney International [82] with permission). (B) Light micrograph of a kidney from a deconditioned rat. This gnotobiotic animal was fed NDGA in a germfree environment for 3 weeks and then exposed to an ambient microbial environment for an additional 3 weeks. Many more dilated to cystic nephrons (arrow) are found throughout the cortex and medulla of this deconditioned animal as compared to the conventional NDGA-treated kidney seen in Fig. 4.4A. (Reprinted from Kidney International [82] with permission). (C) Light micrograph from the kidney shown in Fig. 4.4B. This cystic collecting tubule (C) possesses numerous polymorphonuclear leukocytes (arrows) located subjacent to a large micropolyp. (D) This light micrograph shows portions of several cysts from a deconditioned NDGA-treated rat. Numerous PMNs (arrows) are located subjacent to areas of irregular hyperplasia and micropolyp formation.

peripheral blood. The tight correlation of cystic change to the number of neutrophils suggested a significant role for the leukocytes in the generation of the cystic lesions. Similar correlations have been demonstrating among circulating and infiltrating neutrophils, micropolyp formation, nephron dilatation, renal pathology, and azotemia in conventional rats fed NDGA and injected with endotoxin[83]. The cyst-promoting effects of endotoxin in combination with NDGA are, therefore, not restricted to the germfree setting.

The morphologic lesion in the NDGA-treated kidney closely resembles that of ADPKD (see Chapter 2), suggesting that similar pathogenic processes may be operative in human cystic disease. The model may have particular value in elucidating the role of specific environmental factors in modulating cyst enlargement.

2.4. Corticosteroids

Since Baxter's original description of cortisone-induced renal cystic changes in young rabbits[21], several glucocorticoids have been utilized to induce glomerular and tubular cysts in newborn rabbit[78,144–147,152,166,167,193], newborn and young rats[52,54,140,197], newborn hamsters[71] and young dogs[140]. Despite interspecies differences, several conclusions can be drawn. With the exception of renal proximal tubular dilatation following repeated injection of 9-fluoroprednisolone acetate in newborn Syrian hamsters[71] and repeated cortisone injections in young rabbits[21], the initial cystic lesions produced by glucocorticoids are localized to developing cortical collecting tubules. In newborn rabbits treated with methylprednisolone acetate, lesions extended at a later stage to glomeruli[144,145,166] and, to a lesser extent, proximal tubules[146]. Similarly, following initial localization to cortical collecting tubules, cystic lesions produced by prednisolone butylacetate in newborn rats extended to glomeruli and proximal tubules[197]. It has become apparent that all of the corticosteroid-induced cystic models are highly influenced, if not directly mediated by hypokalemia and electrolyte imbalance. Thus, Perey et al.[152] showed that corticosteroid-induced cystic disease in newborn rabbits correlated directly with mineralocorticoid effects and consequent hypokalemia, and was largely prevented by co-administration of potassium chloride. Though a less direct relationship was present in the other glucocorticoid-induced models, hypokalemia was an important modulating factor of corticosteroid-induced cyst formation in the various rat, hamster and dog models[52,54,71,140,197]. This is of particular interest given the reported effects of hypokalemia in producing renal tubular dilatation in several species[28,73,149,173,181].

The morphologically most completely studied glucocorticoid model has been that in which 9-fluroprednisolone acetate or methylprednisolone acetate was administered to newborn rabbits[152]. Renal microdissection and light and electron microscopic analysis revealed three distinct stages of cyst development[78,144–147,166,167]. An initial stage of decreased nephrogenesis was followed by accelerated tubular cell death without significant inflammation or cellular infiltration. Enlargement and cyst formation of cortical collecting tubules was accompanied by preservation of normal principal to intercalated cell ratios and elongation of cortical proximal tubular segments. These changes occurred with persistence of patterned cell death in tubular cyst walls and the continued absence of a cortical nephrogenic zone. Glomerular cyst formation was then accompanied by partial regression of tubular cysts. The glomerular cysts were unique in that the parietal epithelial layer underwent transformation to podocytes.

Although the precise mechanisms of cyst-formation and progressive enlargement in the corticosteroid models are unknown, the regular production of cystic lesions at different sites along the nephron makes these models potentially useful for studying the differential susceptibility of specific nephron segments to cyst formation. Further, the reproducibility of cyst formation following corticosteroid administration permits study of environmental factors that might modulate cyst formation or enlargement. The corticosteroid models may also be of value in the study of renal epithelial differentiation and the assembly of the glomerular filtration surface[145,158,166]. A major drawback to the corticosteroid-induced whole animal models is the well-known multiple effect of corticosteroids on renal and cellular physiology, growth, differentiation, the inflammatory response and the metabolism of extracellular matrix[22,148,178].

2.5. 5,6,7,8 Tetrahydrocarbazole-3-acetic acid

During toxicity testing of a new anti-inflammatory compound, AH 2835 Poyncer et al. [156] noted the development of bilateral cystic kidneys in rats. Subsequent studies confirmed the cyst-promoting effects of the agent in rats of varying ages[126–128]. Microdissection studies localized the earliest cystic changes to the proximal convoluted tubule, with less prominent effects on distal and collecting tubules[128]. AH 2835 produced most significant changes in male rats of younger ages. Cyst formation was accompanied by hyperplasia of tubular epithelial cells and intercellular vacuolization. These features and changes in Na–K ATPase activity in treated animals led McGeoch et al. [126,127] to hypothesize that intrauterine increases in renal Na–K ATPase activity might trigger tubular epithelial hyperplasia and promote cystic changes. Due to methodologic limitations, their hypothesis could not be tested through direct measurement of enzyme activity in fetal kidneys. The removal of AH 2835 from production precluded further experimental work, but this model was the first to link altered tubular transport energetics with epithelial hyperplasia in producing tubular cystic changes. The relationship of transtubular solute transport (with consequent fluid accumulation) to epithelial hyperplasia in tubular cyst formation and progressive enlargement remains an active area of current investigation[2,80] (see Chapter 5).

2.6. Other agents

Many agents have been reported to cause renal tubular dilatation or frank cyst formation (Table 4.1). In general, renal cyst formation has not been the major pathologic finding produced by these compounds and thus has remained incompletely characterized. This precludes analysis of the role of such chemicals in the production of useful experimental models of renal cystic disease.

3 In vivo models: Mechanically-induced experimental renal cystic disease

Cystic renal changes have been produced in fetal and adult experimental animals by surgical maneuvres such as obstruction[23,70,184,187] or reduction in renal mass with hyperfiltration[113] (Table 4.2).

Table 4.2. Mechanically-induced experimental renal cystic disease

Experimental Procedure	Species	Reference
Fetal ureteral ligation	Lamb	23,184
	Rabbit	70,187
5/6 nephrectomy	Rat	113

3.1. Fetal nephron obstruction

Nephron obstruction, with increased intraluminal hydrostatic pressure, has been implicated as an important pathogenic factor in most proposed theories of renal cyst formation and cyst growth[2,67,80,93,182,195].

Experimental models of hydronephrosis have been produced by ureteric obstruction[100,176], but Beck was the first to demonstrate that intrauterine urinary obstruction in fetal lambs produced a surgical model of renal cystic disease[23]. Both early fetal age and contralateral nephrectomy were required to produce cystic changes. Although microdissection and special histologic studies were not performed, the cystic malformation appeared to be localized to proximal convoluted tubules. Additional studies have confirmed that the renal pathology produced by fetal ureteric obstruction is largely determined by the timing and nature of the experimental procedure. Thus, while urethral obstruction in third trimester fetal lambs produced hydronephrosis[98,99], early midtrimester ureteral obstruction produced renal dysplasia[88,89].

A similar model of renal cystic disease has been produced in the fetal rabbit following *in utero* unilateral ligation of the ureter[70,187]. Contralateral nephrectomy was not a necessary condition for cyst formation, and the severity of cystic lesions was inversely proportional to fetal gestational age at the time of surgery. By microdissection, cysts, although present in all nephron segments, were most prominent in the loops of Henle and collecting tubules[70]. The induction of renal abnormalities by fetal obstruction is highly-species dependent, as shown by production of only hydronephrosis by obstruction of chick ureters from early through late gestation[25].

Experimental models of fetal urinary obstruction demonstrate that physical factors such as increased intratubular pressure may be cystogenic only at certain stages of nephron development. Although it has been theorized that nephron susceptibility to cyst formation may be a simple function of differences in intratubular pressure generated along the nephron[150], this has not been confirmed by segmental intratubular pressure measurements. The theory fails to explain the necessity of contralateral nephrectomy for cyst formation in the lamb model, unless it is assumed that unilateral nephrectomy leads to increased filtration, fluid flow, and intratubular pressure within the remaining kidney. Perhaps renotropic factors, which are known to be produced following reduction in renal mass and are known mediators of cellular hyperplasia and hypertrophy[72], also have pathogenic significance in renal cyst formation.

3.2. *Reduction in renal mass: 5/6 nephrectomy (Fig. 4.5A–B)*

In studying the effects of protein intake on renal function and structure in partially nephrectomized rats, Kenner *et al.* [113] described the production of renal cyst formation. Animals subjected to 5/6 nephrectomy developed cortical and outer medullary cysts. Cystic changes were more prominent in animals fed a high protein diet and were most prominent in proximal and collecting tubules. Cyst formation was associated with morphologic evidence of hyperplasia and hypertrophy in affected nephron segments and was paralleled by significant interstitial nephritis.

While the mechanisms of tubular cyst formation in the 5/6 nephrectomy model have not been clearly delineated, the features of hypertrophy and hyperplasia with intratubular polyp formation suggest that uncontrollable tubular cell growth might cause intermittent tubular obstruction[67]. The extreme degree of cellular infiltration present in this model and the potential mitogenic effect of macrophage-dependent cytokines[84] suggest that the 5/6 nephrectomy model might be useful in the future study of growth factor modulation of cystogenesis. The exacerbation of the cystic changes by high- protein intake suggests that physical factors such as hyperfiltration may promote cyst formation under conditions of increased tubular transport[72] or vulnerability to toxic injury[33].

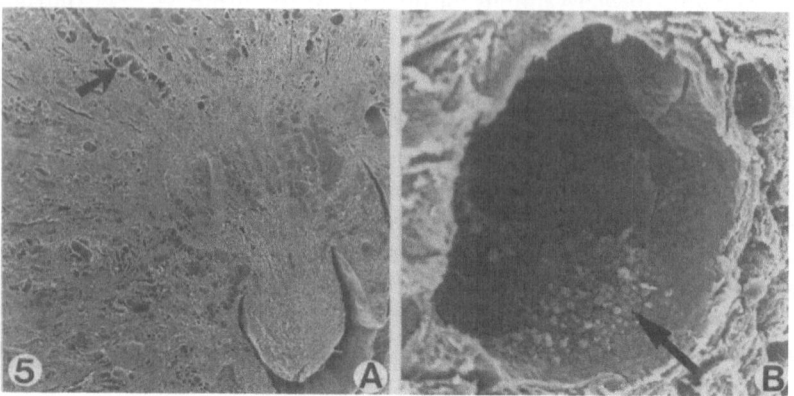

Figure 4.5A–B. Cyst formation following 5/6 nephrectomy. (A) Scanning electron micrograph of a remnant (5/6 nephrectomy) kidney from an animal on a high protein diet. The kidney is grossly enlarged with a spongy, cystic (arrow) appearance. These animals were in chronic renal failure. (B) Scanning electron micrograph showing a dilated proximal tubule from the same kidney illustrated in Fig. 4.5A. Hyperplasia is obvious by the enlarged diameter of this tubule; however, an area of irregular hyperplasia (arrow) is also seen. (Reprinted from Kidney International [113] with permission).

4. In vivo models: genetically transmitted experimental renal cystic disease

Renal cysts have been described as sporadic pathologic findings in cats[20,116,142,175,177], coyotes[165], gerbils[170], monkeys[19,133,174], goldfish[137,172], and skunks[170]. In all such reports, cysts were isolated to individual animals, were not transmitted to offspring, and might have been secondary to environmental toxins[137,165,170,172]. Several genetically transmitted renal cystic diseases have also been described (Table 4.3). The study of cyst formation and enlargement in genetically transmitted animal models has the potential of identifying both specific cystogenic gene products and biological and environmental factors that modulate cyst formation. Of the genetically transmitted animal models, three have been well characterized: the C57BL/6J–CPK (CPK) mouse[7,18,47,49,63,77,87,94,131,141,143,154,169]; the CFW$_{wd}$ mouse[94,196]; and the CBA/CaH–KD mouse[69,110–112,118,139]. The first two are described in greater detail here, while the CBA/CaH–KD mouse, a model of autoimmune interstitial nephritis and medullary cystic disease, is described in detail in Chapter 3.

Table 4.3. Genetically-transmitted renal cystic disease

Species	Strain or Breed	Inheritance	Reference
Antelope	Springbox	AR	105
Cat	Mixed breed	AR (?)	56
Dog	Cairn terrier	AR (?)	129
Mouse	KK/CY	AR	183
	PM/Se	AR	161–163
	SA	AR (?)	91
	C57	AR (?)	91
	C57BL/6J-JPK	AR	75
	C57BL/6J-CPK	AR	7,12,18,47,49,63,87,94,131,141,143,154,169
	DBA/2J-CPK	AR	77
	DA	AR	168
	CBA/CaH-KD	AR	69,110–112,118,139
	CFW$_{wd}$	AD	94,196
	SV Tag 188	Transgenic	130
Pig	Mixed breed	AR	136
	Mixed breed	AD	199
Rabbit	III vo	AR	74
Rat	Not described	?	179
	Gunn	AD	117

4.1. The CPK mouse

In 1977, a spontaneous mutation (CPK) in C57BL/6J mice at Jackson Laboratories, Bar Harbor, Maine produced an autosomal recessive polycystic kidney disease[169]. The CPK strain has subsequently been maintained in several laboratories through controlled breeding of obligatory heterozygotes. CPK animals, which appear normal at birth, develop progressive lethargy and abdominal protuberance and die in renal failure at 3–4 weeks of post-natal age with massively enlarged kidneys[87,131,154]. Although abnormalities are limited to the kidneys in affected CPK mice[154], obligatory heterozygotes for the cystic gene have been reported to develop focal biliary cystic dilatation[49]. The cystic gene has produced pancreatic and hepatic fibrosis and ductal dilatation when crossbred into the basic DBA/2J strain[77]. Therefore, the CPK mouse has been suggested as an animal model of human autosomal recessive polycystic kidney disease[7,49,131,154].

The morphology and ontogeny of tubular cyst formation in the CPK mouse have been studied by light and transmission electron microscopy and intact nephron microdissection[7,77,87,141,154]. The earliest morphologic alterations consist of tubular dilatation and early cyst formation in the distal proximal tubular anlagen of S2 and S3 segments in 17-day fetuses (Fig. 4.6B)[7,87,141]. Cysts occur as outpouchings of proximal tubular segments and remain in continuity with glomeruli, recurrent loops and distal nephron segments.

Transmission electron microscopy analysis of the earliest abnormality reveals widening of the tubular intercellular spaces, without other evidence of cell injury[7].

The site of involvement shifts to cortical and outer medullary collecting tubules as the disease progresses (Table 4.4). Avner *et al.* [7] localized the majority of cystic proximal tubules to the juxtamedullary zone, as opposed to the mid- and sub-capsular zones of active nephrogenesis in CPK kidneys, and

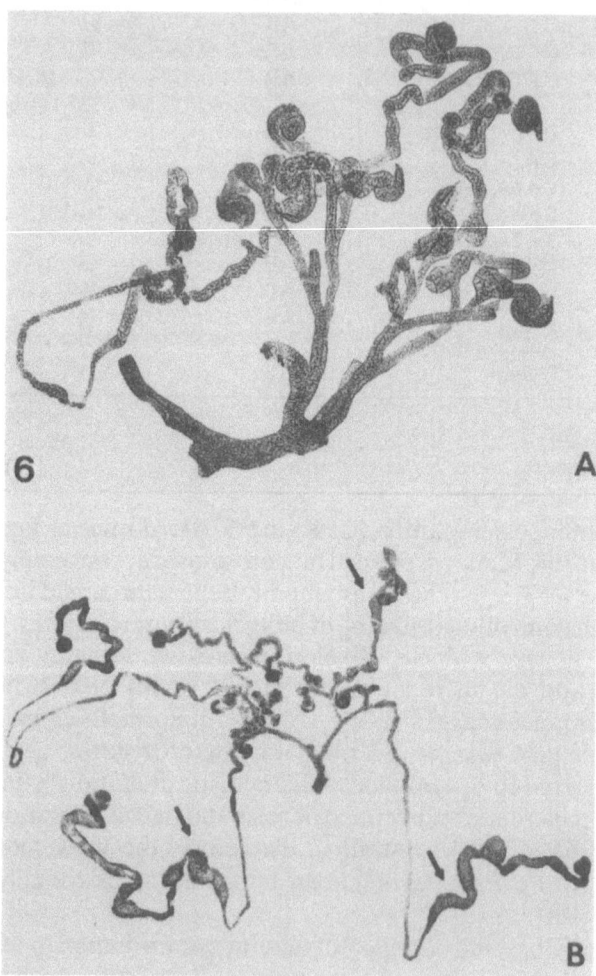

Figure 4.6 (A–B) Microdissection of fetal murine nephrons at 17 days gestation (Reprinted from The Journal of Pediatric Nephrology[7] with permission). (A) Control kidney shows nephrons in various stages of development in normal relation to collecting tubules. (B) CPK kidney displays tubular dilatation and cyst formation in the distal portion of proximal tubules (arrows) in a subpopulation of nephrons which shares normal collecting tubules with non-cystic nephrons.

Table 4.4. Ontogeny of tubular cyst formation in the CPK mouse

Stage	Proximal tubules[a]					Collecting tubules[a]		
	Cystic percentage of total proximal tubules	Cortical location of cysts (percentage of total proximal tubules in each zone)			Cyst volume (mm^3x10^{-3}, M range)	Cystic, percentage of total collecting tubules (M + SD)	Generations-involved by cysts (VI > XV)	Cyst volume (mm^3 x10^{-3}, M, range)
		Sub-capsular	Mid	Juxta-medullary				
Fetal day 17	54 ± 6	10	50	70	4.6 (2.1– 5.9)	0	0	0
Newborn	81 ± 10[b]	30	90	100	3.2 (1.9– 5.7)	4 ± 3	X > XV	1.1 (0.2– 1.4)
Postnatal day 5	52 ± 9[b]	18	78	93	6.2 (4.1– 7.3)[b]	36 ± 9[c]	VIII > XV	6.9 (5.2– 8.6)[c]
Postnatal day 12	43 ± 5	20	30	75	9.8 (7.7–12.6)[b]	79 ± 7[c]	VI > XV	53.5 (36.7– 73.3)[c]
Postnatal day 21	31 ± 4[b]	20	40	50	27.3 (21.8–38.6)[c]	100[c]	VI > XV	386.1 (302.3–511.4)[c]

a n = 90–120 for each stage analyzed
b vs. previous stage, $p < 0.025$
c vs. previous stage, $p < 0.001$
Reprinted from The Journal of Pediatric Nephrology [7] with permission

suggested that proximal tubular cysts were acquired lesions in a population of nephrons formed during the earliest stages of organogenesis. Collecting tubular abnormalities were initially localized to the terminal five generations of collecting tubules in newborn CPK kidneys, and progressed to diffuse involvement of outer medullary and cortical collecting ducts by day 21 post-natally. The formation and enlargement of collecting duct cysts was not associated with a characteristic ultrastructural abnormality. From post-natal day 5 onward, progressive proximal tubule and collecting duct cystic enlargement occurred with prominent tubular cell hyperplasia[7,87]. Quantitative analysis of nephron dimensions revealed that cyst formation was not associated with abnormal patterns of differentiation or alterations in basic renal architecture[7].

Avner et al. correlated the earliest phases of proximal tubular cyst formation with increased whole kidney Na–K ATPase activity[18], and, in a preliminary report, localized increased enzyme activity specifically to proximal tubules[12]. Increased renal Na–K ATPase activity occurred before significant epithelial hyperplasia and without abnormalities in tubular basal lamina glycoprotein expression, suggesting that increased Na–K ATPase activity with consequent tubular epithelial hyperplasia were early markers of CPK gene expression[18]. Ion and fluid transport, with epithelial proliferation, might then mediate cyst formation[2,80,195]. The hypothesis is supported by *in vitro* studies of proximal tubular cyst formation in explants of CPK kidneys[10,11].

The late stages of cyst formation in CPK kidneys have been associated with abnormalities in glucocorticoid metabolism[49,143], abnormal regulation of basal lamina gene expression[63] and elevated protooncogene expression[47]. Crocker et al. [49] reported elevated corticosterone levels, and suggested a pathogenic role for dysregulation of post-natal steroid metabolism. CPK animals treated with an experimental compound that binds to glucocorticoid cytoplasmic receptors without agonist activity exhibited prolonged survival[143]. Glucocorticoids increase renal Na–K ATPase activity[13,86,106] and stimulate tubular luminal Na$^+$-hydrogen antiport, with consequent intracellular alkalinization. Such elevated intracellular pH is a proven stimulus to cellular proliferation[76,155].

Ebihara et al. [63] studied the expression of type 4 collagen and laminin in CPK kidneys at 1–3 weeks of post-natal age. Although confirming previous reports that immunohistologic expression of basement membrane components was normal in tubular cyst walls at 1 week[18], focal decreases in basement membrane antigen expression were later demonstrated in enlarged cysts[63]. The immunohistologic findings were inversely correlated with whole kidney mRNA levels for type 4 collagen and laminin. Thus, while decreased message levels were associated with immunohistologically normal antigen expression, increased message levels were associated with focal decreases in immunohistologic expression of these components. These alterations may be meaningless if the viscoelasticity (a measure of deformability) of tubular basement membranes from CPK kidneys does not differ from those of controls[94].

Cowley et al. [47] described elevated c-myc protooncogene expression in

CPK kidneys during the latter stages of cystogenesis. Up to 30-fold increases in oncogene expression appeared to be disproportional to the relative rate of cell division in CPK kidneys measured by histone H_4 expression, suggesting that abnormal c-myc expression may somehow be involved in cystogenesis.

Although the mechanism of cyst formation and the shift in site of nephron involvement from proximal to collecting tubules have not been clearly delineated, studies in the CPK model have the potential for unravelling the molecular mechanisms by which certain genes and their products direct cystogenesis.

4.2. The CFW$_{wd}$ mouse

In 1984 Werder et al. [196] described a new mutation in the CFW strain of inbred AKR mice, which developed a form of autosomal dominant renal cystic disease (CFW$_{wd}$). Affected animals developed progressive bilateral renal enlargement and died with progressive uremia by 16–24 months of age. Renal cysts were predominantly localized to glomeruli and also occurred with regular frequency in the distal tubules and cortical collecting tubules. However, papillary necrosis preceded cyst-formation and caused epithelial hyperplasia within the medullary collecting ducts. There were also progressive interstitial nephritis and renal amyloidosis. Approximately 15% of the affected mice that died with cystic kidneys also had hepatic cysts, and an unspecified proportion developed thoracic aortic aneurysms. Additional studies demonstrated that in contrast to almost 100% mortality from cystic disease at age 24 months following exposure to a clean conventional environment, only 4% of CFW$_{wd}$ animals that lived their entire lives in a germfree environment developed cystic kidneys. Movement of animals from the germfree to clean conventional environment at any stage increased the mortality. The CFW$_{wd}$ model provides dramatic evidence of environmental modulation of a cystic disease, although it still is not clear whether the cystic disease is genetically determined or secondary to papillary necrosis and obstruction.

5. In vitro models of renal cystic disease

Because of the uncontrolled variables inherent in the study of *in vivo* cyst formation, several investigators have recently turned to the *in vitro* study of cystic renal tubular epithelium. *In vitro* studies, which include cyst-induction in renal organ culture (Table 4.5) and cell culture of cyst-derived tubular epithelia and established epithelial cell lines (Table 4.6), permit highly controlled experimental conditions. *In vitro* models thereby permit precise study of abnormalities of cellular metabolism and function that promote cyst development.

Table 4.5. Organ culture models of renal cystic disease

Source of renal tissue	Gestation	Cyst induction	Reference
SW Albino mouse	Fetal, 13 d	Cis-platinum	8
		Glucocorticoids	6,9,13,14
		Triiodothyronine	9,17
Unspecified mouse	Fetal, 11–18 d	Hypokalemia(?)/95% O_2	55,159
C57BL/6J-CPK mouse	Newborn	Genetic/Triiodothyronine	10,11,16
Long Evans rat	Fetal, 15–18 d	Spontaneous	135
Human	Fetal, 5–12 wk	Hypokalemia(?)/95% O_2	48

Table 4.6. Cell culture of cystic renal epithelia

Source of renal tissue	Culture system	Reference
C57BL/6J-CPK mouse	Monolayer	202
Human ADPKD	Monolayer	201,203,204
	Explant/Collagen-gel	119
MDCK cell line	Collagen-gel	120–124,190

5.1. In vitro models: renal organ culture

Organ culture methodology is particularly suited to controlled studies of renal cystogenesis because cyst formation can be induced in a tissue undergoing advanced organotypic differentiation[3–5,15]. Tubular cysts can be experimentally produced in renal explants incubated in chemically defined, serum-free medium in the absence of vascularization, perfusion, or urine production[6,8–11,13,14,16,17]. Thus, the processes of cyst formation and progressive enlargement are experimentally isolated from the influences of glomerular filtration and flow-related phenomena, endothelial–mesangial cell interaction, and the effects of growth factors and transport substrates present in mammalian serum or urine. Crocker and others[48,55,159] were the first to utilize organ culture in the study of renal cystic disease. Experimental manipulation of potassium concentration produced abnormal branching of ureteric buds, poor induction of metanephric tissue and occasional dilatation of the ureteric bud[48,55]. Monie *et al.* [135] described spontaneous tubular cyst formation in cultured fetal rat kidneys. Although these investigations were limited by their dependence on uncharacterized growth medium[48,55,135] and although oxygen toxicity was subsequently determined to be the major cause of abnormalities produced *in vitro*[159], they demonstrated the potential of organ culture methodology.

Avner *et al.* subsequently demonstrated that proximal tubular cyst formation could be induced in developing metanephric organ culture tissue under completely defined conditions by *cis*-dichlorodiammine II platinum[8], glucocorticoids[6,14] and triiodothyronine[17]. Proximal tubular cyst formation was produced in the metanephric culture system amid a background of normal organotypic epithelial differentiation (Fig.4.7A–C). Cyst induction in the glucocorticoid and triiodothyronine models was directly mediated by increases in Na–K ATPase activity and was completely inhibited by specific Na–K ATPase blockade with ouabain[13,17]. Subsequent studies suggested that the mechanism of cyst formation in these models involved increases in meta-nephric organic anion uptake driven by sodium gradients, with intratubular sequestration of osmotically active substances obligating net intratubular fluid accumulation[9]. Abnormal transtubular transport under these experimental conditions led to net fluid secretion in discrete nephron segments, playing a significant role in cyst-formation and enlargement.

Avner et al.[16] showed that cystic lesions of CPK renal explants undergo complete regression when cultured under defined environmental conditions in serum-free organ culture medium. In vitro tubular cyst regression in CPK explants was directly correlated with increases in explant Na–K ATPase activity and could be directly modulated by experimental stimulation of Na–K ATPase activity with triiodothyronine or by blockade of Na–K ATPase activity with ouabain[11]. Experimental modulation of tubular cyst regression and formation in this model was effected without alterations in tubular epithelial hyperplasia or tubular basal lamina composition. As in the organ culture studies of normal fetal murine tissue, preliminary studies have demonstrated that sodium pump-dependent alterations in transtubular organic anion transport promote proxi-mal tubular cyst enlargement[10]. Thus, organ culture studies have delineated certain mechanisms by which cysts may be produced in normal developing tubules as well as a genetically-programmed renal cystic disease.

5.2. In vitro models: Renal cell culture

In several recent investigations, tubular epithelial cells have been cultured from cyst walls of ADPKD[119,201,203,204] and CPK[202] kidneys. In addition, MDCK cells form epithelial cysts when grown in hydrated collagen gels[120–124,190] (Table 4.6).

5.2.1 Human ADPKD epithelia

Cell culture of human renal cyst epithelia holds promise for the development of experimental model systems that express critical characteristics of the cystic renal tubule. Cultured cells that retain features of cyst epithelia provide a tool to characterize the ion and solute transport systems, the proliferative capacity, and the epithelial response of cystic tubules. The overlying objective of isolating cells from cyst walls is to obtain a population of cells functionally and struc-turally representative of the site of origin. Although several isolation

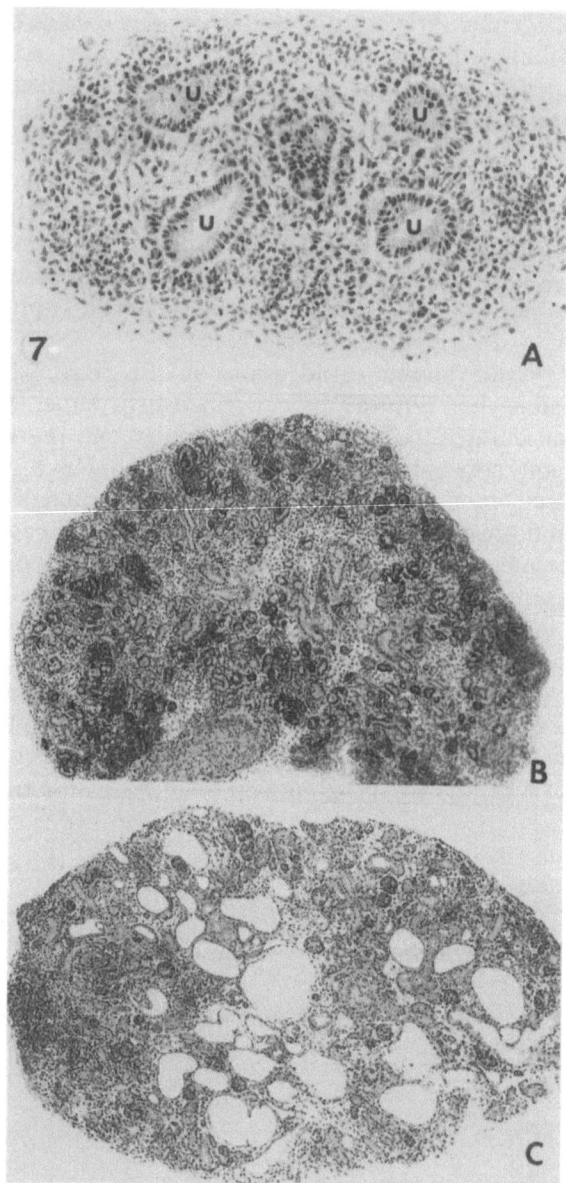

Figure 4.7A–C. Organ culture of fetal Swiss Webster albino murine metanephros. (A) At the time of explantation into organ culture (13±0.4 days gestation), metanephric tissue consists of aggregations of metanephric blastema and early tubular forms surrounding distal ramifications of the ureteric bud (U). (B) Following 120 hours of culture in defined serum-free medium, control explants demonstrate extensive organotypic tubulogenesis and formation of epithelial glomeruli. (C) Following 120 hours of culture in control medium supplemented with triiodothyronine 2×10^{-8}, explants demonstrate extensive proximal tubular cyst formation amid a background of normal *in vitro* organogenesis.

procedures have been devised to allow propagation of cyst lining cells, none as yet satisfies all criteria of the ideal ADPKD cultured cell model.

Human cyst wall presents, in one respect, an ideal specimen for explant or primary culture. The lining epithelium lying along the free surface of the tissue has unhindered access for harvest by enzymatic dissociation, but the use of proteolytic enzymes carries the risk of altering the characteristics of the isolated cell population[103,191,200]. This is a concern sufficient to encourage the use of cell isolation methods that do not involve enzymes. Two methods have been described for the culture of epithelial cells as outgrowths from ADPKD cyst wall explants positioned on underlying substrates: monolayer culture and suspension culture in hydrated collagen gel.

Wilson et al. [204] adapted a technique of propagating cells from isolated segments of renal tubule. Cells migrated from explants within 5–7 days and subsequently proliferated to form a cytokeratin-positive, polarized epithelial monolayer. Studies comparing cultured ADPKD cells with cells of various normal nephron segments revealed several differences in the morphology of the basal lamina and the enzyme-staining activity of the plasma membrane[204]. Cultured ADPKD cells produced a thickened basal lamina with unusual ultrastructural properties (P.D. Wilson, unpublished data). When the cells were grown atop type I collagen, they deposited submicron, ruthenium red-positive, proteinaceous spheroids subjacent to the basal plasma membrane. When the cells were raised atop a layer of Matrigel™ (containing laminin, fibronectin, type IV collagen and entactin), the cells formed amorphous fibrils, which were present also within intracellular vacuoles. Cultured ADPKD cells also demonstrated increased incorporation of [^{35}S]sulphate into basal lamina glycoproteins, indicating that abnormalities of the tubular basal lamina and extracellular matrix are inherent features of cystic lesions in certain experimental and human diseases[38,40,42,63,108].

Wilson and colleages[201] examined ADPKD cells in monolayer culture cytochemically to determine activity of the membrane-associated enzymes Na–K ATPase and gamma-glutamyl transpeptidase. The cells did not stain for the proximal tubule brush border enzyme, but were highly reactive for Na–K ATPase. Na–K ATPase in the normal renal tubule is limited to the basolateral membrane, but staining in ADPKD cyst walls and cultured ADPKD cells was predominantly at the apical membrane. These observations support the notion that altered ion and solute transport by ADPKD epithelium may be involved in fluid accumulation within renal cysts. ADPKD cells also showed an abnormal pattern of lectin binding at the plasma membrane (P.D. Wilson, unpublished data). Whereas normal proximal tubule cells stain positively for wheat germ agglutinin and cortical collecting duct cells for both *Ulex europeus I* and peanut agglutinin, ADPKD cells were positive for both wheat germ and peanut but negative for Ulex agglutinins. This pattern of lectin staining is not characteristic of any identifiable renal cell type, but it may only reflect selective dedifferentiation or loss of cell organelles in dilated tubules.

Additional studies by Wilson and coworkers[203,204] examined cell growth and hormone responsiveness of ADPKD cells in monolayer culture. ADPKD cells had a diminished cAMP response to vasopressin, parathormone and forskolin, compared to normal proximal tubule and cortical collecting tubule epithelium, perhaps reflecting the partially dedifferentiated nature of cyst lining cells. ADPKD cells grew more rapidly than did cells derived from normal tubules, indicating the proliferative capacity of the cyst wall epithelium, otherwise expressed as papillary and polypoid hyperplasia in the enlarging renal cyst[66,67]. In addition, ADPKD cells showed different requirements for medium composition and extracellular matrix for optimal growth, compared to cells from the normal kidney. This finding may represent an intrinsic alteration in the regulatory mechanism of cell growth.

A second method of isolating and growing ADPKD epithelium involves medium-hydrated collagen gel as the culture substrate[119] (Fig. 4.8 and Fig. 4.9A–E). Pieces of cyst wall are planted within type I collagen gel and cells migrate from the explant to form a polarized epithelium. The cells are typically cuboidal and bear short apical microvilli, but occasionally possess elongated microvilli characteristic of brush border. The outgrowth of cells results in the formation of a confluent epithelial sheet directly opposing the explant. This cell layer, atop its collagen substrate, then pulls away from the explant, leaving a fluid-filled interspace. ADPKD cyst wall explants maintained in culture for an extended period (3–6 weeks) frequently show formation of small diameter (200–500 μm) cysts. The cells of the mural cysts are similar in morphology to the cells that lined major cysts, and are generally not characteristic of identifiable renal cell types.

Cells derived from human ADPKD kidney following hydrated collagen gel culture have yet to be fully characterized. Aspects of the *in vitro* behavior of these cells are, however, suggestive of specific characteristics of renal cysts. For example, fluid accumulation within the interspace between the cyst wall explant and its confluent epithelial outgrowth may be evidence that net basal to apical fluid movement occurs across the renal cyst wall. In addition, the formation of small mural cysts within the wall of renal cyst explants may be related to the events involved in tubular enlargement and cyst dilation in ADPKD.

5.2.2. The MDCK cyst

The MDCK cyst is a cultured cell model in which polarized epithelial cysts are raised within a three-dimensional collagen gel substrate[120–123]. The growth of MDCK cysts involves cell proliferation and fluid accumulation, and thereby mimics two consistent features (e.g., epithelial hyperplasia and fluid accumulation) of renal cyst enlargement in experimental and human cystic diseases[2,80,95]. Only a small percentage of the cells (1–10%, depending upon

EXPLANT CULTURE OF HUMAN
RENAL CYST WALL

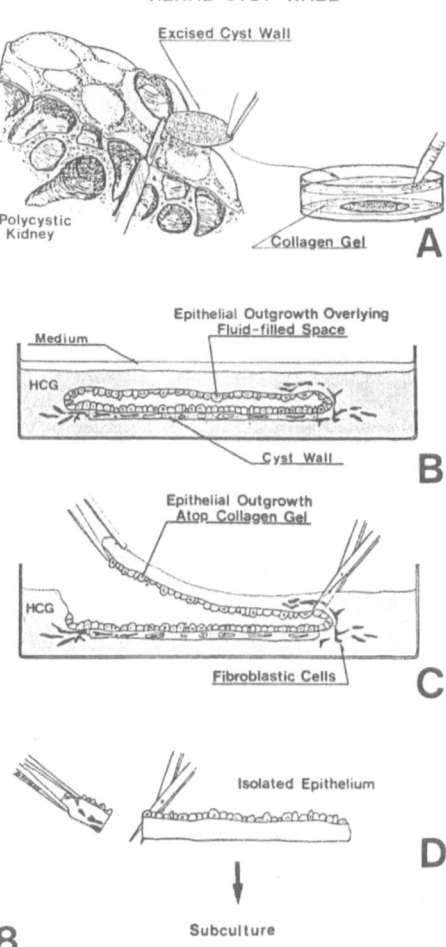

Figure 4.8. Explant culture of human ADPKD renal cyst-wall. This drawing illustrates the method of explant culture used to isolate epithelial cells derived from individual renal cysts. (A) Explantation of renal cyst wall. Broad portions of cyst-wall are excised and embedded (fully submerged) within medium-hydrated collagen gel. (B) Formation of epithelial outgrowth. Epithelial cells migrate from the explant to populate the surface of the collagen gel in contact with the cyst lining. The outgrowth of cyst-lining cells is accompanied by the formation of an epithelial sac that accumulates fluid within its lumen. (C) Collecting of epithelial outgrowth. Sheets of cyst-derived epithelium are harvested by excising areas of the collagen substrate bearing the primary cell-outgrowth. (D) Isolation and subculture of cyst-derived epithelium. Once the primary epithelial sheet is collected, areas free from fibroblastic outgrowth can be isolated for subculture. (Reprinted from McAteer JA, Carone FA, Grantham JJ, Kempson SA, Gardner KD Jr, Evan AP, Explant culture of human polycystic kidney, Lab Invest, 59, 126–136, 1988, (C) by US and Canadian Acad of Pathology[119]).

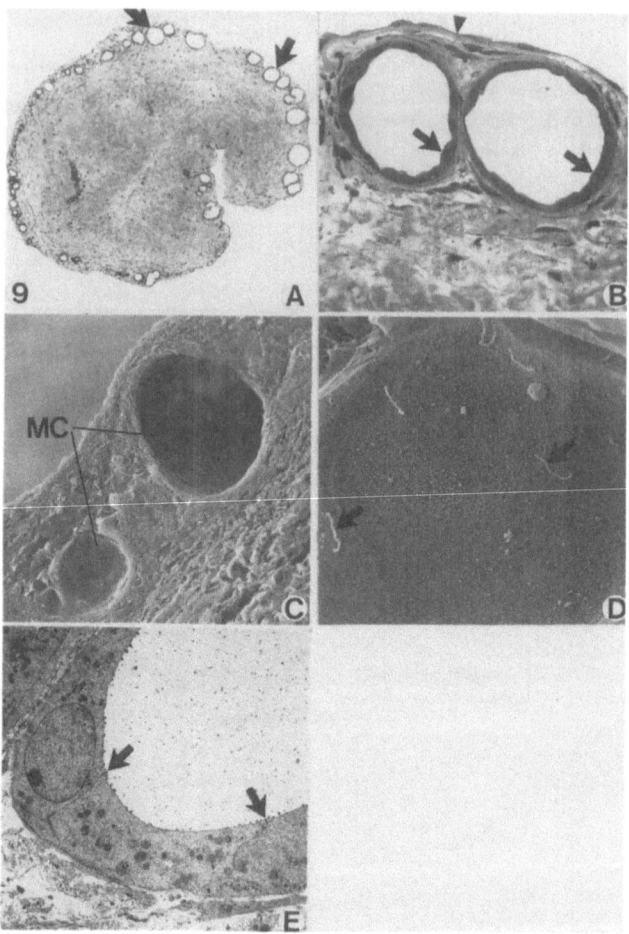

Figure 4.9A–E. Morphology of mural cysts within human ADPKD cyst wall explants. (A) This light micrograph of a tissue section shows the structure of a renal cyst wall explant cultured 18 days in fluid submersion culture. Numerous spherical cysts (arrows) populate the periphery of the explant. The core of the explant is densely-collagenous and does not appear to contain epithelial tubules. (B) This light micrograph shows a pair of mural cysts located close to the surface of an explant. The cysts are lined by a single cuboidal epithelium (arrows) that does not show tubule-specific identifying characteristics. The surface of the explant is lined by an attenuated epithelium (arrowhead) overlying a thickening basement membrane. (C) This is a scanning electron micrograph of the cryofractured surface of a submersion-cultured cyst-wall explant. Two mural cysts (MC) are surrounded by a dense collagenous interstitium. (D) This scanning electron micrograph shows the surface features of epithelial cells lining the smaller of the two cysts shown in Fig. 4.9C. The cells bear an irregular apical contour lined by short microvilli. Most of the cells possess a solitary cilium (arrows). (E) This transmission electron micrograph shows a portion of the wall of a mural cyst. The cells are simple-cuboidal in form, are joined by apical tight junctions (arrows), and bear only a small number of microvilli at their apical surface. The tubule segment of origin of these cells is not apparent by their morphology. (Figs. 4.9A–E reprinted from Reference 119, with permission).

culture conditions) proliferate to form isolated colonies in the form of epithelial cysts[166]. The cells are organized as a simple epithelium with the apical surfaces facing the lumen and the basolateral surfaces resting in contact with the surrounding collagen lattice (Fig. 4.10). The cells replicate the histotypic orientation of the kidney tubule or a renal cyst.

MDCK cysts demonstrate several specific morphologic features[122] (Fig. 4.11A–C). The cells are typically cuboidal to moderately attenuated in shape, have apical tight junctions, a solitary cilium and numerous short apical microvilli. The cells also produce a ruthenium red-positive basal lamina. Cultures of MDCK cysts are not entirely homogenous. Most cysts possess a simple, relatively uniform epithelium, but a small percentage (< 1%) form irregular walls with multilayered epithelium[164]. The formation of multilayered cysts is stimulated by treatment with ouabain (see below). MDCK cysts enlarge with continued culture. Cyst enlargement follows a sigmoid growth curve in which the rate of growth (increase in diameter) is influenced by culture conditions, including seeding density, medium composition and collagen concentration in the gel substrate[124]. Cysts may achieve a diameter of 500–2000 μm before cessation of growth. The rate of cyst enlargement can be stimulated by supplemental hormones and growth factors (J.J. Grantham, unpublished data) and by agents that regulate ion and solute transport[189,190]. Growth will cease unless individual MDCK cysts are explanted to monolayer culture, suggesting that the cyst culture environment and the organization of cells in cyst configuration have influences on cell proliferation.

As a closed epithelial sac, the MDCK cyst resembles those renal cysts that have lost their connections with the nephron. Ultrastructural studies of ADPKD, for example, have demonstrated that isolated cysts make up the majority of cysts in endstage kidneys[95]. It is likely, however, that isolated cysts continue to enlarge after they have lost connection with the renal tubules. Fluid accumulation within a solitary cyst, whether *in vivo* or *in vitro*, necessarily involves transepithelial fluid movement. The MDCK cyst thus offers a model for investigating fluid accumulation through regulation of ion and solute transport across the epithelium[189,190]. The system presents both methodologic and conceptual challenges. Cells configured as a cyst and surrounded by a collagen lattice are not readily accessible to direct manipulation, but isolated cysts can be impaled with micropipettes or microelectrodes and cyst growth can be monitored microscopically. The direction of net fluid movement across the wall of the MDCK cyst (basal to apical) is opposite that which occurs in fluid-transporting epithelia in monolayer culture or in the normal renal tubule, suggesting that selected transport systems may be altered or that the polarity of transporters may be abnormal. Perhaps the properties of the MDCK cyst epithelium that allow fluid movement in a basal to apical direction are similar to characteristics of the ADPKD epithelium responsible for fluid accumulation within renal cysts.

Measures of the osmolality of cyst fluid collected by micropuncture indicate that fluid within the lumens of MDCK cysts is slightly hypoosmotic to the tissue culture medium (318 ± 13 versus 328 ± 6 mosm/kg H_2O) that bathes the basolateral cell surface. Although the reason for this difference is not clear, the difference indicates that cyst fluid composition is influenced by the epithelial activity. Fluid accumulation within the lumens of renal cysts may occur through a passive process secondary to chloride secretion. Measurements of intracellular chloride activity in MDCK cysts indicate that chloride is accumulated in the cells at a level three times higher than that predicted for passive distribution of chloride.

Measurements of intraluminal hydrostatic pressures in renal cysts in both ADPKD and animal models show that cyst walls may be under elevated tension[29,85,107]. If so, the lining epithelium may be subjected to a physical stress that serves as a stimulus to cell proliferation[36]. If, in turn, elevated intraluminal pressure is due to net fluid secretion (basal to apical fluid transport), the fluid secretory activity of the epithelium may be driving cell proliferation.

MDCK cysts exhibit an elevated transmural pressure that is 6.7 mmH$_2$O greater than that in the surrounding medium[132]. Grantham (unpublished data) has shown that MDCK cysts raised in hyperosmotic medium enlarge at rates comparable to cysts in isosmotic medium, suggesting that luminal volume and pressure may not influence cyst enlargement. However, it has not been determined if the MDCK cyst epithelium, which apparently exhibits unusual transport properties, also functions in a predictable manner when cultured in a hypertonic environment.

Grantham and colleagues[189,190] have demonstrated that the enlargement of MDCK cysts can be regulated by inhibitors of active solute transport. Amiloride and several amiloride analogues administered at submaximal concentrations slowed the rate of cyst enlargement, possibly by affecting both cell proliferation and fluid secretion. The degree of retardation of cyst growth was related to the inhibitory activity of these agents on Na^+-dependent Ca^{2+}-transport (determined in a variety of other cell types). Treatment with ouabain, an inhibitor of Na–K ATPase, reduced fluid accumulation within cysts but did not fully inhibit cell proliferation. As a result, ouabain-treated cysts exhibited multilayering of the epithelium. These data suggest that cyst enlargement can be manipulated with agents that influence transepithelial fluid movement.

MDCK cyst cultures may prove useful in examining the role of the extracellular matrix in renal cyst formation and growth. As previously noted, data from both experimental and human cystic diseases suggest tht alterations of the tubular basal lamina accompany renal cysts. Factors derived from the renal interstitium may directly influence epithelial cell behavior in the nephron, driving the events that result in cyst formation and growth. Since it is possible to manipulate the composition of the collagen gel substrate that surrounds MDCK cysts, this culture system may be uniquely suited for investigating the influence of the various extracellular matrix components on epithelial behavior in cyst formation and enlargement.

MDCK-CYST GROWTH IN VITRO

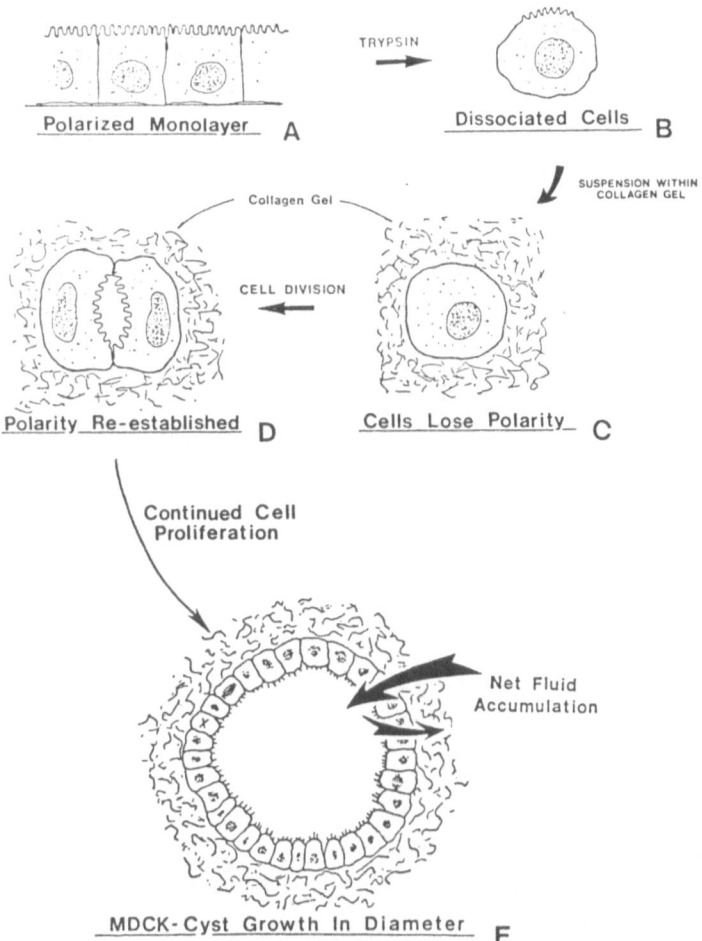

Figure 4.10. Morphogenetic clonal growth of kidney epithelial cell-line MDCK. This drawing illustrates the events involved in the formation and growth of polarized epithelial cysts by MDCK-cells cultured within medium-hydrated collagen gel. (A) Substrate-dependent mono-layer cultures of cell-line MDCK (ATCC CCL 34) are raised on conventional culture-grade plastic. (B) The cells are dissociated by a routine method (Trypsin–EDTA). Although cell–cell interactions have been disrupted, the individual cells retain some morphologic features charac-teristic of a polarized cell. (C) A monodispersed suspension of MDCK cells is mixed with collagen gel and incubated at 37 °C. The cells are fully surrounded by collagen. Within this environment, the cells likely lose polarity. (D) Polarity is re-established when the cell undergoes mitotic division. When division occurs, the daughter cells likely remain contiguous. The region of contact between cells creates a collagen-free area of the cell surface, and provides an interface against which the cells can polarize. (E) Subsequent cell proliferative activity adds polarized epithelial cells to the cyst wall. The net basal-to-apical transport of fluid (derived from the surrounding medium) results in fluid accumulation within the lumen. The MDCK-cyst grows in diameter.

86

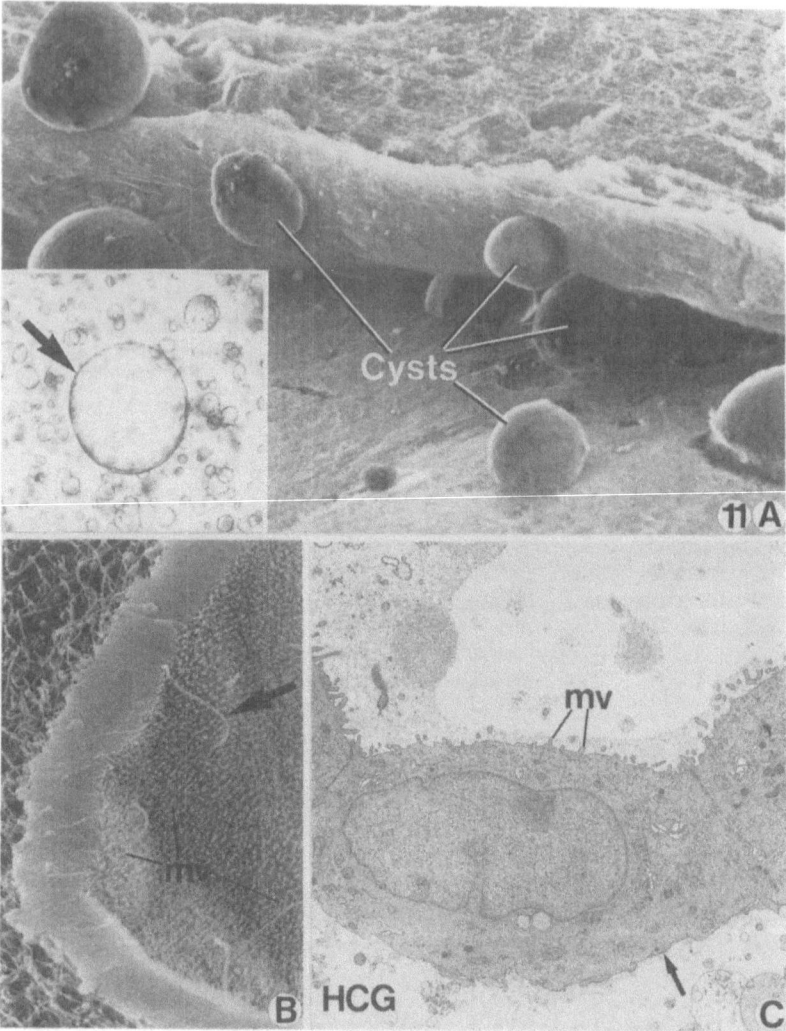

Figure 4.11A–C. Morphology of MDCK-cyst cultures. (A) Scanning electron micrograp showing MDCK-cysts at the interface between the base and overlying layers of collagen gel. This
specimen was prepared by stripping away the upper collagen layer prior to fixation. Inset: light
micrograph of living culture (10 days), showing numerous spherical cysts of various sizes. A large
cyst (arrow) near the centre of the field measures approximately $800\,\mu$m in diameter. (B)
Scanning electron micrograph of a cryofractured MDCK-cyst shows abundant microvilli (mv) at
the apical cell surface. Each cell also bears a long filamentous single cilium (arrow). (C)
Ultrastructure of MDCK-cyst wall. Transmission electron micrograph shows portions of three
cells. The apical surface bears microvilli (mv), while lateral and basal surfaces are relatively
simple. Golgi stacks and smooth-surfaced vesicles appear polarized towards the cell apex. Basal
lamina is not abundant, although patches of apparent extracellular material are present (arrow).
The lumen contains a flocculent precipitate. Collagen-gel (HCG). (Figures 4.11A–C reprinted
from Reference 122, with permission).

6. The relationship of experimental models to human cystic disease states

6.1. Theories of renal cyst formation

Experimental studies on the models noted above have identified tubular hyperplasia, distal nephron obstruction, abnormalities of the basement membrane and fluid accumulation (tubular secretion) as potential pathogenic mechanisms in renal cyst formation. What is the evidence that any of these mechanisms is significant in the pathophysiology of human renal cystic diseases? Tubular hyperplasia is a central morphologic feature of all described human renal cystic diseases[26,27,66,67]. In ADPKD for example, hyperplasia of epithelial cells lining cyst walls was noted as early as the late 19th century[138]. More recent studies have shown both tubular epithelial hyperplasia and discrete intratubular micropolyps, identical to those found in chemically-induced experimental diseases[67]. Hyperplasia, with expansion of tubular wall segments to accommodate an increased cellular mass, and partial obstruction from intratubular polyps are strongly implicated as pathogenic factors in ADPKD. Similar findings have been reported for acquired cystic disease in endstage kidneys. Indeed, hyperplasia, which in some fashion escapes regulatory control, may potentiate malignancy in such kidneys[26,27,32,96]. As previously noted, tubular cells from ADPKD cysts have abnormally high proliferative indices when compared to normal tubular epithelia[119,203,204].

There is little to support the idea that abnormal compliance of the tubular basement membrane is a primary event in any specific human renal cystic disease. However, ultrastructural studies of the very early stages of ADPKD have revealed glomerular as well as tubular basal lamina abnormalities[134], and epithelial cells from ADPKD cysts appear to produce abnormal basement membrane-like material in vitro [203,204]. ADPKD kidneys have decreased expression of heparan sulphate core protein in cyst wall basal laminae and increased expression of fibronectin in peritubular and interstitial regions[40]. Additional studies directed towards the specific biochemical composition of the tubular basement membrane at different stages in development of human cystic diseases and molecular studies of the genetic control of basal lamina production in human diseases states may clarify the role of abnormal extracellular matrices in renal cystic diseases.

Fluid accumulation by the cystic nephron is a strong indication that abnormal fluid transport is involved in cyst formation and enlargement. If it were not for the accumulation of fluid, there would only be solid nests of hyperplastic cells. The long-held perception that the transport functions of renal cyst walls mimic their segment of origin[35,57,79,104,107,153] may be incorrect. Morphologic analysis has shown that over 70% of renal cysts in late-stage ADPKD lack patent connections to the nephron[95]. Tracer studies have demonstrated abnormal transtubular transport of various markers into ADPKD renal cysts, suggesting that active basolateral transport of osmotically active substances plays a role in progressive cystic enlargement[24,198]. A similar process of organic anion transport obligating fluid secretion may be a factor in the growth of acquired cysts in the endstage kidney[92,93]. Cyst fluid accumulation involves net transepithelial secretion, a conclusion supported by *in vitro* models of cyst enlargement in which cyst growth can be altered by experimental manipulation of transport processes[9–11,13,17,121–124,190,198].

6.2. *From theories to hypothesis: the pathogenesis of renal cyst formation*

It should be obvious that the theories of renal cyst formation generated in experimental models are not mutually exclusive, and that they are largely complementary. On the basis of mathematical models it has been suggested that if tubular epithelial hyperplasia is present any additional factor or combination of factors such as obstruction, abnormal tubular basement membrane compliance, or fluid secretion, is sufficient to explain the observed kinetics of cyst growth in ADPKD[195] (see Chapter 5). Thus, a hypothesis has been generated to interrelate such factors in experimental renal cyst formation and to provide a theoretical framework for future investigations[2] (Fig. 4.12). In this hypothesis, a mutant gene or certain environmental factors can directly lead to alterations in tubular epithelial metabolism. Further, environmental factors can modulate the expression of a mutant gene or directly lead to tubular cell death. An induced alteration in tubular cell metabolism may subsequently lead directly to abnormal extracellular matrix production or to the production of

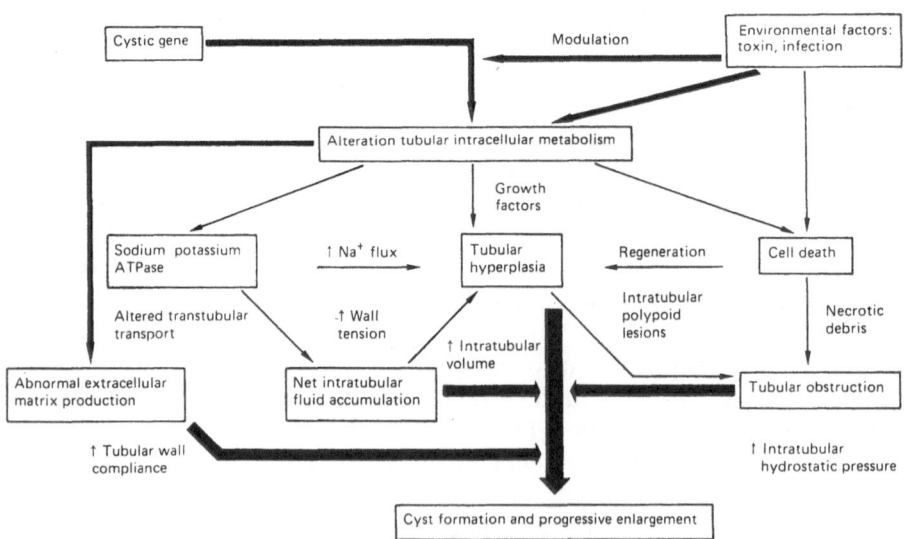

Figure 4.12. Hypothetical scheme of the pathogenesis of renal cyst formation and progressive enlargment. (Reprinted from Nephron [2] with permission, S. Karger AG, Basel).

growth factors mediating tubular hyperplasia. Induced changes in transtubular transport energetics may lead to hyperplasia secondary to increased transmembrane sodium flux, while programmed cell death may lead to further hyperplasia secondary to tubular regeneration. Alterations in sodium pump-mediated transtubular transport could lead to net intratubular fluid accumulation. Subsequent increases in tubular wall tension may further increase stimulation of epithelial proliferation, leading to tubular hyperplasia. The presence of a particular pattern of tubular hyperplasia and necrotic debris from cell death could lead to partial tubular obstruction. Finally, abnormal extracellular matrix production with increased tubular wall compliance, net intratubular fluid accumulation leading to increased intratubular volume, and tubular obstruction with increased intratubular hydrostatic pressure could, in the presence of tubular hyperplasia, lead to cyst formation and progressive cyst enlargement. Such a hypothesis of renal cyst formation appropriately focuses future investigations on the molecular mechanisms by which tubular epithelial hyperplasia is controlled and tubular metabolism is altered in both experimental and human cystic diseases.

References

1. Ambrose AA, Booth AN, DeEds F and Cox AJ. A toxicological study of biphenyl, a citrus fungistate. Food Research 1960, 25, 328–336.
2. Avner ED. Renal cystic disease: insights from recent experimental investigations. Nephron 1988, 48, 89–93.
3. Avner ED, Ellis D, Temple T and Jaffe R. Metanephric development in serum-free organ culture. In Vitro Cell Developmental Biology 1982, 18, 675–682.
4. Avner ED, Jaffe R, Temple T, Ellis D and Chung AE. The development of renal basement membrane glycoproteins in metanephric organ culture. Laboratory Investigation 1983, 48, 263–268.
5. Avner ED, Piesco NP, Sweeney WE and Ellis D. Renal epithelial development in organotypic culture. Pediatric Nephrology 1988, 2, 92–99.
6. Avner ED, Piesco NP, Sweeney WE, Studnick FM, Fetterman GH and Ellis D. Hydrocortisone-induced cystic metanephric maldevelopment in serum-free organ culture. Laboratory Investigation 1984, 50, 208–218.
7. Avner ED, Studnick FE, Young MC, Sweeney WE, Piesco NP, Ellis D and Fetterman GH. Congenital murine polycystic kidney disease. I. The ontogeny of tubular cyst formation. Pediatric Nephrology 1987, 1, 587–596.
8. Avner ED, Sweeney WE and Ellis D. Cyst formation in metanephric organ culture induced by cis-dichlorodiammine platinum (II). Experientia 1983, 39, 74–76.
9. Avner ED, Sweeney WE and Ellis D. Increased organic anion uptake mediates proximal tubular cyst formation in metanephric organ culture. Kidney International 1987, 31, 159 (abstract).
10. Avner ED, Sweeney WE and Ellis D. Transtubular organic anion transport mediates congenital murine renal tubular cyst formation in vitro. Clinical Research 1988, 36, 782a (abstract).
11. Avner ED, Sweeney WE and Ellis D. In vitro modulation of tubular cyst regression in murine polycystic kidney disease. Kidney International 1988, 34 (in press).
12. Avner ED, Sweeney WE and Ellis D. Isolated proximal tubules and proximal tubular cysts

of CPK mice have increased Na–K ATPase activity. Kidney International 1989, 35 (in press) (abstract).

13. Avner ED, Sweeney WE, Finegold DN, Piesco NP and Ellis D. Sodium–potassium ATPase activity mediates cyst formation in metanephric organ culture. Kidney International 1985, 28, 447–455.

14. Avner ED, Sweeney WE, Piesco NP and Ellis D. A new model of glucocorticoid-induced cystic metanephric maldevelopment. Experientia 1984, 40, 489–490.

15. Avner ED, Sweeney WE, Piesco NP and Ellis D. Growth factor requirements of metanephric differentiation in serum-free murine organ culture. In Vitro Cell Developmental Biology 1985, 21, 297–304.

16. Avner ED, Sweeney WE, Piesco NP and Ellis D. Regression of genetically-determined polycystic kidney disease in murine organ culture. Experientia 1986, 42, 77–80.

17. Avner ED, Sweeney WE, Piesco NP and Ellis D. Triiodothyronine-induced cyst formation in metanephric organ culture: the role of increased Na–K ATPase activity. Journal of Laboratory and Clinical Medicine 1987, 109, 441–454.

18. Avner ED, Sweeney WE, Young MC and Ellis D. Congenital murine polycystic kidney disease. II. Pathogenesis of tubular cyst formation. Pediatric Nephrology 1988, 2, 210–218.

19. Baskin GB, Roberts JA and McAfee RD. Infantile polycystic renal disease in a Rhesus Monkey. Laboratory Animal Science 1981, 31, 181–183.

20. Battershell D and Garcia JP. Polycystic kidney in a cat. Journal of the American Veterinary Medical Association 1969, 154, 665–666.

21. Baxter TJ. Cortisone-induced renal changes in the rabbit: a microdissection study.

22. Beauwens R and Crabbè J. Biochemistry of hormone action. In: Kinne RKH, ed., Renal Biochemistry. Amsterdam: Elsevier, 1985, 273–335.

23. Beck AD. The effect of intrauterine urinary obstruction upon the development of the fetal kidney. Journal of Urology 1971, 105, 784–789.

24. Bennett WM, Wickre CG and Muther RS. Movement of organic molecules into cysts. In: Cummings B and Klahr S, eds, Chronic Renal Disease. New York: Plenum Press, 1985, 89–94.

25. Berman DJ and Maizels M. The role of urinary obstruction in the genesis of renal dysplasia. Journal of Urology 1982, 128, 1091–1096.

26. Bernstein J, Evan AP and Gardner KD Jr. Epithelial hyperplasia in human polycystic kidney disease. American Journal of Pathology 1987, 129, 92–101.

27. Bernstein J, Evan AP and Gardner KD Jr. Human cystic diseases: epithelial hyperplasia in the pathogenesis of cysts and tumors. Pediatric Nephrology 1987, 3, 393–396.

28. Biava CG, Dyrda I, Genest J and Bencosme SA. Kaliopenic nephropathy. Laboratory Investigation 1963, 12, 443–453.

29. Bjerle P, Lindquist B and Michaelson G. Pressure measurements in renal cysts. Scandinavian Journal of Clinical Investigation 1971, 27, 135–138.

30. Booth AN, Ambrose AM, DeEds F and Cox AJ. The reversible nephrotoxic effects of biphenyl. Toxicology and Applied Pharmacology 1961, 3, 560–567.

31. Boyland E, Dukes CE, Grover PL and Mitchley BCV. The induction of renal tumors by feeding lead acetate to rats. British Journal of Cancer 1962, 16, 283–288.

32. Breton PN, Busch MP, Hricak H and Williams RD. Chronic renal failure: A significant risk factor in the development of acquired renal cysts and renal cell carcinoma. Cancer 1986, 57, 1871–1879.

33. Brezis M, Rosen S, Silva P, Spokes K and Epstein FH. Polyene toxicity in renal medulla: injury mediated by transport activity. Science 1984, 244, 66–68.

34. Bricker NS. Experimental polycystic renal disease and susceptibility to pyelonephritis. In: Bricker NS, ed., Angiontensin Systems and Experimental Renal Diseases. Boston: Little Brown, 1963, 180–204.

35. Bricker NS and Patton JF. Cystic disease of the kidneys. American Journal of Medicine 1955, 18, 207–219.

36. Brunete DM. Mechanical stretching increases the number of epithelial cells synthesizing DNA in culture. Journal of Cell Science 1984, 69, 35–45.
37. Burk D and Woods M. Hydrogen peroxide, catalase, gluthione peroxidase, quinones, nordihydroguaiaretic acid, and phosphopyridine nucleotides in relation to x-ray action on cancer cells. Radiation Research 1963, 3, 212–228.
38. Butkowski RJ, Carone FA, Grantham JJ and Hudson BG. Tubular basement membrane changes in 2-amino 4,5-diphenylthiazole induced polycystic disease. Kidney International 1985,28, 744–751.
39. Carone FA. Functional changes in polycystic kidney disease are tubulo–interstitial in origin. Seminars in Nephrology 1988, 8, 89–93.
40. Carone FA, Makino H and Kanwar YS. Basement membrane antigens in renal polycystic disease. American Journal of Pathology 1988, 130, 466–471.
41. Carone FA, Ozono S, Samma S, Kanwar YS and Oyasu R. Renal functional changes in experimental cystic disease are tubular in origin. Kidney International 1988, 33, 8–13.
42. Carone FA, Rowland RG, Perlman SG and Ganote CE. The pathogenesis of drug-induced renal cystic disease. Kidney International 1974, 5, 411–421.
43. Carone FA, Stolarczk J, Krumlovsky FA, Perlman SG, Roberts TH and Rowland RG. The nature of drug-induced renal concentrating defects in rats. Laboratory Investigation 1975, 31, 658–664.
44. Chesterman FC, Franks LM, Knudsen ET and Williams PC. Possible aldosteronism in stilbesterol-treated guinea pigs. Lancet 1956, 1192–1193.
45. Christensen S, Ottosen PD and Olsen S. Severe functional and structural changes caused by lithium in the developing rat kidney. Acta Pathologica Microbiologica Immunologica Scandinavica 1982, 90, 257–267.
46. Courtney KD, Gaylor DW, Hogan MD and Falk HL. Teratogenic evaluation of 2,4,5-T. Science 1970, 168, 864–866.
47. Cowley BD, Smardo FL, Grantham JJ and Calvet JP. Elevated c-myc protooncogene expression in autosomal recessive polycystic kidney disease. Proceedings of the National Academy of Sciences (USA) 1987, 84, 8394–8398.
48. Crocker JFS. Human embryonic kidneys in organ culture: abnormalities of development induced by decreased potassium. Science 1973, 181, 1178–1179.
49. Crocker JFS, Blecher SR, Givner ML and McCarthy SC. Polycystic kidney and liver disease and corticosterone changes in the CPK mouse. Kidney International 1987, 31, 1088–1091.
50. Crocker JFS, Brown DM, Borch RF and Vernier RL. Renal cystic disease induced in newborn rats by diphenylamine derivatives. American Journal of Pathology 1972, 66, 343–350.
51. Crocker JFS, Brown DM and Vernier RL. Developmental defects of the kidney: a review of renal development and experimental studies of maldevelopment. Pediatric Clinics of North America 1971, 18, 355–376.
52. Crocker JFS and McDonald ATJ. Effects of lithium chloride and ethacrynic acid on experimental polycystic kidney disease. Clinical Investigative Medicine 1988, 11, 16–21.
53. Crocker JFS, Safe SH and Alcott P. Effects of chronic phthalate exposure on the kidney. Journal of Toxicology and Environmental Health 1988, 23, 433–444.
54. Crocker JFS, Stewart AG, Sparling JM and Bruneau RT. Steroid-induced polycystic kidneys in the newborn rat. American Journal of Pathology 1976, 82, 373–380.
55. Crocker JFS and Vernier RL. Fetal kidney in organ culture: abnormalities of development induced by decreased amounts of potassium. Science 1970, 169, 485–487.
56. Crowell WA, Hubbell JJ and Riley JC. Polycystic renal disease in related cats. Journal of the American Veterinary Association 1979, 175, 286–288.
57. Cuppage FE, Huseman RA, Chapman A and Grantham JJ. Ultrastructure and function of cysts from human adult polycystic kidneys. Kidney International 1980, 17, 372–381.
58. Darmady EM, Offer J and Woodhouse MA. Toxic metabolic effect in polycystic disease of kidney. Lancet 1970, 1, 547–550.

59. deVos JG and Koeman JH. Comparative toxicological study with polychlorinated biphenyl in chickens with special reference to porphyria, edema formation, liver necrosis and tissue residues. Toxicology and Applied Pharmacology 1970, 17, 656–663.

60. Dobyan DC. Long-term consequence of *cis*-platinum-induced renal injury: a structural and functiona study. Anatomical Record 1985, 212, 239–245.

61. Dobyan DC, Hill D, Lewis T and Bulger RE. Cyst formation in rat kidney induced by *cis*-platinum administration. Laboratory Investigation 1981, 45, 260–268.

62. Dousa TP, Rowland RG and Carone FA. Renal medullary adenylate cyclase in drug-induced nephrogenic diabetes insipidus. Proceedings of the Society for Experimental Medicine 1973, 142, 720–722.

63. Ebihara I, Killen PD, Laurie GW, Huang T, Yamada Y, Martin GR and Brown RS. Alterend mRNA expression of basement membrane components in a murine model of polycystic kidney disease. Laboratory Investigation 1988, 58, 262–269.

64. Evan AP and Gardner KD Jr. Comparison of human polycystic and medullary cystic kidney disease with diphenylamine-induced cystic disease. Laboratory Investigation 1976, 35, 92–101.

65. Evan AP and Gardner KD Jr. Nephron obstruction in nordihydroguaiaretic acid-induced renal cystic diseases. Kidney International 1979, 15, 7–19.

66. Evan AP and Gardner KD Jr. Morphology of polycystic kidney disease in man and experimental models. In: Cummings B and Klahr S, eds, Chronic Renal Disease. New York: Plenum Press, 1985, 55–68.

67. Evan AP, Gardner KD Jr and Bernstein J. Polypoid and papillary epithelial hyperplasia: A potential cause of ductal obstruction in adult polycystic disease. Kidney International 1979, 16, 743–750.

68. Evan AP, Hong SK, Gardner KD Jr, Park YS and Itagaki R. Evolution of the collecting tubular lesion in diphenylamine-induced renal disease. Laboratory Investigation 1978, 38, 244–252.

69. Fernandes G, Yunis EJ and Miranda M. Nutritional inhibition of genetically determined renal disease and autoimmunity with prolongation of life in kdkd mice. Proceedings of the National Academy of Sciences (USA) 1978, 75, 2888–2898.

70. Fetterman GH, Ravitch MM and Sherman FE. Cystic changes in fetal kidneys following ureteral ligation: Studies by microdissection. Kidney International 1974, 5, 111–121.

71. Filmer RB, Carone FA, Rowland RG and Babcock JR. Adrenal corticosteroid-induced renal cystic disease in the newborn hamster. American Journal of Pathology 1973, 72, 461–472.

72. Fine L. The biology of renal hypertrophy. Kidney International 1986, 29, 619–634.

73. Fourman P, McCance RA and Parker RA. Chronic renal disease in rats following a temporary deficiency of potassium. British Journal of Experimental Pathology 1956, 37, 40–43.

74. Fox RR, Krinsky WL and Crary DD. Hereditary cortical renal cysts in the rabbit. Journal of Heredity 1971, 62, 105–109.

75. Fox S and Eicher EM. Juvenile polycystic kidneys (jpk). Mouse Newsletter 1970, 58, 47–51.

76. Freiberg JM, Kinsella J and Sacktor B. Glucocorticoids increased the $Na^+–H^+$ exchange and decrease the Na^+ gradient-dependent phosphate-uptake systems in renal brush border membrane vesicles. Proceedings of the National Academy of Sciences (USA) 1982, 79, 4932–4936.

77. Fry JL, Koch WE, Jennette JC, McFarland E, Fried FA and Mandel J. A genetically determined murine model of infantile polycystic kidney disease. Journal of Urology 1985, 134, 828–833.

78. Garcià-Porrero JA, Ojeda JL, Hurlè JM. Cell death during the postnatal morphogenesis of the normal rabbit kidney and in experimental renal polycystosis. Journal of Anatomy 1978, 126, 303–318.

79. Gardner KD Jr. Composition of fluid in twelve cysts of a polycystic kidney. New England Journal of Medicine 1969, 281, 985–988.

80. Gardner KD Jr. Cystic kidneys. Kidney International 1988, 33, 610–621.
81. Gardner KD Jr and Evan AP. Renal cystic disease induced by diphenylthiazole. Kidney International 1983, 24, 43–52.
82. Gardner KD Jr, Evan AP and Reed WP. Accelerated renal cyst development in deconditioned germ-free rats. Kidney International 1986, 29, 1116–1123.
83. Gardner KD Jr, Evan AP and Reed WP. Azotemia and nephropathology correlate in the experimental cystic nephropathy of endotoxin-injected conventional rats. Kidney International 1988, 33, 375 (abstract).
84. Gardner KD Jr, Reed WP, Evan AP, Zedalis J, Hylarides MD and Leon AO. Endotoxin provocation of experimental renal cystic disease. Kidney International 1987, 32, 329–334.
85. Gardner KD Jr, Solomon S, Fitzgerrel WW and Evan AP. Function and structure in the diphenylamine-exposed kidney. Journal of Clinical Investigation 1976, 57, 796–806.
86. Garg LC, Narang N and Wingo CS. Glucocorticoid effects on Na–K-ATPase in rabbit nephron segments. American Journal of Physiology 1985, 248, F487–F491.
87. Gattone VH, Calvet JP, Cowley BD, Evan AP, Shaver TS, Helstadter K and Grantham JJ. Autosomal recessive polycystic kidney disease in a murine model: a gross and microscopic description. Laboratory Investigation 1988 (in press).
88. Glick PL, Harrison MR, Adzick NS, Noall RA and Villa RL. Correction of congenital hydronephrosis *in utero* IV: *In utero* decompression prevents renal dysplasia. Journal of Pediatric Surgery 1984, 19, 649–657.
89. Glick PL, Harrison MR, Noall RA and Villa RL. Correction of congenital hydronephrosis *in utero* III. Early mid-trimester ureteral obstruction produces renal dysplasia. Journal of Pediatric Surgery 1983, 18, 681–687.
90. Goodman T, Grice HC, Becking GC and Salem FA. A cystic nephropathy induced by nordihydroguaiaretic acid in the rat. Laboratory Investigation 1970, 23, 93–107.
91. Gorer PA. Renal lesions found in pure lines of mice. Journal of Pathology and Bacteriology 1940, 50, 25–30.
92. Grantham JJ. Studies of organic anion and cation transport in isolated segments of proximal tubules. Kidney International 1982, 22, 519–525.
93. Grantham JJ. Polycystic kidney disease: A Predominance of giant nephrons. American Journal of Physiology 1983, 244, F3–F10.
94. Grantham JJ, Donoso VS, Evan AP, Carone FA and Gardner KD Jr. Viscoelastic properties of tubule basement membranes in experimental renal cystic disease. Kidney International 1987, 32, 187–197.
95. Grantham JJ, Geiser JL and Evan AP. Cyst formation and growth in autosomal dominant polycystic kidney disease. Kidney International 1987, 31, 1145–1152.
96. Grantham JJ and Levine E. Acquired cystic disease. Replacing one kidney disease with another. Kidney International 1985, 28, 99–105.
97. Grice HC, Becking G and Goodman T. Toxic properties of nordihydroguaiaretic acid. Food and Cosmetic Toxicology 1968, 6, 155–161.
98. Harrison MR, Nakayama KD and Noall R. Correction of congenital hydronephrosis *in utero* II. Decompression reverses the effects of obstruction on the fetal lung and urinary tract. Journal of Pediatric Surgery 1982, 17, 965–974.
99. Harrison MR, Ross N, Noall R and deLorimer AA. Correction of congenital hydrophrenosis *in utero* I. The model: fetal ureteral obstruction produces hydronephrosis and pulmonary hypoplasia in fetal limbs. Journal of Pediatric Surgery 1983, 18, 247–256.
100. Hinman F and Hepler AB. Experimental hydronephrois: the effect of changes in blood pressure and in blood flow on its rate of development. Archives of Surgery 1925, 11–19.
101. Hirata M, Inamitsu T, Hashimoto T and Koga T. An inhibitor of lipozygenase, nordihydroguaiaretic acid, shortens actin filaments. Journal of Biochemistry 1984, 95, 891–894.
102. Hjelle JT, Hjelle JJ, Maziasz TJ and Carone FA. Diphenylthiazole-induced changes in renal ultrastructure and enzymology: toxicologic mechanisms in polycystic kidney disease. Journal of Pharmacology and Experimental Therapeutics 1987, 243, 758–766.
103. Horster M. Hormonal stimulation and differential growth response of renal epithelial cells

cultured *in vitro* from individual nephron segments. International Journal of Biochemistry 1980, 12, 29–35.

104. Huseman R, Grady A, Welling D and Grantham J. Macropuncture study of polycystic disease in adult human kidneys. Kidney International 1980, 18, 375–385.

105. Iverson WO, Fetterman GH, Jacobson ER, Olsen JH, Senior DF and Schobert EE. Polycystic kidney and liver disease in Springbok: I. Morphology of the lesions. Kidney International 1982, 22, 146–155.

106. Igarashi Y, Aperia A, Larsson L and Zetterstrom R. Effect of betamethasone on Na–K-ATPase activity and basal and lateral cell membranes in proximal tubular cells during early development. American Journal of Physiology 1983, 245, F232–F237.

107. Jacobsson K, Linduist B, Michaelson G and Bjerle P. Fluid turnover in renal cysts. Acta Medica Scandinavica 1977, 202, 327–329.

108. Kanwar YS and Carone FA. Reversible changes of tubular cell and basement membrane in drug-induced renal cystic disease. Kidney International 1984, 26, 35–43.

109. Kanwar YS, Makino H and Carone FA. Basement membrane proteoglycans of the kidney. Seminars in Nephrology 1985, 5, 307–313.

110. Kelly CJ, Korngold R, Mann R, Clayman M, Haverty T and Neilson EG. Spontaneous interstitial nephritis in kdkd mice. II Characterization of a tubular antigen-specific, H-2K-restricted lyt-2 + effector T cell that mediates destructive tubulointerstitial injury. Journal of Immunology 1986, 136, 526–531.

111. Kelly CJ and Neilson EG. Contrasuppression in autoimmunity. Abnormal contrasuppression facilitates expression of nephritogenic effect T cells and interstitial nephritis in kdkd mice. Journal of Experimental Medicine 1987, 165, 107–123.

112. Kelly CJ and Neilson EG. Medullary cystic disease: an inherited form of autoimmune interstitial nephritis? American Journal of Kidney Disease 1987, 10, 389–395.

113. Kenner CH, Evan AP, Blomgren P, Aronoff GR and Luft FC. Effect of protein intake on renal function and structure in partially nephrectomized rats. Kidney International 1985, 27, 739–750.

114. Kime SW, McNamara JJ, Luse S, Farmer S, Silbert C and Bricker NS. Experimental polycystic renal disease in rats: electron microscopy, function, and susceptibility to pyelonephritis. Journal of Laboratory and Clinical Medicine 1962, 60, 64–78.

115. Lee CS, Mauer SM, Brown DM, Sutherland DER, Michael AF and Najarian JS. Renal transplantation in diabetes mellitus in rats. Journal of Experimental Medicine 1974, 139, 793–801.

116. Lettow E and Dammrich K. Congenital polycystic liver and kidney lesions in a cat. Kleintier-Prax 1967, 12, 34–43.

117. Lozzio BB, Chernoff AI, Machado ER and Lozzio CB. Hereditary renal disease in a mutant strain of rats. Science 1967, 156, 1742–1744.

118. Lyon MF and Hulse EV. An inherited kidney disease of mice resembling human nephronophthisis. Journal of Medical Genetics 1971, 8, 41–48.

119. McAteer JA, Carone FA, Grantham JJ, Kempson SA, Gardner KD Jr and Evan AP. Explant culture of human polycystic kidney. Laboratory Investigation 1988, 59, 126–136.

120. McAteer JA, Dougherty GS, Gardner KD Jr and Evan AP. Scanning electron microscopy of kidney cells in culture: surface features of polarized epithelia. Scanning Electron Microscopy 1986, III, 1135–1150.

121. McAteer JA, Dougherty GS, Gardner KD Jr and Evan AP. Polarized epithelial cells *in vitro*: a review of cell and explant culture systems that exhibit epithelial cyst formation. Scanning Electron Microscopy 1988, 2, 1739–1763.

122. McAteer JA, Evan AP and Gardner KD Jr. Morphogenetic clonal growth of kidney epithelial cell line MDCK. Anatomical Record 1987, 217, 229–239.

123. McAteer JA, Evan AP Vance EE and Gardner KD Jr. MDCK-cysts: an *in vitro* model of epithelial cyst formation and growth. Journal of Tissue Culture Methods 1986, 10, 245–248.

124. McAteer JA, Welling DJ, Evan AP, Connors BA and Welling LD. Determination of

growth rate for MDCK cysts cultured within collagen gel. Federation Proceedings 1985, 44, 1039 (abstract).

125. McCune EL, Savage JE and O'Dell BL. Hydropericardium and ascites in checks fed a chlorinated hydrocarbon. Poultry Science 1962, 41, 295–299.

126. McGeoch JEM and Darmady EM. Enzyme changes in experimental renal microcystic disease. British Journal of Experimental Pathology 1973, 54, 555–565.

127. McGeoch JEM and Darmady EM. Polycystic disease of kidney liver, and pancreas; a possible pathogenesis. Journal of Pathology 1976, 119, 221–228.

128. McGeoch JEM, Woodhouse MA and Darmady EM. Experimental infantile polycystic kidney in rats: the influence of age and sex. British Journal of Experimental Pathology 1972, 53, 322–340.

129. McKenna SC and Carpenter JL. Polycystic disease of the kidney and liver in the Cairn Terrier. Veterinary Pathology 1980, 17, 436–442.

130. MacKay K, Striker LJ, Pinkert CA, Brinster RL and Striker GE. Glomerulosclerosis and renal cysts in mice transgenic for the early region of SV 40. Kidney International 1987, 32, 827–837.

131. Mandell J, Koch WK, Nidess R, Premlinger GM and McFarland E. Congenital polycystic kidney disease. American Journal of Pathology 1983, 113, 112–114.

132. Mangoo-Karim R and Grantham JJ. Water permeability of MDCK cell cysts in hydrated collagen gel. 1988, FASEB Journal, 2, A1727 (abstract).

133. Maruffo CA and Cramer DC. Congenital renal malformation in monkeys. Folia Primatologia 1967, 5, 305–311.

134. Milutinovic J and Agoda LY. Potential causes and pathogenesis in autosomal dominant polycystic kidney disease. Nephron 1983, 33, 139–144.

135. Monie IW and Morgan JR. Cysts in cultured fetal rat kidneys. Teratology 1975, 11, 143–152.

136. Mullaney TP, Reindel JF, Matzat P and Padgett GA. Animal model: the mode of inheritance of polycystic disease in pigs. American Journal of Medical Genetics 1988 (in press).

137. Munkittrick KR, Moccia RD and Leatherland JF. Polycystic kidney disease in goldfish (*Carassius auratus*) from Hamilton Harbour, Lake Ontario, Canada. Veterinary Pathology 1985, 22, 232–237.

138. Nauwerck C and Huischmid K. Über das Multicoloculare Adenokystom der Niere Beitr. Path Anat Allgemeine Pathologie 1983, 12, 1–32.

139. Neilson EG, McCafferty E, Feldman A, Clayman MD, Zakheim B and Korngold R. Spontaneous interstitial nephritis in kdkd mice. I. An experimental model of autoimmune renal disease. Journal of Immunology 1984, 133, 2560–2565.

140. Newberne PM. Caridorenal lesions of potassium depletion on steroid therapy in the rat. American Journal of Veterinary Research 1964, 1256–1260.

141. Nidess R, Koch WE, Fried FA, McFarland E and Mandell J. Development of the embryonic murine kidney in normal and congenital polycystic kidney disease: characterization of a proximal tubular degenerative process as the first observable light microscopic defect. Journal of Urology 1984, 131, 156–162.

142. Northington JW and Juliana MM. Polycystic kidney disease in a cat. Journal of Small Animal Practice 1977, 18, 663–666.

143. Ogborn MR, Crocker JFS and McCarthy SC. RU 38486 prolongs survival in murine congenital polycystic kidney disease. Journal of Steroid Biochemistry 1987, 28, 783–784.

144. Oikarinen AI, Uitto J and Oikarinen J. Glucocorticoid action on connective tissue. Medical Biology 1986, 64, 221–230.

145. Ojeda JL, Barbosa E and Gomez-Bosque P. Morphological analysis of renal polycystosis induced by corticoids. Journal of Anatomy 1972, 111, 399–413.

146. Ojeda JL and Garcià-Porrero JA. Structure and development of parietal podocytes in renal glomerular cysts induced in rabbits with methylprednisole acetate. Laboratory Investigation 1982, 167–176.

147. Ojeda JL and Garcià-Porrero JA. Proximal tubule changes in polycystic kidney induced by methyl prednisolone acetate in the newborn rabbit. Experientia 1981, 37, 894–896.

148. Ojeda JL, Ros MA and Garcià-Porrero JA. Polycystic kidney disease induced by corticoids. Nephron 1986, 42, 240–248.

149. Oliver J, MacDowell M, Welt LG, Holliday W Jr, Winters RW, Williams TF and Segar WE. The renal lesions of electrolyte imbalance. Journal of Experimental Medicine 1957, 106, 563–573.

150. Osathanondh V and Potter EL. Pathogenesis of polycystic kidneys: Type 4 due to urethral obstruction. Archives of Pathology 1964, 77, 502–509.

151. Percy DH. Teratogenic effects of the pyrimidine analogues 5-iododeoxyuridine and cystosine arabinoside in late fetal mice and rats. Teratology 1975, 11, 103–118.

152. Perey DYE, Herdman RC and Good RA. Polycystic renal disease: a new experimental model. Science 1967, 158, 494–496.

153. Perrone RD. *In vitro* function of cyst epithelium from human polycystic kidney. Journal of Clinical Investigation 1985, 76, 1688–1691.

154. Preminger GM, Koch WE, Fried FA, McFarland E, Murphy ED and Mandell J. Murine congenital polycystic kidney disease: a model for studying development of cystic disease. Journal of Urology 1982, 127, 556–560.

155. Pouyssègur J, Franchi A, L'Allemain G, Magnaldo I, Paris S and Sardet C. Genetic approach to structure function, and regulation of the Na^+/H^+ antiporter. Kidney International 1987, 32 (Suppl 23), S144–S149.

156. Poyneer D, Selway S and Spurling NW. The effect on an anti-inflammatory compound (AH 2835) on the rat kidney. Proceedings of the European Society for the Study of Drug Toxicity 1968, 181, 191–203.

157. Radomski JL, Fuyat HN, Nelson AA and Smith PK. The toxic effects, excretion, and distribution of lithium chloride. Journal of Pharmacology and Experimental Therapeutics 1950, 100, 429–444.

158. Reeves WH, Kanwar YS and Farquhar MG. Assembly of the glomerular filtrations surface. Journal of Cell Biology 1980, 85, 735–753.

159. Resnick JS, Brown DM and Vernier RL. Oxygen toxicity in fetal organ culture. Laboratory Investigation 1973, 28, 437–445.

160. Resnick JS, Brown DM and Vernier RL. Normal development and experimental models of cystic renal disease. In: Gardner KD Jr, ed, Cystic Diseases of the Kidney. New York: Wiley, 1976, 221–242.

161. Ribacchi R. Rene policistico congenito in topi PM/Se. Lav Anat Pat Perugia 1975, 35, 81–85.

162. Ribacchi R. Ipoplasia del time e della milza nei topi PM/Se con rene policistico congenito. Lav Anat Pat Perugia 1976, 36, 43–46.

163. Ribacchi R. Riduzione progressiva della fosfatasi alcaline e della adenosintri–fosfatasi mg-dipendente nel rene policistico congenito dei topi PM/Se. Lav Anat Pat Perugia 1977, 37, 9–14.

164. Richardson JCW, Scalera V and Simmons NL. Identification of two strains of MDCK cells which resemble separate nephron tubule segments. Biochimica Biophysica Acta 1981, 673, 26–36.

165. Roher DP and Nielsen SW. Polycystic kidneys in a western coyote. Journal of the American Veterinary Medical Association 1983, 183, 1276–1277.

166. Ros MA, Garcìa-Porrero JA and Ojeda JL. Duplication of slit diaphragms in the cystic glomeruli of rabbits treated with methylprednisolone acetate. Acta Anatomica 1987, 130, 362–365.

167. Ros MA, Ojeda JL and Garcìa-Porrero JA. Vascular architecture modifications in the steroid-induced kidney. Nephron 1985, 40, 332–340.

168. Rupple BM. Congenital polycystic disease of the kidney occurring in mice. Journal of the National Cancer Institute 1955, 5, 1183–1187.

169. Russell ES and McFarland EC. Cystic kidneys. Mouse Newsletter 1977, 56, 40–43.

170. Ryan CP. Polycystic disease of the kidneys. Veterinary Medicine 1981, 76, 1351–1354.
171. Safouh M, Crocker JFS and Vernier RL. Experimental cystic disease of the kidney. Laboratory Investigation 1970, 23, 392–400.
172. Schlumberger HG. Polycystic kidney in the goldfish. Archives of Pathological Laboratory Medicine 1950, 50, 400–410.
173. Schwartz WB and Relman AS. Effects of electrolyte disorders on renal structure and function. New England Journal of Medicine 1967, 276, 383–389.
174. Scott HH and Camb H. Congenital malformations of the kidney. Proceedings of the Zoological Society Land 1925, 2, 1259–1270.
175. Sehic M and Bauer M. Bilateral cystic renal disease in a cat. Veterinary Archives 1970, 40, 152–154.
176. Shimamura T, Kissane JM and Gyorkey F. Experimental hydronephrosis: nephron dissection and electron microscopy of the kidney following obstruction of the ureter and in recovery from obstruction. Laboratory Investigation 1966, 15, 629–640.
177. Silvestro D. Bilateral polycystic kidneys in a cat. Aca Medica Vet (Napoli) 1970, 13, 349–361.
178. Slater EP, Andersen T, Cattini P, Issacs R, Birnbaum MJ, Gardner DG, Eberhardt NL and Baxter JD. Mechanisms of glucocorticoid hormone action. Advances in Experimental Med Biol 1986, 196, 67–80.
179. Soloman S. Inherited renal cysts in rats. Science 1973, 181, 451–452.
180. Sondergaard D and Blom L. Polycystic changes in rat kidney induced by biphenyl fed in different diets. Archives of Toxicology 1979, Suppl. 2, 499–502.
181. Spargo B. Kidney changes in hypokalemic alkalosis in the rat. Journal of Laboratory and Clinical Medicine 1954, 43, 802–814.
182. Striker GE and Striker IMM. Pathogenesis of renal cysts in polycystic kidney disease. Contr Nephrol 1985, 48, 169–177.
183. Takahashi H, Ueyama Y, Hibino T, Kuwahara Y, Suzuki S, Hioki K and Tamaoki N. A new mouse model of genetically transmitted kidney disease. Journal of Urology 1986, 135, 1280–1283.
184. Tanagho EA. Surgically induced partial urinary obstruction in the fetal lamb: III. Ureteral obstruction. Investigative Urology 1972, 10, 35–52.
185. Thomas JO, Cox AJ and DeEds F. Kidney cysts produced by diphenlamine. Stanford Medical Bulletin 1957, 15, 90–93.
186. Thomas JO, Ribelin WE, Wilson RH, Keppler DC and DeEds F. Chronic toxicity of diphenylamine to albino rats. Toxicology and Applied Pharmacology 1967, 10, 362–374.
187. Thomasson BH, Esterly JR and Ravitch MM. Morphologic changes in the fetal rabbit kidney after intrauterine ligation. Investigative Urology 1970, 8, 261–272.
188. Torres VE, Berndt TU, Okamura M, Nesbit JW, Holley KE, Carone FA, Knox FG and Romero JC. Mechanisms affecting the development of renal cystic disease induced by diphenylthiazole. Kidney International 1988, 33, 1130–1139.
189. Uchic ME, Donoso VS, Kornhaue J, Cragoe EJ and Grantham JJ. Alteration of MDCK cyst enlargement in hydrated collagen gel by inhibitors of solute transport. Kidney International 1988, 33, 386 (abstract).
190. Uchic M, Kornhaus J, Grantham JA, McAteer J, Cragoe EJ Jr and Granthan JJ. Amiloride and amiloride analogues retard the enlargement of MDCK cysts grown in hydrated collagen gel. Kidney International 1987, 31, 184 (abstract).
191. Valentich JD and Stokols MF. An established cell line from mouse medullary thick ascending limb. I. cell culture techniques, morphology and antigenic expression. American Journal of Physiology 1986, 251, C299–311.
192. Vargas L, Friederici HHR and Maibenco HC. Cortical sponge kidneys induced in rats by alloxan. Diabetes 1970, 19, 33–44.
193. Vlachos JD. A new experimental model of polycystic kidneys. American Journal of Diseases of Childhood 1972, 123, 118–120.
194. Von Ardenne M, Chaplain RA and Reitnauer RG. *In vitro* Messungen zur Schadigung

98

von Krebszellen in guter Versorgungslage durch die Attackenkomination Nordihydro-guajaretasure + 40 °C-Hyperthermie ohne und mit der Strahlendosis 1000 r. Archiv für Geschwulstforschung 1969, 34, 1–26.

195. Welling IW and Welling DJ. Kinetics of cyst development in cystic renal disease. In: Cummings NB and Klahr S, eds, Chronic Renal Disease. New York: Plenum, 1985, 95–104.

196. Werder AA, Amos MA, Nielsen AH and Wolfe GH. Comparative effects of germ-free and ambient environments on the development of cystic kidney disease in CFM_{wd} mice. Journal of Laboratory and Clinical Medicine 1984, 103, 399–407.

197. Whitehouse RW, Lendon RG and Lendon M. Renal polycystosis in the rat induced by prednisolone tertiary butylacetate. Experientia 1980, 36, 244–245.

198. Wickre CG and Bennett WM. Renal cyst epithelial transport in non-uremic polycystic kidney disease. Kidney International 1983, 23, 514–518.

199. Wijeratne WVS. Inherited renal cysts in pigs: results of breeding experiments. Veterinary Record 1980, 107, 484–488.

200. Wilson PD, Dillingham MA, Breckon and Anderson RJ. Defined human renal tubular epithelia in culture: growth characterization, and hormonal response. American Journal of Physiology 1985, 248, F436–443.

201. Wilson PD and Hreniuk D. Altered polarity of Na–K ATPase in epithelia with a genetic defect and abnormal basement membrane. Journal of Cell Biology 1987, 105, 176a (abstract).

202. Wilson PD, Hreniuk D and Avner ED. Cellular and transport-related defects in cultures of congenital murine polycystic kidney disease epithelia. Kidney International 1987, 31, 394 (abstract).

203. Wilson PD, Hreniuk D and Gabow PA. Relationship between abnormal extracellular matrix and excessive growth of human adult polycystic kidney disease epithelia. Laboratory Investigation 1989 (in press).

204. Wilson PD, Schrier RW, Breckon RD and Gabow PA. Human polycystic kidney disease epithelia in culture. A new method for studying abnormalities and pathogenesis. Kidney International 1986, 30, 371–378.

205. Wilson RH and DeEds F. Toxicity studies on the antioxidant 6-ethoxy-1,2-dihydro-2,2,4-trimethyquinoline. Journal of Agriculture and Food Chemistry 1959, 7, 203–211.

206. Woodhouse MA, Offer J and Darmady EM. Diphenylamine induced polycystic kidneys compared with human polycystic kidneys: electron microscopic observations. Nephron 1965, 4, 253–254.

5
Pathogenesis of Cysts and Cystic Kidneys

L.W. Welling

Abstract

Although the formation of fluid-filled renal cysts is a fairly common event that has received attention for more than a century, the mechanisms involved in their development are not well understood. In this chapter we consider a series of model explanations to which we add or subtract until we arrive at one with the greatest number of favorable traits. It is agreed that renal cysts develop in pre-existing nephrons and collecting ducts, and that they can develop in the absence of distal tubule obstruction, large transmural pressure or solute gradients, abnormally stretchable basement membranes, or permanent connection to their tubule of origin. It is decided, however, that there is an absolute requirement for diffuse hyperplasia of the lining epithelium that keeps pace exactly with the enlarging surface area of the cyst cavity. At the same time, the cyst cavity is always filled with fluid, and that probably requires the new development of a net secretory mechanism. As to the question of which comes first, the cellular proliferation or the accumulation of fluid, the two in fact must occur simultaneously and are perhaps consequences of the same cause.

Key words   Renal cysts;
Polycystic kidney disease;
Balloon model;
Hyperplasia model;
Hyperplasia–net secretion model;
Obstruction–hyperplasia model;
Saturation model.

1. Introduction

Renal cystic diseases and their pathogenesis have been considered in the medical literature for well over 100 years. They have always been controversial topics, and the rise and fall of the considerable number of conflicting or complementary classifications and theories make for a fascinating tour of practically all aspects of renal physiology, embryology and pathology.

Historically, the possibility of a neoplastic origin of cysts was raised several times and discarded in favor of some form of urinary obstruction as the underlying mechanism. It was thus implied that distally obstructed nephrons and ducts could accumulate fluid, presumably by continuing glomerular filtration or by tubule secretion, and dilate like so many balloons. It was frequently observed that sufficient epithelial hyperplasia occurred to accommodate the increasing surface area of the cyst wall. The earliest proposed causes of the initial obstruction included crystal deposition or post-infectious scarring, sometimes with complete isolation of a tubule segment from its original afferent and efferent connections. With wider understanding of the embryology and dual origin of the kidney, however, it became popular to think of the obstructions and the disconnected segments as having been caused by a failure of the nephrons and collecting systems to connect, to remain properly connected, or even to degenerate appropriately during renal organogenesis[40,46,47].

In the 1960's, the emphasis shifted away from the possibility of a single mechanism and, perhaps more importantly, away from the idea that all varieties of cysts might represent a single disease state or be explained by a single mechanism. In their extensive microdissection studies, Osathanondh and Potter[41–44,46] found no evidence of embryologic non-connections or of any other consistent form of tubule isolation or intrarenal obstruction. They rejected most of the earlier theories and concluded that nearly all renal cystic diseases could be categorized into four types, each reflecting different degrees or different timings of *defective interaction between the two* anlagen of the developing kidney. That defect might be primary, perhaps genetic, or secondary, perhaps due to toxins or to extrarenal obstruction with a damaging elevation of hydrostatic pressure. It resulted in an abnormality of the products of metanephric development, the nephrons and collecting ducts, that eventually led to secondary enlargement and cyst formation. The exact mechanism was not further specified, but did not include intrarenal malconnections or obstructions of the types previously considered. Even though some patterns of cyst formation (Types II and IV) were associated with dysplastic changes, particularly abnormal duct branchings[42,44], and other patterns (Types I and III) were not[41,43], the overall effect of this viewpoint was an abandonment of the earlier theories or a refocusing of those theories into the context of developmental abnormalities. Regardless of the type of the cystic disease or whether it manifested itself in the newborn period or in later adult life, it always was seen as a congenital anomaly.

Since the 1960's, there has been considerable activity in the field. In addition to further, conflicting microdissection studies that have either found[33] or not found[4] duct branching abnormalities or other evidence of maldevelopment in human cystic disease, renal cystic disease has been induced in otherwise normal animals by a variety of chemicals[48] and has been found to occur in humans as an acquired disorder[17]. Clearly, therefore, cystic disease is not always a developmental abnormality. Furthermore, cystic disease has also been observed and studied in rats, mice and other animals, with several patterns of inheritance, allowing a new experimental approach not previously possible. The result has been a general re-evaluation of the genesis of cysts with a de-emphasizing of the role of renal embryologic maldevelopment. In fact, only a few of the earlier concepts have survived recent close scrutiny. As was suggested by many early workers, there now is little doubt that all renal cysts arise from pre-existing normal or at least non-cystic nephrons and collecting duct segments. Also as suggested earlier, there is now considerable evidence that cellular hyperplasia is an important factor, at least insofar as there is clearly a greater number of cells available to line the increasing surface areas of cyst walls. Finally, there is now confirmation of the old histologic and microdissection studies showing that many cysts eventually lose communication with their nephron or duct of origin. Continuing growth of such cysts implies some form of secretion into the cyst cavity, either by continuing glomerular filtration or by transtubular, transepithelial volume flow. The role of obstruction, however, has otherwise remained uncertain, and there is yet to be a single theory that can explain the development of any cyst from its earliest stimulus to its final form. Our purpose, therefore, cannot be to provide a final answer. Rather, it is to review the available information and to point toward directions of promise. We do this by considering first the basic mechanisms and then a series of models to which we add or subtract until we arrive at one with the greatest number of favorable traits.

2. Basic mechanisms

Renal cysts are always filled with fluid. The fluid has generally been thought of as urine, or at least as a glomerular filtrate or tubule secretion. It has long been recognized to show the effects of water, urea and glucose absorption[37], and more recently it has been reported to resemble, in composition, the fluid normally found in proximal or in distal tubule segments[22,34]. The cysts are lined with an epithelium in which cells are increased in number at least to the extent that they maintain approximately normal dimensions and density even though the cysts have surface areas many times greater than those of normal nephron or duct segments. This feature, too, has long been recognized (Bialestock[7] quotes a source from 1908), but has been emphasized only recently[29]. The epithelium may also be focally hyperplastic to the extent of polyp formation, a phenomenon that also was observed quite early (Potter[46] quotes late 19th century sources), but only recently emphasized[6,19,20,29,31].

The facts just stated, namely that the cysts are always filled with fluid and always lined with epithelium, brings us immediately to the most basic question about cyst genesis: does the abnormality leading to cyst formation lie principally in the growth properties of the limiting epithelial membrane or in the forces leading to fluid accumulation? That is, does epithelial growth come first and, either by producing cells with the capacity for net fluid secretion or by forcing, through proliferation, an increase in the surface area of a cylindrical or spherical shell, somehow generate forces sufficient to keep the shell filled with ambient fluid or, alternatively, does the accumulation of fluid in a pre-formed tissue space (nephron or duct segment) somehow stretch and induce the limiting epithelial layer to grow in surface area just sufficiently to keep up with increasing cyst volume? In theory at least, the growth-first possibility should be easily separable from the fluid-first possibility on the basis of fairly simple observations[12,53].

2.1. Cell proliferation

Let us consider first the possibility that a previously stable epithelial layer is induced to grow further, or that a normally developing epithelial layer fails to stop growing on reaching normal size. The latter might be the case, for example, in a congenital cystic disease such as autosomal recessive polycystic kidney disease (ARPKD), in which marked saccular or uniform generalized enlargement of collecting ducts in the kidneys of newborns has been attributed to "secondary hyperplasia"[42,46]. Using ARPKD as an example, we may assume further that epithelial cells usually maintain a fairly constant size and that the proliferating epithelium remains predominantly a single layer structure. We also assume, for the moment at least, that the epithelium forms neither surface folds nor polyps of significant size and does not produce multilayered tumour masses. With these provisions, the pattern of growth of an ideal spherical cyst can be predicted to be exponential[53,54], because the surface area of a cyst is proportional to the number of cells present at any given time. Therefore, if cell division were a primary event, the time rate of change of the number of cells and the time rate of change of cyst wall surface area would be proportional to the number and area at that time. The resulting growth curve for cyst outer surface area (A) thus would be of the form $A_0 \exp(kt)$, where A_0 is the initial area and k is the rate constant. That rate constant is related to the time (t) required for the number of cells to double, and in turn might be influenced by environmental circumstances such as resistance to cyst enlargement afforded by the surrounding matrix or interstitial tissue. Nonetheless, if cyst growth is a result of such cell multiplication, it still follows that the radius, surface area and volume of the cyst would be exponential functions of time whose rate constants would be $k/2$, k, and $3k/2$, respectively. The example would thus have unique characteristics, and, to confirm the possibility that such an example exists *in vivo*, we would need only to observe a cyst for some period of time and to find that cyst radius, surface area and volume all varied with time in the required exponential manner.

2.2. Fluid accumulation

Consider now the alternative, second possibility in which fluid accumulation is the primary event in cyst formation, with cell growth following only as a consequence. The cyst growth patterns are again predictable in theory. Namely, if fluid accumulation were driven by osmotic or hydrostatic forces and if those forces remained constant with time, the radius of a spherical cyst would increase as a linear function of time while the surface area and volume would be quadratic and cubic functions of time, respectively[53,54]. The time (t) required to achieve a given cyst volume (V) under these conditions is given by the equation,

$$t = (V - V_0) / (J_{Vin} - J_{Vout} + J_{Vs} - J_{Vab})$$

in which V_0 is the starting normal volume of a renal tubule or duct, about 10^{-5} ml. If the initial osmotic forces were conceived to decay with time (e.g., by dilution of intracystic osmotic solutes) or to increase with time (e.g., by continuing enzymatic breakdown of trapped macromolecules) or if the hydrostatic forces were changed by increases or decreases in glomerular filtration or tubule secretion into the cyst cavity, the growth curves would become asymptotic or non-linear. Similar effects might result from changes in the deformability of the paracystic matrix. It is unlikely, however, that a combination of driving forces for or resistance to fluid accumulation could persist for sufficient time to generate an exponential growth curve. Again, these possibilities might be investigated by simple *in vivo* observations.

Having developed the means for dissecting the mechanisms involved in cyst formation, the next logical step normally would be to examine the reported observations on cyst growth characteristics and to reach some logical conclusions. Unfortunately, however, we have few data about naturally occurring and experimentally induced renal cystic disease *in vivo*. Perhaps surprisingly, the data on cyst growth rates are simply not available. Nonetheless, it is possible to exclude certain mechanisms.

3. Models of cyst development

The hypothetical conditions under which a fluid-filled renal cyst develops *in vivo* [53,54] are summarized in Fig. 5.1. The several arrows represent volume flows and their direction. J_{Vin} is the proximal inflow and, for a given tubule or collecting duct segment, is equal to the single nephron glomerular filtration rate plus or minus any secretory or reabsorptive volume flux that may have occurred upstream. Mostly because of upstream reabsorption, reasonable values for J_{Vin} range from about 5 to about 50 nl/min in the normal kidney. If connection to a functional glomerulus is lost, of course, proximal inflow may be zero.

At the opposite, downstream end of the tubule or duct, J_{Vout} is simply the distal outflow. It will range from zero during complete outlet obstruction to values greater than or less than J_{Vin} depending upon intervening fluid absorp-

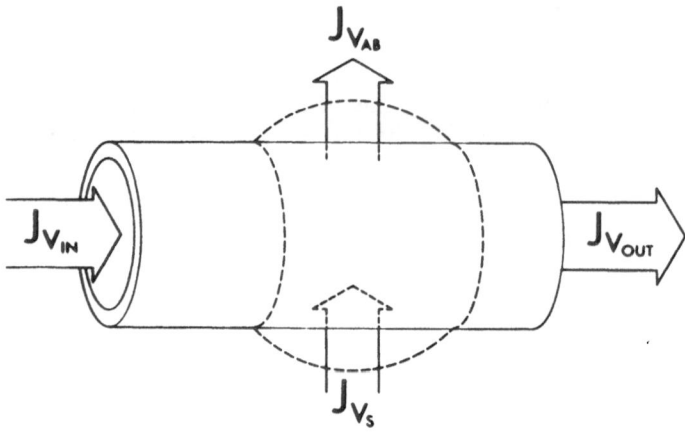

Figure 5.1. Hypothetical nephron segment predisposed to cystic dilation. Arrows represent volume flows and directions. (Reproduced from ref. 53, with permission).

tion out of the lumen, J_{Vab}, or fluid secretion into the lumen, J_{Vs}. Typical values of J_{vout} range from 2 to 20 nl/min in the normal kidney. In any case, the net effect of the several volume flows can be summarized by the equation

$$(J_{Vin} - J_{Vout} + J_{Vs} - J_{Vab}) = dV/dt$$

in which the change in cyst volume (V) with time (t) is simply the algebraic sum of the several independent volume flows.

Not shown in Figure 5.1 are the forces that might be generated if cell division or cell hypertrophy in the cyst wall caused an increase in both the surface area and the diameter of the cyst. Also not shown are those forces that might be generated in the paracystic matrix or renal interstitium to retard or to facilitate cyst enlargement.

3.1. Balloon model

The most logical explanation of cyst formation has been thought historically to be some form of distal obstruction of a renal tubule or collecting duct in the face of a continuing glomerular filtration or tubule secretion. On occasion, the cyst-forming tubule segment was thought to be entirely sequestered (i.e., to have lost all connection to its tubule or duct of origin) and presumably to gain fluid entirely by secretory flux. In either case, cyst formation was analogous to the filling of a balloon.

Let us examine what would happen if a tubule or duct segment were in fact totally obstructed distally and if the wall of the developing cyst were impermeable and inert. Clearly, this is a fluid-first type of situation, and, if the glomerular filtration rate and the net secretory and reaborptive fluxes were truly constant with time, the cyst volume would grow linearly with time, as shown by the solid line in Fig. 5.2. The, if J_{Vin} were on the order of 5 nl/min, as seems reasonable for distal tubule and collecting duct segments under otherwise normal conditions, spherical cysts of volume 0.1, 1, 10, and 100 ml could be produced in about 14 days, 140 days, 3.8 years, and 38 years, respectively, as shown in Table 5.1. If J_{Vin} were on the order of 50 nl/min, as seems reasonable for proximal tubule segments, cysts of the various sizes could be produced 10 times faster.

Table 5.1. Linear cyst growth

	Time	
Cyst volume (ml)	dV/dt: 5 nl/min	50 nl/min
0.1	14 days	1.4 days
1	140 days	14 days
10	3.8 years	140 days
100	38 years	3.8 years

As it turns out, all of these times are reasonable, both in some human renal cystic diseases and in some experimental cystic diseases in animals[12,19,27]. Furthermore, if one does not require the maintenance of a strictly constant absorptive flux during cyst wall stretching and allows instead a progressive decrease in transport function, zero transport or even cell death, the result might be a faster-than-linear growth pattern (the dotted curve in Figure 5.2) or a linear pattern with a slope greater than in the original constant flux situation. The end result would be cysts larger than predicted in Table 5.1 or perhaps a mixture of smaller and larger cysts, as actually seen in cystic kidneys.

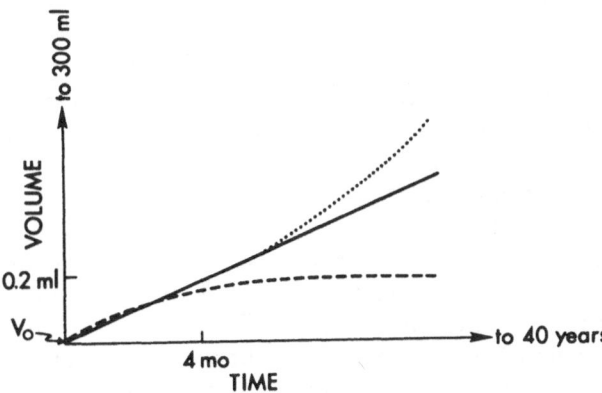

Figure 5.2. Possible cyst growth patterns; linear, faster than linear, and "saturation". The times and volumes are arbitrary. (Reproduced from ref. 53, with permission).

Before these calculations are taken as evidence favoring the fluid-first theory of cyst formation, however, there are several other factors that must be considered.

First, when a balloon is stretched, its surface area increases at the expense of wall thickness. Thus, if the cell and basement membrane mass were to remain constant during cyst formation, the original cell height of about 7.5 μm and the original basement membrane thickness of about 0.25 μm (Table 5.2) would become attenuated to about 0.25 and 0.01 μm, respectively, in cysts only 1 mm in diameter, and would be attenuated by an additional factor of 10 in cysts just 1 cm in diameter. Numerous observations, both recent and old, however, have shown the epithelial cells of many cysts not to be thinner than normal, but similar in size to the normal lining cells of nephrons and collecting ducts[5,7,12,15,19,29,31,41]. Furthermore, the tubule basement membrane is found more often to be normal or even increased in thickness than to be thinned. It must be concluded, therefore, that cysts cannot result from a simple, balloon-like stretching of a pre-existing tubule segment. For a fluid-first situation actually to be effective, some connection must be made between stretching and a degree of cell growth sufficient to maintain reasonably normal cell and basement membrane dimensions.

Table 5.2. Attenuation of constant cell and basement membrane (BM) mass

Tubule OD (mm)	Cell height (μm)	BM thickness (μm)
0.04	7.5	0.25
1	0.25	0.01
10	0.025	0.001

Second, the normal renal tubule has a limited stretchability, mostly because of its basement membrane. This is true and the tubule distensibility is similar both for isolated tubules in vitro[51,52] and for tubules surrounded by normal renal tissue in vivo[13,35]. The result is that a change in outer tubule diameter of nearly 40%, from about 35 to about 50 μm, can be accomplished by changes in transtubular hydrostatic pressure within a physiological range of about 5–40 cm H_2O. However, as indicated by the solid line in Fig. 5.3, the diameter–pressure curve flattens off near the latter pressure, and a further significant tubule enlargement would require unphysiologic hydrostatic pressures far larger than the small ones frequently observed in the context of cyst formation[1,8,16,19,24,27,34]. Furthermore, even if the basement membrane is histologically[15,39] and biochemically[10,11,18,32,36] abnormal and is assumed as a consequence to be abnormally stretchable[12,39] (the broken line in Fig. 5.3), we are still required to find some connection between stretching and new growth both of cells and of basement membrane. In any case, recent studies indicate that basement membrane stretchability probably is not abnormal in the walls of renal cysts[28].

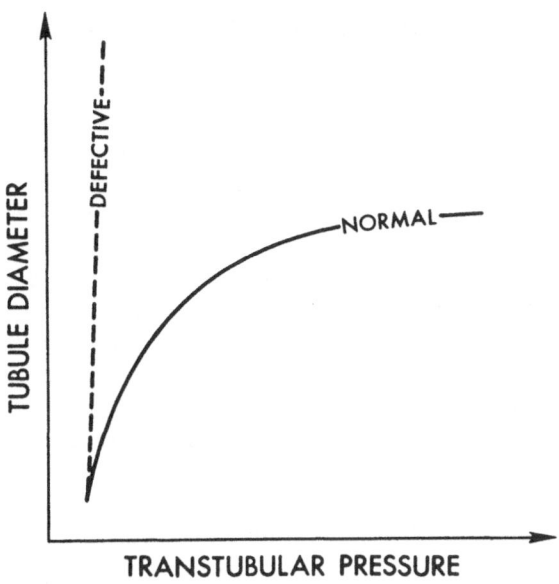

Figure 5.3. Comparison of compliance for normal and hypothetical abnormal tubule basement membrane. (Reproduced from ref. 53, with permission).

Hyperplasia model

As just explained, closer examination of a simple balloon model soon indicates that cellular proliferation and basement membrane production must be important aspects of cyst formation in the kidney. However, whether that knowledge helps in choosing between the fluid-first hypothesis and the cell growth-first hypothesis of cyst formation remains to be seen.

There is ample evidence that cellular growth occurs during cyst formation. In addition to the numerous observations that the epithelial cells of the cyst wall are often of approximately normal size and density (number per unit area), and in addition to the arguments just stated in the discussion of the balloon model, there are reports of micropapillary hyperplasia in the cyst wall epithelium[6,17,20,29,31]. Micropolyps clearly show the propensity of the epithelium to proliferate, at least focally. At the same time, the polyps have been observed at the distal ends of fusiform spaces and in positions that might cause outlet obstruction[19,20]. It is not clear, therefore, which event is the more important to the eventual formation of the cyst, the proliferation itself or the obstruction with fluid accumulation. Furthermore, even if there were no obstructive aspect to the cellular hyperplasia, it is not apparent how proliferation alone could generate the forces necessary to expand a spherical or cylindrical shell of cyst epithelium.

First, although labelled thymidine uptake may be appreciable in some cystic disease models[19], the paucity of mitotic figures to be found in the wall of most cysts suggests that whatever mechanical forces might result from cell division (two cells wedging into the space of one), they probably cannot be distributed evenly throughout the shell. Why then are cysts usually seen to be symmetrically spherical or cylindrical? It might even be asked why they are cysts at all, rather than solid masses of cells as occur in adenomas.

Second, as the cyst enlarges the adjacent tissue must be displaced. While that might not be so difficult in a soft and presumably plastic kidney of a developing fetus or newborn, or even at the subcapsular or parapelvic surface of an adult kidney, newly developing cysts are not uncommon within the mass of an adult kidney (e.g., simple cysts), and cysts are known to develop fairly rapidly even in the scarred and shrunken endstage kidneys of patients on dialysis (i.e., acquired cystic disease[17]).

Third, even though one might think of the proliferating epithelium as a highly permeable membrane able to allow a spontaneous transepithelial flow sufficient to keep the growing cyst filled with ambient fluid[54], even a slowly percolating flow requires a favorable osmotic or hydrostatic gradient. In fact, suitable osmotic gradients have not generally been found, and the hydrostatic pressure gradients, instead of being slightly lumen-negative as would be expected if expansion of the shell were the only active process in cyst enlargement, usually are lumen-positive and in the wrong direction for passive filling of the cyst cavity. Finally, when growing epithelial cells are put into a situation in which they must push laterally against a resistance (e.g., confluent culture cells filling and encountering the sides of a Petri dish), cell division is inhibited[21]. Pushing against neighboring cells in order to increase cyst wall area and thus to increase cyst diameter against a resistive medium seems to be a similarly inhibiting situation.

Therefore, just as the balloon model was found above to be untenable unless additional factors were considered, the hyperplasia model also seems to be untenable in its pure form. At a minimum, what seems to be needed is a way to assure an approximately symmetrical cyst cavity (i.e., a symmetrically distributed force for cyst enlargement) and a means to prevent or reverse contact inhibition within the growing and expanding epithelial sheet of the cyst wall.

3.3. Obstruction–hyperplasia model

Just as the balloon hypothesis can be salvaged to some extent if cell growth is added, the hyperplasia model also can be salvaged to some extent if one adds to it some mechanism for fluid accumulation and an increase in hydrostatic pressure[53]. Outflow obstruction would provide such a mechanism. Hydrostatic pressure within the cyst lumen would be symmetrically distributed, and, if it caused a stretching of the cyst wall with a consequent lateral (circumferential) stretching of the epithelial sheet, it would tend actually to facilitate cell proliferation[18,21].

The proposed interplay between obstruction with fluid accumulation and cellular hyperplasia is depicted in Fig. 5.4. In the left panel is the normal situation with eight cells around the circumference of a renal tubule at a transmural hydrostatic pressure of 10 cm H_2O. In the middle panel a distal obstruction has caused a moderate increase in the tubule diameter that is well within the range allowed by normal basement membrane stretchability. Note, however, that the cells are now both flattened and stretched, a situation known from cell culture work to facilitate cellular proliferation[18,21]. The right panel shows the effect of such proliferation, there now being nine rather than eight cells per tubule circumference. The more important effect, however, is that each of the nine cells have reverted to approximately normal dimensions and perhaps to a normal nuclear–cytoplasmic volume ratio[9], thus both reducing the presumed stimulus for proliferation and, by increasing the cellular and presumably also the basement membrane mass, decreasing the basement membrane stretch and allowing the transmural pressure to return to normal. The stage is set, therefore, for a repetition of the cycle. Because the triggering of this cycle of events is an accumulation of fluid with a consequent increase in hydrostatic pressure, the model is clearly a fluid-first situation.

At first sight the obstruction–hyperplasia model would seem to have only good features. If the cause of the original increase in luminal pressure remained in place, for example, the cycle of pressure increase, cell stretching, cell division and return toward normal pressure might continue indefinitely, with the result of continuing enlargement in the absence of unacceptable degrees of wall attenuation or hydrostatic pressure. The model also leaves open and can easily accommodate (even with some advantage) the possibilities that the stretchability of the basement membrane might in fact be increased and that the epithelial cells might be more susceptible than normal to stimuli promoting cell division. That is, if the tubule or cyst wall were more stretchable than

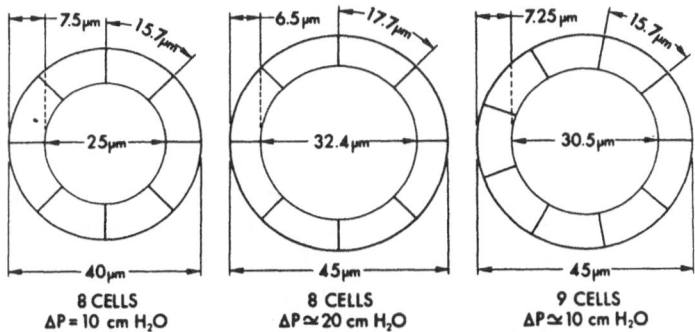

Figure 5.4. Suggested manner of tubule cell growth induced by tubule dilation. (Reproduced from ref. 53, with permission).

normal and responded to a given luminal pressure increase with a greater than normal increase in area, the threshold for stretch-induced cell division might be achieved with only a trivial increase in luminal pressure. Similarly, if the cells themselves had a lower threshold for the initiation of stretch-induced cell division, cell division might again be achieved with only small pressure fluctuations. Such a lowered threshold might reflect a genetic predisposition, as is perhaps demonstrated by the increased growth rate of cyst epithelial cells in culture[56], or abnormal environmental conditions induced perhaps by corticosteroids[2,13,14], or the renin–angiotensin system[49], or the effects of endotoxin[25,26]. On closer examination, however, we soon find that none of these cycles is likely to continue for long without a fundamental change in cellular properties not yet mentioned in our discussion. These properties have to do with the intrinsic ability of the cells to transport fluid by either absorption or secretion.

3.4. Saturation model

The scenarios considered thus far have assumed that the fluid flow into the cystic spaces is constant, as if by a constant glomerular filtration, and that the outflow is zero, as if by total distal obstruction of an inert tubule segment. However, the cells that lined the originally normal segment most typically would have had a considerable capacity for fluid reabsorption, and there is ample evidence that the epithelium of cysts maintains some physiologic function[2,22,34,37,45]. Thus, if at least some of the absorptive capacity per unit area of the original epithelium were maintained as the epithelium proliferated to cover the ever enlarging inner surface area of the cyst cavity, a point eventually would be reached at which all inflow into the cyst cavity would be entirely reabsorbed across the cyst wall and no further growth of the cyst size could occur.

This circumstance, a modified fluid-first situation that we previously have termed "saturation"[53], is shown by the dashed line in Fig. 5.2 and is described by the equation

$$(J_{Vin} - J_{Vout} + J_{Vs}) = (J_{Vab}/A_0)A$$

Sample calculations are shown in Table 5.3. Thus, if the flows into cysts of proximal tubule and collecting duct origins are 50 and 5 nl/min, respectively, and if J_{Vab}/A_0 values are 10 and 1 nl/min per cm tubule length (about 10 and 1 nl/min per mm^2 luminal surface area) in the two segments, it can be predicted that cysts of proximal tubule and collecting duct origin might stabilize or "saturate" at volumes not larger than about 0.002 and 2.0 ml, respectively, and at diameters of 1.4 and 14 mm. Of course, smaller inflows would lead to smaller cysts and smaller reabsorptive capacities would lead to larger cysts. Nonetheless, the predicted sizes are not unreasonable for several of the human cystic diseases and reported animal models.

Table 5.3. Saturation cyst growth

(J_{Vab}/A_o) (nl/min per cm tubule length)	Volume (diameter)	
	1 cm Cylinders	Spheres
10	3×10^{-4} ml (0.2mm)	1.4×10^{-3} ml (1.4mm)
1	3×10^{-2} ml (2 mm)	1.4 ml (14 mm)
0.1	3 ml (20 mm)	1400 ml (140 mm)

On the other hand, it is not uncommon in human material to encounter much larger sizes, even among cysts which by the composition of their fluid are consistent with proximal tubule origin[34], and to find large cysts that are apparently sequestered and isolated[4,29,37]. Cysts without the possibility of glomerular filtration are also observed in experimental systems such as cultured metanephros[2,3] and MDCK cell clones in 3-dimensional hydrated collagen gel matrix[38]. We come again, therefore, to the need to add modifying factors and circumstances to yet another model, the need here being the possibility for a net secretory volume flux.

3.5. Hyperplasia–net secretion model

The properties of this model are identical to those of the obstruction–hyperplasia model except that the source of flow into the cyst cavity must eventually be independent of the usual sources, such as glomerular filtration (J_{Vin}), and must eventually exceed both the reabsorptive capacity (J_{Vab}) of the epithelium and the usual outflow (J_{Vout}) through a connected downstream segment. Since significant reabsorptive flux would be a function of the number of epithelial cells and the surface area of the cyst (as in the saturation model), the secretory flux must also be a function of the number of cells and presumably, therefore, an intrinsic property of those cells.

To avoid the problems of wall thinning, asymmetry of cysts and excessive luminal pressure in the face of cyst walls of limited stretchability, a cycle similar to that described with the obstruction–hyperplasia model would also be necessary, the periodic build-up of cyst cavity pressure now being generated by volume secretion in excess of outflow. Only two questions remain to be answered. First, can volume secretion of the required magnitude seriously be proposed for a simple epithelium[15,29], derived presumably from a normal tubule or duct epithelium having no history of large secretory volume flux and apparently generating no appropriate gradients[34,45]? Second, can a decision be made in choosing between the growth-first possibility and the fluid-first possibility?

To the question of the plausibility of a significant secretory flux, a variety of recently reported data suggest that the answer is probably yes. Although cyst walls *in vitro* exhibit fluid movement in an absorptive rather than secretory direction[45] and net secretion has yet to be demonstrated in human cystic kidneys[23], considerable support for the possibility of secretion by cyst wall epithelium does come from model systems. For example, proximal tubule cyst formation may be induced in organ cultures of developing metanephros in the absence of glomerular filtration. This is directly mediated by increases in Na–K ATPase, is blocked by ouabain, and involves sodium-gradient driven increases in organic anion uptake with intratubular sequestration of osmotically active substances obligating net intratubular fluid accumulation[2]. A related type of secretion also occurs in isolated segments of adult proximal tubule under suitable conditions[30], and the active basolateral transport of endogenous anions such as hippurates, with sequestration inside cysts, has been suggested as playing a role in the process of cyst growth[55]. Also pertinent is a new model in which transformed cells of distal tubule origin (MDCK) form clonal, cyst-like spherical shells when cultured in hydrated collagen gel[38]. In this system, preliminary evidence is consistent with a pharmacologically sensitive secretory mechanism acting across an epithelium of limited permeability[50].

Regarding the question of growth-first versus fluid-first, if the hyperplasia-net secretion model is simply a modification of the obstruction–hyperplasia model it certainly is a fluid-first situation. On the other hand, net volume secretion is not an usual property of proximal tubule or collecting duct epithelium and presumably must represent, in these cases, the acquisition of a new capability. Furthermore, the new cells that line the enlarging surface of the growing cyst must all have such a capacity if secretion into the cyst cavity is to remain greater than absorption or other means of outflow from the cyst cavity. Do these cells thus represent a new or at least different from normal line of cells that have inherited or acquired a different genetic message? Perhaps so, but the answer is not yet known. If yes, the cellular modification would precede the fluid accumulation mechanisms and the situation would be a growth-first situation. On the other hand, cell growth alone is not sufficient, as we have seen, and in the present case must be very closely associated with fluid secretion. It seems logical to suggest, therefore, that while separate growth-first and fluid-first viewpoints might be of value in dissecting the requirements of cyst development, one finally comes to the understanding that both must be present simultaneously.

4. Summary and conclusions

In exploring some logical means for evaluating the mechanisms of cyst growth it is found that too few data are available to reach firm conclusions. Nonetheless, from a stepwise examination of circumstantial evidence it seems highly probable that cell growth and basement membrane growth are both absolute requirements, as is, apparently, the acquisition by the cyst wall epithelium of a capability for net secretory volume flow. The question of which comes first, the cellular growth or the accumulation of fluid, probably has no correct answer. The apparent need for both simultaneously suggests that they are in fact consequences of the same cause. That cause, in turn, would seem most likely to be an inherited or acquired, perhaps environmentally induced, change in the genetic message of renal tubule epithelial cells or change in the way those cells interpret an otherwise normal message. Cysts result when the cells proliferate to cover the inner surface of a tubule space that is supplied by fluid sufficient to keep the cyst cavity filled at ambient or slightly increased hydrostatic pressure. Although that fluid might in some cases derive predominantly from natural sources such as glomerular filtration in excess of tubule outflow, in the final analysis it must be the proliferating cells themselves that, by some mechanism of net secretion, supply the cyst with fluid sufficient in quantity to overcome any reabsorptive flux or outflow by a patent downstream connection. Outflow obstruction would be pertinent only insofar as it enters into that equation. In this final viewpoint, then, blocking either the stimulus for cell proliferation or the stimulus for net secretion would be sufficient to block the continuing growth of cysts.

References

1. Amis ES Jr, Cronan JJ, Yoder IC, Pfister RC and Newhouse JH. Renal cysts: curios and caveats. Urological Radiology 1982, 4, 199–209.
2. Avner ED. Renal cystic disease. Insights from recent experimental investigations. Nephron 1988, 48, 89–93.
3. Avner ED, Piesco NP, Sweeney WE, Studnicki FM, Fetterman GH and Ellis D. Hydrocortisone-induced cystic metanephric maldevelopment in serum-free organ culture. Laboratory Investigation 1984, 50, 208–218.
4. Baert L. Hereditary polycystic kidney disease (adult form): A microdissection study of two cases at an early stage of the disease. Kidney International 1978, 13, 519–525.
5. Baxter TJ. Cysts arising in the renal tubules. A microdissection study. Archives of Diseases in Childhood 1965, 40, 464–473.
6. Bernstein J, Evan AP and Gardner KF Jr. Human cystic kidney diseases: epithelial hyperplasia in the pathogenesis of cysts and tumors. Pediatric Nephrology 1987, 1, 393–396.
7. Bialestock D. The morphogenesis of renal cysts in the stillborn studied by micro-dissection techniques. Journal of Pathology and Bacteriology 1956, 71, 51–59.
8. Bjerle P, Lindqvist B and Michaelson G. Pressure measurements in renal cysts. Scandinavian Journal of Clinical Laboratory Investigations 1971, 27, 135–138.

9. Brunette DM. Mechanical stretching increases the number of epithelial cells synthesizing DNA in culture. Journal of Cellular Science 1984, 69, 35–45.

10. Butkowski RJ, Carone FA, Grantham JJ and Hudson BG. Tubular basement membrane changes in 2-amino-2,4-diphenylthiazole-induced polycystic disease. Kidney International 1985, 28, 744–751.

11. Carone FA, Makino H and Kanwar YS. Basement membrane antigens in renal polycystic disease. American Journal of Pathology 1988, 130, 466–471.

12. Carone FA, Rowland RG, Perlman SG and Ganote CE. The pathogenesis of drug-induced renal cystic disease. Kidney International 1974, 5, 411–421.

13. Cortell S, Gennari FJ, Davidson M, Bossert WH and Schwartz WB. A definition of proximal and distal tubule compliance: Practical and theoretical implications. Journal of Clinical Investigation 1973, 52, 2330–2339.

14. Crocker JFS, Blecher SR, Givner ML and McCarthy SC. Polycystic kidneys and liver disease and corticosterone changes in the cpk mouse. Kidney International 1987, 31, 1088–1091.

15. Cuppage FE, Huseman RA, Chapman A and Grantham JJ. Ultrastructure and function of cysts from human adult polycystic kidneys. Kidney International 1980, 17, 373–381.

16. Derezic D and Cecuk L. Hydrostatic pressure within renal cysts. Journal of Urology 1982, 54, 93–94.

17. Dunnill MS, Millard PR and Oliver D. Acquired cystic disease of the kidneys: a hazard of long-term intermittent maintenance hemodialysis. Journal of Clinical Pathology 1977, 30, 868–877.

18. Ebihara I, Killen PD, Laurie GW, Huang T, Yamada T, Martin GR and Brown KS. Altered mRNA expression of basement membrane components in a murine model of polycystic kidney disease. Laboratory Investigation 1988, 58, 262–269.

19. Evan AP and Gardner KD Jr. Nephron obstruction in nordihydroguaiaretic acid-induced renal cystic disease. Kidney International 1979, 15, 7–19.

20. Evan AP, Gardner KD Jr and Bernstein J. Polypoid and papillary epithelial hyperplasia: a potential cause of ductal obstruction in adult polycystic disease. Kidney International 1979, 16, 743–750.

21. Folkman J and Moscona A. Role of cell shape in growth control. Nature 1978, 273, 345–349.

22. Gardner KD Jr. Composition of fluid in twelve cysts of a polycystic kidney. New England Journal of Medicine 1969, 281, 985–988.

23. Gardner KD Jr. Pathogenesis of human cystic renal disease. Annual Review of Medicine 1988, 39, 185–191.

24. Gardner KD and Evan AP. Renal cystic disease induced by diphenylthiazole. Kidney International 1983, 24, 43–52.

25. Gardner KD Jr, Evan AP and Reed WP. Accelerated renal cyst development in deconditioned germ-free rats. Kidney International 1986, 29, 1116–1123.

26. Gardner KD Jr, Reed WP, Evan AP, Zedalis J, Hylarides MD and Leon AA. Endotoxin provocation of experimental renal cystic disease. Kidney International 1987, 32, 329–334.

27. Gardner KD Jr, Solomon S, Fitzgerald WW and Evan AP. Function and structure in the diphenylamine-exposed kidney. Journal of Clinical Investigation 1976, 57, 796–806.

28. Grantham JJ, Donoso VS, Evan AP, Carone FA and Gardner KD Jr. Viscoelastic properties of tubule basement membranes in experimental renal cystic disease. Kidney International 1987, 32, 187–197.

29. Grantham JJ, Geiser JL and Evan AP. Cyst formation and growth in autosomal dominant polycystic kidney disease. Kidney International 1987, 31, 1145–1152.

30. Grantham JJ, Qualizza PB and Irwin RL. Net fluid secretion in proximal straight renal tubules *in vitro*: Role of PAH. American Journal of Physiology 1974, 266, 191–197.

31. Gregoire JR, Torrest VE, Holley KE and Farrow GM. Renal epithelial hyperplastic and neoplastic proliferation in autosomal dominant polycystic kidney disease (ARPKD). American Journal of Kidney Disease 1987, 9, 27–38.

32. Haverty TP and Neilson EG. Basement membrane gene expression in polycystic kidney disease. Laboratory Investigation 1988, 58, 245–248.
33. Heggo O. A microdissection study of cystic disease of the kidneys in adults. Journal of Pathology and Bacteriology 1966, 91, 311–315.
34. Huseman R, Grady D, Welling D and Grantham J. Macropuncture study of polycystic disease in adult human kidneys. Kidney International 1980, 18, 375–385.
35. Jensen PK and Steven K. Influence of intratubular pressure on proximal tubular compliance and capillary diameter in the rat kidney. Pflugers Archiv 1979, 382, 179–187.
36. Kanwar YS and Carone FA. Reversible changes of tubular cell and basement membrane in drug-induced renal cystic disease. Kidney International 1984, 26, 35–43.
37. Lambert PP. Polycystic disease of the kidney. A review. Archives of Pathology 1947, 44, 34–58.
38. McAteer JA, Evan AP and Gardner KD. Morphogenetic clonal growth of kidney epithelial cell line MDCK. Anatomical Record 1987, 217, 229–239.
39. Milutinovic J and Agodoa LY. Potential causes and pathogenesis in autosomal dominant polycystic kidney disease. Nephron 1983, 33, 139–144.
40. Norris RJ and Herman L. The pathogenesis of polycystic kidneys: Reconstruction of cystic elements in four cases. Journal of Urology 1941, 46, 147–176.
41. Osathanondh V and Potter EL. Pathogenesis of polycystic kidneys: Type 1 due to hyperplasia of interstitial portions of collecting tubules. Archives of Pathology 1964, 77, 466–473.
42. Osathanondh V and Potter EL. Pathogenesis of polycystic kidneys: Type 2 due to inhibition of ampullary activity. Archives of Pathology 1964, 77, 474–484.
43. Osathanondh V and Potter EL. Pathogenesis of polycystic kidneys: Type 3 due to multiple abnormalities of development. Archives of Pathology 1964, 77, 485–502.
44. Osathanondh V and Potter EL. Pathogenesis of polycystic kidneys: Type 4 due to urethral occlusion. Archives of Pathology 1964, 77, 502–509.
45. Perrone RD. *In vitro* function of cyst epithelium from human polycystic kidney. Journal of Clinical Investigation 1985, 76, 1688–1691.
46. Potter EL. Normal and abnormal development of the kidney. Chicago Year Book Medical Publishers, Inc., 1972.
47. Rall JE and Odel HM. Congenital polycystic disease of the kidney: Review of the literature, and data on 207 cases. American Journal of Medical Sciences 1949, 218, 399–407.
48. Resnick JS, Brown DM and Vernier RL. Normal development and experimental models of cystic renal disease. In: Gardner KD Jr, ed, Cystic Diseases of the Kidney. New York: John Wiley & Sons, 1976, 221–241.
49. Torres VE, Berndt TJ, Okamura M, Nesbit JW, Holley KE, Carone FA, Knox FG and Romero JC. Mechanisms affecting the development of renal cystic disease induced by diephenylthiazole. Kidney International 1988, 33, 1130–1139.
50. Uchic ME, Donoso VS, Kornhaus J, Cragoe EJ and Grantham JJ. Alteration of MDCK cyst enlargement in hydrated collagen gel by inhibitors of sodium transport. (abstract) Kidney International 1988, 33, 386.
51. Welling LW and Grantham JJ. Physical properties of isolated perfused renal tubules and tubular basement membranes. Journal of Clinical Investigation 1972, 51, 1063–1075.
52. Welling LW and Welling DJ. Physical properties of isolated perfused basement membranes from rabbit loop of Henle. American Journal of Physiology 1978, 234, F54–F58.
53. Welling LW and Welling DJ. Kinetics of cyst development in cystic renal disease. In: Cummings NB and Klahr S, eds, Chronic Renal Disease. New York: Plenum Medical Book Company, 1985, 95–103.
54. Welling LW and Welling DJ. Theoretical models of cyst formation and growth. Scanning Electron Microscopy 1988, 2, 1097–1102.
55. Wickre CG and Bennett WM. Renal cyst epithelial transport in non-uremic polycystic kidney disease. Kidney International 1983, 23, 514–518.

56. Wilson PD, Schrier RW, Breckon RD and Gabow PA. A new method for studying human polycystic kidney disease epithelia in culture. Kidney International 1986, 30, 371–378.

6
The Genetics of Renal Cystic Disease

S.T. Reeders

Abstract

We are beginning to understand the underlying molecular pathology of inherited renal cystic disease. The development of techniques for manipulating large DNA molecules, combined with rapid progress in gene mapping strategies, has offered a new approach to the molecular pathology of human disease. These methods focus attention on the genetics of cystic disease rather than on the morphology and distribution of cysts. In this chapter, inherited renal cystic diseases are classified according to genetic principles, and the molecular genetic approach to autosomal dominant polycystic kidney disease is discussed in detail.

1. Introduction

In some renal cystic diseases, such as autosomal dominant polycystic kidney disease (ADPKD), it is likely that almost all of the features of the disease can be explained by a single mutation in each case. In a subset of these diseases, it is also likely that the mutation causing the disease is the same in every case. In other disorders, different mutations in the same gene may be responsible for the disease. The phenotypes produced by the different mutations may nor may not be distinguished clinically. In addition, cases with similar or identical phenotypes may be caused by mutations in different genes. It has recently been discovered, for example, that mutations in more than one gene can lead to ADPKD. In each individual family, of course, mutations in one gene are responsible and hence the term "single gene disorder" can be applied, indicating a Mendelian mode of inheritance.

It is clear, even for a well-defined disorder such as ADPKD, that a number of different genetic determinants may need to be characterized in order to arrive at a complete predictive description of the disease. Furthermore, patients must exist, though they may be rare, in which two or more disease-producing mutations coexist. The combination of mutations may produce new syndromes or may lead to syndromes that are indistinguishable from those caused by either mutation alone. Given that such complex genetic patterns exist, it is not surprising that exceptions to the expected patterns of inheritance and phenotypes exist within each of the major disease categories. The resolution of these exceptional cases must await an understanding of hereditary renal cystic disease at the level of DNA.

Most of the hereditary disorders to be discussed below are known to be single gene disorders. There are a few congenital but sporadic renal cystic disorders that may represent either the chance coexistence of several mutations at different loci in one individual or a "contiguous gene syndrome", produced when a large deletion, translocation, or other major genetic rearrangement simultaneously disrupts the expression of more than one gene. A contiguous gene syndrome may have a phenotype in which a number of distinct diseases can be identified as, for example, in certain X-chromosome deletions that produce Duchenne muscular dystrophy, retinitis pigmentosa and glycerol kinase deficiency[27]. Other mutations of contiguous genes may produce more complex phenotypes in which a set of common features are found, but in which, because of the varying extent of the mutations, almost every individual has a unique array of clinical findings. Currently, only some of the major chromosomal rearrangements that produce contiguous gene syndromes can be resolved by cytogenetics. These include certain trisomies of chromosomes 13 and 18, in which renal cystic change is a relatively common feature. Other contiguous gene syndromes are produced by submicroscopic rearrangements. As the map of the human genome progresses to completion, it is likely that methods will become available to detect these submicroscopic mutations, and that the phenotype will be predicted precisely from a knowledge of the constituents of the disturbed region.

Even though genes are the key to an understanding of hereditary renal disease, the methods of classical genetics have hitherto contributed little to our knowledge of the underlying mechanisms of cyst formation. Classical methods have, however, provided a system of classifying cystic diseases and, even though a genetic nosology offers no better understanding of the molecular pathology of cystic disease than does a morphological system, it does offer an alternative means of defining disease entities for clinical study. Moreover, knowledge of classical genetics of hereditary cystic disease is extremely important in diagnosis and genetic counselling. Recently, the development of recombinant DNA technology has brought a major new impetus to the genetic analysis of hereditary diseases such as renal cystic disease[92]. It will eventually be possible to explain all of these syndromes, however complex, in terms of alteration in the genetic code at the level of DNA. This will provide the ultimate nosology, one based on the primary molecular pathology.

2. Single gene disorders

2.1. Polycystic disease of the kidney

2.1.1. Classification

From the geneticist's viewpoint, the most powerful potential method of classification of the polycystic kidney diseases is according to the molecular defect of the mutated gene(s). But, since no polycystic disease mutations have yet been characterized, the mode of inheritance is often used as an alternative primary classifier. This is an effective system for the polycystic kidney diseases, since the two major clinical varieties have different modes of inheritance: in general, "adult polycystic kidney disease" corresponds to ADPKD, whereas "infantile polycystic kidney disease" corresponds to autosomal recessive polycystic kidney disease (ARPKD). As with any classification system not founded on etiology or pathophysiology, this system is not foolproof. For example, we now know that mutations in at least two genes may lead to ADPKD; classification based simply on mode of inheritance makes no use of this information. It does, however, overcome the considerable problems of classification caused by childhood onset of "adult-type" disease and the survival into adulthood of patients with the "infantile" form. Furthermore, a method of classification based on genetics highlights information that is important in the genetic counselling of families. In this chapter, the polycystic diseases will be classified according to their genetics in order to emphasize the benefits of this method.

2.1.2. Autosomal dominant polycystic kidney disease:

2.1.2.1. Incidence. The frequency of ADPKD mutations in Caucasian populations has been estimated in several studies. Estimates vary widely, presumably because of differences in sampling and diagnostic criteria. Despite these limitations, a consensus has emerged, based largely on the studies of Dalgaard[18] and Iglesia *et al.* [50]. For a detailed analysis the reader is referred to a review by Torres *et al.* [90].

Dalgaard, in a study of the population of Copenhagen, found the lifetime risk of symptomatic ADPKD to be ~ 0.8 per 1,000. A more recent study of the residents of Olmsted County, Minnesota recorded a lifetime risk of 1.18 per 1,000 for symptomatic disease[50]. Both of these figures are substantially less than the autopsy frequencies observed in many other studies. In Minnesota, for example, the frequency of ADPKD rises to ~ 2.5 per 1,000 if cases detected at autopsy are taken into account.

There are several possible explanations for the greater frequency of disease observed at autopsy. First, it has been found that some patients diagnosed at autopsy have been symptomatic and have, in retrospect, a family history suggestive of autosomal dominant polycystic kidney disease[42]. Presumably, these cases represent instances of failure to diagnose the disease during life. Second, multiple bilateral "simple" cysts may account for a few cases diagnosed at autopsy. Hatfield and Pfister[42] excluded such cases by insisting on the presence of both renal and hepatic cysts for the diagnosis of ADPKD. Nevertheless, they still found a large number of cases at autopsy. It appears, therefore, that a substantial fraction of the autopsy cases represent asymptomatic ADPKD. Only one in 32 asymptomatic autopsy cases had a family history of ADPKD[42]. It is unclear whether the lack of family history was due to mild and, therefore, undetected disease in other family members or due to truly sporadic disease. For this reason further study of the natural history is required to determine what fraction of the cases detected at autopsy represents ADPKD as opposed to some other form of polycystic disease. In the interim, the available evidence points to the fact that there is a substantial number of undetected cases with "mild ADPKD" and a good prognosis. This has become increasingly apparent with the availability of sensitive non-invasive cyst imaging methods such as ultrasonography[16]. If the excess of cases seen at autopsy can largely be explained by asymptomatic ADPKD, then as many as half the cases with the morphological features of ADPKD may have a normal lifespan.

Although almost all reports of ADPKD refer to Caucasian populations, the disease has been seen in patients with origins in Africa, the Indian subcontinent, Southeast Asia, Japan and China. The relative frequencies of ADPKD in these populations are not known with any precision. It appears, however, that the frequency of ADPKD in North American[78] and South African blacks[32] is significantly less than in Caucasians.

2.1.2.2. Spontaneous mutation rate. Dalgaard[18] estimated the spontaneous mutation rate in ADPKD to be $6.5 - 12 \times 10^{-5}$ mutations per gene per generation. However, this estimate was based on population genetic theory and incorporates many assumptions. Estimates based on literature surveys are almost certainly inflated by failure to detect the disease retrospectively in the parents of patients, and by the failure to allow for the occasional instance where the nominal father is not the true father. Dalgaard found one unequivocal mutation in his survey. In a study of patients seen at the renal unit in Oxford, England, I was able to find only one *de novo* case of proven paternity in a general population of ~250,000 (unpublished data). This is probably a minimum estimate, as there were several patients who could not be counted as having new mutations since asymptomatic ADPKD in their deceased parents could not be ruled out.

2.1.2.3. Molecular genetics of autosomal dominant adult polycystic kidney disease. In most families of Northern European origin, the mutation that gives rise to ADPKD disrupts a gene on the distal third of the short arm of chromosome 16, in close genetic linkage with the genes for the alpha chain of human hemoglobin[70,73]. This localization was established when genetic linkage was found between ADPKD and a highly polymorphic region at the 3' end of the alpha-globin cluster (3'HVR) in nine families of English and Dutch origin. Alpha-globin had previously been localized to the distal half of the short arm of chromosome 16 (16p), thereby localizing the gene for ADPKD in these families to the same region. This localization was confirmed by the demonstration of genetic linkage between ADPKD and the polymorphic protein, phosphoglycolate phosphatase (PGP), which had also previously been localized to 16p[71].

Reeders et al. [73] carried out a study of 28 families of English, Dutch, Scottish and Finnish origin to determine whether linkage to alpha-globin is a common finding in ADPKD families or whether mutations in a second gene, unlinked to alpha-globin, can lead to a similar disease. The authors concluded that, in populations of Northern European origin at least, mutations of the same single gene are probably responsible for all ADPKD cases. Several other investigators have also demonstrated linkage between ADPKD and 3'HVR in patients of Welsh, English, French, Italian and German origin[2,10,20,60]. These studies confirmed that ADPKD mutations predominantly affect a single chromosome 16 gene or cluster of genes. At the *Eighth Human Gene Mapping Workshop* (Helsinki, 1985), the locus name "PKD1" was assigned to the ADPKD gene that had been shown to lie on the short arm of chromosome 16.

Just as it was becoming apparent that ADPKD was a disorder of a single gene, PKD1, Kimberling et al. [56] reported that they were unable to confirm genetic linkage between alpha-globin and ADPKD in a large family of Italian extraction residing in Colorado, USA. This family is so large that the authors were able to exclude linkage to alpha-globin with a very high degree of certainty. Romeo et al. [77] also described an Italian family from Bologna in which genetic linkage markers on both sides of the PKD1 gene were used[75]. Such "flanking markers" enhance the power of linkage analysis by defining a small genetic interval in which the disease gene lies. Therefore, despite the fact that the Bolognese family is much smaller than the Colorado family and, therefore, less powerful for linkage analysis, Romeo et al. [77] were able to show that the mutation did not map to the interval containing the PKD1 locus, thereby confirming the finding of Kimberling et al. [56] that mutations in at least two separate genes can lead to ADPKD. In neither of the two studies were the authors able to distinguish the clinical disease pattern seen in the "unlinked families" from the pattern seen in other families in which the disease is clearly linked to alpha-globin. It appears, therefore, that ADPKD is a true example of genetic heterogeneity in that mutations of at least two distinct genes can lead to indistinguishable ADPKD phenotypes. Despite the fact that mutations in two genes can cause it, ADPKD is a 'single gene disorder'. This term refers to the fact that, in any given family, mutations of a single gene segregate with the disease phenotype.

It is unlikely that the unlinked form is confined to families from the southern Mediterranean region, since preliminary study of Danish families strongly suggests genetic heterogeneity within the Danish population (Søren Nørby, Copenhagen, personal communication). The true fraction of families that are unlinked has not been measured with any accuracy since sampling of families has not been random. Nevertheless, a crude estimate, based on the published literature, suggests that approximately 2% of mutations are unlinked. The genetic localization of the unlinked mutations has not been determined.

The following discussion of the molecular genetics of ADPKD pertains to the linked form, that is the form in which mutations affect PKD1, the locus closely linked to alpha-globin. The term ADPKD refers to the consensus phenotype, that is, a form of polycystic kidney disease that is autosomal dominant and can be caused by mutations in either PKD1 or other genes.

2.1.2.4. The molecular genetics of the PKD1 locus. Initial studies placed PKD1 at a recombination fraction of ~ 5% from alpha-globin[70]. The mapping of PKD1 gene in this region acted as a spur to further refinement of the subchromosomal localization of the alpha-globin cluster itself since the cluster was to be the anchor point of attempts to place PKD1 on an extended linkage map.

A number of naturally-occurring chromosomal translocation breakpoints were used to divide 16p into segments based on its chromosomal banding pattern. Breuning *et al.* [11] studied cells from a fetus that had been aborted because of an unbalanced translocation between chromosomes 16 and 4 (46(XY), –16, + {16qter – 16p 13.3::4q31.1 – 4qter}). The fetal cells contained a normal chromosome 16 and an aberrant chromosome 16 in which the most distal (telomeric) band on the short arm (16p13.3) was replaced by most of chromosome 4. When DNA from fetal tissue was blotted by Southern's method and hybridized with 3'HVR probe representing the alpha-globin cluster, it was clear that only one allele of the 3'HVR had been inherited by the fetus. Breuning *et al.* were, therefore, able to conclude that the portion of chromosome 16p beyond the breakpoint contains the alpha-globin cluster and that alpha-globin resides within the 16p13.3 band. Simmers *et al.* [83] used *in situ* hybridization to show that the alpha-globin genes lie within the distal third of the 16p13 region, probably within 16p13.2 or 16p13.3.

The more precise localization of the alpha-globin genes suggested that PKD1 is distally placed on the chromosome. On average, 5% recombination corresponds to approximately 5×10^6 base-pairs of DNA, which represents about 5% of the total DNA of chromosome 16. This places PKD1 within one cytogenetic band of alpha-globin, that is within 16p13.2 or 16p13.3. There is, however, marked variation in the relationship between recombination rate and physical length of DNA from one region of the human genome to another. Moreover, the linkage of PKD1 to a single precisely mapped marker, alpha-globin, does not by itself indicate the orientation of PKD1 with respect to that marker either in the chromosome (telomeric or centromeric) or in relation to DNA sense (3' or 5'). For these reasons, linkage to a single marker still allowed a region of up to 20×10^6 bp in which the PKD1 gene might lie.

Further refinement of the localization of PKD1 necessitated the identification of genetic markers on both sides of the gene. Such "flanking markers" have the advantage that they define not only the genetic map interval in which the PKD1 gene lies, but also the physical limits of the map location of the disease gene. At the commencement of studies to identify flanking markers, the map of chromosome 16 was very sketchy with only two genes, alpha-globin and PGP, having been assigned to the short arm. Therefore, a genetic map of the chromosome had to be constructed before further study of the PKD1 locus could be initiated: a number of new polymorphic DNA probes had to be isolated and their relative positions on the chromosome had to be determined. As a result of this effort, more than 30 polymorphic DNA segments were added to the map of the distal third of 16p between 1985 and 1987. Several of these probes were shown to reside on the proximal (centrometric) side of the PKD1 locus, whereas alpha-globin was mapped distal (telomeric) to PKD1[74]. A composite map of the region is based on Breuning et al. [10], Reeders et al. [74,75], Keith et al. [55], and Harris et al. [40] (Figure 6.1). This map also contains some unpublished data, kindly made available by these authors and their colleagues. For further details of the probes themselves, their origins and the polymorphic systems which they recognize, the reader is referred to the above papers and to The Human Gene Mapping Library, Howard Hughes Medical Institute, 25 Science Park, New Haven, Connecticut 06514, USA, where data on all published and many unpublished loci are stored.

2.1.2.5. Phenotypic heterogeneity of ADPKD: molecular genetic analysis. Several authors have documented the marked variation that exists in the clinical pattern and prognosis of ADPKD between one individual and another within the same family and between individuals in different families. These differences could be due to the effects of different mutations in the same gene, the effects of mutations in different genes, or the effects of other environmental or genetic influences on the expression of the mutated genes. The question of heterogeneity is most easily resolved by the study of the pattern of expression within families rather than by the study of populations of unrelated individuals. If variation is due to the effects of different ADPKD mutations at the same locus, then intrafamilial variation should not be marked; if due to mutation at different loci, then the prognosis in each member of a given family should be similar, but the genetic linkage relationships of the disease will vary from family to family; if phenotypic variation is due to other environmental or genetic influences, then prognosis should vary markedly within each family. Unfortunately, in the interval since Dalgaard[18] first addressed this issue, few investigators have paid attention to the clinical study of family units. Dalgaard found that the age at diagnosis of members of a particular sibship tends to be similar. However, members of a sibship do share other genetic and environmental influences, as the author points out. Study of more distantly related patients within extended families overcomes this problem.

In a study of 241 members of 15 families identified from 19 index cases attending the Oxford Renal Unit, I observed a marked intrafamilial similarity in the age of presentation of first symptoms and at age of development of endstage renal disease (ESRD). Concordance between members of the same

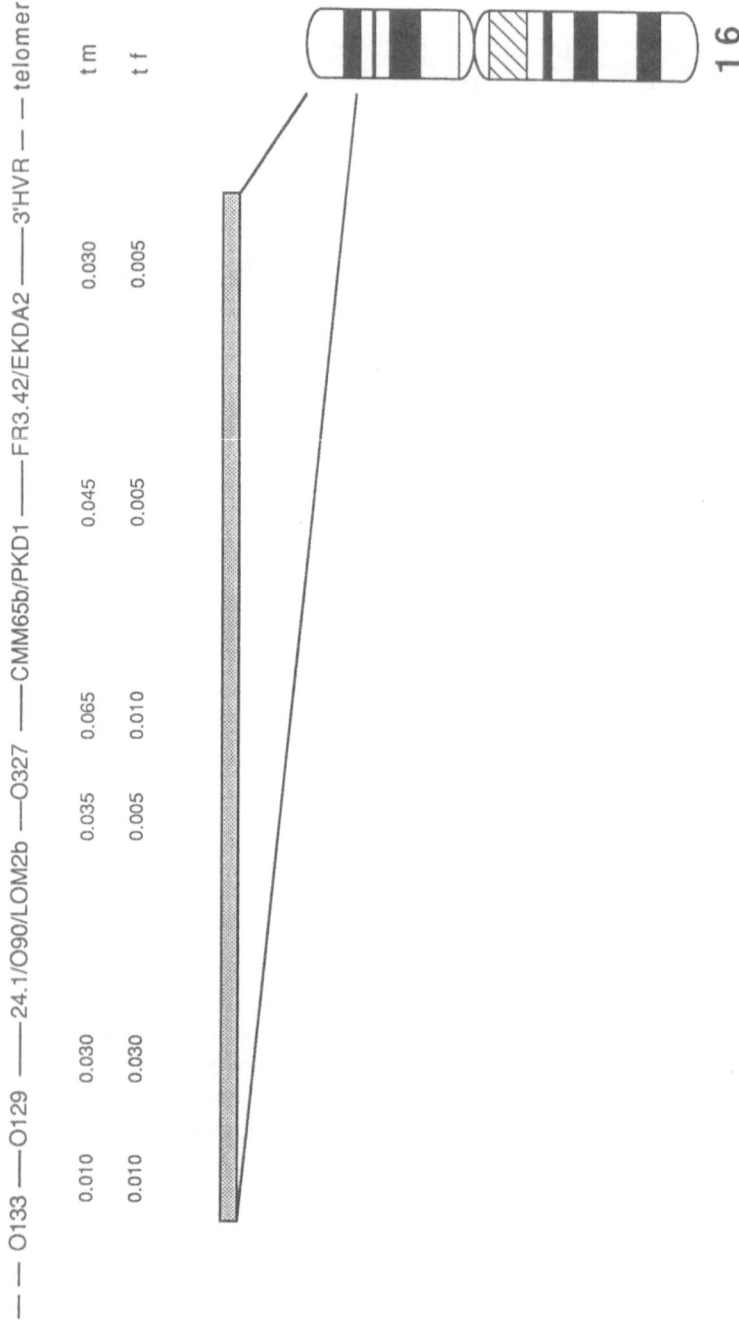

Figure 6.1. Map of the region of the ADPKD gene (PKD1). The position of the PKD1 gene is shown with respect to an array of arbitrarily-named polymorphic DNA segments. The centromere is on the left. Recombination frequencies between the loci are given for male (tm) and female (tf) meioses. The order of those loci separated by oblique lines cannot be determined genetically since recombination has not, as yet, been observed between them. The six proximal (centromeric) genetic markers closest to PKD1 are shown. Ten other proximal markers of use in linkage analysis have been described (see text). Probes CMM65b and EKDA2 were isolated by Y. Nakamura (Howard Hughes Medical Institute, Salt Lake City); FR3.42 was isolated by Guang-hui Xiao and Gerd Scherer (Albert-Ludwigs-Universität, Freiburg). Details of these probes are on file with the *Human Gene Mapping Library*.

family (excluding siblings) was significantly different from concordance between members of different families (unpublished data). These observations suggest that the characteristics of different mutations at a single locus (shown to be PKD1 in five of the families tested) determine the prognosis of the disease, and that the genetic and environmental background play a minor role. Onset of ADPKD in childhood appears to be the exception to this rule, as discussed below.

Study of the molecular genetics of the PKD1 locus has also been used to address the question of heterogeneity. For example, the possibility that mutations in different genes were responsible for the differences in clinical expression seen in 28 Northern European families was excluded by Reeders et al. [73]. Ryynanen et al. [79] studied a Finnish family in which the morphological changes characteristic of ADPKD were not associated with functional renal impairment. The disease in this family (FINPK1) was found to have the same linkage relationships as in other families in which renal failure was a frequent occurrence, suggesting that different mutations in the same gene (PKD1) were responsible for the differences in clinical features.

2.1.2.6. Childhood onset of ADPKD. A flurry of reports over the last 20 years has clearly documented the occurrence of symptomatic ADPKD in childhood. With the advent of non-invasive imaging techniques such as ultrasonography, asymptomatic children from ADPKD families are also being investigated with increasing frequency. The detection of the disease in asymptomatic at-risk children has led to confusion concerning the epidemiology of childhood onset ADPKD. This has been compounded by the failure of many authors to note the age of first symptoms in relatives of probands with early-onset ADPKD. Such data is extremely important for genetic counselling since it is needed to establish whether clustering of early-onset cases occurs. Moreover, a true understanding of the epidemiology of childhood onset ADPKD may help to unravel its molecular mechanism. In this section, *childhood onset ADPKD* will be used to denote a clinically significant renal disease with impaired renal function occurring within a family in which classical autosomal dominant polycystic kidney disease is segregating.

Sedman et al. [80] studied 154 children under 18 years of age from 83 ADPKD families. Twenty-three children had clearcut ultrasound changes of ADPKD, but few of these had symptoms which could confidently be ascribed to the disease. Three children developed endstage renal disease, giving a frequency of ~ 2% for childhood onset of ADPKD. Unfortunately, the method of ascertainment of families in this study is not well documented and there may be ascertainment bias. In addition, the full family history of these cases is not presented.

Kääriäinen and her colleagues[52,53,54,69] used a variety of ascertainment methods to obtain a frequency of 1 in 43,000 for childhood onset of ADPKD in the Finnish population. About half of these were symptomatic. Because

Kääriäinen studied the families of her cases, she was able to address the question of familial clustering of childhood onset cases. In these families, as in those published previously and listed by Kääriäinen, there is a clear tendency for early manifestation to recur in a sibship. The frequency of such events is difficult to measure because there is a tendency for the asymptomatic sibs of affected children to be investigated and for the asymptomatic cysts to be discovered many years before they might otherwise become apparent. There are thus, at present, insufficient data to determine the likely mechanism for familial clustering of early onset cases.

Zerres has concentrated on the study of families in which at least one child has had symptomatic ADPKD, usually with functional renal impairment (personal communication). Many of Zerres' families are too small to allow linkage to chromosome 16 markers to be demonstrated independently[95]. However, taken as a whole, the data are consistent with the hypothesis that mutations of PKD1, rather than of a second gene, are responsible for the disease in these families. Since, in each family, a number of individuals with classical features of the disease coexist with one or more early onset cases, it is unlikely that specific mutations of the PKD1 gene cause the disease to manifest early.

Taitz et al. [88] have forwarded the hypothesis that an interaction between an ADPKD mutation and a coincidental heterozygous mutation for ARPKD is responsible for the more severe early-onset cases. The cumulative published data are, as yet, insufficient to allow the use of segregation analysis to test this hypothesis. As Kääriäinen[52] points out, the existence within one sibship of four early-onset ADPKD cases with the same affected mother and two fathers makes it unlikely that a genetic contribution from the unaffected parent is responsible for early onset. A contribution from the unaffected (non-ADPKD) parent is implicit in the model put forward by Taitz et al. [88].

2.1.2.7. Diagnostic applications of DNA probes in PKD1. The discovery of genetic linkage markers has provided a diagnostic test of considerable utility in the management of ADPKD[10,72,75]. The basis of the test is that, in any given family in which a mutant PKD1 gene is responsible for the disease, specific variants of the marker loci will be inherited along with the disease mutation.

The NDM-H family illustrates the use of the test (Fig. 6.2). In NDM-H, AG, RG, TG, PG and LR have symptomatic cystic renal disease with multiple bilateral cysts detected by ultrasound. The 3'HVR probe[70], which detects more than 20 different 3'HVR variants (alleles), was used as a diagnostic genetic marker. Six alleles, given the arbitrary identifying names *A–F*, were detected in this family. The family shown is part of a much larger kindred in which linkage between ADPKD and 3'HVR was unequivocally established. RG inherited the disease from his father along with 3'HVR allele *A*; TG, PG and LR have inherited the disease along with allele *A*. LG, who is asymptomatic at the age of 31 and has had two negative ultrasound examinations, has inherited the 3'HVR allele *B* along with the normal PKD1 gene from his father. The linkage

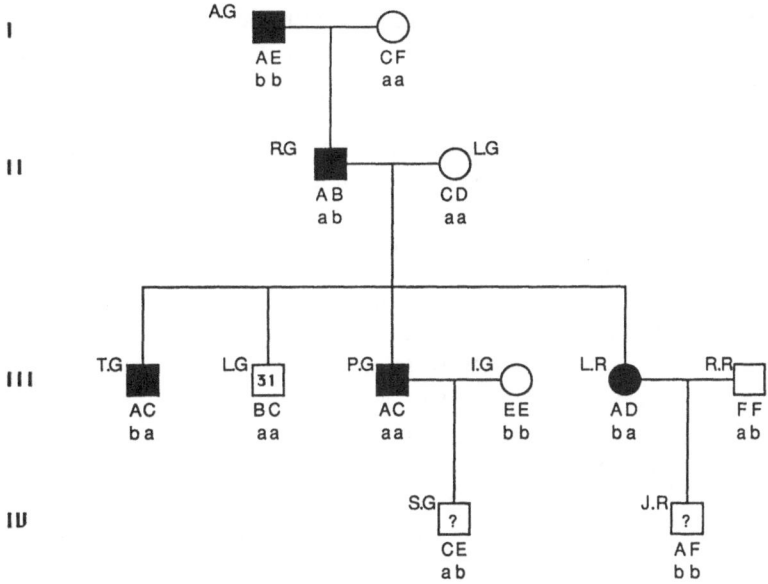

Figure 6.2. Pedigree of family NDM-H. Filled symbols indicate ADPKD patients. Numbers within empty symbols refer to the age of last 'normal' renal ultrasound examination. Empty symbols without numbers represent subject in whom cyst imaging (ultrasound, computed tomography, excretory urography) has not been performed. Upper case letters (*A–F*) refer to 3'HVR alleles. Lower case letters (*a,b*) refer to O90 alleles.

between 3'HVR allele *A* and the disease can be used to predict the disease status of SG and JR in the following way. PG has passed on the allele *C* to his son and, therefore, the likelihood is that SG has not inherited the PKD1 mutation. However, there remains the possibility of genetic recombination between PKD1 and 3'HVR, which occurs with a frequency of ~ 7% in male meioses (that is when the affected parent is the father)[75]. It is impossible to detect whether recombination has occurred between disease locus and marker during this particular meiosis, and, therefore, there is a 7% chance of an incorrect prediction of the disease status of SG. In the case of LR's son, JR, it is predicted that the PKD1 mutation has been inherited from his mother, since he has inherited allele *A* at the 3'HVR locus. Again genetic recombination leads to the possibility of misdiagnosis. The recombination rate between PKD1 and 3'HVR is, however, only 2% in female meiosis so that the error rate is less, as in this case, when the affected parent is the mother. The sex-specific difference in recombination rates, which is observed on both sides of the PKD1 locus, has not been explained[75].

There are certain limitations to the power of tests based on genetic linkage analysis of DNA sequence polymorphisms. The most important of these relates to the "informativeness" of the polymorphism. If an allele of a marker locus is to be traced from a parent to a child along with the disease mutation then the parent must be heterozygous (informative) for the marker locus. Conversely, if the parent is homozygous for a particular allele then the allele inherited by normal children will be indistinguishable from that inherited by affected children and no diagnosis will be possible. The polymorphism information content (PIC) of a marker is the fraction of a large number of random matings for which the marker is informative. The PIC of 3′HVR is ~ 96%, whereas the PIC of a second marker, O90, is only ~ 50%. Sets of closely linked markers such as those in Fig. 6.1 may be combined to increase the overall PIC and thereby increase the power of diagnosis.

A second limitation of DNA-based diagnosis relates to the determination of "phase of linkage". In the NDM-H family, (Fig. 6.2) the PKD1 mutation is in phase with 3′HVR allele A in RG, i.e. allele A is on the same chromosome as the PKD1 mutation. We know this because allele A was coinherited with the disease from AG. If we had studied RG in isolation, however, the phase of linkage would not be known – we would not know whether allele A had been inherited from the normal mother or the affected father. If we studied TG as well as his father, we might deduce that the phase of linkage is with allele A in RG. There would be a significant chance of error, however, if recombination had occurred between the marker and disease genes, displacing the disease mutation from the chromosome containing allele B (in RG) to the chromosome containing 3′HVR allele A in TG. Clearly, the greater the number of family members available for study, the greater the probability of correctly deducing the phase of linkage. Incorrect determination of phase leads to an incorrect diagnosis and is a second cause of error in this method.

In practice, genetic counselling requires the consideration of all types of predictive information. In the case of presymptomatic diagnosis, for example, diagnostic imaging and other clinical information should be combined with genetic linkage test data to provide a more precise risk estimate. One of the practical problems of using cyst imaging and clinical evaluation in the diagnosis of ADPKD is that they depend heavily on the age of the patient for their interpretation[3]. The lack of a "gold standard" for diagnosis of ADPKD has limited the value of single time-point studies of the "accuracy" of cyst imaging methods. Long-term longitudinal studies would be required for accurate interpretation of these data. Fortunately, the discovery of flanking markers for the PKD1 locus offers a virtual "gold standard" for the diagnosis in most ADPKD patients who have mutations in the PKD1 gene. Preliminary data[75], based on flanking markers, suggests a false positive error rate of ~ 2% and a false negative error rate of ~ 2% for ultrasound imaging. These estimates are for the age-group 15–65 years. Further studies are required to determine the age-dependency of sensitivity and specificity of ultrasound using genetic analysis as a "gold standard".

2.1.2.8. Flanking markers in DNA-based diagnosis of ADPKD. The availability of two closely linked flanking markers (Fig. 6.1) reduces the diagnostic error rate in ADPKD by at least an order of magnitude compared with the use of a single marker. Fig. 6.3 illustrates the use of one pair of flanking markers, O90 and 3'HVR. Each marker has a recombination rate (female) of ~ 2% with PKD1. There are four possible outcomes of meiosis. The most likely is that neither marker will recombine (cross over) with the disease. In this case the diagnosis based on either marker will be correct. There is a 2% chance that O90 alone will crossover with the disease locus. In this case O90 will give the wrong diagnosis, but 3'HVR will give a correct prediction. It will be apparent that a crossover has occurred between the two marker loci, but it will not be apparent which marker has crossed over. Therefore diagnosis will not be possible but diagnostic error will be avoided.

There is also a 2% chance that 3'HVR will crossover and, again, diagnosis will not be possible. There is a small, but finite, chance that both markers will recombine with the disease gene. In this case it will not be apparent from the marker studies that recombination has occurred since there is no net recombination between the marker loci, the two crossovers having cancelled each other out. An incorrect diagnosis will be made. Such double crossover events occur with a frequency which is approximately equal to the product of the frequencies of the independent crossover events (2% × 2% = 0.04%).

Double crossovers are probably even rarer because of interference, the reduction of the frequency of crossing over in a particular interval caused by the occurrence of a second crossover close by. Thus, the use of flanking marker

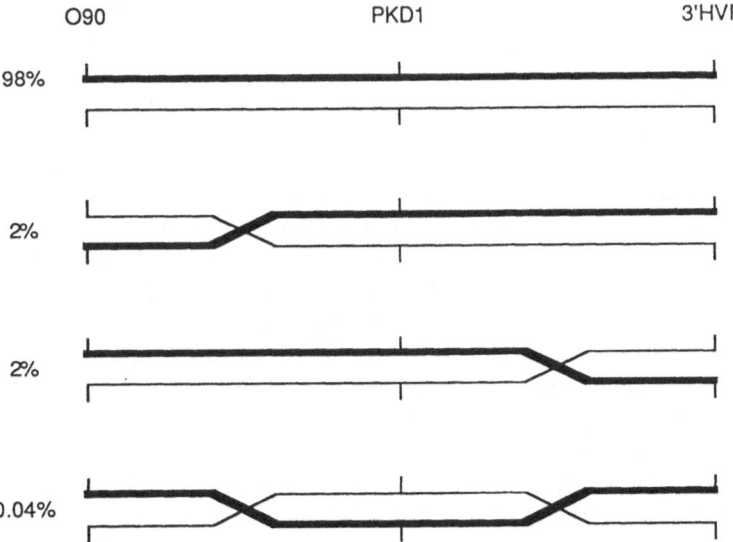

Figure 6.3. One pair of flanking markers, O90 and 3'HVR are placed in the order determined by Reeders *et al.* [75]. The approximate recombination frequencies between O90 and PKD1 and between PKD1 and 3'HVR are 2% during female meiosis. The four possible outcomes of meiosis are shown with their relative frequencies on the left.

loci offers a means of DNA-based diagnosis with an error rate of a fraction of 1%. The power of the test is, however, limited by the same factors that have been discussed for the use of single genetic markers above. Moreover, the limitations are frequently greater, since both markers must be informative and the phase of linkage must be determined for both. The 3'HVR and O90 markers, for example, are both informative in only 48% of meioses. These limitations can, however, be overcome by the combined use of several markers. The use of all the markers shown in Fig. 6.1 gives the method an informativeness greater than 95% and an accuracy greater than 99.9%. Nevertheless, in about 10% of informative cases, a confident prediction will not be possible, because, as was discussed above, markers on one side of the PKD1 gene recombine with the disease locus. In summary, a confident diagnosis is possible in ~ 90% of cases where the family is large enough for phase to be determined; the accuracy of the diagnoses in these cases will be > 99.9%.

The NDM-H family (Fig. 6.2) illustrates some of the principles of diagnosis based on the use of flanking markers. RG has inherited the disease, 3'HVR allele A, and O90 allele b from his father. These three alleles (two marker alleles and a disease allele) must, therefore, lie on the same chromosome in RG. In each of his children it is possible to determine which of the two paternal O90 alleles were inherited, since the mother (LG) is homozygous for allele a and must, therefore, have passed this allele on to all her children. Thus it can be said that the children are informative for paternal inheritance of O90. Since 3'HVR-A and O90-b are in phase in RG, we would expect these two alleles to be co-inherited in all his offspring. This is true for all except PG, who has inherited 3'HVR-A with O90-a, indicating that there must have been a crossover (recombination) between these two loci. There is unequivocal evidence that PG has inherited the disease, which is linked in him (as in the others) to 3'HVR-A. The crossover must, therefore, have occurred between O90 and both 3'HVR and PKD1. If, however, we had not had access to clinical diagnostic information, we would not be able to predict the disease status of PG from genetic marker data, since we would not know whether the crossover occurred between 3'HVR and PKD1 or between O90 and PKD1. Whatever the case, PG has inherited the disease, 3'HVR-A and O90-a from his father and these must, therefore, all lie on the same chromosome. However, we cannot use this information for diagnosis of SG, because PG is homozygous for O90 (i.e SG will inherit O90-a whichever paternal chromosome he inherits). O90 is said to be non-informative in this case and contributes nothing to the diagnosis.

LR has inherited 3'HVR-A, and O90-b and the disease together from her grandfather. She has transmitted 3'HVR-A and O90-b to her son, JR. There is, therefore, a > 99.9% probability that JR has inherited the disease mutation. The probability that he is normal is equal to the probability of two crossovers, one between O90 and ADPKD, and one between 3'HVR and ADPKD, a very rare occurrence.

2.1.2.9. Prenatal diagnosis of ADPKD. The discovery of genetic markers for PKD1 mutations has led to the first method for diagnosis of ADPKD during fetal life. Diagnosis can be made from any source of fetal tissue, including cultured amniocytes and chorionic villus biopsy samples. An example of this method was reported by Reeders *et al.* [72] using the 3'HVR probe. The diagnosis was confirmed by the observation of renal cystic change in the fetal kidneys at 11 weeks of gestation.

2.1.2.10. The place of genetic linkage analysis in the management of ADPKD. The role of accurate presymptomatic or prenatal diagnosis in the management of a genetic disease that has its onset in adult life is a complex issue; in the case of ADPKD, considerable further study will be required to assess the value of genetic linkage methods. The National Kidney Foundation of the United States is preparing a set of guidelines for the use of these tests until such time as systematic evaluation of their contribution to management is reported.

2.1.2.11. Pathophysiology of ADPKD. Neither classical biochemistry nor reverse genetics has, as yet, identified the underlying biochemical defect in ADPKD. However, recent advances in understanding of some other genetic diseases[38] suggest a mechanism that may explain some of the features of the pathology of ADPKD. One of the striking features of the disease is that, despite the fact that all renal cells contain the ADPKD mutation, the cystic change is focal, affecting only a part of each of a limited number of nephrons. Moreover, the cysts may occur at any point in the nephron. These features suggest that, in addition to the presence of the heritable mutation, a second sporadic event must occur at the points where cysts arise. One possibility is that somatic mutations, occurring at the same locus as the inherited germline mutation, lead to homozygosity for a defect that leads to clonal hyperplasia of tubular epithelium. The occurrence of hyperplasia in both human and experimental polycystic kidney disease has been demonstrated by Evan *et al.* [24] The proof of the hypothesis must await the molecular analysis of both germline and somatic mutations in ADPKD.

2.1.3. Autosomal recessive polycystic kidney disease

The term ARPKD designates several overlapping clinical syndromes, principally of childhood, having a common mode of inheritance, similar renal pathology and distinctive hepatic lesions. Other recessive cystic diseases of childhood, which enter into the differential diagnosis ARPKD, are described below. Kissane[58] and Bernstein[4] have distinguished these other diseases pathologically and Blyth and Ockenden[9] have set out a number of clinical and pathological criteria whereby the category of "polycystic disease of kidneys and liver presenting in childhood" – which is a clinical classification broadly corresponding to ARPKD – can be distinguished from other cystic diseases of childhood.

Blyth and Ockenden[9], in one of the largest studies of this disorder, concluded that it exists in at least four forms: perinatal, neonatal, infantile and juvenile. These forms differ according to the degree of renal involvement, age of onset, prognosis and extent of hepatic involvement, as summarized in Table 6.1. One of the striking claims of Blyth and Ockenden was that the same form of disease is seen in members of the same sibship. The authors stated that this observation provides evidence for four separate genetic forms of the disease and went on to suggest that "the most likely inheritance mechanism is that a separate autosomal recessive gene is responsible in each group". Even if we accept their observation, the conclusions are incorrect. The correct conclusion from their observations is that, in each family, the phenotype depends on mutation at a single locus rather than on the interaction of other genetic or environmental influences with the major disease-producing locus. This is important for genetic counselling since it implies that affected children within each sibship are likely to have similar prognoses.

Not everyone agrees with Blyth and Ockenden's[9] classification of ARPKD or with the observation that the disease runs true in families. In Kääriäinen's[52,53,54,69] study, for example, cases could not easily be classified according to the outline set out in Table 6.1. She found that when death occurs in the neonatal period there was concordance between affected sibs for prognosis in 11 of 14 families. In three other sibships, however, the ages at death were 0 and 4, 0.3 and 8, 0.8 and 23. Zerres et al. [95] listed a number of other studies in which cases from within the same sibship belonged to different categories as defined by Blyth and Ockenden[9]. Zerres et al. concluded that "multiple allelism with only a few different alleles would account for the great variety of manifestations in different families, particularly with regard to a possible compound heterozygosity, and would explain the relatively high intra-familial constancy in manifestation as well". A true explanation of the phenotypic variability in ARPKD must await the molecular genetic analysis of this condition at the level of DNA.

2.1.3.1. Molecular genetics of ARPKD. Three independent studies have demonstrated that mutations leading to ARPKD are not allelic with ADPKD mutations[2,68,93]. The genetic localization of ARPKD mutations has not been established.

2.1.4. Autosomal dominant single gene disorders:

2.1.4.1. von-Hippel Lindau syndrome (VHL). VHL is a multisystem disorder inherited as an autosomal dominant characteristic. Renal cysts and tumors are a common feature occurring in about 28% and 25% of affected individuals,

Table 6.1. Division of ARPKD into four clinicopathological groups.

Group	Age of presentation	Mode of presentation	Typical progress	Typical survival	Pathology		
					Kidneys	Liver	
					Proportion of dilated renal tubules	Proportion of dilated and infolded bile ducts	Extent of periportal fibrosis
Perinatal	at birth	Bilateral huge renal masses	Early decease or rapid progression of uraemia and death	1 d	>90%	All affected	Minimal
Neonatal	1 d–1 m	Bilateral large kidneys	Progressive renal failure	1 y	~60%	All affected	Mild
Infantile	3–6 m	Bilateral large kidneys; hepatosplenomegaly	Chronic renal failure; systemic and portal hypertension	3–10 y	~25%	All affected	Moderate
Juvenile	1–5 y	Hepatomegaly	Portal hypertension, often necessitating portocaval shunt	>10 y	<10%	All affected	Gross

Based on Blyth and Ockenden[9] with modifications and simplifications.

respectively[35,48]. Bernstein et al. [7] considered both the neoplastic and cystic elements to be manifestations of the same epithelial hyperplasia. The renal lesions of VHL rarely, if ever, lead to endstage renal failure.

VHL mutations have been localized to the short arm of chromosome 3 by genetic linkage to the human homologue of the RAF1 oncogene, which maps to chromosome 3p25[81]. The underlying biochemical defect in VHL is not known. Renal cell carcinomas have been found to be associated with the loss of regions of chromosome 3p, and the common finding of renal cell carcinomas in VHL was the spur to the localization of the VHL mutations to chromosome 3. In addition, a renal cell carcinoma from a VHL patient has been shown to contain a chromosome 3p deletion[57].

2.1.4.2. Tuberous sclerosis (TS). TS is an autosomal dominant multisystem disorder with a prevalence estimated at between 1 in 15,000 and 1 in 1,000,000, depending on the population studied and the criteria of diagnosis. Gomez[34] has devised a list of primary and secondary diagnostic criteria. The former, of which one is required for diagnosis, include cortical tubers, subependymal glial nodules, and retinal hamartomas, facial angiofibromas, ungual fibromas, forehead/scalp fibrous plaques and multiple renal angiomyolipomas. The second set of criteria, of which two are required for diagnosis, include infantile spasms, myoclonic, tonic, or atonic seizures, hypomelanotic macules, shagreen patches, peripapillary retinal hamartoma indistinguishable from drusen, gingival fibromas, dental enamel pits, multiple renal tumours, renal cysts, cardiac rhabdomyoma, pulmonary lymphangiomyomatosis, radiographic "honeycomb" lungs, wedge-shaped cortical–subcortical calcification, multiple subcortical hypomyelinated lesions and an immediate relative with TS. Renal angiomyolipomas are the commonest renal abnormalities[15,86]. These are benign, slow-growing tumours which are frequently bilateral. Renal cysts, adenomas and carcinomas occur less frequently. Bernstein et al. [7] consider the cysts and tumours of TS to be manifestations of the same epithelial hyperplastic process.

In a population of 274 TS patients, Stillwell et al. [86] found renal cysts in 10% of the 51 patients who had had renal evaluation. Polycystic kidneys may be the presenting feature of TS and overshadow the cutaneous and neurological signs[22,59]. Nimr et al. [65] suggest that when cystic disease is prominent, renal failure is more likely to accompany the renal manifestations of TS. The renal lesions of TS are reviewed by Bernstein et al. [6].

Bundey and Evans[12] estimated the new mutation rate to be 86%. The variable phenotypic expression of the disease probably leads to an overestimation of mutation rate since mild disease in the parents may be overlooked.

A gene for TS has recently been assigned to chromosome 9 by linkage to the ABO blood group[28]. Nineteen British families were studied with a number of genetic markers. In addition to linkage between TS and ABO, weak evidence was found for linkage between the disease and adenylate kinase (AK1) which had previously been linked to ABO. The same families have also been studied using a restriction fragment length polymorphism detected by a DNA probe from the v-abl oncogene[17]. Close linkage was observed between the locus for the human homologue of this oncogene and TS, confirming the assignment of TS to the long arm of chromosome 9.

2.1.4.3. Medullary cystic disease. Medullary cystic disease is an autosomal dominant disorder that is morphologically similar to autosomal recessive juvenile nephronophthisis. Both of these disorders are considered together below.

2.1.5. Autosomal recessive single gene disorders:

2.1.5.1. Asphyxiating thoracic dystrophy (Jeune syndrome). Jeune syndrome is a rare autosomal recessive disorder manifested by a generalized osteochondrodysplasia predominantly affecting the thoracic cage. Short ribs cause reduced thoracic capacity with a restrictive respiratory defect that frequently leads to death within the first few years of life. The long bones and pelvis are also affected, and the extremities are shorter than normal. The spectrum of disease, radiology and differential diagnosis have been discussed by Herdman and Langer[44].

Several abnormalities have been found in association with the skeletal abnormalities. Clinical findings include isolated proteinuria, hypertension, renal failure, proximal tubular defects, concentrating defects and ureterovesical obstruction[23,44,82]. Histopathologic studies have shown a chronic tubulointerstitial nephritis with secondary glomerular sclerosis and occasional cystic transformation[5,37,44,82]. Donaldson et al.[21] consider the renal lesion of Jeune syndrome in older subjects to be indistinguishable from that of familial juvenile nephronophthisis. Molecular analysis at the DNA level will ultimately be required to determine the relationship between these syndromes.

2.1.5.2. Cerebro–hepato–renal syndrome (Zellweger syndrome). Zellweger syndrome is an autosomal recessive disorder with cerebral, hepatic, ocular, facial and skeletal abnormalities, in addition to renal and lower urinary tract dysmorphology. Renal involvement is common, affecting at least 80% of cases. The principal renal abnormality is multiple, mainly small, cortical cysts, which are found under microscopic examination to be cysts of Bowman's space[66]. These abnormalities are associated with mild proteinuria in the absence of azotemia. The tubules are normal.

Goldfischer et al.[33] found that peroxisomes are absent in the liver and kidney of patients with Zellweger syndrome and that the mitochondria are abnormal. More recently, abnormalities of the pathways for glycerolipid and glycerol–ether lipid biosyntheses, which are located in the peroxisomes, have been detected by Datta et al.[19]. These findings are consistent with the observation of reduced amounts of the plasmalogen class of glycerol–ether lipids in tissues of patients[46]. Dihydroxy-acetone phosphate (DHAP) acyltransferase levels were significantly reduced in the leukocytes, fibroblasts and erythrocytes of patients. The levels of glycerophosphate acyltransferase and alkyl DHAP synthase were also reduced, but the activity of acyl/alkyl DHAP:NADPH reductase was not altered in patients. The primary abnormality responsible for the reduction in activities of these enzymes has not been elucidated.

2.1.5.3. Meckel syndrome (dysencephalia splanchnocystica). Meckel syndrome is an autosomal recessive disorder consisting of cerebral, facial, splanchnic and digital abnormalities, as well as polycystic kidneys. Although there are clinical similarities with trisomy 13, chromosomal aberrations have not been observed in Meckel syndrome.

Renal abnormalities are the most common feature of the syndrome, cystic changes occurring in almost all cases[49]. The renal abnormality is a form of renal dysplasia, comprising abnormal lobar differentiation, reduced nephrogenesis and cysts[5,63]. The cysts arise in abnormally differentiated collecting ducts. The cystic kidneys lead to massive abdominal enlargement that may hinder delivery. Oligohydramnios and neonatal death from renal insufficiency are common. Horseshoe kidney, hypoplastic kidney, medullary sponge kidney and dilated ureters have also been observed in Meckel syndrome[36,49].

2.1.6. Nephronophthisis/medullary cystic disease

"Nephronophthisis" is the term originally given by Fanconi *et al.* [25] to a familial syndrome in which the kidneys are severely shrunken and often contain medullary cysts. "Medullary cystic disease" was coined by Hogness and Burnell[47] to describe a condition with similar pathology in adults. There has been considerable controversy as to whether these are really the same disease with different ages of onset. An understanding of the molecular pathology of these disorders will ultimately be required to define the relationship between them and resolve this question. Nevertheless, there are good reasons to believe that they are indeed separate entities, despite the similarity in clinical and pathological features. Perhaps the best reason is that the genetics of the juvenile- and adult-onset forms are different: disease presenting in the first and second decades (nephronophthisis) is usually inherited in an autosomal recessive fashion, whereas disease presenting in the third or subsequent decades (medullary cystic disease) usually follows an autosomal dominant or sporadic pattern[13,29]. Gardner listed the ages of onset and death of published cases classified according to the apparent mode of inheritance. Autosomal dominant cases from two families studied in detail[13,29] had a mean age of onset of 26.7 y (14.0–48.2). Autosomal recessive cases had a mean age of onset of 10.5 y (0.5–27.0). Steele *et al.* [85] reported that recessive cases had a mean age of 11.7 y

(5–29). The difference in age of onset in the two modes of inheritance is highly significant, and the mode of inheritance is, therefore, useful in predicting prognosis. The pattern of inheritance in the majority of published families makes it unlikely that juvenile and adult onset forms represent different doses of the same mutation. This does not, of course, exclude the possibility that the two forms are allelic (i.e, that they are different mutations of the same gene).

Two families have been described with juvenile onset autosomal dominant cystic disease of the medulla. In one of these families the inheritance of the nephropathy is not entirely consistent with an autosomal dominant pattern[30]. In the second[62], the clinical features suggest a different disorder, as discussed by Chamberlain et al. [13]. Inevitably, there are reported cases, many of them sporadic, in which a clear pattern of inheritance cannot be established. Recessive disease will appear to be sporadic when a single child is affected within a sibship. Sporadic cases of adult onset, on the other hand, may represent de novo mutations. Gardner[29] reviewed the published sporadic cases and found a range of ages of onset consistent with his interpretation that this group represents a mixture of de novo dominant and isolated recessive cases. He also speculated that some sporadic medullary cystic disease may be acquired rather than inherited.

The histological features of nephronophthisis and medullary cystic disease were each found in different individuals of the same family[87]. However, most authors are unable to make a clear histological distinction between the two disease categories, as both may include medullary cysts, and this finding does not, therefore, refute the hypothesis that there are two different diseases with characteristic modes of inheritance and ages of onset. Wrigley et al. [94] described a family with adult-onset autosomal dominant medullary cystic disease in which age of onset was later than average and progression of disease was relatively slow. The relationship between this and other examples of medullary cystic disease may be difficult to establish until the molecular pathology of these disorders is studied.

Lirenman et al. [61] report a frequency of 1 in 50,000 live births for the recessive form. Estimates based on reported cases suggest a frequency of less than 1 in 100,000 for the dominant form.

Medullary cystic disease has frequently been found in association with red and blond hair[89]. Tapeto–retinal degeneration has also been described by a number of authors[8,26,43,67]. Skeletal abnormalities, hepatic fibrosis, cerebellar ataxia and mental retardation have been reported. Donaldson et al.[21] have reviewed the relationship between these associated disorders, nephronophthisis and Jeune syndrome.

2.1.7. Other single gene disorders

Renal cysts are occasionally found in a number of rare autosomal and X-linked disorders (Table 6.2). The renal abnormalities in these syndromes are variable and not characteristic. Cystic change is not usually an important part of their clinical picture and renal functional impairment rarely occurs.

2.2 Renal cystic dysplasia

It is doubtful whether renal dysplasia with cyst formation is ever inherited as an isolated entity. It does, however, form part of a large number of familial syndromes which are inherited in Mendelian fashion and of certain syndromes associated with chromosomal rearrangements. One of the characteristics of these syndromes is that the phenotypes are very variable, and there has consequently been great difficulty in their classification. Since the emphasis of this chapter is on the genetics rather than morphology, the Mendelian dysplastic disorders have been classified with other cystic diseases according to their mode of inheritance.

Table 6.2. Rare inherited disorders associated with renal cysts

---

Autosomal dominant
Exomphalos–macroglossia–gigantism[51]
Syndrome (Beckwith–Wiedemann)[91]

Autosomal recessive
Fanconi's anemia[31]
Laurence–Moon–Bardet–Biedl syndrome[1,39]
Roberts Syndrome[45]
Short rib–polydactyly syndromes
　　Saldino–Noonan type[76]
　　Majewski type[14,64]

X-linked
Orofaciodigital syndrome[41]

Selected references describe the occurrence of renal cystic disease in each syndrome.

2.3. Renal cysts in chromosomal aneuploidy

Multiple renal cysts are a common feature of trisomies involving the whole of chromosome 13, occurring in 30% of one series[91]. Genital anomalies and urinary tract duplication also occur frequently. Partial trisomy 13 has a somewhat different phenotype in which cystic renal disease is not a prominent feature. In trisomy 18, cystic kidneys are less common (10%) than horseshoe kidneys (21%) and urinary tract duplications (26%)[91]. Cystic kidneys are rare in Down syndrome and Turner syndrome.

Acknowledgements

I thank the Polycystic Kidney Research Foundation, NIDDK and Howard Hughes Medical Institute for their generous support.

References

1. Ammann F. Investigations cliniques et genetiques sur le syndrome de Bardet-Biedl en Suisse. Journal de Genetique Humaine 1970, Supplement 18.
2. Bachner L, Albouze G, Ferran C, Vinet MC, Julier C, Grunfeld JP and Kaplan JC. Family studies of adult dominant polycystic kidney disease (PKD1 locus) using the highly polymorphic probe 3′HVR at HBA locus. Independent locus for the neo-natal recessive disease? Cytogenetic Cell Genetics 1987, 46, 574.
3. Bear JC, McManamon P, Morgan J et al. Age at clinical onset and at ultrasonographic detection of adult polycystic kidney disease – data for genetic counselling. American Journal of Medical Genetics 1984, 18, 45–53.
4. Bernstein J. A classification of renal cysts. In: Gardner KD ed., Cystic Diseases of the Kidney. New York: John Wiley, 1976, 7–30.
5. Bernstein J, Brough AJ and McAdams AJ. The renal lesion in syndromes of multiple congenital malformations – cerebrohepatorenal syndrome; Jeune asphyxiating thoracic dystrophy; tuberous sclerosis; Meckel syndrome. Birth Defects Original Article Series 1974, 10, 35.
6. Bernstein J, Robbins TO and Kissane JM. The renal lesions of tuberous sclerosis. Seminars in Diagnostic Pathology 1986, 3, 97–105.
7. Bernstein J, Evan AP and Gardner KD Jr. Epithelial hyperplasia in human polycystic kidney diseases. Its role in pathogenesis and risk of neoplasia. American Journal of Pathology 1987, 129, 92–101.
8. Betts PR and Forrest-Hay I. Juvenile nephronophthisis. Lancet 1973, 3, 475.
9. Blyth H and Ockenden BG. Polycystic disease of the kidneys and liver presenting in childhood. Journal of Medical Genetics 1971, 8, 257–284.
10. Breuning MH, Reeders ST, Brunner H, Ijdo JW, Saris JJ, Verwest A, Van Ommen GJB and Pearson PL. Improved early diagnosis of adult polycystic kidney disease with flanking DNA markers. Lancet 1987, 2, 1359–1361.
11. Breuning MH, Madan K, Verjaal M, Wijnen JT, Meera Khan P and Pearson PL. Human α-globin maps to pter-p13.3 in chromosome 16 distal to PGP. Human Genetics 1987, 76, 287–289.
12. Bundey S and Evans K. Tuberous sclerosis: a genetic study. Journal of Neurology, Neurosurgery and Psychiatry 1969, 32, 591.
13. Chamberlain BC, Hagge WW and Stickler GB. Juvenile nephronophthisis and medullary cystic disease. Mayo Clinic Proceedings 1977, 52, 485–491.
14. Chen H, Yang SS, Gonzalez E, Fowler M and Al Saadi A. Short rib-polydactyly syndrome, Marjewski type. American Journal of Medical Genetics 1980, 7, 215.
15. Chonko AM, Weiss SM, Stein JH and Ferris TF. Renal involvement in tuberous sclerosis. American Journal of Medicine 1974, 56, 124.
16. Churchill DN, Bear JC, Morgan J, Payne EH, McManamon PJ and Gault MH. Prognosis of adult onset polycystic kidney disease re-evaluated. Kidney International 1984, 26, 190–193.
17. Connor JM, Pirrit LA, Yates JR, Fryer AE and Ferguson-Smith MA. Linkage of the tuberous sclerosis locus to a DNA polymorphism detected by v-abl. Journal of Medical Genetics 1987, 24, 544–546.

18. Dalgaard OZ. Bilateral polycystic disease of the kidneys. A follow up of 284 patients and their families. Acta Medica Scandinavica 1957, 328, 1–233.

19. Datta NS, Wilson GN and Hajra AK. Deficiency of enzymes catalyzing the biosynthesis of glycerol–ether lipids in Zellweger syndrome. New England Journal of Medicine 1984, 311, 1080–1083.

20. del Senno L, Castagnoli A, Zamorani G, Maestri I, De Paoli Vitali E, Storari A, Limone GL, Farinelli A, Marchetti G and Bernardi F. Use of a genetic marker for the diagnosis of adult polycystic kidney disease in Northern Italy. Prot Biological Fluids 1987, 35, 63–66.

21. Donaldson MDC, Warner AA, Trompeter RS, Haycock GB and Chantler C. Familial juvenile nephronophthisis, Jeune's syndrome, and associated disorders. Archives of Diseases of Childhood 1985, 60, 426–434.

22. Durham DS. Tuberous sclerosis mimicking adult polycystic kidney disease. Australian and New Zealand Journal of Medicine 1987, 17, 71–73.

23. Edelson PJ, Spackman TJ, Belliveau RE and Mahoney MJ. A renal lesion in asphyxiating thoracic dysplasia. Birth Defects Original Article Series 1974, 10, 51.

24. Evan AP, Gardner KD and Bernstein J. Polypoid and papillary epithelial hyperplasia: A potential cause of ductal obstruction in adult polycystic disease. Kidney International 1979, 16, 743–750.

25. Fanconi G, Hanhart E, von Albertini A, Uhlinger E, Dolivo G and Prader A. Die familiare juvenile Nephronophthise. (die idiopathische parenchymatose Schrumpfniere.) Helvetica Paediatrica Acta 1951, 6, 1.

26. Fillastre JP, Guenel J, Riberi P, Marx P, Whitworth JA and Kunh JM. Senior–Loken syndrome (nephronophthisis and tapeto–retinal degeneration): a study of 8 cases from 5 families. Clinical Nephrology 1976, 5, 1–14.

27. Francke U. Microdeletions and Mendellian phenotypes. In: Vogel F and Sperling K eds, Human Genetics. Berlin: Springer, 1987.

28. Fryer AE, Conor JM, Povey S, Yates JRW, Chalmers A, Fraser I, Yates AD and Osborne JP. Evidence that the gene for tuberous slcerosis is on chromosome 9. Lancet 1987, 659–661.

29. Gardner KD Jr. Evolution of clinical signs in adult-onset cystic disease of the renal medulla. Annals of Internal Medicine 1971, 74, 47–53.

30. Giangiacomo J, Monteleone PL and Witzleben CL. Medullary cystic disease vs nephronophthisis: a valid distinction? Journal of the American Medical Association 1975, 232, 629–631.

31. Gmyrek D and Syllm-Rapoport I. Zur Fanconi–Anamie (FA). Analyse von 129 beschriebenen Fällen. Zeitschrift für Kinderheilkunde 1964, 91, 297.

32. Gold CH, Isaacson C and Levin J. The pathological basis of end-stage renal disease in Blacks. SA Mediese Tydskrif 1982, 20, 263–265.

33. Goldfischer S, Moore CL, Johnson AB et al. Peroxisomal and mitochondrial defects in the cerebro–hepato–renal syndrome. Science 1973, 182, 62–64.

34. Gomez MR. Tuberous Sclerosis, 2nd Edn. New York: Raven Press, 1988.

35. Freen JS, Bowmer MI and Johnson GJ. Von Hippel–Lindau disease in a Newfoundland kindred. Canadian Medical Association Journal 1986, 134, 133–146.

36. Gresham GA. Chromosomal sex determination in a male internal pseudohermaphrodite. Journal of Pathology and Bacteriology 1955, 70, 546.

37. Gruskin AB, Baluarte HJ, Cote ML and Elfenbein IB. The renal disease of thoracic asphyxiant dystrophy. Birth Defects Original Article Series 1974, 10, 44.

38. Hansen MF and Cavenee WK. Retinoblastoma and the progression of tumor genetics. Trends in Genetics 1988, 4, 125–128.

39. Harnett JD, Green JS, Cramer BC, Johnson G, Chafe L, McManamon P, Farid NR, Pryse-Phillips W and Parfrey PS. The spectrum of renal disease in Laurence–Moon–Biedl syndrome. New England Journal of Medicine 1988 (In Press).

40. Harris PC, Reeders ST, Stroh H, Dolata MM, Tanzi R, Neve R and Latt SA. Linkage

analysis of DNA markers from 16p and adult polycystic kidney disease. American Journal of Human Genetics 1987 (Supplement), 41, 499.

41. Harrod MJ, Stokes J, Peede LF and Goldstein JL. Polycystic kidney disease in a patient with the oral–facial digital syndrome – Type I. Clinical Genetics 1976, 9, 183.

42. Hatfield PM and Pfister RC. Adult polycystic disease of the kidneys (Potter type 3). Journal of the American Medical Association 1972, 222, 1527–1531.

43. Herdman RC, Good RA and Vernier RL. Medullary cystic disease in two siblings. American Journal of Medicine 1967, 43, 335–344.

44. Herdman RC and Langer LO. The thoracic asphyxiant dystrophy and renal disease. American Journal of Diseases of Childhood 1968, 116, 192–201.

45. Hermann J and Opitz JM. The SC phocomelia and the Roberts syndrome: nosologic aspects. European Journal of Pediatrics (Berlin) 1977, 125, 117.

46. Heymans HSA, Schutgens RBH, Tan R, Van den Bosch H and Borst P. Severe plasmalogen deficiency in tissues of infants without peroxisomes (Zellweger syndrome). Nature 1983, 306, 69–70.

47. Hogness JR and Burnell JM. Medullary cysts of kidneys. American Medical Association Archives of Internal Medicine 1954, 93, 355.

48. Horton WA, Wong V and Eldridge R. Von Hippel–Lindau disease: clinical and pathological manifestations in nine families with 50 affected members. Archives of Internal Medicine 1976, 136, 769.

49. Hsia YE, Bratu M and Herbordt A. Genetics of the Meckel syndrome (dysencephalia splanchnocystica). Pediatrics 1971, 48, 237–247.

50. Iglesias CG, Torres VE, Offord KP, Holley KE, Beard CM and Kurland LT. Epidemiology of adult polycystic kidney disease, Olmsted County, Minnesota: 1935–1980. American Journal of Kidney Disease 1983, 2, 630–639.

51. Irving IM. Exomphalos with macroglossia: A study of eleven cases. Journal of Pediatric Surgery 1967, 2, 499–507.

52. Kääriäinen H. Polycystic kidney disease in children: a genetic and epidemiological study of 82 Finnish patients. Journal of Medical Genetics 1987, 24, 474–481.

53. Kääriäinen H. Polycystic Kidney Disease in Children: Differential Diagnosis Between the Dominantly and Recessively Inherited Forms. Department of Medical Genetics, Vaestoliitto, the Finnish Population and Family Welfare Federation; Department of Medical Genetics, University of Helsinki; Children's Hospital, University of Helsinki: Academic Dissertation, 1988.

54. Kääriäinen H, Koskimes O and Norio R. Dominant and recessive polycystic kidney disease in children: evaluation of clinical features and laboratory data. Pediatric Nephrology 1988, 2, 296.

55. Keith T, Green P, Reeders ST, Brown VA, Phipps P, Bricker A, Knowlton R, Nelson C and Donis-Keller H. A linkage map of chromosome 16 with 41 RFLP markers. Human Gene Mapping 9, Paris Conference. Cytogenetics and Cell Genetics 1987, 46, 638.

56. Kimberling WJ, Fain PR, Kenyon JB, Goldgar D, Sujansky E and Gabow PJ. Linkage heterogeneity of autosomal dominant polycystic kidney disease. New England Journal of Medicine 1988, 319, 913–918.

57. King CR, Schimke RN, Arthur T, Davoren B and Collins D. Proximal 3p deletion in renal cell carcinoma cells from a patient with von Hippel–Lindau disease. Cancer Genetics and Cytogenetics 1987, 27, 345–348.

58. Kissane JM. Congenital malformations. In: Heptinstall RH ed., Pathology of the Kidney. Boston: Little, Brown and Company, 1966, 63–117.

59. Kristal C, Berant M and Alon U. Polycystic kidneys as the presenting feature of tuberous sclerosis. Helvetica Paediatrica Acta 1987, 42, 29–33.

60. Lazarou LP, Davies F, Sarfarazi M, Coles GA and Harper PS. Adult polycystic kidney disease and linked RFLPs at the α globin locus: a genetic study in the South Wales population. Journal of Medical Genetics 1987, 24, 466–473.

142

61. Lirenman DS, Lowry RB and Chase WH. Familial juvenile nephronophthisis: experience with eleven cases. Birth Defects Original Article Series 1974, 10, 32.
62. Makker SP, Grupe WE, Perrin E *et al*. Identical progression of juvenile hereditary nephronophthisis in monozygotic twins. Journal of Pediatrics 1973, 82, 773–779.
63. Moerman P, Verbeken E, Fryns JP, Goddeeris P and Lauweryns JM. The Meckel syndrome. Pathological and cytogenetic observations in eight cases. Human Genetics 1982, 62, 240–245.
64. Motegi T, Kusonoki M, Nishi T *et al*. Short rib-polydactyly syndrome, Majewski type, in two male siblings. Human Genetics 1979, 49, 269.
65. Nimr AB, Patel PJ, Tongia RK and Tamizuddin F. Chronic renal failure and tuberous sclerosis: a rare association. Postgraduate Medical Journal 1987, 63, 811–813.
66. Poznanski AK, Nosanchuk JS, Baublis J and Holt JF. The cerebro–hepato–renal syndrome (CHRS) (Zellweger's syndrome). American Journal of Roentgenology 1970, 109, 313–322.
67. Price JDE and Pratt-Johnson JA. Medullary cystic disease with degeneration. Canadian Medical Association Journal 1970, 102, 165–167.
68. Ramsay M, Reeders ST, Thompson PD, Milner LS, Lazarous L, Barratt TM, Yau A, Lehmann OJ and Jenkins T. Mutations for the autosomal recessive and autosomal dominant forms of polycystic kidney disease are not allelic. Human Genetics 1988 (In Press).
69. Rapola J and Kääriäinen H. Morphological diagnosis of recessive and dominant polycystic disease in infancy and childhood. APMIS 1988, 96, 68–76.
70. Reeders ST, Breuning MH, Davies KE, Nicholls DR, Jarman AJ, Higgs DR, Pearson PL and Weatherall DJ. A highly polymorphic DNA marker linked to adult polycystic kidney disease on chromosome 16. Nature 1985, 317, 542–544.
71. Reeders ST, Breuning MH, Corney G, Jeremiah SJ, Meera Khan P, Davies KE, Hopkinson DA, Pearson PL and Weatherall DJ. Two genetic markers closely linked to adult polycystic kidney disease on chromosome 16. British Medical Journal 1986, 292, 851–853.
72. Reeders ST, Zerres K, Gal A, Hogenkamp T, Propping P, Schmidt W, Waldherr R, Dolata MM, Davies KE and Weatherall DJ. First prenatal diagnosis of autosomal dominant polycystic kidney disease using a DNA probe. Lancet 1986, 2, 6–7.
73. Reeders ST, Breuning MH, Ryynanen MA, Wright AF, Davies KE, Kily AW, Watson ML and Weatherall DJ. A study of genetic linkage heterogeneity in adult polycystic kidney disease. Human Genetics 1987, 76, 348–351.
74. Reeders ST, Keith TP, Green P, Dolata MM, Barton NJ, Collier PS, Brown VA, Phipps P, Bricher A and Donis-Keller H. Linkage studies and physical mapping of the autosomal dominant polycystic kidney disease mutation (PKD1). Human Gene Mapping 9, Paris Conference. Cytogenetics and Cell Genetics 1987, 46, 680.
75. Reeders ST, Keith T, Green P, Germino GG, Barton NJ, Lehmann OJ, Brown VA, Phipps P, Morgan J, Bear JC and Parfrey P. Regional localisation of the autosomal dominant polycystic kidney disease locus. Genomics 1988, 3, 150–155.
76. Richardson MM, Beaudet AL, Wagner ML, Malini S, Rosenberg HS and Lucci JA. Prenatal diagnosis of recurrence of Saldino-Noonan dwarfism. Journal of Pediatrics 1977, 91, 467.
77. Romeo G, Costa G, Catizone L, Germino GG, Weatherall DJ, Devoto M, Roncuzzi L, Zucchelli P, Keith T and Reeders ST. A second genetic locus for autosomal dominant polycystic kidney disease. Lancet 1988, 2, 7–10.
78. Rostand SG, Kirk KA, Rutsky EA *et al*. Racial differences in the treatment for end-stage renal disease. New England Journal of Medicine 1982, 306, 1276–1279.
79. Ryynanen M, Dolata M, Lampainen E and Reeders ST. Localisation of a mutation producing autosomal dominant polycystic kidney disease without renal failure. Journal of Medical Genetics 1987, 24, 462–465.
80. Sedman A, Bell P, Manco-Johnson M, Schrier R, Warady BA, Heard EO, Butler-Simon

N and Gabow P. Autosomal dominant polycystic kidney disease in childhood: A longitudinal study. Kidney International 1987, 31, 1000–1005.

81. Seizinger BR, Rouleau GA, Ozelius LJ, Lane AH, Farmer GE, Lamiell JM, Haines J, Yuen JW, Collins D, Majoor-Krakauer D et al. Von Hippel–Lindau disease maps to the region of chromosome 3 associated with renal cell carcinoma. Nature 1988, 332, 268–269.

82. Shokeir MHK, Houston CS and Awen CF. Asphyxiating thoracic chondrodystrophy: Association with renal disease and evidence for possible heterozygous expression. Journal of Medical Genetics 1971, 8, 107–112.

83. Simmers RN, Mulley JC, Hyland VJ, Callen DF and Sutherland GR. Mapping the human α globin gene complex to 16p 13.2 pter. Journal of Medical Genetics 1987, 24, 761–766.

84. Smith DW, Opitz JM and Inhorn SL. A syndrome of multiple developmental defects including polycystic kidneys and intrahepatic biliary dysgenesis in two siblings. Journal of Pediatrics 1965, 67, 617.

85. Steele BT, Lirenman DSA and Beattie CW. Nephronophthisis. American Journal of Medicine 1980, 68, 531–537.

86. Stillwell TJ, Gomez MR and Kelalis PP. Renal lesions in tuberous sclerosis. Journal of Urology 1987, 138, 477–481.

87. Sworn MJ and Eisinger AJ. Medullary cystic disease and juvenile nephronophthisis in separate members of the same family. Archives of Diseases in Childhood 1972, 47, 278.

88. Taitz LS, Brown CB, Blank CE and Steiner GM. Screening for polycystic kidney disease: Importance of clinical presentation in the newborn. Archives of Diseases in Childhood 1987, 62, 443–444.

89. Thorn GW, Keopf GF and Clinton M Jr. Renal failure simulating adrenocortical insufficiency. New England Journal of Medicine 1944, 231, 76–85.

90. Torres VE, Holley KE and Offord KP. General features of autosomal dominant polycystic kidney disease. In: Grantham JJ and Gardner KD eds, Epidemiology. Problems in Diagnosis and Management of Polycystic Kidney Disease. 1985, 49–69.

91. Warkany J, Passarge E and Smith LB. Congenital malformations in autosomal trisomy syndromes. American Journal of Diseases in Childhood 1966, 112, 502–517.

92. Weatherall DJ (ed.). The New Genetics and Clinical Practice. Oxford: Oxford University Press, 1985.

93. Wirth B, Zerres K, Fischbach M, Claus D, Neumann HPH, Lennert T, Brodehl J, Neugebauer M, Muller-Wiefel DE, Geisert J and Gal A. Autosomal recessive and dominant forms of polycystic kidney disease are not allelic. Human Genetics 1987, 77, 221–222.

94. Wrigley KA, Sherman RL, Ennis FA and Becker EL. Progressive hereditary nephropathy: a variant of medullary cystic disease? Archives of Internal Medicine 1973, 131, 240–244.

95. Zerres K, Volpel MC and Weiss H. Cystic kidneys: genetics, pathologic anatomy, clinical picture, and prenatal diagnosis. Human Genetics 1984, 68, 104–135.

Section 3

7
A Classification of Renal Cysts

J. Bernstein

Abstract

Renal cystic diseases are a mixed lot, comprising heritable, developmental and acquired disorders. This classification has been developed, as have several others in the past, to incorporate radiographic, functional and genetic information, and to provide a basis for clinicopathologic correlations. Its major categories are as follows: (1) polycystic kidney diseases, autosomal recessive and autosomal dominant; (2) renal cysts in hereditary syndromes, including tuberous sclerosis, orofaciodigital syndrome and von Hippel–Lindau disease; (3) glomerulocystic kidney disease, a descriptive category of considerable heterogeneity; (4) localized segmental and unilateral renal cysts, and solitary and simple renal cysts; (5) acquired cystic disease, usually resulting in end-stage kidneys; (6) medullary cysts, occurring both as medullary sponge kidney and as an accompaniment of hereditary tubulointerstitial nephritis; (7) renal dysplasia, including multicystic dysplasia and diffuse cystic dysplasia; and (8) extraparenchymal cysts. This classification has remained essentially unchanged for more than a decade and has served its purposes satisfactorily.

Key words   Acquired renal cystic disease;
Extraparenchymal renal cysts;
Glomerulocystic kidney disease;
Hereditary syndromes;
Localized and segmental renal cysts;
Medullary cysts;
Polycystic kidney disease;
Renal dysplasia.

1. Introduction

Renal cysts are relatively common radiographic, clinical and morphologic abnormalities. Considerable progress has been made during the last decade in reaching a consensus, with common terms and usages, among nephrologists, urologists, radiologists and pathologists. Standard terminologies and classifications have been proposed by international bodies[21], and an increasing degree of uniformity is evident in the literature.

Table 7.1. Classification of renal cysts

I.   *Polycystic kidney disease*
      A. Autosomal recessive polycystic kidney disease
          (1) Polycystic disease of newborns and young infants
          (2) Polycystic disease of older children and adults
              (a) Medullary ductal ectasia
              (b) Congenital hepatic fibrosis
              (c) Caroli syndrome
      B. Autosomal dominant polycystic kidney disease
          (1) Glomerulocystic disease of newborn (in part)
          (2) Classic polycystic disease of older children and adults
              (a) Dominant polycystic disease linked to chromosome 16
              (b) Dominant polycystic disease not linked to chromosome 16

II.   *Renal cysts in hereditary malformation syndromes*
      A. Tuberous sclerosis
      B. von Hippel–Lindau syndrome
      C. Zellweger cerebrohepatorenal syndrome
      D. Jeune asphyxiating thoracic dysplasia
      E. Orofaciodigital syndrome I
      F. Brachymesomelia–renal syndrome

III. *Glomerulocystic kidney disease*
      A. Infantile-onset dominant polycystic kidney disease
      B. Syndromal glomerular cystic disease
      C. Non-syndromal glomerular cysts

IV.   *Localized, segmental and unilateral renal cysts*
      A. Simple renal cysts, solitary and multiple
      B. Localized cystic disease

V.   *Acquired renal cystic disease*

VI.   *Renal medullary cysts*
      A. Medullary sponge kidney
      B. Hereditary tubulointerstitial nephritis
          (1) Familial juvenile nephronophthisis
          (2) Medullary cystic disease
          (3) Renal–retinal dysplasia complex

VII. *Renal cystic dysplasia*
      A. Multicystic kidney
      B. Cystic dysplasia associated with lower urinary tract obstruction
      C. Diffuse cystic dysplasia, syndromal and non-syndromal

VIII. *Extraparenchymal renal cysts*
      A. Pyelogenic cyst (pyelocalyceal diverticulum)
      B. Parapelvic lymphangiectasia
      C. Perinephric cyst

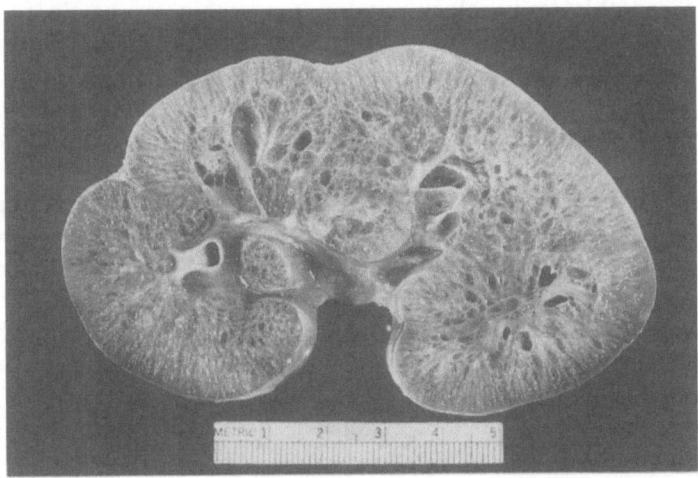

Figure 7.1. Neonatal autosomal recessive polycystic kidney disease. Despite being greatly enlarged, the kidneys retain a reniform configuration. The parenchyma has a spongy appearance because of diffuse collecting duct dilatation. The cortical collecting ducts are elongated, narrow sacs, running from corticomedullary junction to periphery; the medullary collecting ducts are more dilated, with a rounded appearance, obscuring the otherwise normally formed medullary pyramids.

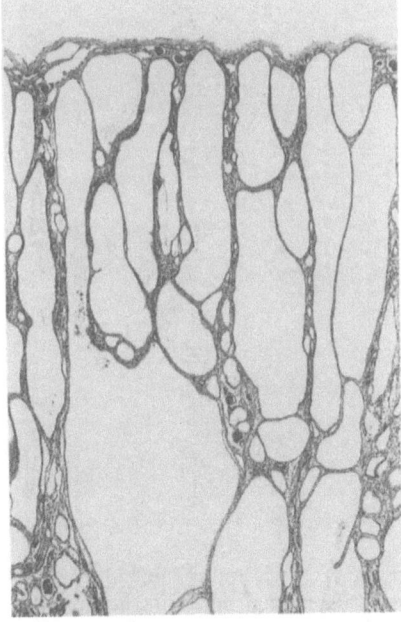

Figure 7.2. Neonatal autosomal recessive polycystic kidney disease. A low-power photomicrograph shows the dilated cortical collecting ducts, with intervening attenuated solid tissue of the cortical labyrinth. There is minimal dilatation of convoluted tubules; glomerular spaces are not dilated. Hematoxylin and eosin ×20.

An acceptable terminology requires terms that are pertinent, have restricted meanings, and enjoy easy usage. The terminology has to account for cysts that have differing patterns of inheritance, differing natural histories, differing prognostic implications and differing therapeutic implications. Accompanying any terminology is a classification that is appropriate clinically, radiographically, genetically and morphologically. The problem in classifying renal cysts is their strong morphologic similarities, despite differences in heredity and pathogenesis. A classification, therefore, needs the contribution of all disciplines[7,8]. The classification that follows was developed first in collaboration with a clinician and a radiologist[12,26]. It is very similar in scope and sense to the classifications developed by Gleason, McAlister and Kissane[32] and Spence[69], and it has been changed but little from the one published in the predecessor to this volume[3]. This classification has been helpful in practical application, but it is subject to change as new evidence of heterogeneity becomes apparent.

Cysts may be hereditary, developmental, or acquired. Although they may arise in any part of the nephron and collecting system, they have a predilection for the loops of Henle and for the collecting tubules and peripheral portions of collecting ducts[58]. Nonetheless, some patterns of cyst formation are charac-

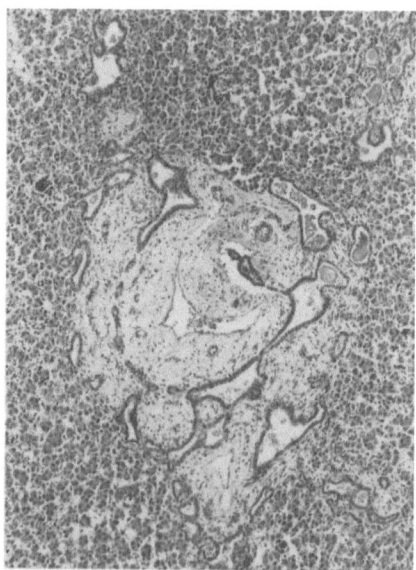

Figure 7.3. Neonatal autosomal recessive polycystic kidney disease. The liver is also involved. The intrahepatic bile ducts are abnormal, appearing in the plane of section to be increased in number and size, as though there were bile duct proliferation. The presence of these elongated, interconnecting biliary structures encircling virtually every portal area of the section indicates, however, that they are flattened sacs rather than ducts, representing arrested and probably abnormal development of the biliary ductal plate. Note also the presence of duct-like structures within the lobules. Hematoxylin and eosin, × 60.

teristic of certain conditions. The cysts in infants with polycystic disease of autosomal recessive type are characteristically located in collecting tubules and ducts[35,58]. Glomerular and tubular microcysts in the peripheral cortex are commonly associated with syndromes of multiple malformations[7]. Dysplastic cysts in the peripheral cortex are commonly associated with lower urinary tract obstruction[4]. That cysts can arise in previously completely formed nephrons and collecting tubules seems to be well established by numerous experimental studies with cystogenic agents and by the clinical development of acquired cystic disease in patients with chronic renal failure. The classification presented (Table 7.1) incorporates clinicopathologic correlations and relies heavily on current genetic information.

2. Polycystic kidney disease

There are two major categories of polycystic disease. The first, with an onset characteristically in childhood and with an autosomal recessive inheritance, has been called *infantile polycystic disease*. It affects both the kidneys and the liver. Very young infants tend to have predominant renal involvement with large

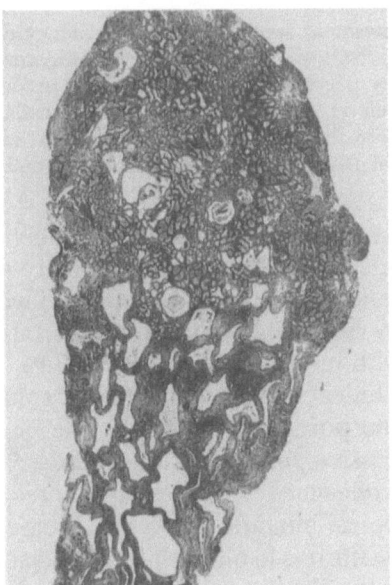

Figure 7.4. Childhood autosomal recessive polycystic kidney disease. A wedge biopsy specimen of cortex and medulla from a child shows the principal site of cyst formation to be in the medulla. This medullary ductal dilatation is frequently confused with medullary sponge kidney, a disease with different clinicopathologic and genetic implications; the abnormality is visualized radiographically as medullary tubular ectasia. The cortex contains scattered collecting duct cysts, more rounded than in the newborn specimen shown in Fig. 7.2. Hematoxylin and eosin, × 13.

152

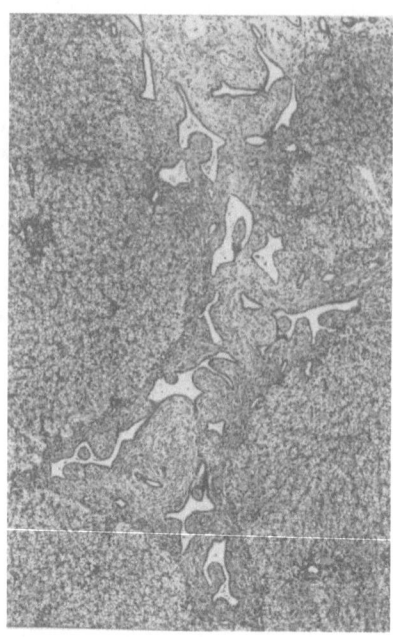

Figure 7.5. Childhood autosomal recessive polycystic kidney disease. The liver is characteristically involved in all patients with recessive polycystic disease. In this specimen of liver from the same child whose kidney specimen is shown in Fig. 7.4, the portal area is enlarged and fibrotic. The abnormality is often referred to as congenital hepatic fibrosis, a term also used for clinical diagnosis. The biliary abnormality, however, is qualitatively the same as that in neonatal cases (see Fig. 7.3), i.e. the ductal plate malformation. Hematoxylin and eosin, × 16.

spongy kidneys (Fig. 7.1) that contain dilated collecting ducts (Fig. 7.2), and there is also involvement of the intrahepatic biliary system (Fig. 7.3). Older children and adults tend to have less severe renal involvement, with a predominance of medullary cysts (Fig. 7.4), and the portal areas contain the same biliary abnormality with increased fibrosis (Fig. 7.5). There is, however, considerable overlap in clinical symptomatology, and some patients develop both renal insufficiency and portal hypertension. The question of heterogeneity within autosomal recessive polycystic kidney disease (ARPKD) is still unresolved. Landing and colleagues[36,47,51] have presented evidence of two genetic subgroups, namely typical infantile polycystic disease in very young children and congenital hepatic fibrosis in older children and adults. Others[19,28,42] have presented evidence of variability amongst sibs, arguing for a continuum of clinical expression without genetic heterogeneity, and Bernstein *et al.* [14] have shown a spectrum in expression of the hepatic abnormality. All are in agreement that the Blyth–Ockenden classification[15] into four subgroups is an overrefinement.

There is, despite a few superficial morphologic resemblances, no real

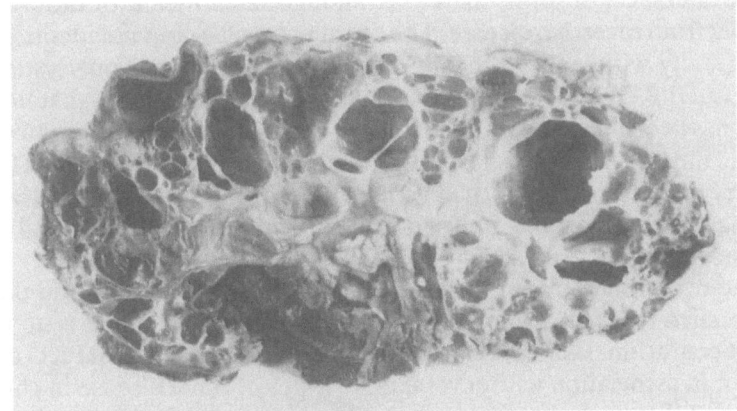

Figure 7.6. Autosomal dominant polycystic kidney disease. An endstage polycystic kidney is greatly enlarged, the parenchyma seemingly replaced by innumerable cortical and medullary cysts, varying in size from millimetres to centimetres. There is little remaining parenchyma.

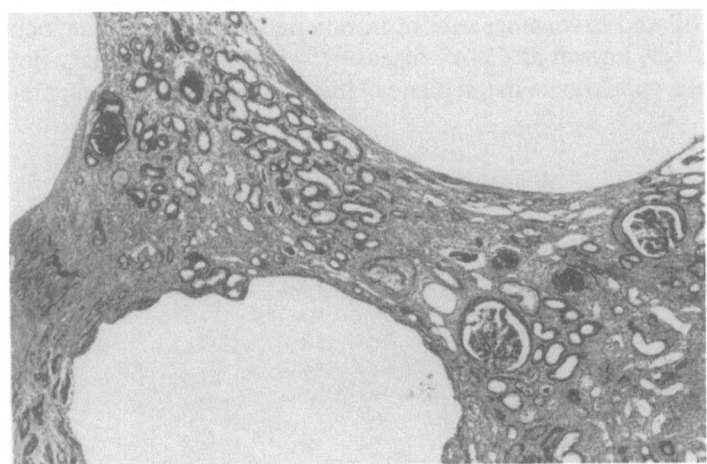

Figure 7.7. Autosomal dominant polycystic kidney disease. Sections show surprisingly abundant attenuated parenchyma among the cysts, with atrophic tubules and sclerotic glomeruli. The nephronic atrophy and interstitial fibrosis, presumably secondary to compression and probable vascular insufficiency, contribute significantly to the development of renal insufficiency. Periodic acid–Schiff × 36.

overlap with the second type of polycystic disease, which typically has its clinical onset in adulthood, is transmitted as an autosomal dominant, and is commonly called *adult polycystic disease* (Figs. 7.6, 7.7). The dominant type may, however, commence in infancy[43,74] or childhood[66] and the recessive type remains asymptomatic into adulthood. Typical infantile-onset recessive disease and infantile-onset dominant disease appear sonographically similar, but the morphologic differences separate the two, even in the absence of a helpful family history.

154

The age at clinical onset is, therefore, an unreliable means of differentiating dominant from recessive disease. The age at onset also does not identify genetic heterogeneity within the category of autosomal dominant polycystic kidney disease (ADPKD). The genetic abnormality in most adult cases that have been studied has been localized through linkage analysis to chromosome 16[60,61], and the same linkage has been shown in a fetus diagnosed prenatally[62]. There was until very recently no evidence of genetic heterogeneity in ADPKD, but a lack of linkage to chromosome 16 has now been demonstrated in several families with otherwise typical dominant disease[65].

The occurrence of intrahepatic biliary alterations in both the dominant and recessive types of polycystic disease is well recognized and is no longer a cause of confusion. Biliary abnormalities similar to those in ARPKD are seen, however, in association with several other types of renal disease in childhood. The same biliary abnormality with mild variation occurs in association with hereditary renal cystic dysplasia and hereditary tubulointerstitial nephritis[5,6]. The biliary abnormality probably stems from arrested development, hence its designation as the ductal plate malformation[40] or biliary dysgenesis[5]. The abnormal biliary passages in many of these disorders, including ARPKD, often become dilated to form a series of intrahepatic communicating ectatic biliary channels[14,40], known as Caroli disease[17]. The failure of biliary development leads to the appearance in the plane of histologic section of elongated, tortuous

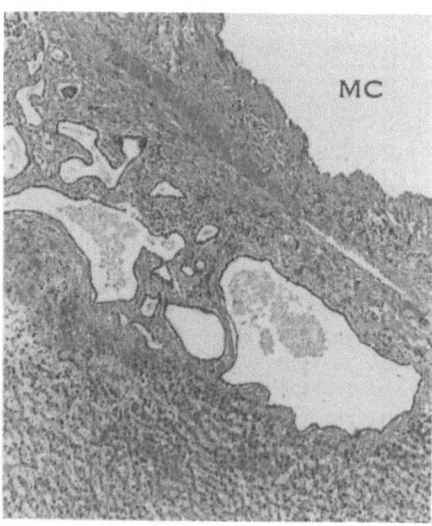

Figure 7.8. Autosomal dominant polycystic kidney disease. The liver is involved less often and more focally than in recessive polycystic disease, and the biliary abnormality consists of clusters of microcystic ducts, each known as a von Meyenburg complex. These ducts, here adjacent to a macrocyst (MC), appear in the plane of section to interconnect, and they contain bile-stained material, indicating communication with the hepatic lobule. Hematoxylin and eosin, × 40.

and anastomosing biliary channels frequently encircling the centrally placed portal vein; the portal areas lack well-formed, centrally placed bile ducts. The appearance of numerous biliary profiles in individual portal areas would on stereologic considerations alone[25] indicate that the biliary passages are not really ducts but that they are in fact flattened, interconnecting sacs, a matter confirmed by reconstruction and microdissection[40,48]. The biliary abnormality in the dominant disease is known also as the von Meyenburg complex (Fig. 7.8). It appears to be a cluster of dilated bile ductules, possibly anastomosing, possibly blind-ended. The livers in ADPKD may also contain gross cysts, sometimes dominating the clinical picture.

The renal lesion in both the recessive and dominant diseases is bilateral, although it may be less than diffuse or apparently unilateral early in the course of dominant disease. Consequently, unilateral and segmental cystic disease[20] must be viewed cautiously in counselling patients. Non-progressive localized cystic disease and multiple simple cysts can in individual cases provide difficult problems in differential diagnosis, and I know of no way to resolve the problem short of long-term follow-up.

3. Renal cysts in hereditary malformation syndromes

Renal cysts are encountered in many hereditary syndromes (Table 7.2), most of them associated with only trivial renal involvement.

Table 7.2. Examples of malformation syndromes associated with renal cortical cysts

Acromandibular syndrome
Autosomal trisomy syndromes, 13 and 18
Chromosomal translocation syndromes
Congenital cutis laxa syndrome
DiGeorge syndrome
Ehlers–Danlos syndrome
Fryns syndrome
Goldenhar syndrome
Jeune asphyxiating thoracic dysplasia syndrome
Lissencephaly syndrome
Marden–Walker (Schwartz–Jampel?) syndrome
Noonan syndrome
Orofaciodigital syndrome
Short rib–polydactyly syndromes
Turner syndrome
Zellweger cerebrohepatorenal syndrome

The abnormality takes the form of peripheral cortical microcysts, affecting predominantly glomeruli and collecting tubules[2,54,58].This abnormality lacks a suitable terminology. The term "microcystic disease" has been taken in con-

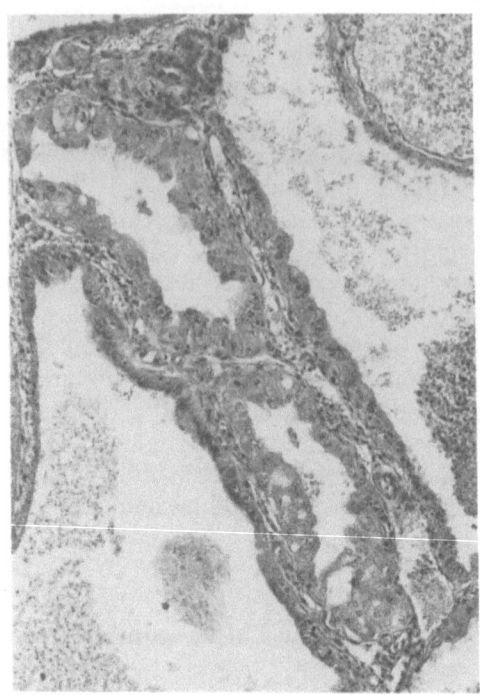

Figure 7.9. Renal involvement in tuberous sclerosis. The renal cysts are lined with a distinctive, perhaps unique, strikingly hyperplastic epithelium that may have arisen from proximal tubular epithelium. The deeply eosinophilic cells are piled up and presumably obstruct lumens to form the cysts. Hematoxylin and eosin, × 180.

nection with the congenital nephrotic syndrome, and the term "multicystic kidney" has been used to designate a particular form of cystic dysplasia. I have suggested the term "pluricystic"[7], but the abnormality lacks sufficient importance to command a proper designation. The important message is not to confuse these minor abnormalities with polycystic kidney disease.

A wider spectrum of cortical cysts has been encountered in *Zellweger syndrome*, encompassing both tiny microcysts and gross cysts that might be visualized radiographically[56,59,68]. We have in a few cases of Zellweger phenotype found generalized cystic dysplasia and have interpreted the severely abnormal metanephric differentiation to be part of the syndrome[9]. A similar spectrum of variability occurs in *Jeune syndrome* of asphyxiating thoracic dysplasia, even though the syndrome is better known for a form of tubulointerstitial nephritis similar to juvenile nephronophthisis.

Severe cystic disease predominantly affecting glomeruli has occurred in patients with orofaciodigital syndrome, type I[71] and the brachymesomelia–renal syndrome[49]. The subject of glomerulocystic disease will be described in greater detail in the next section, with particular attention to its heterogeneity. Renal cystic disease has been associated with Ehlers–Danlos syndrome, perhaps as an inherent part of the syndrome, perhaps as coincidental polycystic disease. Apparently coincidental polycystic disease has also been observed in association with myotonic dystrophy, Peutz–Jeghers syndrome, and hereditary spherocytosis.

An important form of renal cystic disease occurs as an inherent part of the *tuberous sclerosis* complex. The renal abnormality in tuberous sclerosis sits apart as a morphologically distinctive, perhaps unique abnormality[13]. The cysts are lined with a remarkable epithelium of deeply eosinophilic, hyperplastic cells that bear some resemblance to proximal tubular epithelium (Fig. 7.9). Cystic abnormalities appear to be less common and are certainly less well-known than renal angiomyolipomas, also part of the tuberous sclerosis complex[73]. The combination of cysts and angiomyolipomas, the two abnormalities recognizable by computed tomography, is for practical purposes diagnosable as tuberous sclerosis[53]. Extensive cystic disease may result in renal insufficiency[55], and a characteristic early manifestation, even in children, has been relatively severe hypertension. The epithelial hyperplasia probably causes both the cysts and the increased risk of renal malignancy observed in these patients[10].

Renal cysts and tumours occur also in *von Hippel–Lindau disease*, in which the cyst epithelium is often hyperplastic and sometimes frankly neoplastic. The occurrence of mural nodules of renal cell carcinoma within cysts suggests that the cysts and tumours have a common pathogenesis[10]. The cysts are usually scattered and discrete, although the cysts are sometimes numerous enough to be confused with polycystic kidney disease[27].

4. Glomerulocystic kidney disease

Glomerular cysts occur in many circumstances, sometimes as isolated findings, more often in well characterized syndromes[41] (Table 7.3). Most examples of glomerulocystic disease have occurred in infants, but the abnormality occurs also in adults. The most common association is with early-onset autosomal dominant polycystic kidney disease. Glomerular cysts are commonly present in infants having diffuse cystic disease and either a family history indicating autosomal dominant transmission or a parent having radiographic evidence of typical "adult" polycystic disease (Fig. 7.10). The demonstration by DNA probe analysis of the chromosome 16 gene linkage in both a fetus with glomerulocystic disease and a mother with typical dominant polycystic disease[62] confirms that glomerulocystic kidneys can be the morphologic expression of early-onset ADPKD. Whether the same linkage holds in the majority of cases is still not established. Also unanswered are questions as to whether the morphologic glomerular abnormality persists or undergoes transformation to the more typical pattern of dominant polycystic disease in surviving infants, and whether

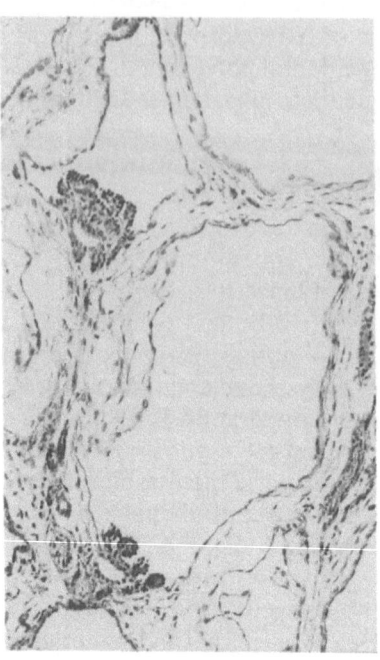

Figure 7.10. Early infantile-onset autosomal dominant polycystic kidney disease. The diffusely cystic kidney of an infant with a family history positive for polycystic disease contains numerous glomerular cysts. Renal cystic disease in the family has all of the features of classical polycystic disease and appears to be inherited as an autosomal dominant. This is the single most common type of glomerulocystic kidney disease. Hematoxylin and eosin, × 94.

Table 7.3. Differential diagnosis of glomerulocystic disease

Autosomal dominant polycystic kidney disease of early infantile onset

Non-syndromal, frequently autosomal dominant glomerulocystic disease

Syndromal glomerulocystic disease
  Major: tuberous sclerosis
         orofaciodigital syndrome, type 1
         brachymesomelia–renal syndrome
  Minor: trisomy 13 syndrome
         Zellweger syndrome

Renal dysplasia

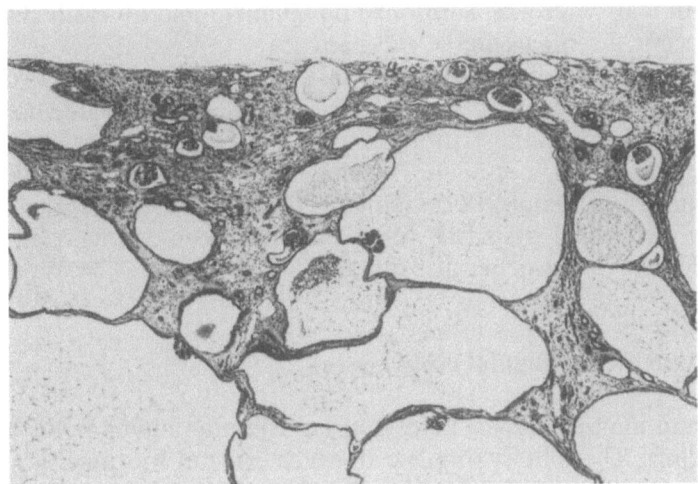

Figure 7.11. Renal involvement in orofaciodigital syndrome. The kidneys were grossly enlarged and diffusely cystic. Sections show the cysts to be concentrated in glomerular spaces, which contain small, relatively ischemic glomerular tufts. Hematoxylin and eosin, × 25.

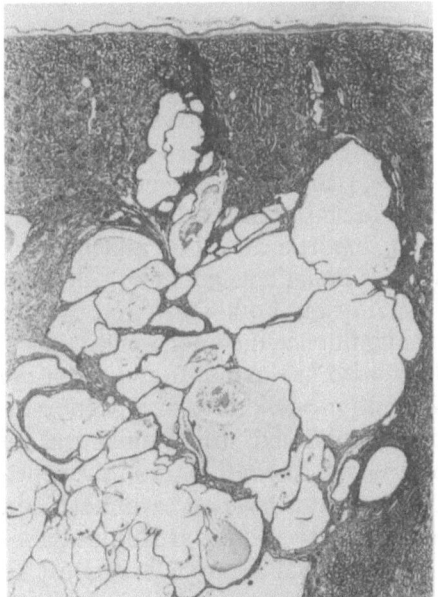

Figure 7.12. Localized cystic kidney disease. One kidney was enlarged, containing an area of cystic transformation microscopically indistinguishable from early involvement in dominant polycystic disease. Microscopic examination shows the cystic area not to be encapsulated, and the cysts are separated by septa of attenuated renal parenchyma. Nonetheless, long-term clinical follow-up failed to show involvement of the other kidney, and the family history was negative for polycystic disease. Hematoxylin and eosin, × 7.5.

adults with non-syndromal autosomal dominant glomerulocystic disease18,63 have the same disease as do the children.

Clear evidence of heterogeneity in glomerulocystic disease comes from the demonstration that significant cystic disease is associated with several malformation syndromes: tuberous sclerosis13,64,72, orofaciodigital syndrome71, and brachymesomelia–renal syndrome49 (Fig. 7.11). Glomerular cysts occur as less important components of trisomy 13 syndrome, Zellweger syndrome and renal dysplasia. Many cases, however, remain as idiopathic glomerulocystic disease, because other associations cannot be identified52,75.

5. Localized and segmental renal cysts

Solitary and multiple *simple renal cysts* are common radiographic and pathologic findings. The solitary simple cyst, which can become quite large, is rarely a problem in differential diagnosis, and the radiographic criteria seem to be well established. Multiple cysts, particularly in middle-aged patients, do present a diagnostic dilemma, namely, the differentiation of non-progressive, non-hereditary cysts from polycystic disease. It hardly seems reasonable merely to resolve the problem simply as polycystic disease, which places a clinical stigma on the patient, but it has undoubtedly been common practice. Most cases of multiple renal cysts are not "early" or incipient polycystic disease, and I doubt very much that these cysts are developmental or congenital. I do think they are acquired, although ascribing them glibly to vascular nephrosclerosis is less than convincing.

Sonography of young people at risk because of family histories of dominant polycystic disease has shown the early changes to consist of isolated and scattered cysts. Greater importance will be attached to a few cysts in such a patient than to a few cysts in patients not at risk. The finding of hepatic cysts and cerebral arterial aneurysms, both known to be associated with polycystic kidney disease, will also influence the interpretation.

Similar difficulties arise in the interpretation of *unilateral* and *localized cystic disease*, in which either one kidney or a portion of one kidney contains multiple cysts. The differentiation of strictly unilateral abnormalities45,50 from polycystic disease must take into consideration the repeated observation that dominant polycystic disease can have an asymmetric onset22. Cystic disease localized to a portion of one kidney is not necessarily familial or progressive20,39, and such segmental abnormalities must be differentiated from multilocular cystadenomas, cystic renal cell carcinomas, and localized cystic renal dysplasia, as well as from dominant polycystic disease (Fig. 7.12). Morphologic examination shows the cysts to be separated by septa of renal parenchyma and the cystic area not to be demarcated or encapsulated. The histopathologic appearance of the cystic lesion strongly resembles the histopathologic appearance of advanced dominant polycystic disease.

6. Acquired renal cystic disease

The development of cysts in the native kidneys of patients with end-stage renal disease of non-cystic cause has been repeatedly confirmed since its description by Dunnill *et al.* [24] barely over a decade ago. Most patients were treated by long-term hemodialysis, and it was quickly obvious that they had acquired renal cysts during the course of their treatment. Subsequent reports have shown that cysts may also occasionally develop in patients treated by peritoneal dialysis, and it appears that the development of cysts correlates directly with the duration of treatment. There has been considerable, unexplained geographic variation in the frequency of acquired cystic disease, but acquired cystic disease is more than a medical curiosity, as the cysts may be associated with hemorrhage, infection and rupture. The cysts are probably secondary to epithelial hyperplasia, and they are often lined with hyperplastic and dysplastic epithelium[10] (Fig. 7.13). The epithelial proliferation may incorporate considerable cytologic atypia, and the proliferations can be regarded as preneoplastic with a high risk of malignancy. The frequency of neoplasia, both benign and malignant, in acquired cystic disease is approximately 20%, and approximately one-quarter of the tumors have been malignant on histopathologic grounds[16,30,31,38]. A few tumors have been clinically malignant.

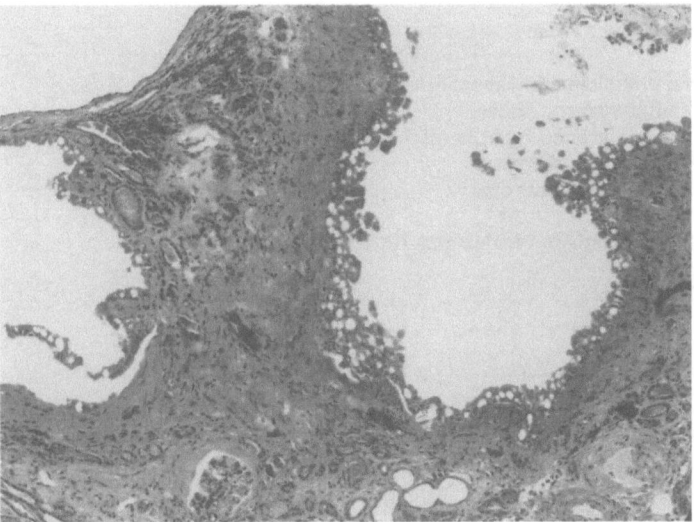

Figure 7.13. Acquired cystic kidney disease. The kidney of a patient under long-term dialysis for renal failure became cystic during treatment. The cysts are lined with hyperplastic and atypical epithelial cells, and multiple epithelial neoplasms were present in the kidney. Hematoxylin and eosin, ×64.

7. Renal medullary cysts

Cystic disorders of the renal medulla include two principal categories, medullary sponge kidney and the uremic medullary cystic diseases, but the differential diagnosis of medullary cysts, as visualized pathologically or radiographically, is somewhat broader (Table 7.4). Dilated medullary ducts, forming small cysts, are also the characteristic feature of autosomal recessive polycystic kidney disease, and they have long been confused with medullary sponge kidney. The literature is replete with examples of this confusion in both children and adults, and the confusion persists in practice. Dilated medullary ducts occur also in Wiedemann–Beckwith syndrome, which has often been labelled as medullary sponge kidney, even though the renal involvement is morphologically a form of medullary dysplasia. Cystic cavitation, frequently re-epithelialized, follows medullary necrosis, renal tuberculosis and nephrolithiasis, constituting a form of acquired medullary cystic disease that can be visualized urographically. Pelvic and calyceal diverticula can also be visualized urographically, and enter the differential diagnosis of medullary cysts.

Table 7.4. Differential diagnosis of medullary cysts

Autosomal recessive polycystic kidney disease

Medullary sponge kidney

Hereditary tubulointerstitial nephritis
    Medullary cystic disease
    Familial juvenile nephronophthisis
    Renal–retinal dysplasia
    Bardet–Biedl syndrome

Medullary dysplasia in Wiedemann–Beckwith syndrome

Medullary necrosis

Pyelogenic cyst

Medullary sponge kidney is predominantly a disease of adults, rarely found in children. It is often regarded as a congenital malformation, but nothing is known of its pathogenesis. Neither a positive family history nor associated hereditary malformations can be identified in the vast majority of cases. The diagnosis is often made as an incidental urographic or sonographic finding in an asymptomatic patient, but complications caused by nephrolithiasis may also lead to the diagnosis[46]. The radiographic findings are customarily diagnostic, despite the confusion with recessive polycystic disease. The condition is usually bilateral; rare cases of unilateral involvement do not necessarily constitute a separate group. There are few histopathologic studies, and the condition seems to be much less common at post-mortem examination than at radiographic examination. The cysts are located in the inner medulla, arising within dilated collecting ducts and reaching a size of 8–10 mm, and are lined with collecting duct epithelium. The ducts contain calcified deposits that become extravasated into the interstitium. Nephrolithiasis occurs in approximately 50% of patients.

The medullary cystic diseases, on the other hand, are heterogeneous, with certain clinical and morphologic features held in common. Despite the frequent emphasis on cysts, the cysts are not regarded as important to the functional abnormality or to the progression of the renal insufficiency. These disorders are better regarded, therefore, as hereditary tubulointerstitial nephritis with three principal subcategories[11]: (1) medullary cystic disease with either sporadic or dominant inheritance and an onset predominantly in adults[29]; (2) familial juvenile nephronophthisis with autosomal recessive inheritance and an onset predominantly in children[77]; and (3) renal–retinal dysplasia with recessive inheritance and retinal degeneration[67]. The same renal abnormality may be associated with cerebellar, skeletal and hepatic abnormalities in different combinations with pigmentary retinopathy[23,77]. Similar renal abnormalities with medullary cysts occur in the Bardet–Biedl syndrome (obesity, mental retardation, retinitis pigmentosa, polydactyly, hypogenitalism)[76] and usually without cysts in Alström syndrome (obesity, blindness, diabetes mellitus, nerve deafness)[33] and in Jeune syndrome (chondrodysplasia with short limbs and narrow chest)[37]. (Jeune syndrome may sometimes be associated with diffuse renal cortical cysts, discussed above.)

The renal abnormality in all of these tubulointerstitial disorders is characterized by urinary concentrating defect and progressive renal insufficiency. Histopathologic examination shows tubular damage out of proportion to glomerular injury. The principal lesions are tubular atrophy with thickening of basement membranes, interstitial and periglomerular fibrosis, and non-specific cellular infiltration. Although the disease is genetically determined, the renal abnormality appears not to be developmental.

8. Renal cystic dysplasia

Renal dysplasia is defined as abnormal parenchymal differentiation. The abnormality is characterized histologically by focal cartilaginous metaplasia of the metanephric blastema and by abnormally differentiated collecting ducts[4]. Abnormal nephronic structures in the form of primitive and rudimentary glomeruli and tubules are also commonly present, but glomerular and tubular alterations can be regressive changes, not necessarily developmental. Dysplastic kidneys are often cystic; conversely, most cystic kidneys in childhood are dysplastic.

Renal dysplasia is frequently associated with obstructive abnormalities of the ureter and lower urinary tract. The frequency of this association and the

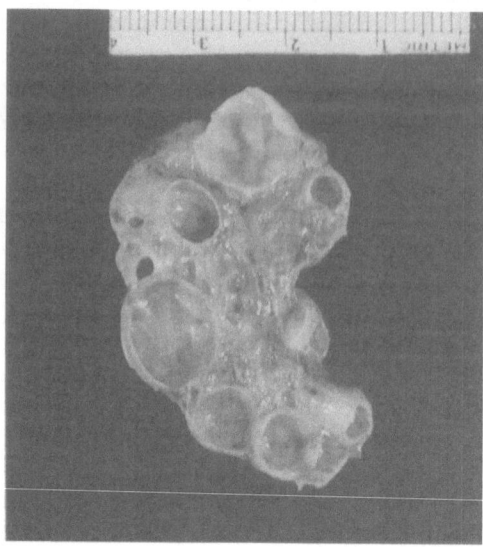

Figure 7.14. Multicystic renal dysplasia. The kidney of a newborn is deformed by multiple cysts that are located predominantly in the periphery of the kidney. The hilar area is solid, with pyelocalyceal occlusion, and the ureter was a thin atretic cord that became detached from the kidney.

relation between renal maldevelopment, on one hand, and the location and severity of the obstructing lesion, on the other, have led us to theorize that dysplasia in such instances is secondary to the urinary tract obstruction[4]. Examples of such associations are cystic dysplasia seen with severe lower urinary tract obstruction, segmental dysplasia seen with renal duplication and ectopic ureterocele and multicystic dysplasia seen with ureteropelvic occlusion. There are many exceptions to the relationship of dysplasia and obstruction; the association holds in about 90% of cases. Renal dysplasia occurs without obstruction in several heritable syndromes of multiple malformation.

The most common form of cystic dysplasia is the enlarged, irregularly and grossly cystic, *multicystic kidney* (Fig. 7.14). The malformation has, in our experience, been invariably associated with ureteropelvic occlusion and ureteral atresia or agenesis, and it is commonly unilateral. The other kidney usually functions well, apart from a relatively high incidence of positional and ureteropelvic abnormalities[44]. Multicystic kidneys are non-functional, but rudimentary lobes of metanephric tissue are usually present and may be visualized by radiographic contrast medium. The kidneys typically contain a central core of relatively solid, dysplastic tissue, with peripherally placed cysts. The cysts can result in considerable renal enlargement and distortion, but the underlying, dysplastic malformation is truly developmental without implication for progressive involvement of the contralateral kidney. Recent serial prenatal

Table 7.5. Diffuse cystic renal dysplasia

Meckel syndrome
    Simopoulos, Goldston and Miranda variants

Jeune syndrome

Zellweger syndrome

Short rib–polydactyly syndrome

Glutaric aciduria, type 2

Renal–hepatic–pancreatic dysplasia

Non-syndromal diffuse cystic dysplasia

---

sonographic studies have shown the multicystic kidney to be in a dynamic state, with changing size and configuration and even complete regression[1,34,57]. Bilateral multicystic dysplasia does occur in newborns and, like agenesis, is a cause of neonatal renal non-function. Multicystic dysplasia is most often a sporadic malformation, but there is a small risk of recurrence because it can be

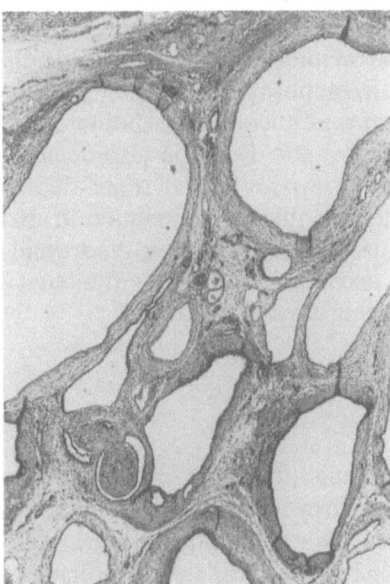

Figure 7.15. Diffuse cystic renal dysplasia. The kidney was reniform in configuration, but gross examination failed to show corticomedullary differentiation. The cortex contains numerous cysts arising in primitive collecting ducts, and there is very little nephronic differentiation. Hematoxylin and eosin, × 20.

a manifestation of the hereditary renal adysplasia syndrome[70]. Syndromal multicystic dysplasia occurs in the VATER association (vertebral defects, anal atresia, tracheo-esophageal fistula, esophageal atresia, radial dysplasia) and the brachio–oto–renal syndrome, and the risks of occurrence are those of the syndromes.

Examples of cystic dysplasia with pyelocalyceal dilatation and lower ureteral occlusion are probably examples of obstructive dysplasia, with cysts in the outer cortex. They are akin to the dysplasia of "giant hydronephrosis" secondary to ureteropelvic obstruction and to the dysplasia with hydrone-phrosis secondary to posterior urethral valves and urethral atresia.

The other principal form of cystic dysplasia is diffuse and non-obstructive, commonly occurring in heritable malformation syndromes (Table 7.5) (Fig. 7.15). The best known is *Meckel syndrome* (microcephaly, posterior encepha-locele, polydactyly, cleft palate and lip, genital abnormalities and hepatic cysts). The brain abnormalities in other closely related syndromes with diffuse renal cystic dysplasia include hydrocephalus (Simopoulos syndrome), Dandy–Wal-ker malformation (Goldston syndrome), and cerebral dysgenesis (Miranda syndrome). Each also includes biliary dysgenesis, an abnormality with a strong resemblance to the hepatic lesion of ARPKD. The similarity has been a source of considerable confusion in evaluating individual cases, but the kidneys are clearly dysplastic and different from those in polycystic disease.

Bilateral cystic dysplasia occurs in *Jeune syndrome* of asphyxiating thoracic dystrophy. The syndrome is actually associated with a spectrum of renal abnor-malities including cortical microcysts, diffuse cystic disease, generalized cystic dysplasia and progressive nephropathy. Similarly, the renal lesion in *Zellweger's cerebrohepatorenal syndrome* encompasses both minor microcystic changes and severe dysplasia. Diffuse cystic dysplasia also occurs in short rib–polydactyly syndrome, glutaric aciduria type 2, and renal–hepatic–pancreatic dysplasia. The renal abnormalities are qualitatively similar in all of them. All of them also include biliary dysgenesis. Isolated or non-syndromal diffuse cystic dysplasia, sometimes with only accompanying biliary dysgenesis, is a rare occurrence; nonetheless, it is probably a recessive trait.

9. Extraparenchymal cysts

This last category is straightforward and requires no special explanations. Pyelogenic cyst, peripelvic cyst and calyceal diverticulum are all synonymous, the last being most accurately descriptive of the abnormality. Parapelvic cyst is often used synonymously with parapelvic lymphatic and parapelvic lymphan-giectasia. Parapelvic lymphangiectasia is common in transplanted kidneys, secondary to lymphatic obstruction. The perinephric cyst is a collection of fluid around the kidney, known variously as hygroma perirenalis, perirenal effusion, hydrocele renalis, and pararenal pseudocyst. Perinephric cysts in childhood are usually subcapsular effusions secondary to urinary tract obstruction. They may in adults lie between the capsule and renal cortex, or between the capsule and perinephric fat. They are believed to result principally from extravasation of urine secondary either to trauma or urinary obstruction.

References

1. Avni EF, Thoua Y, Lalmand B, Didier F, Droulle P and Schulman CC. Multicystic dysplastic kidney: Evolving concepts. *In utero* diagnosis and post-natal follow-up by ultrasound. Annals of Radiology (Paris) 1986, 29, 663–668.
2. Bartman I and Barraclough G. Cystic dysplasia of the kidneys studied by microdissection in a case of 13–15 trisomy. Journal of Pathology 1965, 89, 233–238.
3. Bernstein J. A classification of renal cysts. In: Gardner KD Jr, ed., Cystic Diseases of the Kidney. New York: John Wiley & Sons Publishers, 1976, 7–30.
4. Bernstein J. Developmental abnormalities of the renal parenchyma: Renal hypoplasia and dysplasia. In: Sommers SC, ed., Pathology Annual 1968. New York: Appleton Century Crofts Publishers, 1968, 213–247.
5. Bernstein J. Hepatic and renal involvement in malformation syndromes. Mount Sinai Journal of Medicine 1986, 53, 421–428.
6. Bernstein J. Hepatic involvement in hereditary renal syndromes. In: Bergsma D, ed., Birth Defects: Original Article Series. New York: March of Dimes Birth Defects Foundation Publishers, 1987, 23, 115–130.
7. Bernstein J. Heritable cystic disorders of the kidney: The mythology of polycystic disease. Pediatric Clinics of North America 1971, 18, 435–444.
8. Bernstein J. The classification of renal cysts. Nephron 1973, 11, 91–100.
9. Bernstein J, Brough AJ and McAdams AJ. The renal lesion in syndromes of multiple congenital malformations: cerebrohepatorenal syndrome; Jeune asphyxiating thoracic dystrophy; tuberous sclerosis; Meckel syndrome. In: Bergsma D, ed., The Fifth Conference on the Clinical Delineation of Birth Defects. Birth Defects: Original Article Series. Baltimore: Williams & Wilkins Publishers, 1945, X/4, 35–43.
10. Bernstein J, Evan AP and Gardner KD Jr. Epithelial hyperplasia in polycystic kidney diseases. Its role in pathogenesis and risk of neoplasia. American Journal of Pathology 1987, 129, 92–101.
11. Bernstein J and Gardner KD Jr. Hereditary tubulo–interstitial nephropathies. Chap. 12. In: Cotran RS, Brenner BM and Stein JH, eds, Contemporary Issues in Nephrology. New York: Churchill Livingstone Publishers, 1983, 335–357.
12. Bernstein J and Meyer R. Parenchymal maldevelopment of the kidney. Chap. 26. In: Kelley VC, ed., Brennemann's Practice of Pediatrics, Vol. 3. Hagerstown, MD: Harper & Row Publishers, 1967, 1–30.
13. Bernstein J, Robbins TO and Kissane JM. The renal lesions of tuberous sclerosis. Seminars in Diagnostic Pathology 1986, 3, 97–105.
14. Bernstein J, Stickler GB and Neel IV. Congenital hepatic fibrosis. Evolving morphology. APMIS 1988 Suppl. 4, 96, 17–26.
15. Blyth H and Ockenden BG. Polycystic disease of kidneys and liver presenting in childhood. Journal of Medical Genetics 1971, 8, 257–284.
16. Bretan PN Jr, Busch MP, Hricak H and Williams RD. Chronic renal failure: A significant risk factor in the development of acquired renal cysts and renal cell carcinoma. Case reports and reviews of the literature. Cancer 1986, 57, 1871–1879.
17. Caroli J, Couinaud C, Soupault R, Porcher R and Etévé J. Une affection nouvelle, sans doute congénitale, des voies biliaires. La dilatation kystique unilobaire des canaux hépatiques. Semaine des Hopitaux de Paris 1958, 34, 496–502.

168

18. Carson RW, Bedi D, Cavallo T and DuBose TD Jr. Familial adult glomerulocystic kidney disease. American Journal of Kidney Diseases 1987, 9, 154–165.
19. Chilton SJ and Cremin BJ. The spectrum of polycystic disease in children. Pediatric Radiology 1981, 11, 9–15.
20. Cho KJ, Thornbury JR, Bernstein J, Heidelberger KP and Walter JF. Localized cystic disease of the kidney: Angiographic–pathologic correlation. American Journal of Roentgenology 1979, 132, 891–895.
21. Churg J, Bernstein J, Risdon RA and Sobin LH, eds, Renal Disease: Classification and Atlas. Part II. Developmental and hereditary diseases. New York: Igaku-Shoin Publishers, 1987, 115–263.
22. Dalgaard OZ. Bilateral polycystic disease of the kidneys: A follow-up study of 284 patients and their families. Acta Medica Scandinavica 1957, 158, (Suppl 328), 1–255.
23. Donaldson MDC, Warner AA, Trompeter RS, Haycock GB and Chantler C. Familial juvenile nephronophthisis, Jeune's syndrome, and associated disorders. Archives of Diseases in Childhood 1985, 60, 426–434.
24. Dunnill MS, Millard PR and Oliver D. Acquired cystic disease of the kidneys: A hazard of long-term intermittent maintenance hemodialysis. Journal of Clinical Pathology 1977, 30, 868–877.
25. Elias H. Three dimensional structure identified from single sections. Science 1971, 174, 993–1000.
26. Elkin M and Bernstein J. Cystic diseases of the kidney. Radiological and pathological considerations. Clinical Radiology 1969, 20, 65–82.
27. Frimodt-Møller P, Nissen HM and Dyreborg U. Polycystic kidneys as the renal lesion in Lindau's diseases. Journal of Urology 1981, 125, 868–870.
28. Gang DL and Herrin JT. Infantile polycystic disease of the liver and kidneys. Clinical Nephrology 1986, 25, 28–36.
29. Gardner KD Jr. Juvenile nephronophthisis and renal medullary cystic disease. In: Gardner KD Jr, ed., Cystic Diseases of the Kidney. New York: John Wiley & Sons Publishers, 1976, 173–185.
30. Gardner KD Jr and Evan AP. Cystic kidneys: An enigma evolves. American Journal of Kidney Diseases 1984, 3, 403–413.
31. Gehrig JJ Jr, Gottheiner TI and Swenson RS. Acquired cystic disease of the end-stage kidney. American Journal of Medicine 1985, 79, 609–620.
32. Gleason DG, McAlister WH and Kissane J. Cystic diseases of the kidney in children. American Journal of Roentgenology 1967, 100, 135–146.
33. Goldstein JL and Fialkow PJ. The Alström syndrome: Report of three cases with further delineation of the clinical, pathophysiological, and genetic aspects of the disorder. Medicine 1973, 52, 53–71.
34. Hashimoto BE, Filly RA and Callen PW. Multicystic dysplastic kidney in utero: Changing appearance on US. Radiology 1986, 159, 107–109.
35. Heggö O and Natvig JB. Cystic disease of the kidneys. Autopsy report and family study. Acta Pathologica Microbiologica Scandinavica 1965, 61, 459–469.
36. Helczynski L, Wells TR, Landing BH and Lipsey AI. The renal lesion of congenital hepatic fibrosis: Pathologic and morphometric analysis, with comparison to the renal lesion of infantile polycystic disease. Pediatric Pathology 1984, 2, 441–445.
37. Herdman RC and Langer LO. The thoracic asphyxiant dystrophy and renal disease. American Journal of Diseases in Childhood 1968, 116, 192–201.
38. Hughson MD, Buchwald D and Fox M. Renal neoplasia and acquired cystic kidney disease in patients receiving long-term dialysis. Archives of Pathology and Laboratory Medicine 1986, 110, 592–601.
39. Hutchins KR, Mulholland SG and Edson M. Segmental polycystic disase. New York State Journal of Medicine 1972, 72, 1850–1852.
40. Jørgensen M. The ductal plate malformation. Acta Pathologica Microbiologica Immunologica Scandinavica [A] 1977, Suppl 257, 1–88.

41. Joshi VV and Kasznica J. Clinicopathologic spectrum of glomerulocystic kidneys. Report of two cases and a brief review of literature. Pediatric Pathology 1984, 2, 171–186.

42. Kaplan BS, Kaplan P, de Chadarevian J-P, Jequier S, O'Regan S and Russo P. Variable expression of autosomal recessive polycystic kidney disease and congenital hepatic fibrosis within a family. American Journal of Medical Genetics 1988, 29, 639–647.

43. Kaplan BS, Rabin I, Nogrady MB and Drummond KN. Autosomal dominant polycystic renal disease in children. Journal of Pediatrics 1977, 90, 782–783.

44. Kleiner B, Filly RA, Mack L and Callen PW. Multicystic dysplastic kidney: Observations of contralateral disease in the fetal population. Radiology 1986, 161, 27–29.

45. Kossow AS and Meek JM. Unilateral adult polycystic kidney disease. Journal of Urology 1982, 127, 297–300.

46. Kuiper JJ. Medullary sponge kidney. In: Gardner KD Jr, ed., Cystic Diseases of the Kidney. New York: John Wiley & Sons Publishers 1976, 151–171.

47. Landing BH, Wells TR and Claireaux AE. Morphometric analysis of the liver lesions in cystic diseases of childhood. Human Pathology 1980, 11, 549–560.

48. Landing BH, Wells TR, Reed GB and Narayan MS. Diseases of the bile ducts in children. In: Gall EA and Mostofi FK, eds, The Liver, Chap. 22. Baltimore: Williams & Wilkins Publishers 1973, 480–509.

49. Langer LO Jr, Nishino R, Yamaguchi A, Ito Y, Ueke T, Togari H, Kato T, Opitz JM and Gilbert EG. Brachymesomelia–renal syndrome. American Journal of Medical Genetics 1983, 15, 57–65.

50. Lee JKT, McClennan BL and Kissane JM. Unilateral polycystic kidney disease. American Journal of Roentgenology 1978, 130, 1165–1167.

51. Lieberman E, Salinas-Madrigal L, Gwinn JL, Brennan LP, Fine RN and Landing BH. Infantile polycystic disease of the kidneys and liver: Clinical pathological and radiological correlations and comparison with congenital hepatic fibrosis. Medicine 1971, 50, 277–318.

52. Melnick SC, Brewer DB and Oldham JS. Cortical microcystic disease of the kidney with dominant inheritance: A previously undescribed syndrome. Journal of Clinical Pathology 1984, 37, 494–499.

53. Mitnick JS, Bosniak MA, Hilton S, Raghavendra BN, Subramanyam B and Genieser NB. Cystic renal disease in tuberous sclerosis. Radiology 1983, 147, 85–87.

54. Mottet NK and Jensen H. The anomalous embryonic development associated with trisomy 13-15. American Journal of Clinical Pathology 1965, 43, 334–347.

55. Okada RD, Platt MA and Fleishman J. Chronic renal failure in patients with tuberous sclerosis: Association with renal cysts. Nephron 1982, 30, 85–88.

56. Passarge E and McAdams AJ. Cerebro–hepato–renal syndrome: A newly recognized hereditary disorder of multiple congenital defects, including sudanophilic leukodystrophy, cirrhosis of the liver, and polycystic kidneys. Journal of Pediatrics 1967, 71, 691–702.

57. Pedicelli G, Jequier S, Bowen A'D and Boisvert J. Multicystic dysplastic kidneys: Spontaneous regression demonstrated with US. Radiology 1986, 160, 23–26.

58. Potter EL, ed., Normal and Abnormal Development of the Kidney. Chicago: Year Book Publishers, 1972.

59. Poznanski AK, Nosanchuk JS, Baublis J and Holt JF. The cerebro–hepato–renal syndrome (CHRS); (Zellweger's syndrome). American Journal of Roentgenology 1970, 109, 313–322.

60. Reeders ST, Breuning MH, Corney G, Jeremiah SJ, Meera Khan P, Davies KE, Hopkinson DA, Pearson PL and Weatherall DJ. Two genetic markers closely linked to adult polycystic kidney disease on chromosome 16. British Medical Journal 1986, 292, 851–853.

61. Reeders ST, Breuning MH, Davies KE, Nicholls ED, Jarman AP, Higgs DR, Pearson PL and Weatherall DJ. A highly polymorphic DNA marker linked to adult polycystic kidney disease on chromosome 16. Nature 1985, 317, 542–544.

62. Reeders ST, Zerres K, Gal A, Hogenkamp T, Propping P, Schmidt W, Waldherr R, Dolata

MM, Davies KE and Weatherall DJ. Prenatal diagnosis of autosomal dominant polycystic kidney disease with a DNA probe. Lancet 1986, 2, 6–8.

63. Rizzoni G, Loriat C, Levy M, Milanesi C, Zachello G and Mathieu H. Familial hypoplastic glomerulocystic kidney. A new entity? Clinical Nephrology 1982, 18, 263–268.

64. Rolfes DB, Towbin R and Bove KE. Vascular dysplasia in a child with tuberous sclerosis. Pediatric Pathology 1985, 3, 359–373.

65. Romeo G, Devoto M, Costa G, Roncuzzi L, Catizone L, Zucchelli P, Germino GG, Keith T, Weatherall DJ and Reeders ST. A second genetic locus for autosomal dominant polycystic kidney disease. Lancet 1988, 2, 8–11.

66. Sedman A, Bell P, Manco-Johnson M, Schrier R, Warady BA, Heard EO, Butler-Simon N and Gabow P. Autosomal dominant polycystic kidney disease in childhood: A longitudinal study. Kidney International 1987, 31, 1000–1005.

67. Senior B. Familial renal–retinal dystrophy. American Journal of Diseases in Children 1973, 125, 442–447.

68. Smith DW, Opitz JM and Inhorn SL. A syndrome of multiple developmental defects including polycystic kidneys and intrahepatic biliary dysgenesis in two siblings. Journal of Pediatrics 1965, 67, 617–624.

69. Spence HM and Singleton R. Cysts and cystic disorders of the kidney: Types, diagnosis, treatment. Urological Survey 1972, 22, 131–158.

70. Squiers EC, Morden RS and Bernstein J. Renal multicystic dysplasia. An occasional manifestation of the hereditary renal adysplasia syndrome. American Journal of Medical Genetics 1987, Suppl 3, 279–284.

71. Stapleton FB, Bernstein J, Koh G, Roy S, III and Wilroy RS. Cystic kidneys in a patient with oral–facial–digital syndrome type I. American Journal of Kidney Diseases 1982, 1, 288–293.

72. Stapleton FB, Johnson D, Kaplan GW and Griswold W. The cystic renal lesion in tuberous sclerosis. Journal of Pediatrics 1980, 97, 574–579.

73. Stillwell TJ, Gomez MR and Kelalis PP. Renal lesions in tuberous sclerosis. Journal of Urology 1987, 138, 477–481.

74. Taitz LS, Brown CB, Blank CE and Steiner GM. Screening for polycystic kidney disease: Importance of clinical presentation in the newborn. Archives of Diseases in Childhood 1987, 62, 45–49.

75. Taxy JB and Filmer RB. Glomerulocystic kidney. Report of a case. Archives of Pathology and Laboratory Medicine 1976, 100, 186–188.

76. Tieder M, Levy M, Gubler MC, Gagnadoux MF and Broyer M. Renal abnormalities in the Bardet–Biedl syndrome. International Journal of Pediatric Nephrology 1982, 3, 199–203.

77. Waldherr R, Lennert T, Weber H-P, Födish HJ and Schärer K. The nephronophthisis complex. A clinicopathologic study in children. Virchows Archiv [Pathol Anat] 1982, 394, 235–254.

8
Radiology of Cystic Kidneys

E. Levine and J.J. Grantham

Abstract

Radiographic techniques that may be used in the evaluation of cystic kidneys include excretory urography, radionuclide scintigraphy, ultrasound, computed tomography (CT), magnetic resonance imaging and renal angiography. Of these, CT and ultrasound have had a most dramatic effect on diagnosis of renal cystic disease and these techniques are emphasized in this chapter. Many types of cystic kidneys demonstrate similar CT and sonographic features. Meticulous attention to subtle radiographic finding is, therefore, essential for reaching a correct diagnosis. Also, radiographic findings should always be carefully correlated with clinical features such as patient age, family history, symptoms, physical findings and renal functional status before a diagnosis is attempted. Radiographic features that require analysis include whether cysts are unilateral or bilateral, renal size and functional status, cyst distribution in the kidneys, and presence of hemorrhagic and calcified renal cysts, solid renal masses, extraparenchymal renal cysts and cysts in adjacent organs. We describe the most common radiographic patterns of the various disorders and an optimal imaging approach for each type of cystic disorder is suggested. Conditions described include renal cortical cysts, multicystic dysplastic kidney, hereditary polycystic kidney disease, cystic kidneys in hereditary syndromes, renal medullary cystic disorders, acquired renal cystic disease, cystic renal neoplasms, unilateral renal cystic disease and extraparenchymal renal cysts.

Key words   Computed tomography;
Kidney;
Cysts;
Ultrasound.

1. Introduction

Cystic kidneys are associated with a variety of diseases. Radiographic studies, particularly computed tomography (CT) and sonography, have made significant contributions to their evaluation. However, radiographic findings *per se* are seldom diagnostic in renal cystic disease and need to be interpreted with knowledge of patient age, family history, symptoms, clinical findings and renal functional status. In this chapter, we discuss the radiographic findings in each of the common renal cystic diseases, and describe how each condition may be distinguished from other disorders with similar findings. We also indicate those radiographic techniques most likely to help in evaluating each type of cystic disease.

Because sonography is quick, sensitive and relatively inexpensive, and because it does not involve the use of intravenous contrast material or ionizing radiation, it is an excellent technique for evaluating many cystic renal disorders, particularly in infants and children. Its main limitation is marked dependency on the skill of the sonographer. CT with contrast enhancement is not operator-dependent, and it provides an excellent method of evaluating most cystic renal disorders. However, it should be avoided in patients with significant renal functional impairment. With the availability of sonography and CT, excretory urography and angiography now have limited roles in evaluating patients with renal cystic diseases. Although magnetic resonance imaging has been applied by some investigators in the study of renal cystic disease, it is an expensive and time-consuming technique that does not usually add information to that provided by sonography and CT. We, therefore, think that it is rarely needed in renal cystic disease and no further discussion of this test will be provided.

Although many cystic kidneys are radiographically indistinguishable from each other, there are certain radiographic findings that help greatly in reaching a diagnosis or differential diagnosis in any individual patient. Questions that should be addressed in reviewing radiographic findings should always include the following:

(1) Are renal cysts unilateral or bilateral?
(2) Are the kidneys small, normal in size or enlarged?
(3) Do cysts affect both the renal cortex and medulla?
(4) Are there cysts in the renal sinus and perinephric tissues?
(5) Are cysts uniformly distributed throughout a kidney or are they localized to part of a kidney?
(6) What is the functional status of the affected kidney or kidneys as determined by excretory urography, radionuclide scans or contrast-enhanced CT?
(7) Do any cysts show evidence of hemorrhage or calcification?
(8) Do the kidneys exhibit solid masses in addition to cysts?
(9) Are there extrarenal cysts involving such organs as the liver, spleen and pancreas?

If an attempt is made to answer all these questions in reviewing abdominal scans, and the radiographic findings are correlated with clinical information, a correct diagnosis of the cystic disorder is usually possible.

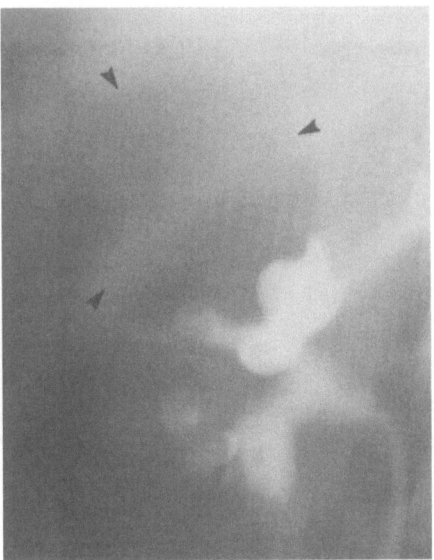

Figure 8.1 Simple cyst (arrowheads) in upper pole of right kidney shown on nephrotomogram during excretory urography. Note low density, sharply defined, smooth, spherical outline and thin wall where cyst protrudes beyond confines of kidney.

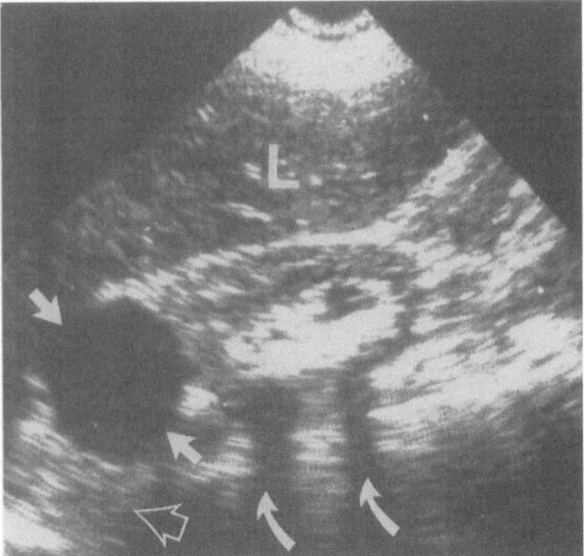

Figure 8.2 Simple cyst (arrows) in upper pole of right kidney demonstrated on longitudinal sonogram. Criteria for diagnosis include absence of internal echoes, spherical outline, sharply marginated, smooth walls and good sound transmission through cyst with resultant posterior acoustical enhancement (open arrow). High amplitude calculi in collecting system cause posterior acoustic shadowing (curved arrows). L = liver.

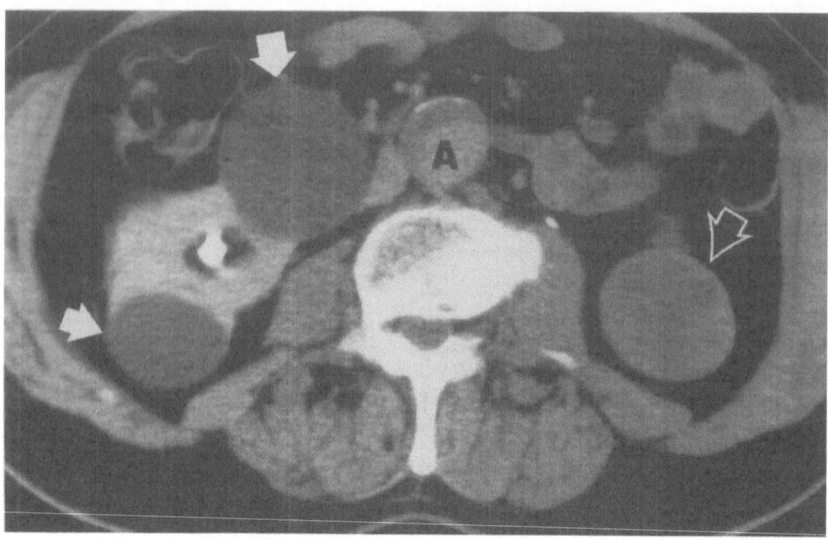

Figure 8.3 Simple cysts (arrows) in right kidney show distinct margins, smooth, round or oval outlines, thin walls and fluid densities (6 and 9 HU). Compare with cystic renal cell carcinoma (open arrow) in left kidney demonstrating thick, irregular wall and attenuation value of 24 HU. A = aortic aneurysm.

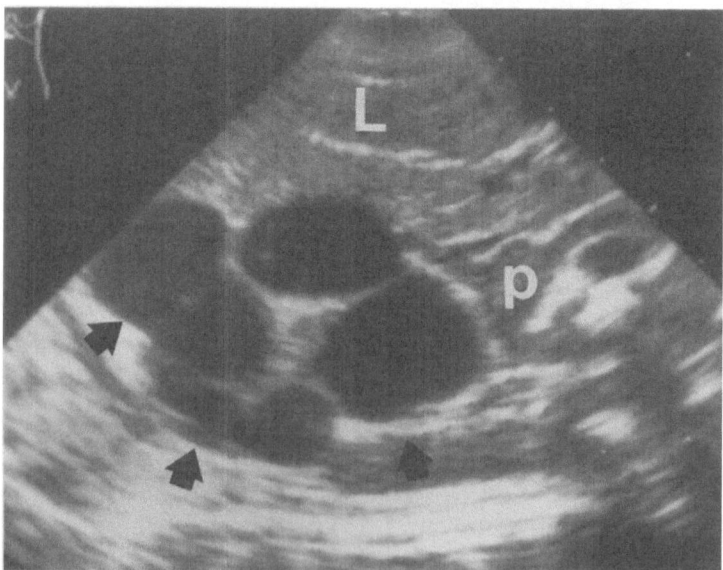

Figure 8.4 Multicystic dysplasia in 3-day-old male shown on transverse sonogram of right kidney (arrows). Note several, variable-sized non-communicating renal cysts. Left kidney was normal. L = liver, p = pancreas.

2. Renal cortical cysts

Simple renal cyst

Simple cysts are the most common renal masses. They may be solitary or multiple and are frequently bilateral. Most are asymptomatic and are discovered incidentally on radiographic studies. Although the diagnosis of simple cyst may be suggested by urographic findings (Fig. 8.1), the diagnosis should be confirmed by sonography or CT which have almost 100% accuracy if all diagnostic criteria are fulfilled[41,48]. Sonographic criteria of a renal cyst include absence of internal echoes, a spherical outline, a sharply marginated, smooth wall and good sound transmission through the mass with resultant posterior acoustical enhancement (Fig. 8.2)[48]. CT criteria of a simple cyst include a smooth, round or oval outline, distinct delineation from adjoining renal parenchyma, no discernible wall thickness, a homogeneous low attenuation value (0–20 Hounsfield units) and no enhancement after intravenous contrast administration (Fig. 8.3)[41]. Simple cysts may also be diagnosed by magnetic resonance imaging, although the accuracy of this test is unknown. Cyst hemorrhage and infection cause atypical sonographic or CT features that may resemble findings in cystic renal neoplasms.

2.2. Glomerulocystic kidney disease (GCKD)

GCKD is a bilateral renal cystic disease that is confined to the renal cortex. Pathologically there are multiple cystic dilatations of Bowman's space containing abortive glomeruli[6]. The condition has been described mainly in infants and children, but may first be diagnosed in young adults[6]. Infants with GCKD sonographically show bilateral nephromegaly, diffuse increase in renal echogenicity and loss of normal demarcation between the renal sinus, medulla and cortex[14,62]. Macroscopic renal cortical cysts are sometimes found[5]. These findings are indistinguishable from those of both ARPKD and ADPKD occurring in infants, and renal biopsy may be necessary for differentiation[5,14,62]. In adults with GCKD, the kidneys are usually normal in size on sonography and there are multiple bilateral small cortical cysts that do not distort the renal contour[6]. Distinction from early ADPKD is usually not possible sonographically and biopsy may be necessary for differentiation[6].

3. Multicystic dysplastic kidney (MDK)

MDK is the most common form of cystic disease in infants, usually presenting as an asymptomatic flank mass. The disorder is associated with ureteral atresia and may be unilateral or bilateral[52]. The unilateral type is more often en-

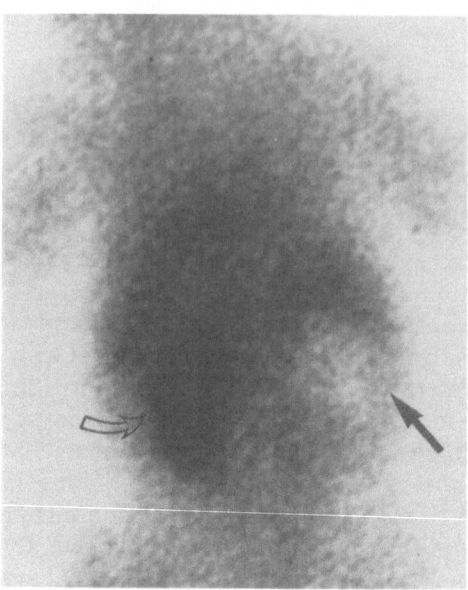

Figure 8.5 Multicystic dysplasia of right kidney in 4-day-old female. Posterior blood-pool image of technetium-99m DTPA scintiscan exhibits photopenic area in right renal fossa (arrow). Left kidney (curved arrow) shows normal tracer activity.

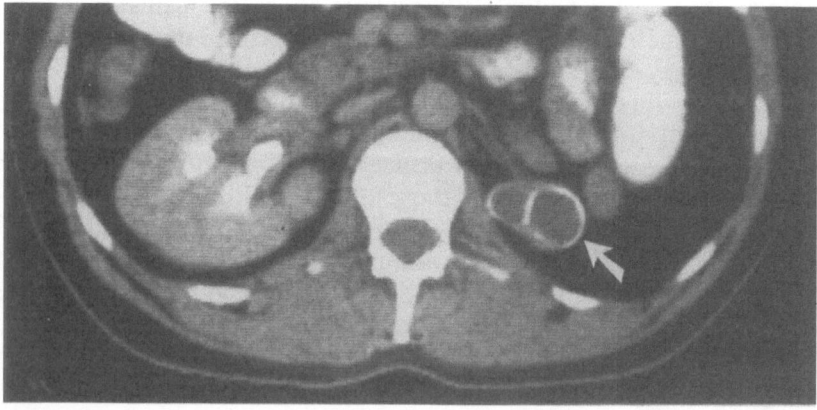

Figure 8.6 Multicystic dysplasia of left kidney in 27-year-old man with microscopic hematuria. CT shows small left kidney composed of cysts with mural calcification (arrow) and compensatory hypertrophy of right kidney.

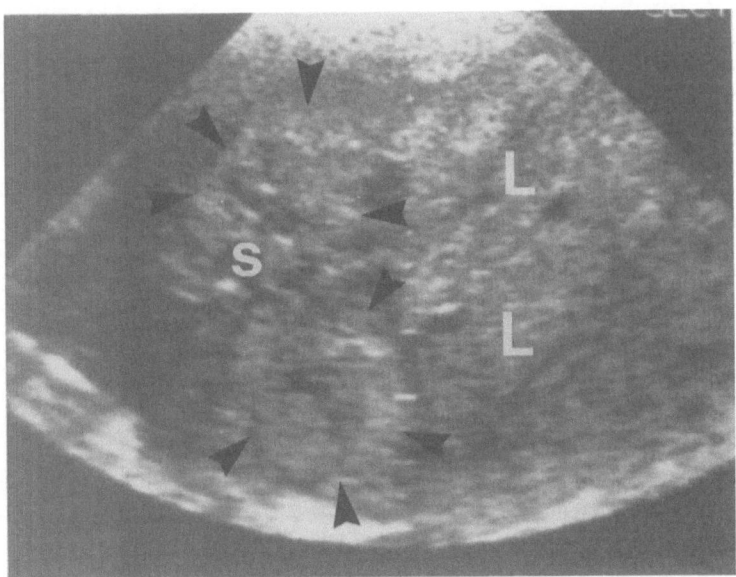

Figure 8.7 Fetal autosomal recessive polycystic kidney disease. Transverse sonogram of fetal abdomen at 26 weeks of gestational age reveals enlarged, diffusely hyperechoic kidneys (arrowheads). s = spine, L = liver.

countered clinically. MDK may be diagnosed by fetal sonography[25,40]. Post-natally, MDK is best evaluated by sonography which shows two types[56]. The classic type (pelvo–infundibular atresia) shows no discernible renal pelvis. The kidney may be small, normal in size or enlarged and contains multiple variable-sized, renal cysts that usually do not communicate (Fig. 8.4)[51]. The hydronephrotic form of the disorder is characterized by dilatation of the renal pelvis and calyces. Differentiation of this type of MDK from simple hydronephrosis is based on the sonographic demonstration of parenchymal cysts that do not communicate with the collecting system[40,46,51].

If sonography suggests the diagnosis of MDK, renal scintigraphy should be done next[56]. Typically this shows non-perfusion of the affected kidney (Fig. 8.5)[56]. Significant contralateral hydronephrosis occurs in about 10% of cases of MDK, and may be secondary to ureteropelvic junction obstruction, ureteral stenosis or vesicoureteric reflux[60]. Accordingly, the contralateral kidney requires evaluation by excretory urography[25,56]. MDK may occasionally first be detected in adults (Fig. 8.6). Many patients with MDK are managed non-surgically and these should be followed by serial sonography[60]. The affected kidney may remain unchanged, but frequently undergoes spontaneous regression[46,60].

178

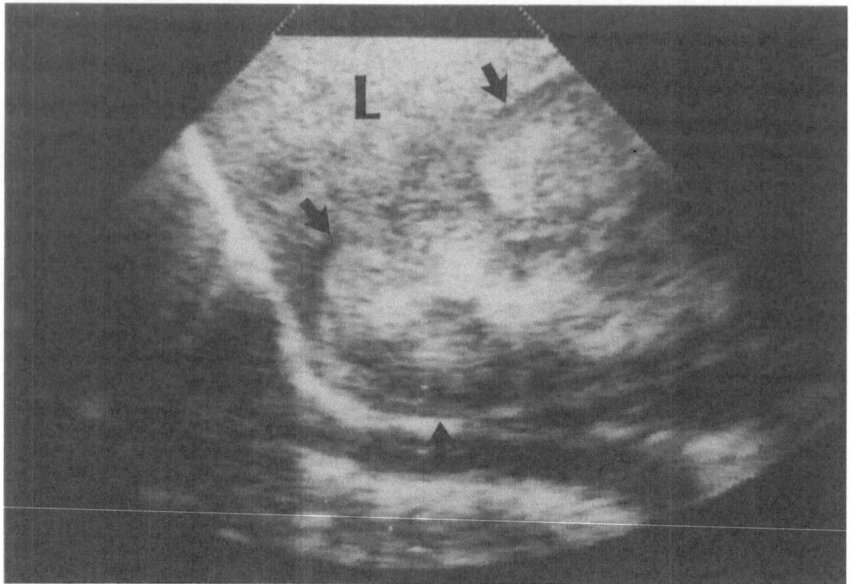

Figure 8.8 Autosomal recessive polycystic kidney disease in neonate with severe respiratory distress and palpable flank masses. Longitudinal sonogram shows markedly enlarged and hyperechoic right kidney (arrows) with loss of delineation between cortex, medulla and sinus. Patient died of respiratory failure 4 days after birth. L = liver.

4. Polycystic kidney disease

Hereditary polycystic kidney disease may be transmitted as an autosomal recessive or autosomal dominant trait.

4.1. Autosomal recessive polycystic kidney disease (ARPKD)

ARPKD is characterized by ectasia of the renal collecting tubules, and variable degrees of portal hepatic fibrosis (congenital hepatic fibrosis) often resulting in portal hypertension[7]. The disorder may be diagnosed by fetal sonography as early as 17 weeks' gestational age (Fig. 8.7)[18]. Impaired function in the fetal kidneys results in severe oligohydramnios and absence of urine in the fetal bladder[15,18]. Neonates with severe ARPKD frequently manifest pulmonary hypoplasia and succumb to pulmonary insufficiency in the first few days of life[18]. Sonography is the best technique for evaluation and shows enlarged, hyperechoic kidneys (Fig. 8.8). The increased echogenicity probably results from reflection of sound waves by innumerable dilated tubules[5].

Patients with milder renal involvement may present at any age from infancy to early adulthood. Excretory urography shows medullary striations

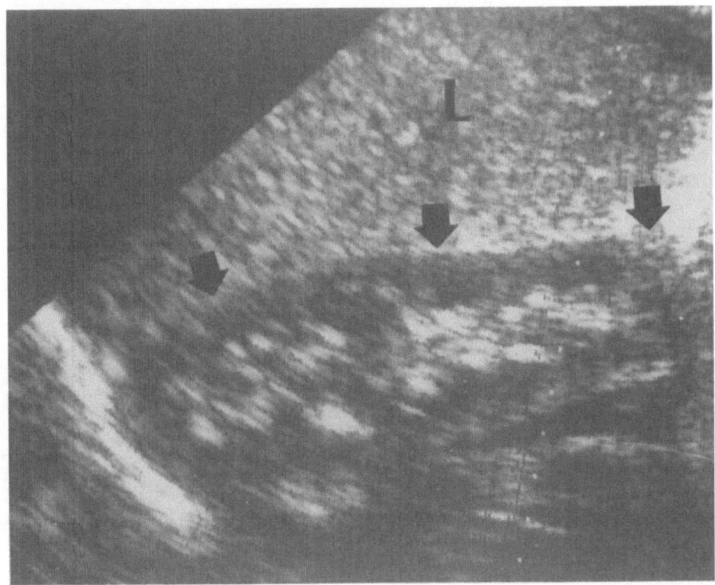

Figure 8.9 Autosomal recessive polycystic kidney disease in 23-year-old man with congenital hepatic fibrosis. Blood urea nitrogen = 17 mg/dl; serum creatinine = 1.2 mg/dl. Longitudinal sonogram of mildly enlarged right kidney (arrows) shows increased echogenicity of renal medulla owing to tubular ectasia. Renal cortical echogenicity is normal. L = liver.

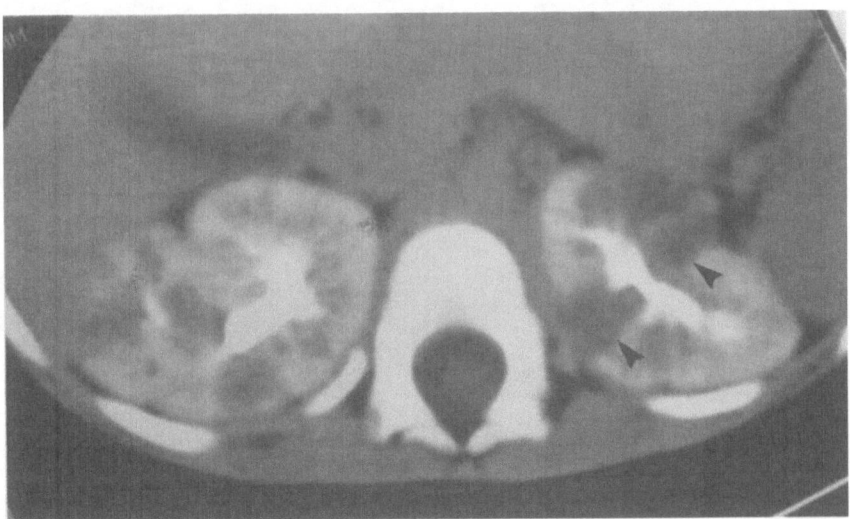

Figure 8.10 Autosomal recessive polycystic kidney disease in 30-month-old female with normal renal function. CT shows dilated collecting ducts in renal medulla bilaterally and relative preservation of renal cortex. Note macroscopic cysts (arrowheads) in left kidney.

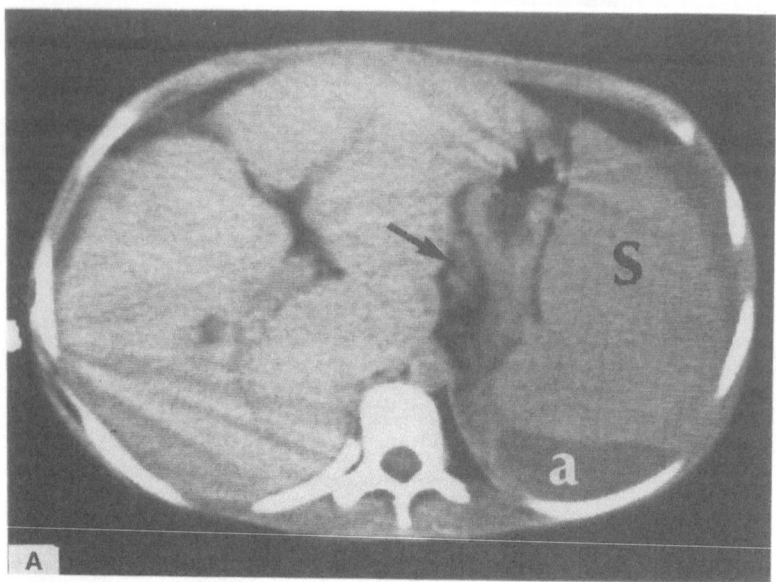

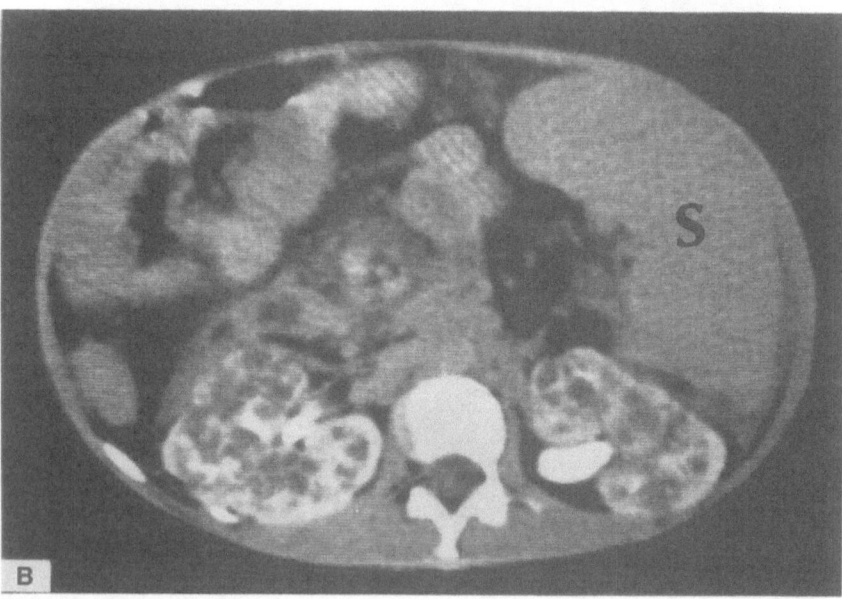

Figure 8.11 Autosomal recessive polycystic kidney disease in 14-year-old female (sister of patient in Fig. 8.9). Blood urea nitrogen = 13 mg/dl; serum creatinine = 0.7 mg/dl. (A) CT shows liver contour irregularity owing to congenital hepatic fibrosis. Spleen (S) is enlarged because of portal hypertension. Note ascites (a) and enlarged left gastric vein (arrow) in hepatogastric ligament. (B) More caudal scan shows mild nephromegaly and multiple medullary cysts with relative preservation of renal cortex. S = spleen. (From Levine E, CRC Critical Reviews in Diagnostic Imaging 1985, 24, 91–200. Copyright, Boca Raton, Florida: CRC Press Inc. With permission.)

owing to tubular ectasia[42]. On sonography, the kidneys are mildly enlarged and show increased medullary echogenicity with normally echogenic renal cortex (Fig. 8.9)[42]. On contrast-enhanced CT, renal tubular ectasia is mainly confined to the renal medulla with only occasional discernible macrocysts (Fig. 8.10). CT may also show evidence of congenital hepatic fibrosis and portal hypertension. The liver contour is often irregular and ascites, splenomegaly and enlarged portal–systemic collateral veins may be seen (Fig. 8.11). Liver cysts are not usually evident. However, some patients show large hepatic cysts of biliary origin due to the presence of Caroli disease[12].

Nephromegaly and increased renal echogenicity on sonography during infancy are not specific for ARPKD and may occur in several other conditions, including infantile autosomal dominant polycystic kidney disease (ADPKD), glomerulocystic kidney disease and renal lymphangiectasia[4,62]. An autosomal dominant pattern of inheritance suggests the diagnosis of infantile ADPKD[62]. Evidence of portal hypertension, e.g. splenomegaly, favors the diagnosis of ARPKD (Fig. 8.11). Sometimes kidney and liver biopsy are necessary for a definitive distinction between infantile ADPKD and ARPKD[55,62]. ARPKD occurring in young adults and adolescents may usually be distinguished from ADPKD by the predominance of cysts in the renal medulla and evidence of portal hypertension in the former condition (Fig. 8.11). In ADPKD, cysts typically involve both renal cortex and medulla.

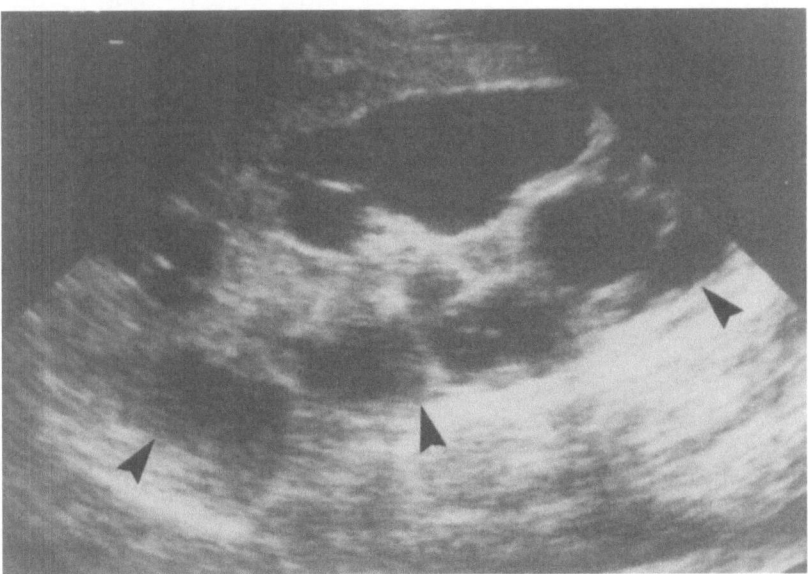

Figure 8.12 Autosomal dominant polycystic kidney disease in 72-year-old woman with hypertension. Longitudinal sonogram shows enlargement of right kidney (arrowheads) and multiple cysts of varying sizes.

4.2. Autosomal dominant polycystic kidney disease (ADPKD)

ADPKD is characterized by multiple bilateral renal cysts that involve both the cortex and medulla. Liver cysts and berry aneurysms of the circle of Willis occur frequently. The disorder typically presents in adult life. However, it may be diagnosed during infancy and childhood[9,50]. Patients with fully-developed ADPKD often show dramatic CT and sonographic findings (Figs. 8.12 and 8.13). CT is particularly helpful for screening asymptomatic progeny of patients with ADPKD (Fig. 8.14)[31]. Individuals at risk older than 20 years without detectable renal cysts have a less than 4% probability of having inherited the gene for ADPKD[44].

Patients with ADPKD frequently complain of flank pain and hematuria, and CT helps determine the origin of such symptoms[31]. Cyst hemorrhage is a common cause of pain in ADPKD. Hemorrhagic cysts have high densities on CT (58–84 HU), are usually subcapsular in location and are often multiple (Fig. 8.15)[33]. They sometimes rupture into the perinephric space, causing large hematomas (Fig. 8.15)[34]. Renal calculi occur in about 12–20% of patients with ADPKD and are well shown by CT[32,58]. Cyst infection is difficult to diagnose on CT, but is suggested by a cyst that is larger than surrounding cysts and that shows thickening and irregularity of its wall, increase in attenuation value of its contents and localized thickening of the adjacent renal fascia (Fig. 8.16)[31].

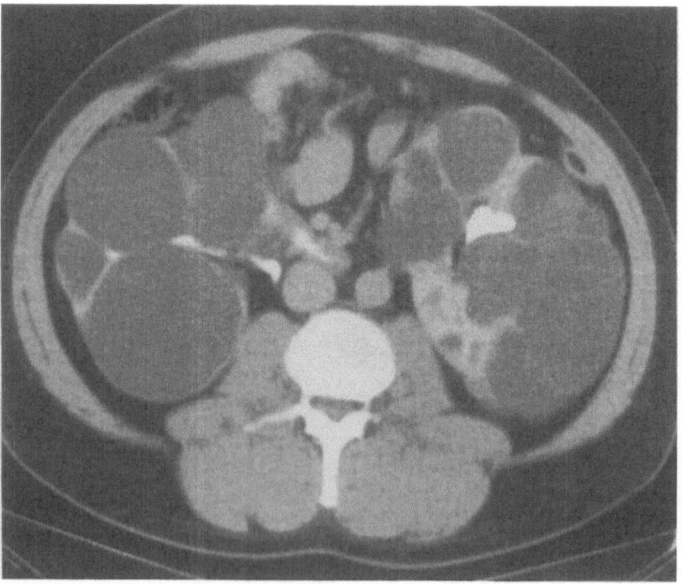

Figure 8.13 Autosomal dominant polycystic kidney disease in 39-year-old man with mild hypertension. Blood urea nitrogen = 28 mg/dl; serum creatinine = 1.9 mg/dl. Post-contrast CT reveals bilateral nephromegaly and large renal cysts with enhancing residual parenchyma between cysts.

Radionuclide scanning using gallium-32 citrate or indium-111 labelled white blood cells may help confirm the diagnosis of cyst infection by demonstrating increased tracer activity at the periphery of the affected cyst (Fig. 8.16)[53,57].

The presence of liver cysts strongly suggests the diagnosis of ADPKD. They occur in about 57% of patients, varying from occasional small cysts (Fig. 8.14) to multiple, large cysts that cause hepatomegaly (Fig. 8.17)[30]. They are

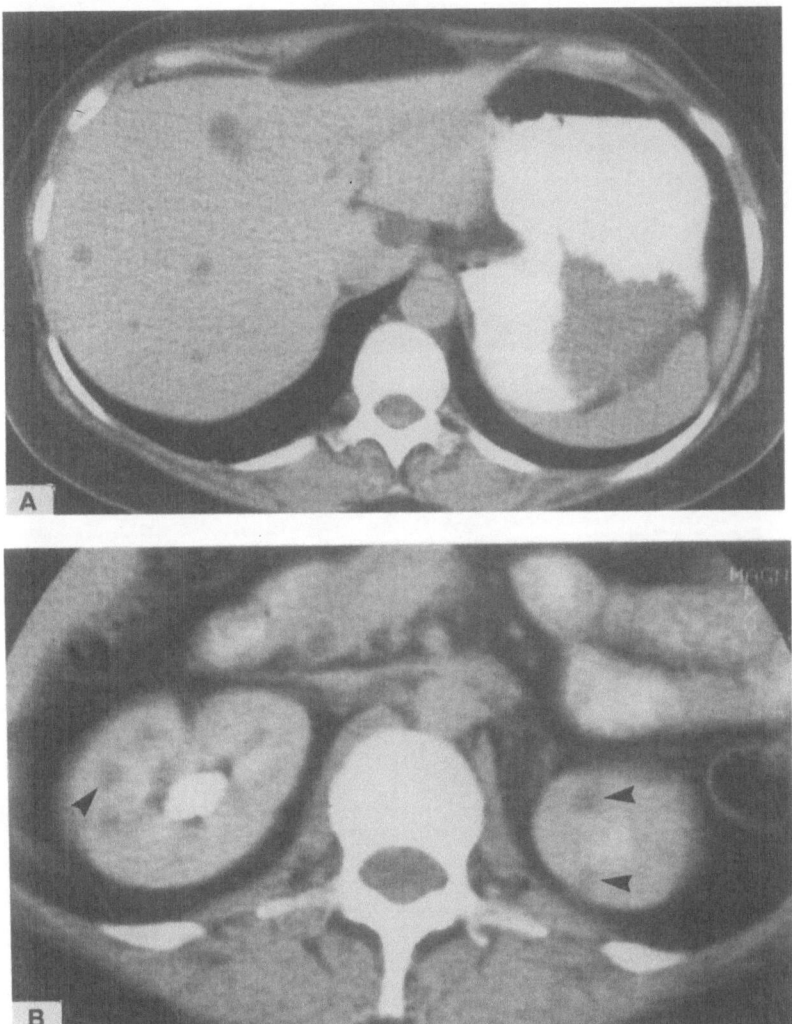

Figure 8.14 Autosomal dominant polycystic kidney disease in asymptomatic 22-year-old woman whose mother has disorder. Excretory urography was normal and sonographic findings were equivocal. (A). CT shows several small liver cysts. (B) Both kidneys exhibit several small cysts (arrowheads).

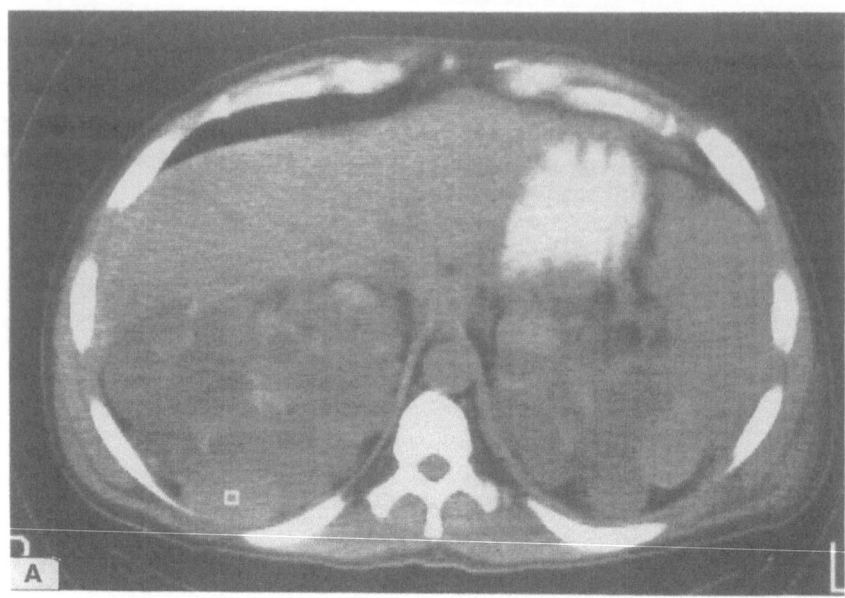

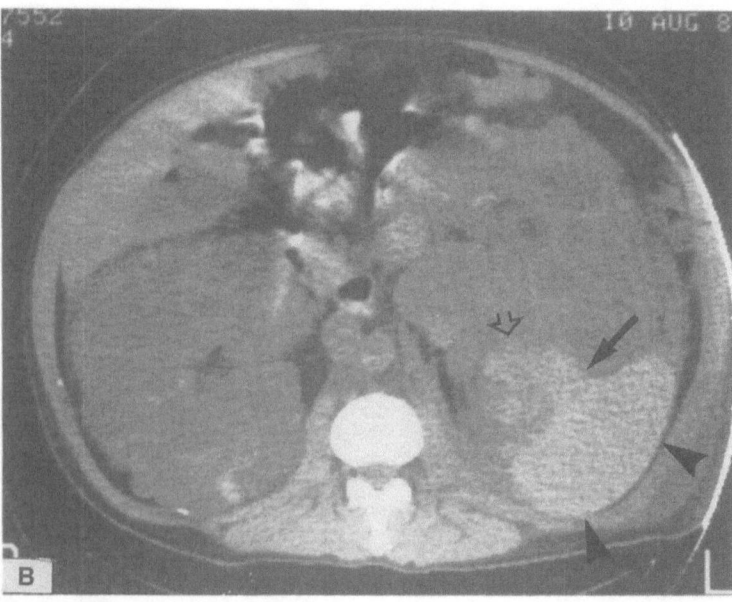

Figure 8.15 Autosomal dominant polycystic kidney disease with cyst hemorrhage in 48-year-old man. Blood urea nitrogen = 120 mg/dl; serum creatinine = 12.9 mg/dl. (A) Unenhanced CT reveals markedly enlarged kidneys replaced by many simple cysts. Note also several high density subcapsular, hemorrhagic cysts. (B) Caudal scan exhibits high-density (55 HU) posterior perinephric hematoma (arrowheads) with anterior displacement of kidney. Ruptured hemorrhagic cyst (open arrow) communicates (arrow) with hematoma. (From Levine E and Grantham JJ. Journal of Computer Assisted Tomography 1987, 11, 108–111. With permission.)

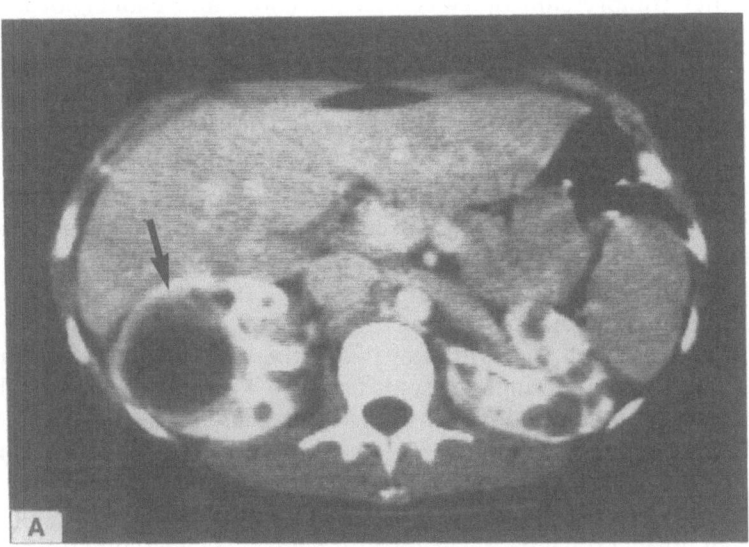

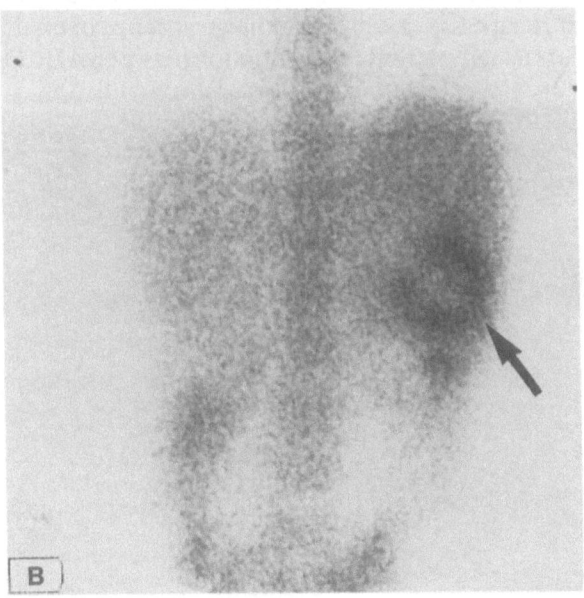

Figure 8.16 Autosomal dominant polycystic kidney disease with cyst infection in 37-year-old woman with right flank pain and urine cultures positive for *Escherichia coli*. (A) CT reveals multiple, small bilateral renal cysts with large thick-walled cyst (arrow) in right kidney. (B) Posterior gallium-67 citrate scan demonstrates intense tracer uptake (arrow) in infected cyst in right kidney. (Courtesy of Bradley Stuewe, MD.)

186

usually asymptomatic and liver function is generally normal[30]. Abnormal liver function studies suggest the development of such complications as common hepatic duct compression by cysts, cyst infection, and cholangiocarcinoma arising from the cyst lining (Fig. 8.18)[30]. The reported prevalence of cerebral aneurysms in patients with ADPKD varies between 10–40%, and rupture of such aneurysms is associated with a high mortality[28,61]. Contrast-enhanced cranial CT may demonstrate aneurysms one centimetre in size or larger, and may be used for screening patients with family histories of cerebral aneurysms[24,59]. MR imaging also has potential for detecting larger aneurysms. Cerebral angiography should not be used for routine screening of patients with ADPKD but should be confined to patients with positive cranial CT or MR scans or with aneurysmal symptoms[28,61].

During the antenatal period and later in neonates and infants, ADPKD, ARPKD and GCKD are sometimes indistinguishable by sonography[62]. ADPKD presenting in younger patients may also be confused with renal cystic disease occurring in tuberous sclerosis[45]. Multiple simple cysts may sometimes be confused with ADPKD. Whereas cysts in typical ADPKD are diffusely distributed throughout the kidneys, which are often enlarged, multiple simple cysts are irregularly distributed in the kidneys and are separated by appreciable amounts of normal renal parenchyma. Uremic ARCD may sometimes closely resemble ADPKD. However, a long history of uremia and dialysis, lack of family history of renal cystic disease and known absence of cystic disease at the onset of the illness usually permit differentiation between ARCD and ADPKD.

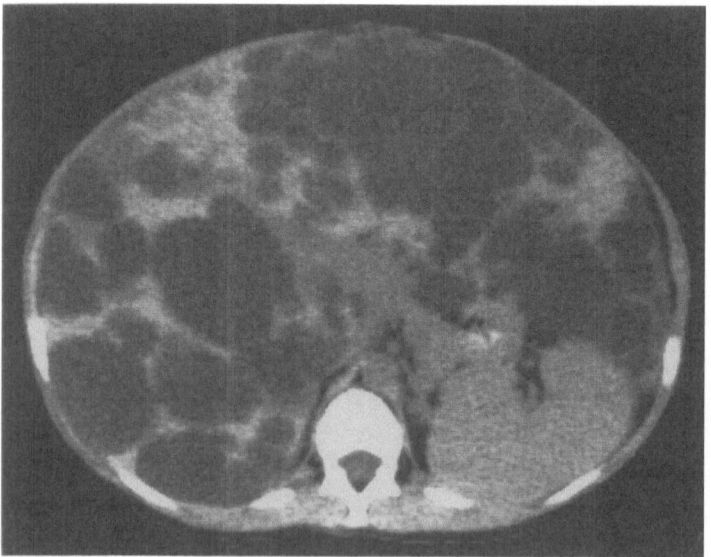

Figure 8.17 Autosomal dominant polycystic kidney disease with marked hepatomegaly owing to liver cysts in 45-year-old woman with normal renal and liver function tests. (From Levine E, Cook LT and Grantham JJ. American Journal of Roentgenology 1985, 145, 229–233. Copyright by American Roentgen Ray Society. With permission.)

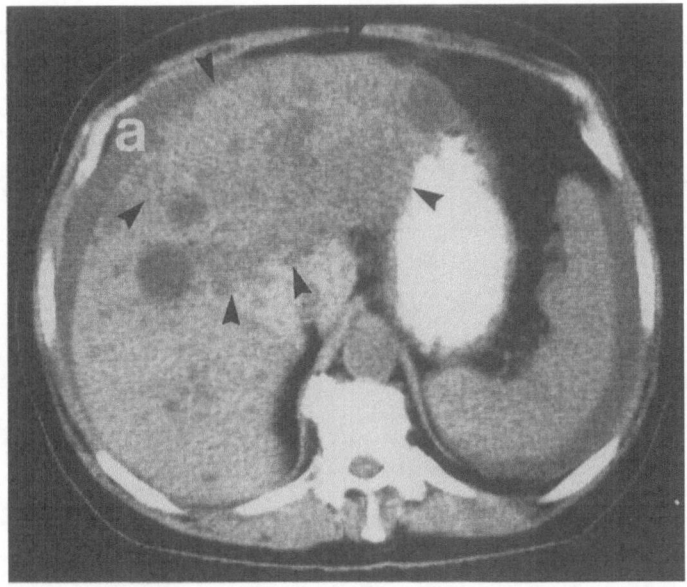

Figure 8.18 Autosomal dominant polycystic kidney disease complicated by cholangiocarcinoma in 69-year-old man complaining of abdominal pain and weight loss. Liver function tests were markedly abnormal. CT demonstrates several cysts in right lobe of liver. Poorly-defined low density mass (arrowheads) involves left lobe and part of anterior segment of right lobe. Ascites (a) is present. Neoplasm was not resectable and patient died of metastatic disease. (From Levine E, Cook LT and Grantham JJ. American Journal of Roentgenology 1985, 145, 229–233. Copyright by American Roentgen Ray Society. With permission.)

5. Renal cystic disease in hereditary syndromes

5.1. Tuberous sclerosis (TS)

TS is characterized by mental retardation, seizures and cutaneous lesions. It may be inherited as an autosomal dominant trait or may occur sporadically[16]. Renal angiomyolipomas, which are usually multiple and bilateral, occur in about 67% of patients[16]. However, renal cystic disease also occurs in TS and may sometimes be the earliest and only clinical manifestation of the disorder in infancy and childhood[1,54]. The kidneys are often markedly enlarged in such patients and are replaced by multiple cysts of varying sizes, some with mural calcification[45]. The cysts usually involve the renal cortex and medulla diffusely (Fig. 8.19)[54], and the findings are similar to those in autosomal dominant polycystic kidney disease[45]. Cranial CT may help establish the diagnosis of TS if it shows typical, small calcified paraventricular lesions (Fig. 8.19)[16]. Also, careful study of the kidneys with thin-section CT may show occasional small fat-containing angiomyolipomas. The combination of cysts and angiomyolipo-

188

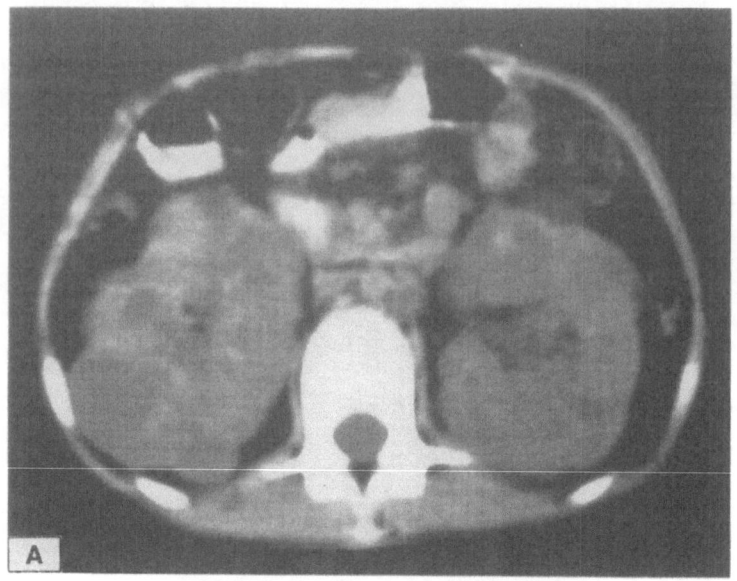

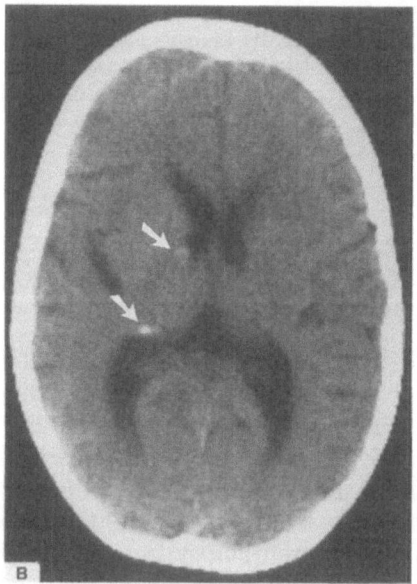

Figure 8.19 Tuberous sclerosis with renal cystic disease in 14-year-old female. Blood urea nitrogen = 28 mg/dl; serum creatinine = 1.3 mg/dl. (A) Unenhanced CT displays enlarged kidneys containing multiple cysts. No fat-containing hamartomas were detected. (B) Cranial CT reveals paraventricular calcifications (arrows) indicating diagnosis of tuberous sclerosis, and permitting differentiation from autosomal dominant polycystic kidney disease.

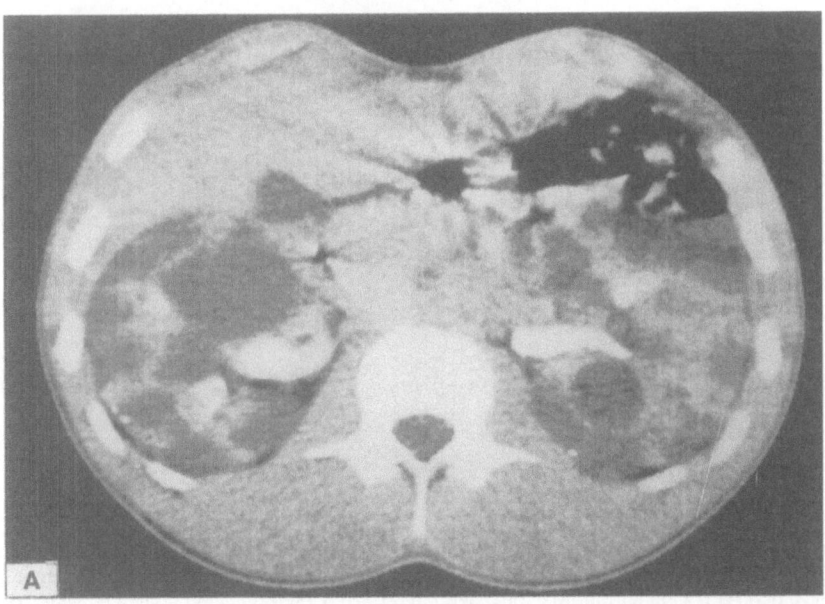

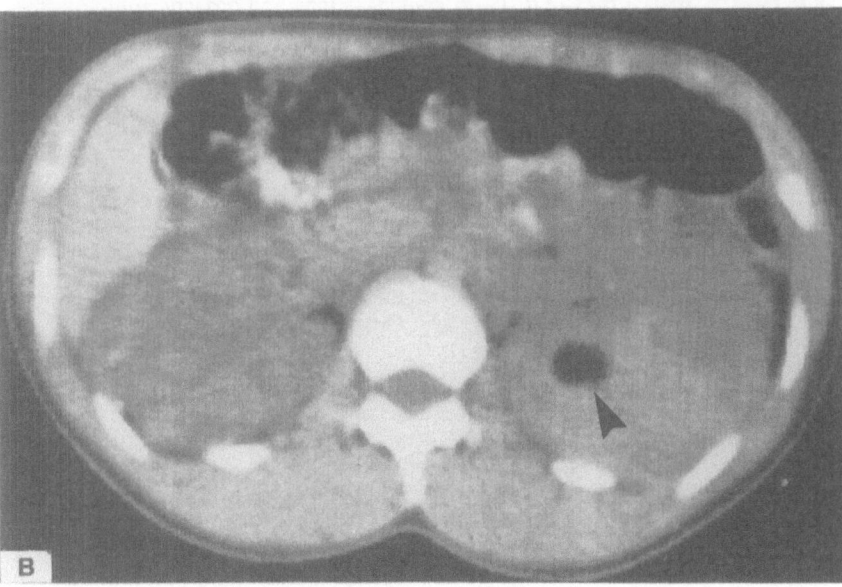

Figure 8.20 Tuberous sclerosis with renal cystic disease in 15-year-old female. (A) Enhanced CT shows enlarged kidneys with multiple fluid-filled cysts. Appearances closely resemble autosomal dominant polycystic kidney disease. (B) Precontrast CT shows 1.9 cm rounded lesion (arrowhead) in left kidney with fat attenuation value (−110 HU). Findings indicate angiomyolipoma and strongly suggest tuberous sclerosis. (From Mitnick JS, Bosniak MA, Hilton S *et al.* Radiology 1983, 147, 85–87. With permission.)

190

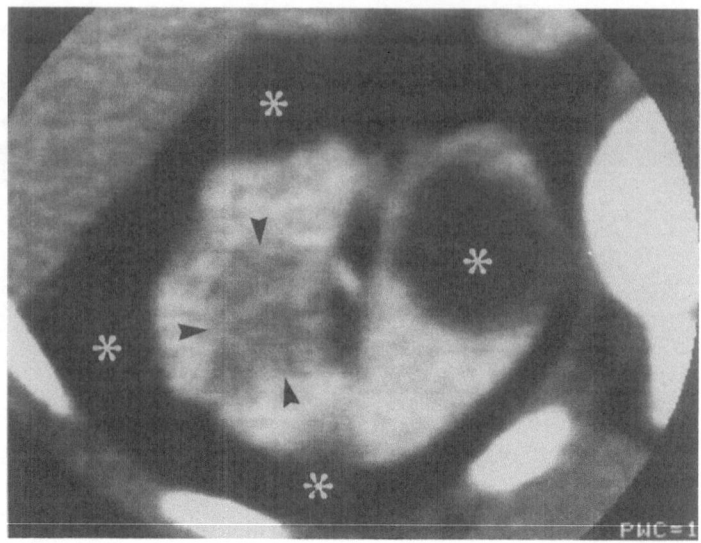

Figure 8.21 von Hippel–Lindau disease with renal cysts and renal cell carcinoma in a 52-year-old man. Post-contrast CT through upper pole of right kidney shows four cysts (*) with attenuation values of 0–6 HU. 3 cm neoplasm with an irregular border (arrowheads) is seen laterally. (From Levine E, Lee KR, Weigel JW and Farber B. Radiology 1979, 130, 703–706. With permission.)

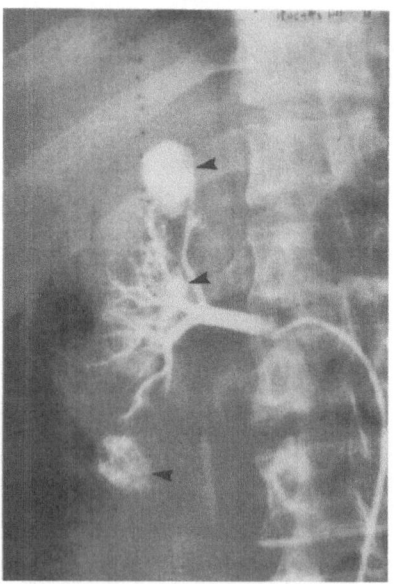

Figure 8.22 von Hippel–Lindau disease with multifocal renal cell carcinomas in a 33-year-old man. CT showed indeterminate small renal masses. Selective angiography after epinephrine injection into renal artery demonstrates three small neoplasms (arrowheads) in right kidney. (Courtesy of DS Hartman, MD, and Armed Forces Institute of Pathology, Washington, DC.)

mas is strongly suggestive of TS (Fig. 8.20)[45]. ARPKD may be distinguished from TS in infancy since the former condition is characterized on imaging studies by medullary tubular ectasia and relatively normal renal cortex with few macroscopic cysts (Fig. 8.10)[7,42].

5.2. von Hippel–Lindau disease (VHLD)

VHLD is transmitted by an autosomal dominant gene. Cerebellar hemangioblastoma and retinal angiomatosis are the most common sources of initial symptoms. At the time of presentation, the abdominal manifestations are generally asymptomatic, but may be detected by CT screening[29]. Small, multiple and bilateral renal cysts are the most common abdominal manifestation occurring in about 76% of patients (Fig.8.21)[29]. Renal cell carcinoma, which is often multicentric and bilateral, occurs in about 36% of patients[13,29]. Such neoplasms may be detected by CT when small and localized to the kidney (Fig. 8.21)[37]. When CT identifies lesions which are likely to be carcinomas, bilateral selective renal angiography should be done to search for additional small tumors that may have been missed by CT and to help plan conservative surgery (Fig. 8.22)[23]. Pancreatic cysts and tumors and adrenal pheochromocytomas also occur in VHLD and are well shown by CT[29].

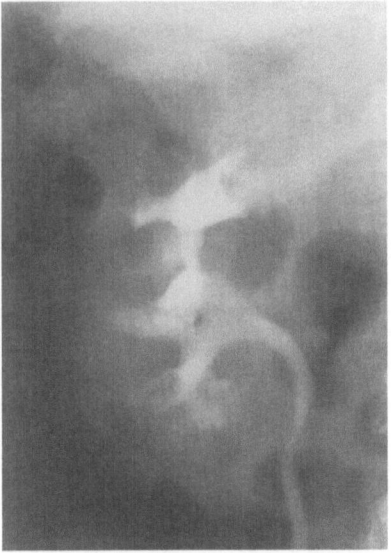

Figure 8.23 Medullary sponge kidney in 59-year-old woman with recurrent urinary tract infections. Excretory urography reveals fine discrete linear striations involving all papillae in right kidney. Enlargement and poor definition of upper pole of kidney were due to acute pyelonephritis.

The multiple renal cysts of VHLD are non-specific in appearance, and similar findings may occur in other disorders such as autosomal dominant polycystic kidney disease. The renal cysts in VHLD are usually fewer and

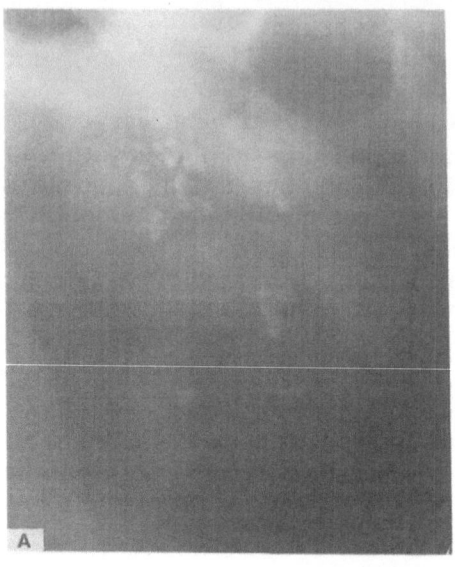

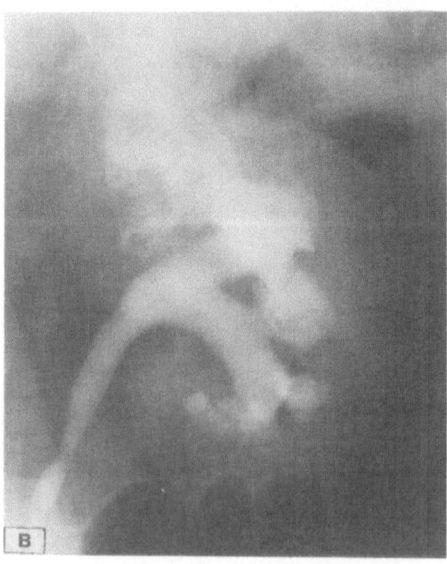

Figure 8.24 Medullary sponge kidney in 65-year-old man with recurrent ureteric colic owing to passage of calculi. (A) Plain film shows multiple small rounded calcifications in left kidney. (B) Excretory urography reveals that calcifications are contained in dilated collecting tubules. Right kidney showed similar appearances.

smaller than those in ADPKD so that renal enlargement in VHLD is less common and renal failure does not occur. However, early ADPKD and VHLD may have similar renal findings. The extrarenal manifestations, particularly the central nervous system and ocular tumors of VHLD, usually permit differentiation.

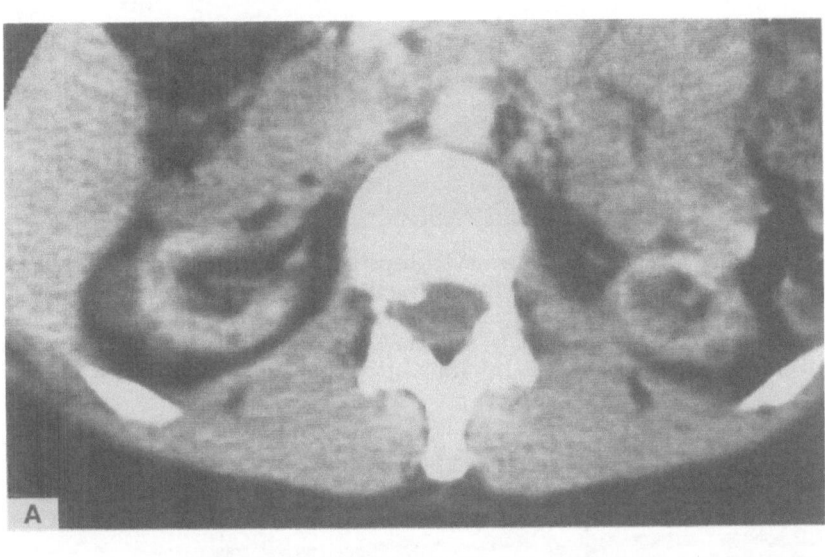

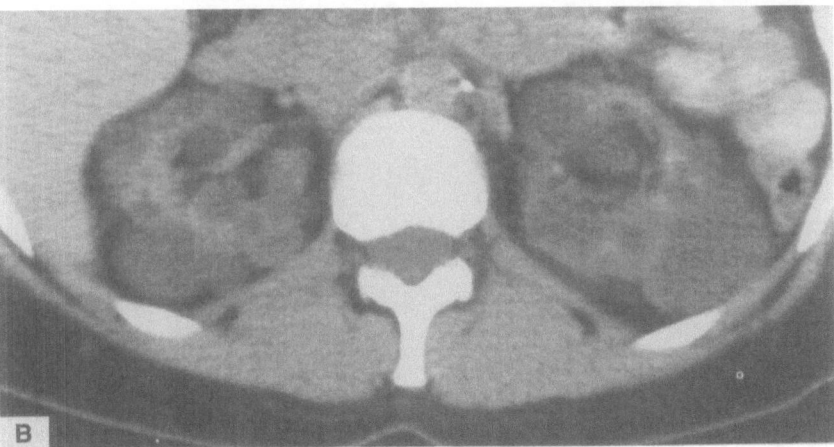

Figure 8.25 Acquired renal cystic disease in 45-year-old man on long-term hemodialysis. (A) CT after 4 years of dialysis shows bilateral small cysts in shrunken kidneys. (B) Follow-up CT 4 years later shows enlargement of cysts and kidneys.

194

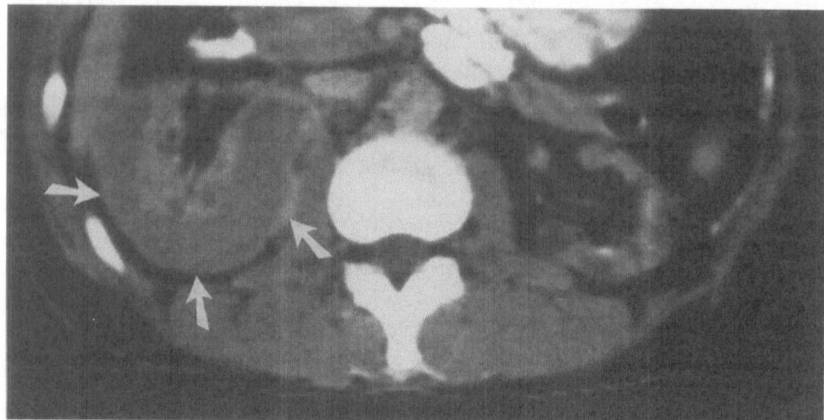

Figure 8.26 Acquired renal cystic disease and right perinephric hematoma in 38-year-old woman managed by hemodialysis for 5 years. Patient had thrombocytopenia owing to systemic lupus erythematosus. CT reveals multiple, small, bilateral renal cysts and right perinephric hematoma (arrows). (From Levine E, Grantham JJ, Slusher SL, Greathouse JL and Krohn BP. American Journal of Roentgenology 1984, 142, 125–131. Copyright by American Roentgen Ray Society.

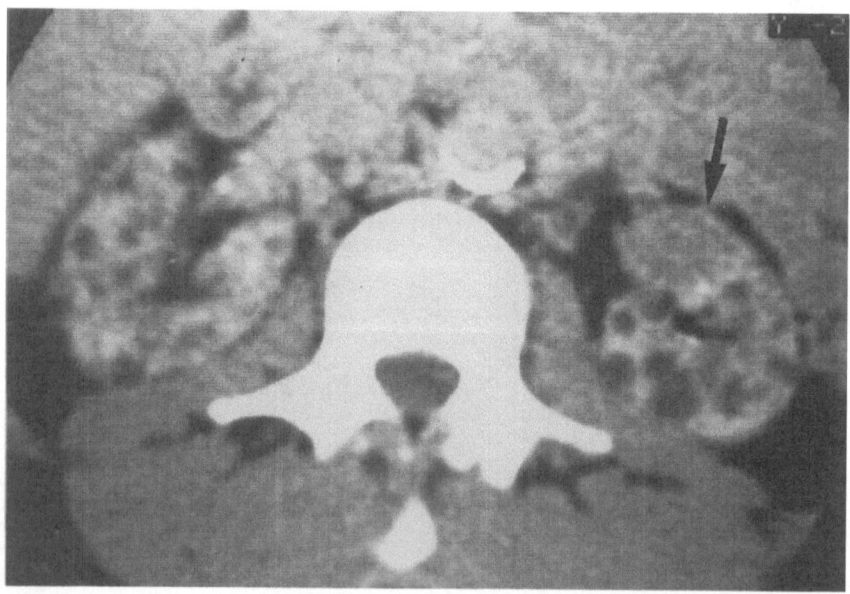

Figure 8.27 Acquired renal cystic disease in patient managed by hemodialysis for 6 years. CT with contrast enhancement demonstrates many small cysts in both kidneys. Note homogeneous, well-marginated 2.7 cm solid mass (arrow) anteriorly in left kidney thought to be small renal neoplasm. Follow-up CT after five years revealed no change in size or appearance of lesion. (From Levine E, Grantham JJ, Slusher SL, Greathouse JL and Krohn BP. American Journal of Roentgenology 1984, 142, 125–131. Copyright by American Roentgen Ray Society. With permission.)

6. Renal medullary cystic disorders

6.1. Medullary sponge kidney (MSK)

MSK is a non-hereditary disorder of unknown cause characterized by dilated collecting ducts in one or more renal pyramids of one or both kidneys[19]. The clinical spectrum varies from an asymptomatic, incidental finding on excretory urography to severe renal calculous disease or urinary tract infection, usually in adult patients[19]. The diagnosis is best established by excretory urography which shows dilated collecting tubules in one or more papillae[11]. These vary from fine discrete linear striations (Fig. 8.23) to small rounded, contrast collections that may contain calculi (Fig. 8.24). The kidneys are usually normal in size. However, renal enlargement may occur when there is diffuse cystic tubular ectasia.

MSK is readily differentiated from other causes of nephrocalcinosis by excretory urography[11]. Calcium disposition in these other disorders occurs in the walls of collecting tubules of normal calibre, whereas in MSK the calcifications lie in cystically dilated collecting tubules. Diffuse linear medullary tubular ectasia may be seen in patients with ARPKD[42]. However, this condition is usually seen in younger patients with positive family histories and evidence of portal hypertension resulting from congenital hepatic fibrosis[42].

6.2. Medullary cystic disease complex

The medullary cystic complex consists of medullary cystic disease and juvenile nephronophthisis. About 73% of patients have medullary cysts and almost all show interstitial nephritis. The major manifestations of the complex are small kidneys and progressive renal failure often in young patients. Sonography shows small smooth kidneys with increased echogenicity[11]. Occasionally small medullary cysts are seen, but often these are too small to be resolved sonographically.

7. Acquired renal cystic disease (ARCD)

Patients with long-standing uremia often develop multiple renal cysts, an entity known as ARCD (Fig. 8.25)[17]. ARCD occurs in about 44% of patients managed by dialysis[17]. The condition is usually asymptomatic, but may be associated with serious complications such as retroperitoneal hemorrhage (Fig. 8.26) and renal neoplasms[17,35,36]. Patients with suspected ARCD are best evaluated by CT[36]. We regard a minimum of five cysts per kidney as being necessary for diagnosis, and both kidneys should be affected[36]. The cysts are best seen on contrast-en-

196

hanced scans (Fig. 8.27)[36]. The affected kidneys are usually small. However, progressive nephromegaly may develop with time (Fig. 8.25)[36].

Renal neoplasms, which are often multiple and bilateral, occur in about 7% of uremic patients[17]. Most are discovered incidentally and are smaller than 3 cm in diameter (Fig. 8.27)[36]. Large locally invasive or metastatic renal cell carcinomas (Fig. 8.28) are less common, having a frequency of 0.33% among dialysis patients[17]. This frequency is somewhat higher than in the general population. Because of their propensity to develop malignant renal neoplasms,

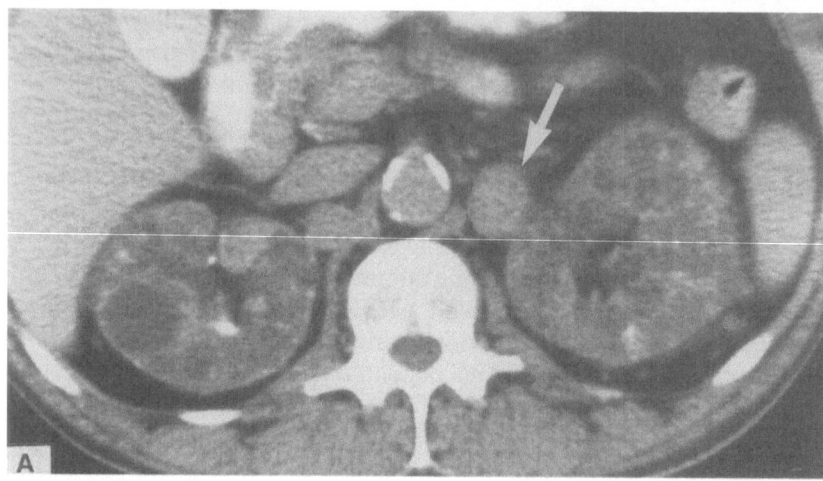

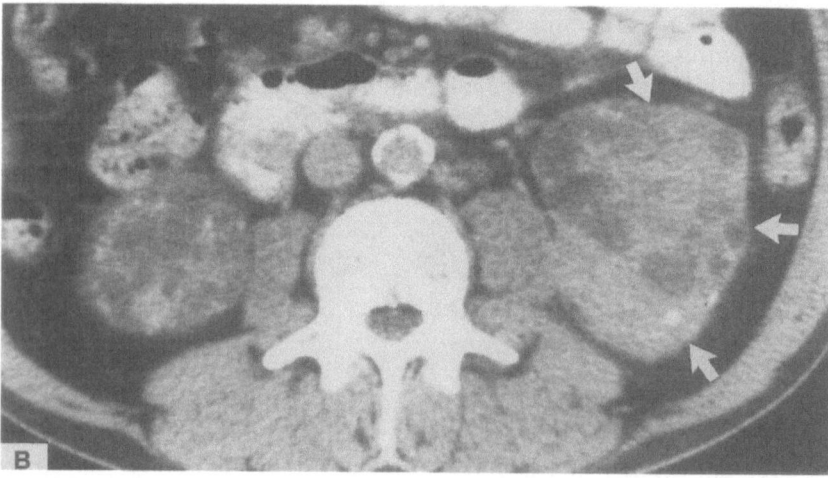

Figure 8.28 Acquired renal cystic disease and metastatic renal cell carcinoma in 46-year-old man managed by hemodialysis for 10 years. Patient developed hematuria. (A) CT exhibits multiple renal cysts and renal enlargement. Note enlarged lymph node (arrow) adjacent to left renal hilum. (B) Caudal CT reveals extensive infiltrating solid mass (arrows) in lower pole of left kidney. Left nephrectomy revealed renal cell carcinoma with metastases to paraaortic lymph nodes.

dialysis patients should have CT evaluation of their native kidneys if they develop flank pain or hematuria[36].

The CT appearances of ARCD are non-specific and may occur in other conditions such as ADPKD, medullary cystic disease, multiple simple cysts and tuberous sclerosis. However, the diagnosis of ARCD can be made with reasonable certainty if a patient's previous studies (biopsy or imaging) showed no cysts, if the original renal disease process was well-documented, if there is no family history of renal cystic disease, and if the patient has been uremic for a significant time period.

8. Miscellaneous parenchymal renal cysts

8.1. Cystic renal neoplasms

Many renal neoplasms contain small cystic areas resulting from necrosis or old hemorrhage. However, the cystic component in cystic neoplasms predominates (Fig. 8.3). Although usually solid, childhood renal neoplasms such as Wilms' tumor, mesoblastic nephroma and clear cell sarcoma may have multiocular configurations[21]. Adult renal cell carcinoma may have a unilocular (Fig. 8.3) or multiocular cystic configuration, and CT may help in diagnosis[20,21].

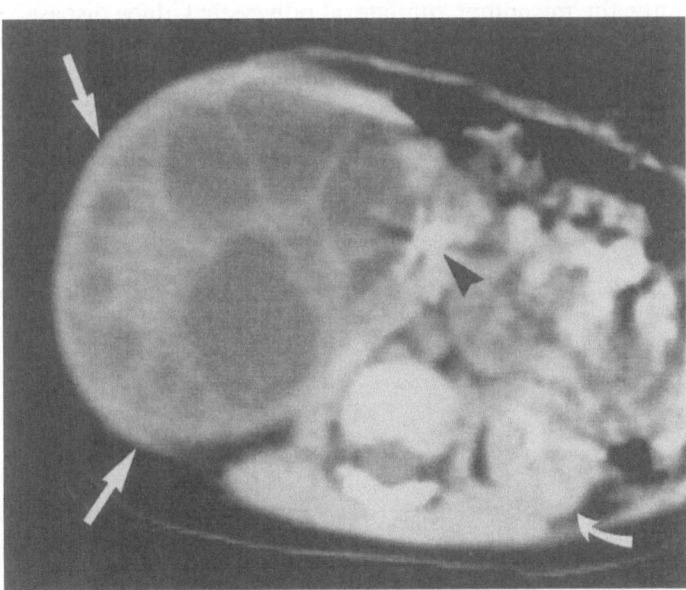

Figure 8.29 Multilocular cystic nephroma in one-year-old male. Note well-circumscribed mass (arrows) in right kidney with thick capsule and multiple prominent septa. Opacified right pelvicaliceal system (arrowhead) is displaced medially. CT appearances are indistinguishable from cystic Wilms' tumor. Left kidney (curved arrow) is normal.

Multilocular cystic nephroma MLCN, also sometimes called multilocular cyst, is a bulky, well-encapsulated, non-infiltrating, usually benign renal tumor[2,39]. It presents in young children as an asymptomatic abdominal mass and in adults with abdominal pain and hematuria[39]. Multilocular cysts, at least in children, may be partially differentiated Wilms' tumors representing the benign end of the spectrum of the neoplasm[3]. MLCN presents on CT or sonography as a non-specific well-defined multilocular renal mass (Fig. 8.29)[2,39]. Contrast excretion by the affected kidney is usually normal[2].

MLCN is often indistinguishable by CT or sonography from other cystic renal neoplasms, particularly cystic Wilms' tumor in children and multilocular cystic renal cell carcinoma in adults[21]. Unilateral renal cystic disease can usually be distinguished from MLCN, because the former lesion lacks encapsulation and the cysts are separated by bands of enhancing normal renal parenchyma. In multicystic renal dysplasia the entire kidney is usually replaced by cysts and the affected kidney is non-functional.

8.2. Unilateral renal cystic disease (URCD)

In URCD most of one kidney is replaced by multiple cysts and the contralateral kidney is normal[8,27]. There is usually no family history of kidney cysts[8], and the condition is not related to autosomal dominant polycystic kidney disease. Consequently, the misnomer "unilateral polycystic kidney disease" should be avoided. Affected patients range in age from childhood to the sixth decade and may have hypertension, flank pain or hematuria[8,26,27]. Sonography reveals multiple simple cysts separated by septa[8,26,27]. On CT, the cysts are separated

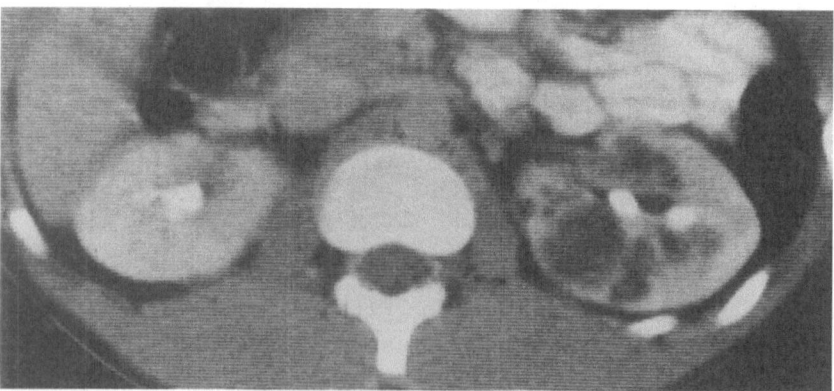

Figure 8.30 Unilateral renal cystic disease in 15-year-old man with history of intermittent gross hematuria starting at 5 years of age. CT through midregion of left kidney reveals partial replacement by many cysts which are separated by bands of enhancing normal parenchyma. Entire kidney showed similar findings. Right kidney is free of cysts and follow-up CT 7 years later showed no change.

by enhancing bands of normal renal parenchyma so that no distinct encapsulated renal mass is identified (Fig. 8.30). The affected kidney may be enlarged and shows normal contrast excretion[8,26,27].

URCD should be differentiated from other causes of unilateral cystic disease. Unlike URCD, cystic renal neoplasms are usually discrete, encapsulated masses and are well-demarcated from adjacent renal parenchyma (Fig. 8.29). Simple cysts may be multiple and unilateral. However, they are seldom as numerous as in URCD[8]. Although the total absence of cysts in the contralateral kidney on CT in adults usually excludes the diagnosis of ADPKD, caution is necessary before making a definitive diagnosis of URCD in children. In ADPKD, renal cysts develop slowly during childhood and may become apparent earlier in one kidney[49]. Accordingly, in children follow-up CT should be performed after an appropriate interval before a final diagnosis of URCD is made.

9. Extraparenchymal renal cysts

9.1. Parapelvic cyst

Parapelvic cysts are benign extraparenchymal cysts that are located in the renal sinus[22]. They are not true renal cysts, but may be lymphatic in origin or arise

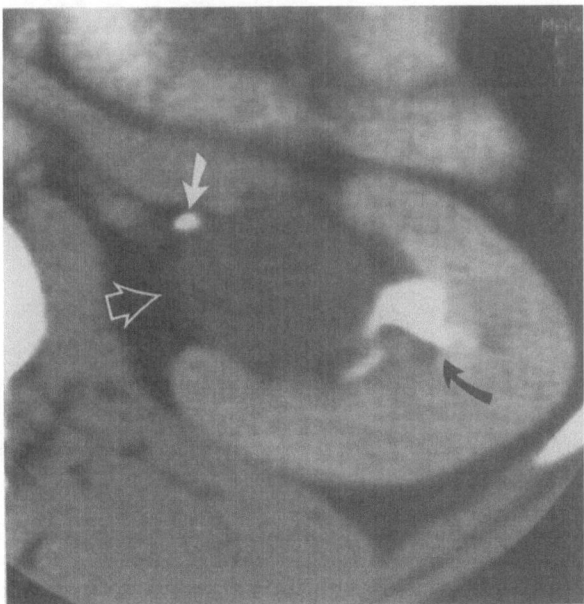

Figure 8.31 Parapelvic renal cyst. Contrast-enhanced CT reveals that cyst (open arrow) is surrounded by a halo of renal sinus fat, indicating its extrarenal origin. Note non-dilated collecting system (curved arrow) and ureter (arrow).

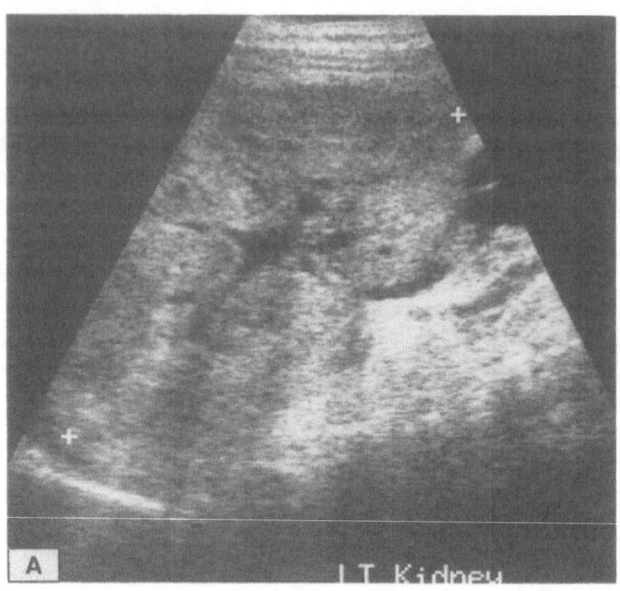

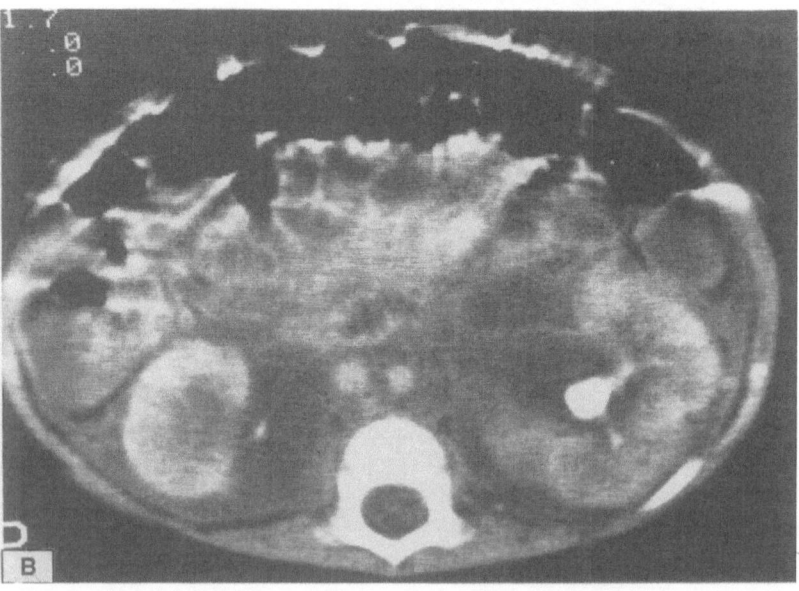

Figure 8.32 Renal lymphangiectasia in 10-month-old boy with abdominal mass on routine physical examination and normal renal function. (A) Longitudinal sonogram of enlarged left kidney shows diffusely hyperechoic renal parenchyma with loss of delineation between renal cortex, medulla and sinus. Appearance is similar to autosomal recessive polycystic kidney disease. (B) Contrast-enhanced CT reveals extensive retroperitoneal lymphatic cysts. (From Blumhagen JD, Wood BJ and Rosenbaum M. Journal of Ultrasound in Medicine 1987, 6, 487–495. With permission.)

from embryological rests[22]. They may be unilocular or multilocular and are often bilateral[22]. They do not communicate with the collecting system[22]. Most are asymptomatic and are discovered incidentally by radiographic studies[22]. On sonography, a parapelvic cyst appears as a well-defined sonolucent renal sinus mass[22]. It is differentiated from a dilated renal pelvis by lack of communication with the calyces[22]. On CT, the characteristic feature of a parapelvic cyst is a surrounding halo of renal sinus fat, indicating its extrarenal origin (Fig. 8.31)[10]. Parapelvic cysts are differentiated by their fluid attenuation values from solid renal sinus masses such as lymphoma and invasive transitional cell carcinoma.

9.2. Renal lymphangiectasia (RL)

RL is probably due to developmental obstruction of the larger lymphatics draining the kidney through the renal pedicle[4,38,47]. The condition is usually bilateral and is characterized by large lymphatic cysts in the renal sinuses and perinephric tissues and diffuse intrarenal lymphangiectasia[4,43]. Patients are usually discovered clinically because of abdominal masses due to nephromegaly[4,47]. In neonates and infants with RL, sonography shows enlargement

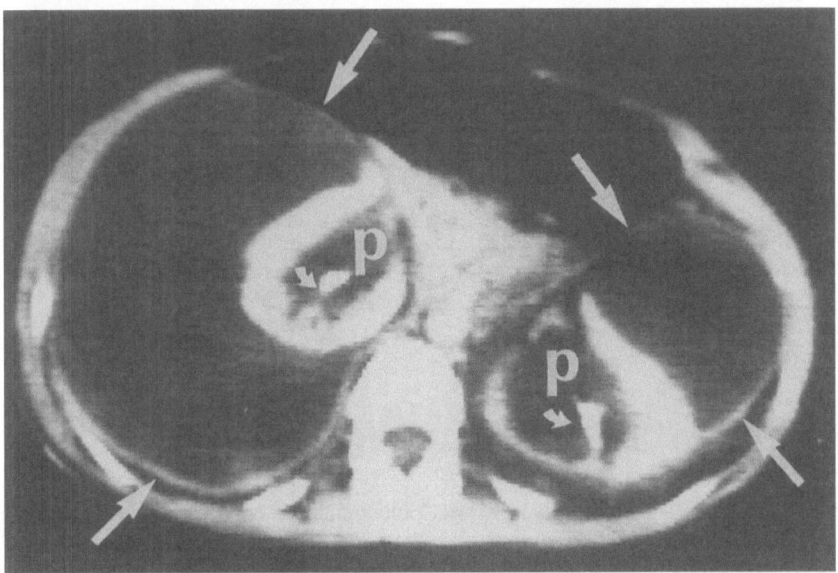

Figure 8.33 Renal lymphangiectasia in 23-year-old woman. Contrast-enhanced CT done shortly after pregnancy. Non-dilated calyces (curved arrows) are attenuated by bilateral parapelvic cysts (p). Note large bilateral perinephric lymph collections (arrows). (From Meredith WT, Levine E, Ahlstrom NG and Grantham JJ. AJR 1988, 151, 965–966. Copyright by American Roentgen Ray Society. With permission.)

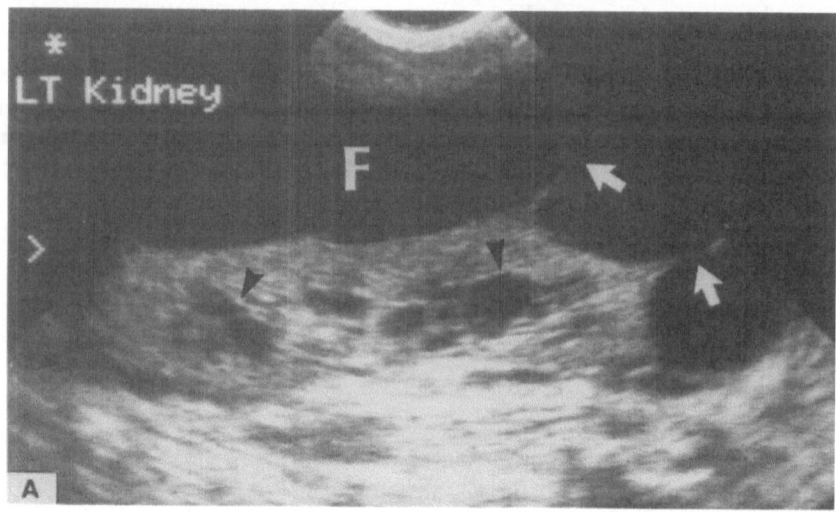

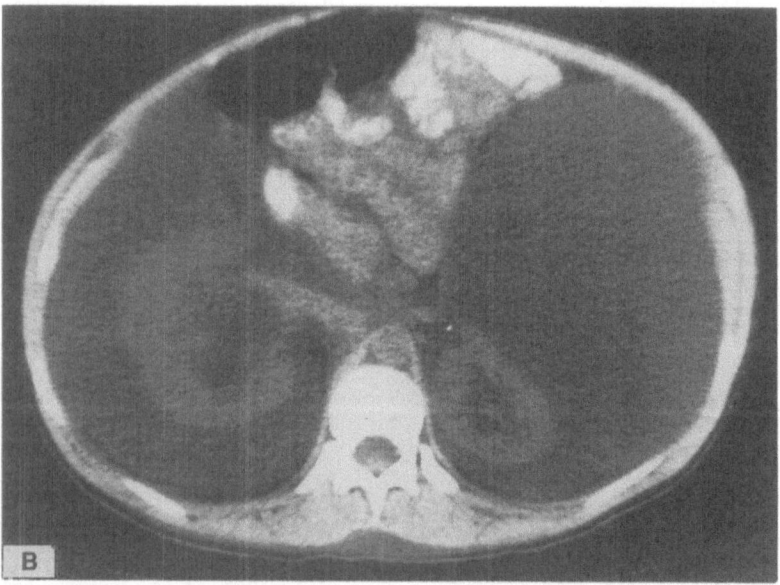

Figure 8.34 Renal lymphangiectasia in 25-year-old woman (sister of patient in Fig. 8.33) who developed severe abdominal distension during pregnancy. (A) Logitudinal coronal sonogram of left kidney during pregnancy. Note prominent pericalyceal cysts (arrowheads) and large perinephric fluid collection (F) with delicate septa (arrows). (B) CT demonstrates large bilateral perinephric fluid collections and parapelvic cysts. (From Meredith WT, Levine E, Ahlstrom NG and Grantham JJ. AJR 1988, 151, 965–966. Copyright by American Roentgen Ray Society. With permission.)

and increased echogenicity of both kidneys, and small parenchymal cysts may be found (Fig. 8.32)[4,47]. These findings are similar to those of ARPKD (Fig. 8.8)[5]. However, the presence on sonography or CT of renal sinus, perinephric or central retroperitoneal cysts sometimes permits distinction between the two conditions (Fig. 8.32)[4]. A diffuse increase in renal echogenicity in RL probably results from multiple dilated intrarenal lymphatics.

Excretory urography in children and adults with RL shows bilateral nephromegaly with calyceal distortion caused by multiple large parapelvic and pericalyceal cysts[4]. These findings may superficially resemble those of ADPKD. However, CT and sonography confirm the predominant pelvic and pericalyceal location of the cysts in RL with only occasional small parenchymal cysts (Figs. 8.33 and 8.34), whereas ADPKD is characterized mainly by prominent parenchymal cysts. RL may be complicated during pregnancy by large perinephric lymph collections and ascites (Figs. 8.33 and 8.34)[43]. These findings may be secondary to lymphatic rupture owing to increased renal lymph flow during pregnancy in the presence of lymphatic obstruction[43].

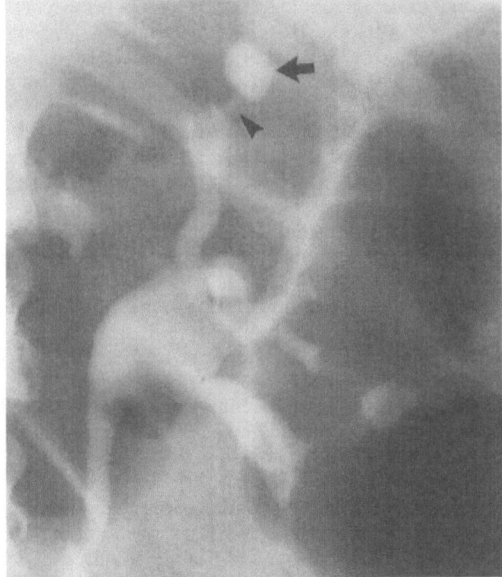

Figure 8.35 Calyceal diverticulum (arrow) demonstrated by excretory urography. Diverticulum is connected to upper pole calyx by narrow isthmus (arrowhead).

9.3. *Calyceal diverticulum*

Calyceal diverticula, also known as pyelogenic cysts, are urepithelium-lined pouches that arise from the collecting system and extend into the adjacent renal parenchyma. They are probably developmental in origin. Most are asymptomatic and are discovered incidentally during excretory urography[11]. Occasionally, there may be associated hematuria, calculi, infection, flank pain or colic which resolve after excision of the diverticulum. Calyceal diverticula communicate with the collecting system and usually opacify during excretory urography (Fig. 8.35). They may contain calculi. Lesions which simulate calyceal diverticula on excretory urography include simple cysts or renal abscesses that have ruptured into the collecting system, localized renal papillary necrosis and focal calyectasis due to infundibular obstruction caused by a neoplasm, calculus or inflammatory process[11].

References

1. Avni EF, Szliwowski H, Spehl M, Lelong B, Baudain P and Struyven J. Renal involvement in tuberous sclerosis. Annals of Radiology 1984, 27, 207–214.
2. Banner MP, Pollack HM, Chatten J and Witzleben C. Multiocular renal cysts: radiologic–pathologic correlation. American Journal of Roentgenology 1981, 136, 239–247.
3. Beckwith JB and Kiviat NB. Multiocular renal cysts and cystic renal tumors. Editorial. American Journal of Roentgenology 1981, 136, 435–436.
4. Blumhagen JD, Wood BJ and Rosenbaum DM. Sonographic evaluation of abdominal lymphangiomas in children. Journal of Ultrasound in Medicine 1987, 6, 487–495.
5. Boak DK and Teele RL. Sonography of infantile polycystic kidney disease. American Journal of Roentgenology 1980, 135, 575–580.
6. Carson RW, Bedi D, Cavallo T and DuBose TD. Familial adult glomerulocystic kidney disease. American Journal of Kidney Disease 1987, 9, 154–165.
7. Chilton SJ and Cremin BJ. The spectrum of polycystic disease in children. Pediatric Radiology 1981, 11, 9–15.
8. Cho KJ, Thornbury JR, Bernstein J, Heidelberger KP and Walter JF. Localized cystic disease of the kidney: angiographic–pathologic correlation. American Journal of Roentgenology 1979, 132, 891–895.
9. Cole BR, Conley SB and Stapleton FB. Polycystic kidney disease in the first year of life. Journal of Pediatrics 1987, 111, 693–699.
10. Crummy AB and Madsen PO. Parapelvic renal cyst: the peripheral fat sign. Journal of Urology 1966, 96, 436–438.
11. Davidson AJ, ed. Radiology of the Kidney. Philadelphia: W.B. Saunders Company, 1985.
12. Davies CH, Stringer DA, Whyte H, Daneman A and Mancer K. Congenital hepatic fibrosis with saccular dilatation of intrahepatic bile ducts and infantile polycystic kidneys. Pediatric Radiology 1986, 16, 302–305.
13. Fill WL, Lamiell JM and Polk NO. Radiographic manifestations of von Hippel–Lindau disease. Radiology 1979, 133, 289–295.
14. Fitch SJ and Stapleton FB. Ultrasonographic features of glomerulocystic disease in infancy: Similarity to infantile polycystic kidney disease. Pediatric Radiology 1986, 16, 400–402.
15. Fong KW, Rahmani MR, Rose TH, Skidmore MB and Connor TP. Fetal renal cystic disease: sonographic–pathologic correlation. American Journal of Roentgenology 1986, 146, 767–773.
16. Gomez R, ed. Tuberous Sclerosis. New York: Raven Press, 1979.
17. Grantham JJ and Levine E. Acquired cystic disease: Replacing one kidney disease with another. Kidney International 1985, 28, 99–105.
18. Habif DV, Berdon WE and Yeh M. Infantile polycystic kidney disease: *In utero* sonographic diagnosis. Radiology 1982, 142, 475–477.
19. Harrison AR and Rose GA. Medullary sponge kidney. Urological Research 1979, 7, 197–207.

20. Hartman DS, Davis CJ, Johns T and Goldman SM. Cystic renal cell carcinoma. Urology 1986, 28, 145–153.
21. Hartman DS, Davis CJ, Sanders RC, Johns TT, Smirniotopoulos J and Goldman SM. The multiloculated renal mass: Considerations and differential features. Radiographics 1987, 7, 29–52.
22. Hidalgo H, Dunnick NR, Rosenberg ER, Ram PC and Korobkin M. Parapelvic cysts: Appearance on CT and sonography. American Journal of Roentgenology 1982, 138, 667–671.
23. Kadir S, Kerr WS and Athanasoulis CA. The role of arteriography in the management of renal cell carcinoma associated with von Hippel–Lindau disease. Journal of Urology 1981, 126, 316–319.
24. Kaehny W, Bell P, Earnest M, Stears J and Gabow P. Family clustering of intracranial aneurysms in autosomal dominant polycystic kidney disease. Kidney International 1987, 31, 204a.
25. Kleiner B, Filly RA, Mack L and Callen PW. Multicystic dysplastic kidney: Observations of contralateral disease in the fetal population. Radiology 1986, 161, 27–29.
26. Kutcher R, Sprayregen S, Rosenblatt R and Goldman M. The sonographic appearance of segmental polycystic kidney. Journal of Ultrasound in Medicine 1983, 2, 425–429.
27. Lee JKT, McClennan BL and Kissane JM. Unilateral polycystic kidney disease. American Journal of Roentgenology 1978, 130, 1165–1167.
28. Levey AS. Cerebral aneurysms. In: Grantham JJ and Gardner KD, eds, Problems in Diagnosis and Management of Polycystic Kidney Disease. Kansas City, Missouri: Intercollegiate Press, 1985, 135–144.
29. Levine E, Collins DL, Horton WA and Schimke RN. CT screening of the abdomen in von Hippel–Lindau disease. American Journal of Roentgenology 1982, 139, 505–510.
30. Levine E, Cook LT and Grantham JJ. Liver cysts in autosomal-dominant polycystic kidney disease: Clinical and computed tomographic study. American Journal of Roentgenology 1985, 145, 229–233.
31. Levine E and Grantham JJ. The role of computed tomography in the evaluation of adult polycystic kidney diseas. American Journal of Kidney Diseases 1981, 1, 99–105.
32. Levine E and Grantham JJ. Complications and radiologic recognition. In: Grantham JJ and Gardner KD, eds, Problems in Diagnosis and Management of Polycystic Kidney Disease. Kansas City, Missouri: Intercollegiate Press, 1985, 34–39.
33. Levine E and Grantham JJ. High-density renal cysts in autosomal dominant polycystic kidney disease demonstrated by CT. Radiology 1985, 154, 477–482.
34. Levine E and Grantham JJ. Perinephric hemorrhage in autosomal dominant polycystic kidney disease: CT and MR findings. Journal of Computer Assisted Tomography 1987, 11, 108–111.
35. Levine E, Grantham JJ and MacDougall ML. Spontaneous subcapsular and perinephric hemorrhage in end-stage kidney disease: Clinical and CT findings. American Journal of Roentgenology 1987, 148, 755–758.
36. Levine E, Grantham JJ, Slusher SL, Greathouse JL and Krohn BP. CT of acquired cystic kidney disease and renal tumors in long-term dialysis patients. American Journal of Roentgenology 1984, 142, 125–131.
37. Levine E, Lee KR, Weigel JW and Farber B. Computed tomography in the diagnosis of renal carcinoma complicating Hippel–Lindau syndrome. Radiology 1979, 130, 703–706.
38. Lindsey JR. Lymphangiectasis simulating polycystic disease. Journal of Urology 1970, 104, 658–662.
39. Madewell JE, Goldman SM, Davis CJ, Hartman DS, Feigin DS and Lichtenstein JE. Multilocular cystic nephroma: a radiographic–pathologic correlation of 58 patients. Radiology 1983, 146, 309–321.
40. Mahony BS, Filly RA, Callen PW, Hricak H, Golbus MS and Harrison MR. Fetal renal dysplasia: sonographic evaluation. Radiology 1984, 152, 143–146.
41. McClennan BL, Stanley RJ, Melson GL, Levitt RG and Sagel SS. CT of the renal cyst: Is cyst aspiration necessary? American Journal of Roentgenology 1979, 133, 671–675.
42. Melson GL, Shackelford GD, Cole BR and McClennan BL. The spectrum of sonographic

findings in infantile polycystic kidney disease with urographic and clinical correlations. Journal of Clinical Ultrasound 1985, 13, 113–119.

43. Meredith WT, Levine E, Ahlstrom NG and Grantham JJ. Exacerbation of familial renal lymphangiomatosis during pregnancy. American Journal of Roentgenology 1988, 151, 965–966.

44. Milutinovic J. Radiologic screening: Impact on genetic counselling. In: Grantham JJ and Gardner KD, eds, Problems in Diagnosis and Management of Polycystic Kidney Disease. Kansas City, Missouri: Intercollegiate Press, 1985, 26–33.

45. Mitnick JS, Bosniak MA, Hilton S, Raghavendra BN, Subramanyam BR and Genieser NB. Cystic renal disease in tuberous sclerosis. Radiology 1983, 147, 85–87.

46. Pedicelli G, Jequier S, Bowen A and Boisvert J. Multicystic dysplastic kidneys: Spontaneous regression demonstrated with ultrasound. Radiology 1986, 160, 23–26.

47. Pickering SP, Fletcher BD, Bryan PJ and Abramowsky CR. Renal lymphangioma: A cause of neonatal nephromegaly. Pediatric Radiology 1984, 14, 445–448.

48. Pollack HM, Banner MP, Arger PH, Peters J, Mulhern CB and Coleman BG. The accuracy of gray-scale renal ultrasonography in differentiating cystic neoplasms from benign cysts. Radiology 1982, 143, 741–745.

49. Porch P, Noe HN and Stapleton FB. Unilateral presentation of adult-type polycystic kidney disease in children. Journal of Urology 1986, 135, 744–746.

50. Pretorius DH, Lee ME, Manco-Johnson ML, Weingast GR, Sedman AB and Gabow PA. Diagnosis of autosomal dominant polycystic kidney disease *in utero* and in the young infant. Journal of Ultrasound in Medicine 1987, 6, 249–255.

51. Sanders RC and Hartman DS. The sonographic distinction between neonatal multicystic kidney and hydronephrosis. Radiology 1984, 151, 621–625.

52. Sanders RC, Nussbaum AR and Solez K. Renal dysplasia: sonographic findings. Radiology 1988, 167, 623–626.

53. Schwab SJ, Bander SJ and Klahr S. Renal infection in autosomal dominant polycystic kidney disease. American Journal of Medicine 1987, 82, 714–718.

54. Stapleton FB, Johnson D, Kaplan GW and Griswold W. The cystic renal lesion in tuberous sclerosis. Journal of Pediatrics 1980, 97, 574–579.

55. Stapleton FB, Magill HL and Kelly DR. Infantile polycystic kidney disease: An imaging dilemma. Urological Radiology 1983, 5, 89–94.

56. Stuck KJ, Koff SA and Silver TM. Ultrasonic features of multicystic dysplastic kidney: Expanded diagnostic criteria. Radiology 1982, 143, 217–221.

57. Sweet R and Keane WF. Perinephric abscess in patients with polycystic kidney disease undergoing chronic hemodialysis. Nephron 1979, 23, 237–240.

58. Torres VE, Erickson SB, Smith LH, Wilson DM and Hattery RR. Th association of nephrolithiasis and autosomal dominant polycystic kidney disease. *Xth International Congress of Nephrology Abstracts*, 1987, 10:44.

59. Torres VE, Forbes GS, Wiebers DO, Erickson SB and Smith LH. Value of routine screening for intracranial aneurysms in autosomal dominant polycystic kidney disease. *Xth International Congress of Nephrology Abstracts*, 1987, 10:45.

60. Vinocur L. Slovis TS, Perlmutter AD, Watts FB and Chang CH. Follow-up studies of multicystic dysplastic kidneys. Radiology 1988, 167, 311–315.

61. Wiebers DO. Management of unruptured intracranial aneurysms. In: Grantham JJ and Gardner KD, eds, Problems in Diagnosis and Management of Polycystic Kidney Disease. Kansas City, Missouri: Intercollegiate Press, 1985, 145–153.

62. Worthington JL, Shackelford GD, Cole BR, Tack ED and Kissane JM. Sonographically detectable cysts in polycystic kidney disease in newborn and young infants. Pediatric Radiology 1988, 18, 287–293.

9
Systemic Manifestations of Renal Cystic Disease

V.E. Torres

Abstract

A host of heterogeneous conditions have in common the presence of cystic kidneys. The recognition of the renal and extrarenal abnormalities as components of the same phenotype may be essential to establish the correct diagnosis. In this chapter, cystic kidneys are considered in three categories, based on their presumed pathogenesis. In the first category, that of cystic kidneys due to abnormal metanephric differentiation, perplexing patterns of renal and extrarenal abnormalities result from specific interferences in the normal inductive interactions between renal and extrarenal primordia during development. The second group of cystic kidneys is characterized by the presence of a hereditary interstitial nephritis, and is often accompanied by a variety of extrarenal manifestations including pigmentary retinopathy, skeletal abnormalities, hepatic fibrosis and abnormalities of the central nervous system. The third category of cystic kidneys, characterized by hyperplasia of the tubular epithelium in the presence of normal metanephric differentiation, includes the most important renal cystic diseases, autosomal recessive polycystic kidney disease (ARPKD) and autosomal dominant polycystic kidney disease (ADPKD). The main extrarenal associations of ARPKD are congenital hepatic fibrosis and Caroli disease. ADPKD has been associated with a variety of extrarenal disorders including hepatic cysts, intracranial aneurysms, other cardiovascular abnormalities, and possibly colon diverticulosis.

Key words   Biliary microhamartomas;
              Congenital hepatic fibrosis;
              Intracranial aneurysms;
              Multiple malformation;
              Multiple malformation syndromes;
              Pigmentary retinopathy.

1. Introduction

Renal cysts are common and usually insignificant. Yet, a host of heterogeneous conditions – congenital, developmental or acquired, with or without a genetic cause, with a variety of extrarenal expressions – have in common the presence of cystic kidneys (Table 9.1). The recognition of the renal and extrarenal abnormalities as components of the same phenotype may be essential to establish the correct diagnosis. The relative contributions of the renal cysts and the extra renal abnormalities to the morbidity and mortality of these diseases

Table 9.1. Cystic diseases of the kidney with extrarenal manifestations.

I. Defects of metanephric differentiation

(1) Sporadic
   (a) Cystic dysplastic kidneys
   (b) De Lange syndrome
   (c) Klippel–Feil syndrome
   (d) VATER association

(2) Single gene mutations
   (a) Dominantly inherited renal adysplasia
   (b) Branchiootorenal dysplasia
   (c) Cryptophthalmos–syndactyly syndrome
   (d) Acrorenal field defect
   (e) Skeletal dysplasias
   (f) Other autosomal recessive metabolic dysplasias and multiple malformation syndromes

(3) Chromosomal aberrations
   (a) Numerical (eg trisomies 21, 18, 13)
   (b) Structural (eg 4p deletion)

(4) Multifactorial
   (a) Neural tube defects

(5) Disruptions
   (a) Radiation
   (b) Teratogenic chemicals (thalidomide, alcohol, trimethadione)
   (c) Metabolic (diabetes mellitus, hypercalcemia, hypoxia)
   (d) Infections (rubella)
   (e) Teratomas (presacral teratoma)

II. Renal cystic diseases with hereditary interstitial nephritis (nephronophthisis–medullary cystic disease complex)

   (1) Senior–Loken syndrome
   (2) Conorenal syndromes
   (3) Nephronophthisis with congenital hepatic fibrosis
   (4) Oculocerebrohepatorenal dysplasia
   (5) Laurence–Moon–Bardet–Biedl syndrome
   (6) Alström syndrome

III. Renal cystic diseases with normal metanephric differentiation and hyperplasia of the tubular epithelium

   (1) Autosomal recessive polycystic kidney disease (ARPKD)
   (2) Autosomal dominant polycystic kidney disease (ADPKD)
   (3) Tuberous sclerosis
   (4) von Hippel–Lindau disease
   (5) Orofaciodigital syndrome type I

are variable. In some, the morbidity of the extrarenal abnormalities may become increasingly important as the mortality from renal failure decreases (e.g hepatic involvement in autosomal dominant polycystic kidney disease). In others, the renal disease may become more relevant as the mortality from major extrarenal involvements is reduced (e.g cystic kidneys in tuberous sclerosis).

2. Cystic kidney disease due to abnormal metanephric differentiation

The kidney, as any other organ, is not developmentally autonomous, but intimately interacts with other contiguous primordia that constitute different developmental fields during embryonic and fetal life[154,155,186]. A developmental field is a region of an embryo responding as a coordinated unit to embryonic interaction and resulting in complex anatomical structures. Morphologic anomalies can result from an intrinsic (*malformation*) or extrinsic (*disruption*) defect in a developmental field, from the abnormal organization of cells into tissue (*dysplasia*), or from mechanical forces (*deformation*). The components of a field are usually closely contiguous (monotopic fields). The components of some fields, however, may end up rather distantly located (polytopic fields). A defect in the development of a polytopic field may result in a puzzling pattern of multiple abnormalities, the common pathogenesis of which may be difficult to recognize (e.g acrorenal field defect).

Sequence, *syndrome* and *association* are terms used to describe other patterns of multiple morphologic defects. A *sequence* is a pattern of multiple anomalies derived from a single known or presumed prior anomaly or mechanical factor. An example is the oligohydramnios or Potter sequence. The Potter sequence is the result of any condition leading to oligohydramnios, such as a lack of fetal urine caused by bilateral renal agenesis, severe dysplasia or cystic disease. It comprises a typical facies, wrinkled skin, compression deformities of the limbs and respiratory distress caused by pulmonary hypoplasia[33,165].

A *syndrome* is a pattern of multiple anomalies thought to be pathogenically related and not known to represent a polytopic field defect or a single sequence. For example, complicated patterns of multiple anomalies may result from a single gene acting at various times on different organs during pre- and postnatal development (e.g branchiootorenal syndrome).

An *association* is a non-random occurrence in two or more individuals of multiple anomalies not known to be a polytopic field defect, a sequence, or a syndrome (e.g the VATER association). A concise review of general embryology and the normal development of the kidney may help in the appreciation of how specific interferences in the normal inductive interactions between different primordia can result in perplexing patterns of renal and extrarenal abnormalities.

Shortly after fertilization, a rapid succession of cell divisions results in the

210

formation of three germ layers: the ectoderm, the mesoderm and the endoderm (Fig. 9.1). By the end of the third week, the mesodermal layer has differentiated into paraxial mesoderm, the intermediate mesoderm and the parietal and visceral mesoderms. The nephrogenic tissue cord with the first primitive glomeruli and tubules develops in the beginning of the fourth week from the intermediate mesoderm, about the time that the neural tube develops in the ectoderm and that the mesenchyma derived from the paraxial mesoderm migrates to form the vertebral column, the branchial arches and the limb buds[156,169,175]. The nephrogenic cord is a continuously developing and degenerating unit that progresses in a cephalocaudal direction. It has completely disappeared at the level of the cervical region (pronephros) by the end of the fourth week. The contribution of the pronephros, however, is necessary for the formation of a duct, which later becomes the mesonephric or wolffian duct and is essential for later stages of development. The mesonephros forms an elongated organ that disappears by the end of the second month. The formation of the metanephros or permanent kidney begins in the fifth week. The ureteral bud arises from the caudal end of the mesonephric duct and penetrates the caudal end of the nephrogenic cord or metanephric blastema. The active growing tip of the ureteral bud or ampulla undergoes repeated dichotomous branching. After the initial 3–5 divisions, the ampullae begin to induce the cells of the metanephric blastema to organize into "S-shaped" bodies that later become glomeruli, proximal tubules, loops of Henle and distal tubules. One limb of the "S-shaped" body, destined to be the distal tubule, attaches to a division of the ureteral bud, which will become a collecting tubule. As the ureteral bud divides and advances, it carries the newly formed nephrons, thus explaining the absence of glomeruli in the renal medulla. The renal pelvis and

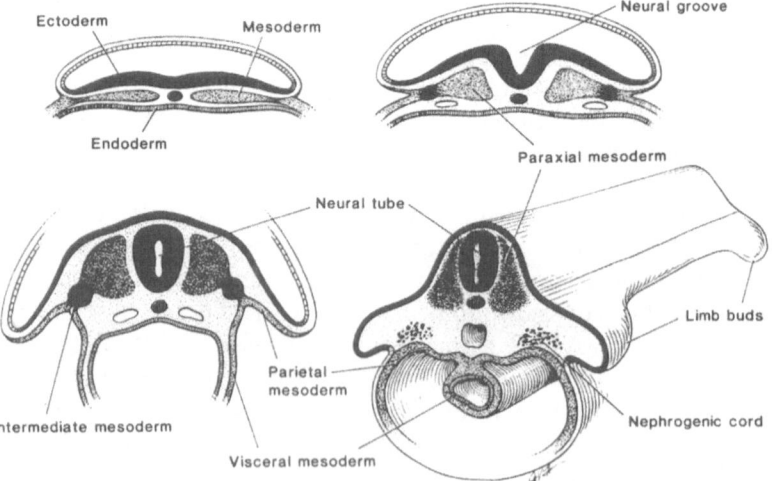

Figure 9.1. Stages of embryonic development during the third and fourth weeks.

calices derive from the first six divisions, while the papillary collecting ducts originate from divisions 6–10. The renal pelvis forms by 10–12 weeks, when the first divisions of the ureteral bud dilate and expand as a result of the pressure of urine excreted by the first few generations of nephrons.

The nature of the interrelations and interactions between the renal and extrarenal primordia at a molecular level are just beginning to be understood. For example, the coexistence of renal and cerebellar anomalies in several syndromes may be due to the defective production of a common cell-adhesion molecule (CAM) or the inability of cell surface receptors to bind these molecules[55]. The simultaneous involvement of the inner ear, the branchial arches and kidneys in the branchiootorenal syndrome probably reflects that differentiation of these organs is under the control of the same inducing or organizing mechanisms[78]. The fact that the spine and kidney develop at approximately the same time, during the fourth week, has been thought to explain the frequent association of congenital renal anomalies and neural tube defects[100]. The close proximity between the pronephros and the developing cervical spine probably accounts for the frequent occurrence of renal anomalies in the Klippel-Feil syndrome[145]. Finally, in the acrorenal field defects, the limb anomalies are thought to be due to the defective production of a limb inductor by the mesonephros. At an early stage of development, the limb buds and nephrogenic cord are in very close proximity, and it is known that mesonephric tissue is required for limb bud cartilage to continue development *in vitro*[116].

2.1. Sporadic defects

2.1.1. Cystic dysplastic kidneys

A spectrum of cystic dysplastic renal abnormalities including multicystic renal dysplasia with ureteral atresia and cystic dysplasia with congenital hydronephrosis results from an interference with metanephric induction and differentiation[15,85,157,159,217]. Most often these abnormalities occur as sporadic events and not as components of recognizable polytopic field defects, syndromes, or associations. Even in these sporadic cases, however, coexisting congenital abnormalities, such as cardiovascular, gastrointestinal and skeletal anomalies, are not rare[85]. Specific etiologies should always be considered and ruled out by careful review of the history and physical examination. Certain combinations of renal and extrarenal abnormalities and patterns of familial aggregation should alert the physician to the correct diagnosis, which may have important implications for prognosis, management and genetic counselling, as illustrated in the following sections.

2.1.2. Sporadic syndromes or associations

Defects of metanephric differentiation may occur as constituents of syndromes or associations without an identifiable cause. The de Lange's syndrome consists of physical and mental retardation, brachycephaly, hypertrophy of brows and lashes, limb abnormalities, a characteristic facies and, frequently, renal abnormalities including cystic dysplasia and hydronephrosis[62]. Significant upper urinary tract abnormalities, including renal agenesis and cystic dysplasia, have been associated with all three types of Klippel–Feil syndrome: type I, fusion of all the cervical and upper thoracic vertebrae; type II, fusion of one or two pairs of cervical vertebrae; and type III, combination of type I or type II with lower thoracic or lumbar fusions[92]. VATER is an acronym used to describe an association of anomalies including V = vertebral or vascular abnormalities; A = anal malformations; TE = tracheo-esophageal fistula, esophageal atresia; and R = radial or renal abnormalities. Certain presentations of the same abnormalities with a definable syndromal identity, such as on certain chromosomal abnormalities (e.g trisomy 18, trisomy 22 or "cat-eye" syndrome) and disruption syndromes (see below), should be distinguished from the usually sporadic VATER association[168].

2.2. Single gene mutations

2.2.1. Dominantly inherited renal adysplasia

Although renal agenesis and related abnormalities are frequently sporadic, many reports of familial clustering of these abnormalities have been published[23,26,138,172]. An autosomal dominant inheritance with incomplete penetrance and variable expression is the most likely pattern of transmission for most familial cases[138].

2.2.2. Branchiootorenal syndrome

The branchiootorenal syndrome is an autosomal dominant disorder manifested by various combinations of preauricular pits, lateral cervical sinuses, cysts or fistulas, structural defects of the outer, middle or inner ear, sensorineural, conductive, or mixed hearing loss, and renal abnormalities including renal agenesis, hypodysplastic and multicystic kidneys and related anomalies[61,64,139]. Preauricular pits are a very common minor anomaly, occurring in about 1% of the white population. Most patients with preauricular pits do not have branchiootorenal syndrome. The estimated risk of profound hearing loss in a child with preauricular pits is 1 in 200 and the risk of branchiootorenal syndrome is 1 in 400. Branchiootorenal syndrome is characterized by a high penetrance (almost all known carriers adequately examined show some manifestation) and variable expressivity, being harmless in a majority of cases. In the reported cases where the kidneys have been examined radiologically, 23% had agenesis or severe dysplasia and 43% had mild asymptomatic dysplasia. If one assumes that agenesis or severe dysplasia were absent when not reported, the estimated risk of severe renal involvement is 6%.

2.2.3. Cryptophthalmos–syndactyly syndrome

Cryptophthalmos is a rare congenital malformation in which the eyelids are fused or replaced by continuous skin[32,63]. Syndactyly and other malformations are frequently associated. Unilateral or bilateral renal agenesis and related renal abnormalities occur in approximately 10% of the cases. The mode of inheritance is usually autosomal recessive, with probable dominant inheritance reported in rare cases.

2.2.4. Acrorenal field defect

The association of renal agenesis or related renal abnormalities and congenital malformations of hands and feet, such as syndactyly, polydactyly and ectrodactyly, in the absence of other malformations has been reported in a small number of patients[37,46]. In one case, described as acrorenal-mandibular syndrome, severe mandibular hypoplasia was also associated[89]. Autosomal dominant and autosomal recessive patterns of inheritance have been suggested.

2.2.5. Skeletal dysplasias

Renal agenesis, cystic dysplasia and related renal abnormalities have been reported in association with a variety of skeletal dysplasias with an autosomal recessive inheritance. The biochemical defects responsible for these disorders have not been identified, but it is known that the rhizomelic type of chondrodysplasia punctata is a peroxisomal disorder closely related to the Zellweger syndrome[77,94]. A detailed description of these conditions is beyond the scope of this chapter[197]. Most of the diseases are lethal at birth or during early childhood, but survival to adulthood is possible in chrondroectodermal dysplasia and in asphyxiating thoracic dysplasia. Chondroectodermal dysplasia or Ellis–Van Creveld syndrome is characterized by acromelic dwarfism, impaired development of teeth, nails and hair, polydactyly, and congenital heart disease[18,174]. Asphyxiating thoracic dystrophy or Jeune syndrome comprises rhizomelic dwarfism and short horizontal ribs that result in a narrow thoracic cage with restricted mobility and respiratory impairment[93,125,178,184] (Fig. 9.2).

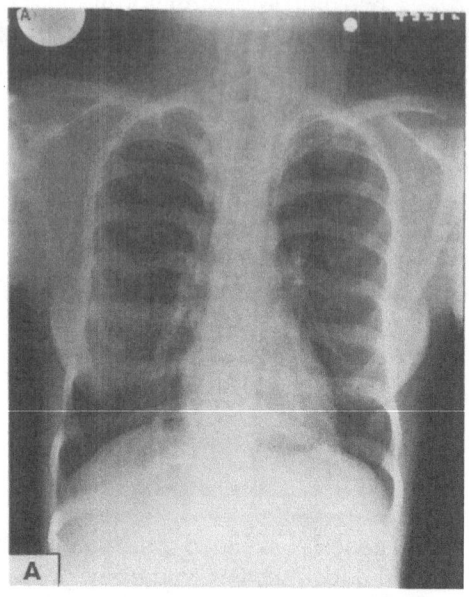

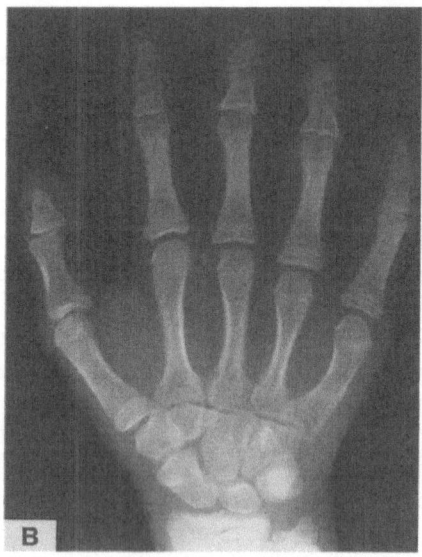

Figure 9.2. 14-year-old renal transplant patient with Jeune syndrome. (A) Narrow thoracic cage with short horizontal ribs. (B) Peripheral dysostosis with short middle and distal phalanges due to premature metaepiphyseal fusion; fusion of the middle and distal phalanges in the second and fifth fingers; the cone shaped epiphyses are no longer apparent.

Many of the patients who survive the respiratory difficulties in infancy develop chronic renal failure later in childhood. Biliary dysgenesis and pancreatic dysplasia are prominent features in some of these diseases[7,8,9]. The renal involvement in some of these conditions overlaps between defects of metanephric differentiation (lobar disorganization, deficient nephronic differentiation and cystic dysplasia) and hereditary interstitial nephritis (dilatation of medullary collecting ducts and infiltration of fibrillar PAS-positive material through ruptured tubules into the interstitium) (see page 221, conorenal syndromes).

2.2.6. Other autosomal recessive metabolic dysplasia and multiple malformation syndromes

Cystic dysplasia and related renal abnormalities occur at varying rates in numerous autosomal recessive multiple malformation syndromes. These conditions have been reviewed in more detail elsewhere[197]. They are usually lethal at birth or during infancy with the exception of the cerebro-oculohepatorenal syndrome. The renal involvement in cerebrooculohepatorenal syndrome overlaps with that seen in the cystic diseases with inherited interstitial nephritis[135]. Glutaric aciduria type II and the Zellweger syndrome deserve special comment. Glutaric aciduria type II is an autosomal recessive disorder characterized clinically by metabolic acidosis, hypoglycemia and excretion of a special group of organic acids in the urine[19,21,95,118]. Patients with glutaric aciduria type II can be separated into two groups, those with a deficiency in electron transfer flavoprotein and those with a deficiency in electron transfer flavoprotein dehydrogenase. Only those with the second type have associated congenital anomalies. The renal abnormality in glutaric aciduria type II consists of numerous 1–2 mm cysts in the cortex and medulla causing variable degrees of renal enlargement. The basic biochemical defect in the cerebrooculohepatorenal syndrome of Zellweger has not yet been identified, but this syndrome has been characterized at an ultrastructural and biochemical level by the absence of peroxisomes and defects in peroxisomal function[39,105,146,173,192,206,214]. The most common renal abnormality in Zellweger syndrome consists of glomerular and tubular microcysts. The term "prenatal metabolic dysplasia" has been suggested to refer to a group of metabolic disorders such as glutaric aciduria type II and the Zellweger syndrome that result in defects of metanephric differentiation[65,95].

2.3. Chromosomal aberrations

Characteristic phenotypes, often including the presence of renal cystic dysplasia and related abnormalities, occur in several numerical or structural chromosomal aberrations[68,76]. Numerical aberrations result from the non-dysjunction of sister chromatids at anaphase resulting in an aneuploid number of chromosomes. If non-dysjunction occurs at an early division of the zygote rather than during gametogenesis, a mosaicism with two or more cell lines with different numbers of chromosomes results. The chromosomal structural abnormalities include deletion, duplication, insertion and translocation. Deletions are the structural abnormalities that most commonly result in abnormal phenotypes. Usually, numerical chromosomal aberrations occur sporadically and the recurrence risk after an affected offspring is low. Exceptions are a mosaic state in a parent without phenotypic expression and certain structural chromosomal rearrangements such as translocations that may increase the risk of non-dysjunction during gametogenesis. The most common chromosomal aberrations with associated defects of ureteral development and metanephric induction and differentiation (renal agenesis, fused kidneys, vesicoureteral reflux, ureteral duplication, ureteropelvic junction obstruction and the spectrum of cystic dysplastic renal abnormalities) include trisomies 21 (Down syndrome), 18 (Edwards), 13 (Patau), 8, 9, 7 and 2q; chromosome X monosomy (Turner); and 4p deletion (Wolf–Hirschorn)[24,117,179,203,216]. These conditions have been recently reviewed elsewhere[68,76].

2.4. Multifactorial defects

2.4.1. Neural tube defects

The association of neural tube defects and congenital renal abnormalities has been known for a long time, but the first detailed study was by Roberts in 1961[171]. Among 140 cases of spina bifida of a major degree, he reported 25 cases or 17.8% with gross structural renal abnormalities. These include fused kidneys (nine cases), unilateral or bilateral renal agenesis or hypodysplasia (five cases) and cystic kidneys (six cases), in addition to ureteric, bladder and urethral abnormalities. In a later study, Wilcock et al. reported a 29% prevalence of gross renal abnormalities in children with meningomyelocele including cystic dysplasia in 6.9% of the patients[213]. It was suggested that as more cases with neural tube defects are salvaged, the associated renal malformations will become more clinically significant. The pattern of abnormalities associated with neural tube defects is related to the level of the lesion in spina bifida as measured by sensory loss to pinprick[209]. Renal agenesis was associated with a sensory level in the dermatomes T5–8, horseshoe kidneys with T9–L1, and duplications predominantly with the sacral dermatomes. In some children with neural tube defects, these associations are somewhat obscured by the occurrence of vesical dysfunction and the equivalent of severe destructive uropathy.

2.4.2. Disruption syndromes including renal agenesis/dysplasia and associated renal abnormalities

The most common disruption syndromes that include renal agenesis/dysplasia and associated renal abnormalities are listed in Table 9.1. Among them, maternal diabetes mellitus is probably the most common. The renal abnormalities may occur as isolated findings, malformations or more frequently as part of multiple malformation syndromes such as "caudal regression syndrome" and the VATER association[87,113]. The frequent occurrence of cystic dysplasia of the kidneys in Williams syndrome has been recognized recently[13]. This syndrome is characterized by growth retardation, microcephaly with variable degrees of mental retardation, typical facial features and personality, and supravalvular aortic stenosis. It is presumed that in many cases it represents a maternal gestational derangement of Vitamin D or calcium metabolism[66].

3. Renal cystic diseases with hereditary interstitial nephritis (nephronophthisis–medullary cystic disease complex)

Nephronophthisis and medullary cystic disease, initially described as two different diseases, are now considered to be synonymous terms that define a heterogeneous group of disorders rather than a single entity[5,72]. The pathogenesis of these disorders is not known. Recently, a primary tubular basement defect and an autoimmune interstitial nephritis have been reported as possible etiopathogenic factors[33,106]. At least two forms are recognized on the basis of inheritance and clinical presentation, a juvenile recessive form and an adult dominant form. In the recessive type, a subclinical form of the disease expressed by a reduced urinary concentrating ability has occasionally been documented in obligate heterozygotes. Sporadic presentations may represent recessive cases in families with few offspring or new dominant mutations. Extrarenal abnormalities such as pigmentary retinopathy, skeletal abnormalities, hepatic fibrosis and abnormalities of the central nervous system may occur in association with the autosomal recessive forms.

3.1. Senior–Løken syndrome

Contreras and Espinoza[35], Senior et al. [182], and Løken et al. [127] first described the association of the nephronophthisis–medullary cystic disease complex and a pigmentary retinopathy. The terms used to describe this pigmentary retinopathy can be confusing[152]. The term most frequently used is retinitis pigmentosa, although this condition is not, as the name implies, inflammatory. Most patients with retinitis pigmentosa do not have nephronophthisis–medullary cystic disease complex. Retinitis pigmentosa is the common pathway of a number of disease processes which are not understood and may range from metabolic defects to autoimmune mechanisms. It is characterized by widespread depigmentation or atrophy of the retinal pigment epithelium with relative macular sparing (bull's eye pattern), intraretinal pigment migration with bone spicule pigment clumps frequently found in the periphery, retinal vessel narrowing and vitreous macular changes (Fig. 9.3). It affects both rods and cones, but in the early stages, the rods usually are more severely affected.

Retinitis pigmentosa can be classified into many subtypes on the basis of genetic, anatomic and clinical findings. Most patients with retinitis pigmentosa become symptomatic between the ages of 5 and 30 years. The usual presenting complaints are difficulty seeing at night, difficulty adjusting from dim to bright illumination and restricted mobility due to tunnel vision. In some patients, the only evidence of retinal involvement may be obtained by electroretinography. Leber's congenital amaurosis is the most severe manifestation of the retinitis process, and the affected individuals are born blind or become blind during the first years of life and have congenital nystagmus. Sectorial retinitis pigmentosa is characterized by the sectorial distribution of the retinal pigment changes and has a better prognosis. Retinitis punctata albescens is characterized by drusen-like deposits in the mid-peripheral fundus, and most likely represents an early or lightly pigmented form of retinitis pigmentosa.

Patients with the renal–retinal syndrome may have any of these presentations[60,79,80,81]. Even within the same family, the type of retinal involvement may change from patient to patient. Electroretinography and visual field assessment are the most important tests for the functional evaluation of these patients. Electroretinographic studies of family members have also indicated

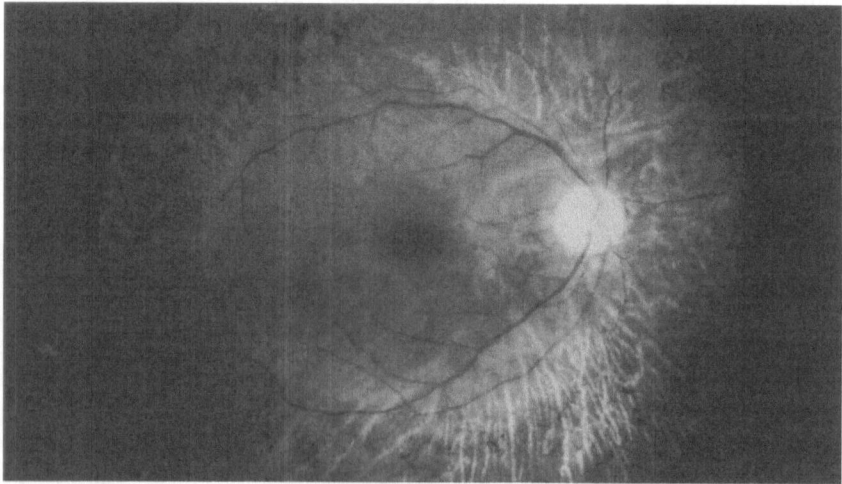

Figure 9.3. Typical fundus appearance of advanced retinitis pigmentosa with pale discs, attenuated retinal vessels and bone spicule pigment formation in the periphery.

that involvement of the kidney and retina may occur together or independently of one another.

Electroretinography may be a useful diagnostic tool in the elucidation of certain cases of renal failure of obscure origin, especially if the nephronophthisis–medullary cystic disease complex is thought to be present[183]. Electroretinographic abnormalities may also be found in some heterozygous gene carriers[96,161]. Keratoconus and mental subnormality with onset in middle childhood have been observed in rare patients with the Senior–Loken syndrome[79]. The association of retinitis pigmentosa and severe congenital sensorineural deafness is referred to as Usher syndrome, and it has not been associated with renal disease. A sporadic case of renal–retinal syndrome with sensorineural hearing loss, nuclear cataracts and diffuse glomerular cysts, in addition to tubular cysts in the corticomedullary region, has been reported[110]. In one family, the nephronophthisis–medullary cystic disease complex was associated with macular degeneration and pendular nystagmus, but retinitis pigmentosa was excluded on the basis of clinical and electroretinographic evidence[163].

3.2. Conorenal syndromes

Giedion has used this term to describe various syndromes characterized by the combination of phalangeal cone-shaped epiphysis of the hands and a chronic renal disease consistent with the nephronophthisis–medullary disease complex[74,75]. These include chondroectodermal dysplasia, asphyxiating thoracic dystrophy, the Saldino–Mainzer syndrome[131,162], and the associations of nephronophthisis and peripheral dysostosis, with or without retinitis pigmentosa[27,47]. Peripheral dysostosis is a dysostosis often affecting only the long bones of the hands. It is characterized by numerous and marked phalangeal changes in the form of cone-shaped epiphyses. Depending on the severity of the con-shaped epiphyseal deformation, the phalanges may grow normally or, by premature meta–epiphyseal fusion, become progressively shortened. Giedion proposed a classification of the cone-shaped epiphysis based on the radiological appearances. Type 28, which is buried deeply in and is broadly connected with the metaphysis, seems to be the most commonly found in the cono-renal syndromes. Irregularities of the femoral neck and small or flattened femoral heads are also frequently found. Chondroectodermal dysplasia and asphyxiating thoracic dystrophy have been discussed on page 215 (Fig. 9.2). The Saldino–Mainzer syndrome comprises nephronophthisis, retinitis pigmentosa, cerebellar truncal ataxia and peripheral dysostosis.

3.3. Nephronophthisis and congenital hepatic fibrosis

The association of the nephronophthisis–medullary cystic disease complex and congenital hepatic fibrosis was first noted by Boichis *et al.* [20] in four children from an interrelated marriage. A fifth sibling had congenital hepatic fibrosis but no evidence of renal disease. Pigmentary retinopathy and skeletal abnormalities may also occur in association with the hepatic fibrosis and the renal disease[48,164]. Portal hypertension in these patients is usually less severe than in autosomal recessive polycystic kidney disease (ARPKD) and congenital hepatic fibrosis.

3.4. Cerebrooculohepatorenal syndrome

The association of congenital Leber's amaurosis, renal disease and maldevelopment of the brain, including agenesis of the cerebellar vermis, was initially described by Dekaban in 1969[41]. Many additional reports have been recently summarised by Matsuzaka *et al.* [135]. These patients share the common clinical manifestation of blindness, severe psychomotor retardation, hypotonia since early infancy and often characteristic facial appearance with unilateral blepharoptosis and telecanthus. Congenital hepatic fibrosis is often present. In some cases, the renal disease was thought to be consistent with nephronophthisis. In other cases, the renal disorder was described as "polycystic kidneys", renal dysplasia and nephrosclerosis[135].

3.5. Laurence–Moon–Bardet–Biedl syndrome

This is an autosomal recessive syndrome characterized by obesity, polydactyly, retinitis pigmentosa, mental retardation and hypogenitalism. Congenital heart disease and renal involvement are also very common. The renal involvement consists of tubulointerstitial nephritis and caliectasis, often with cystic spaces communicating with the collecting system[84,124,187]. Visual impairment usually occurs in the second and third decades of life. Hepatic fibrosis is rare.

3.6. Alström syndrome

A slowly progressive chronic tubulointerstitial nephropathy can also occur in this rare autosomal recessive syndrome characterized by obesity, diabetes mellitus, retinitis pigmentosa and nerve deafness[2,25].

4. Renal cystic diseases with normal metanephric differentiation and hyperplasia of the tubular epithelium

Under this category is included a heterogeneous group of disorders which have to be considered in the differential diagnosis of bilateral cystic disease of the kidney. The cysts originate from completely formed nephrons, and there is no evidence of an abnormal metanephric differentiation. Cyst growth in these diseases is, at least on theoretical considerations, dependent on the production of new epithelial cells[208]. They are caused by single gene mutations of pleiotropic genes as indicated by the frequency and importance of the extrarenal manifestations. The nature of these extrarenal associations is poorly understood, as the basic defect at a molecular level and pathogenetic mechanism are not known for any of these diseases.

4.1. Autosomal recessive polycystic kidney disease (ARPKD)

The main extrarenal associations of ARPKD are congenital hepatic fibrosis and Caroli disease. Choledocal cysts are rarely present. The association with intracranial aneurysms is not as well established as in ADPKD. The association of ARPKD and Ehlers–Danlos syndrome has been reported in one patient[136].

The term congenital hepatic fibrosis refers to a developmental abnormality of the liver that is ordinarily associated but not restricted to ARPKD, occurring also as an isolated abnormality and in association with renal dysplasia and hereditary tubulointerstitial nephritis[12]. It consists of enlarged and fibrotic portal areas with an apparent proliferation of bile ducts, absence of central bile ducts, hypoplasia of the portal vein branches, and, sometimes, prominent fibrosis around the central veins. These histologic features are very different from those in ADPKD and may help in the differential diagnosis of these two conditions which in infancy and childhood is not always easy[166,190]. ARPKD is invariably associated with biliary dysgenesis, while the liver histology in children with ADPKD is usually normal.

The severity of the renal and hepatic involvement in ARPKD appears to be inversely related. The spectrum of the hepatic disease ranges from minimal hepatic involvement in newborns to congenital hepatic fibrosis in adolescents or adults having minimal renal involvement[17]. Some authors have argued that the clinical presentations of ARPKD are genetically different, but this is not supported by the observation of patients with different presentations of the disease within the same family[71,122].

Hepatosplenomegaly and portal hypertension are the common presentations of congenital hepatic fibrosis (Fig. 9.4). The hepatic involvement may become more apparent in the patients with ARPKD after successful renal transplantation. On the other hand, hepatosplenomegaly and portal hypertension may bring the patients to the attention of a physician, and the polycystic kidneys and chronic renal insufficiency may become more important at a later date following successful portal shunting. Liver function tests are usually normal, but mild elevations of the serum alkaline phosphatase and transaminase can occur. A rare complication is the development of a cholangiocarcino-

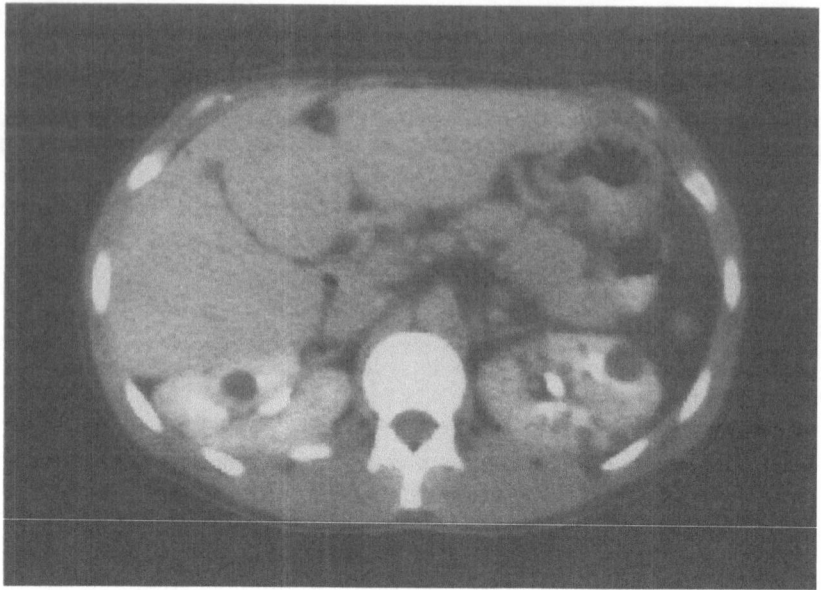

Figure 9.4. Polycystic kidney (ARPKD), enlargement of the caudate and left lobes of the liver consistent with congenital hepatic fibrosis, and surgical absence of the spleen.

ma[16,137]. The patients with symptomatic portal hypertension are excellent candidates for portal systemic shunting procedures, the portal caval shunting being preferred by some[107].

Caroli disease or non-obstructive intrahepatic biliary dilatation occurs as an isolated abnormality or in association with congenital hepatic fibrosis with or without ARPKD[200]. The diagnosis can be suspected by ultrasound and CT scanning and established by endoscopic or percutaneous cholangiography. It may be diffuse or involve only one hepatic lobe. As long as the dilated intrahepatic bile ducts remain uninfected, the patient is asymptomatic. The most common presentation is with a recurrent cholangitis. Gallstones may form in the dilated ducts. Rare complications are steatorrhea[111], secondary amyloidosis[4], and bile duct carcinoma, usually adenocarcinoma and less often squamous cell carcinoma[28,180]. Moderate elevations of serum alkaline phosphatase, transaminase and bilirubin can occur. The treatment consists of antibiotic therapy. Partial hepatectomy can be considered in the cases where the dilatation of the intrahepatic bile ducts is segmental[147].

4.2. Autosomal dominant polycystic kidney disease (ADPKD)

A variety of extrarenal disorders have been associated with ADPKD. Because of the better survival of ADPKD patients in recent years due to improvements in the general medical care and to the availability of dialysis and renal transplantation, the morbidity and mortality related to these associated disorders is likely to become more important[29,43,69,196]. Not for all these disorders has an association been definitely established. Coexistence by chance of two relatively common disorders can be expected and, therefore, associations based on case reports or even a small series of patients should be viewed with caution. Associations of ADPKD and other inherited diseases have been reported in some families. These associations are more likely fortuitous and include familial polyposis of the colon, Peutz–Jeghers syndrome, hypertrophic pyloric stenosis, myotonic dystrophy, lattice-corneal dystrophy, Darier disease, hereditary spherocytosis, carotid glomus tumor, alpha$_1$ antitrypsin deficiency and Marfan syndrome[30,42,49,52,56,108,126,160,181,210]. There have been two reports of the association of neurofibromatosis and "adult" polycystic kidney disease, one of the cases with an associated renal cell carcinoma[185,202]. ADPKD has also been observed in association with hemihypertrophy[59,170].

4.2.1. Hepatic cysts

The association of hepatic cysts and ADPKD is well established. These cysts are lined by a cuboidal or flattened epithelium and contain fluid resembling the bile independent fraction of bile[88]. They are thought to result from progressive dilatation of biliary microhamartomas (von Meyenburg complexes), which are small clusters of bile ducts surrounded by fibrous tissue, commonly connected to the portal tracts and occasionally containing bile[205]. Preliminary observations suggest that the cyst epithelium is an active secretory epithelium responsive to hormones, such as secretin, which normally affect the biliary epithelium[57]. In a recent study, biliary fibroadenomatosis, which is characterized by fibrosis of the portal tracts with an excessive number of more or less dilated bile ducts, was observed with a surprisingly high frequency in patients with ADPKD[88]. The liver histopathologic changes in ADPKD, however, are very different from those observed in congenital hepatic fibrosis, which consists of diffuse biliary fibroadenomatosis. The biliary fibroadenomas in ADPKD are less prominent and less diffuse, and there is no hypoplasia of the portal vein branches. The hepatic cysts in ADPKD usually develop later than the renal cysts, and their number increases with age and the development of renal insufficiency[142]. Nevertheless, severe polycystic liver disease is sometimes seen with but minimal renal involvement. Women with ADPKD tend to have more severe liver cystic disease than men. A correlation between the number of cysts and the number of pregnancies has been suggested, indicating that estrogens might influence the development of hepatic cysts[103].

Despite their frequency, the hepatic cysts in ADPKD usually cause minimal morbidity. Severe, but transient, pain may result from hemorrhage into a cyst. Rarely, these cysts may become infected, especially following renal transplantation or in dialysis patients[73]. Obstructive jaundice due to compression of the bile ducts by the cysts can occur[36,98,205]. It is a rare complication and other causes of obstructive jaundice should be ruled out[1]. Several authors have reported the association of polycystic kidney disease in the adult and congenital hepatic fibrosis[31,53,70,133,193]. In most of these reports, a family history consistent with autosomal dominant inheritance was not documented or very little information was provided. In a recent study, DeVos et al. [45] presented two families with proven transmission of ADPKD from a mother to several children. Two of the children in these families have ADPKD only, four have ADPKD and congenital hepatic fibrosis, and one has congenital hepatic fibrosis only. Whether the polycystic kidney disease and the congenital hepatic fibrosis are expressions of the same genetic defect in these families is uncertain. Very rarely, portal hypertension in the absence of hepatic fibrosis, presumably due to compression of the portal vein by cysts, can be observed in ADPKD[44,167]. A small subset of patients with polycystic liver disease may become incapacitated by mechanical problems and pain produced by massively enlarged polycystic livers. Incapacitating abdominal distention with dyspnea and early satiety can be the main complaints. Rarely, a massively enlarged liver can compress the inferior vena cava and cause ascites and lower extremity edema. Compression of the inferior vena cava may also cause severe hypotension during hemodialysis. Pain and abnormal liver function tests may be the presenting symptom in the rare complication of a cholangiocarcinoma in a polycystic liver. Clinically recognizable hepatocellular dysfunction, if it indeed occurs, is exceedingly rare. This may be due to focal distribution of cystic disease, with sparing of some liver segments and preservation of parenchymal volume despite massive cystic enlargement[148]. When the liver function tests are abnormal, a complication or an unrelated liver disease should be suspected.

Most often, the hepatic involvement in ADPKD requires no treatment. Computed tomography, magnetic resonance imaging and gallium and indium-labelled white blood cell scans may be helpful in the diagnosis of an infected liver cyst. The treatment consists of drainage and prolonged antibiotic therapy. There is no information available on the penetration of antibiotics in the liver cysts. In some patients, abdominal fullness and pain may be due to only one or a few large dominant hepatic cysts. Percutaneous aspiration and sclerosis of the cysts by instillation of alcohol can provide a permanent therapeutic benefit[6,198].

Surgery may play a role in the treatment of patients with highly symptomatic polycystic liver disease. Lin et al.[123] initially described a fenestration procedure consisting of extensive unroofing of superficial cysts and transcystic excision of common cyst walls to decompress and drain into the peritoneal cavity cysts located deeper within the substance of the liver. They reported the use of this technique without complications in three patients with large polycystic livers. The successful use of this technique in small numbers of patients was subsequently reported by several authors[58,99,130,158]. Paliard et al. [158] found that cimetidine reduces the secretion rate by unroofed cysts, possibly by inhibiting gastric acidity and the secretin secretion. van Erpecum *et al.* [201] recently reported the largest experience using this fenestration procedure. Of nine patients with highly symptomatic polycystic liver disease, one died pre-operatively due to irreversible shock. The abdominal complaints disappeared post-operatively in seven of the other eight patients. Obstructive jaundice with esophageal varices resolved in the three patients with these complications. A decrease of the liver size, however, was uncommon.

The combined use of cyst fenestration and segmental hepatectomy has been rarely reported. Armitage and Blumgart[3] performed this surgery in one woman with massive polycystic liver disease. The major operative and post-operative problem encountered was massive fluid losses, but the liver function tests remained normal, the patient claimed that her life had been transformed and that she felt and looked completely normal. Successful use of partial hepatectomy for the treatment of massive polycystic liver disease was also reported by Lanson *et al.* [115] and by Wittig *et al.* [215] in individual patients. On the other hand, two of the three patients reported by Turnage *et al.* [200] died following combined fenestration/segmental hepatectomy. These authors recommend preoperative identification of the cysts responsible for the patient's symptoms, and treatment directed to the unroofing of these cysts only to limit morbidity and mortality. In our experience, a combined fenestration–segmental hepatectomy procedure has provided satisfactory results with minor complications in six patients (Fig. 9.5). A seventh patient with massive polycystic liver disease and ascites following renal transplantation died as a result of intracranial hemorrhage after surgery complicated by severe bleeding and severe hypotension and a prolonged post-operative course with massive fluid losses, jaundice and bacteremia[149]. Until the place of surgery is better defined, careful weighing of the risks and benefits, frank discussion with the patient, and selection of the surgical approach to achieve the desired result with the least risk to the patient are recommended.

4.2.2. Intracranial aneurysms

The association of intracranial aneurysms and ADPKD has been established on the basis of large retrospective autopsy studies[14,22,191,196]. The overall prevalence of intracranial aneurysms in the general population ranges in several large autopsy studies from 0.2 to 9.9%; the more recent studies indicate a frequency of approximately 5%. The observed frequency of coexisting intracranial aneurysms and ADPKD has been significantly higher than expected from chance association alone (Fig. 9.6). Approximately 20% of ADPKD patients have intracranial aneurysms at autopsy. In the Olmsted community study, intracranial aneurysms were found in 19% of the patients, and rupture resulting in subarachoid hemorrhage was the immediate cause of death in 7%. Two small angiographic studies of ADPKD patients in Japan have been published. Wakabayashi *et al.* [204] found asymptomatic, unruptured intracranial aneurysms in 41% of the patients (7 out of 17), suggesting that the frequency of unruptured aneurysms in ADPKD might have been underestimated in autopsy studies. Matsumara *et al.* [134] found aneurysms in three out of five patients with ADPKD.

From studies in the general population, it is known that the vast majority

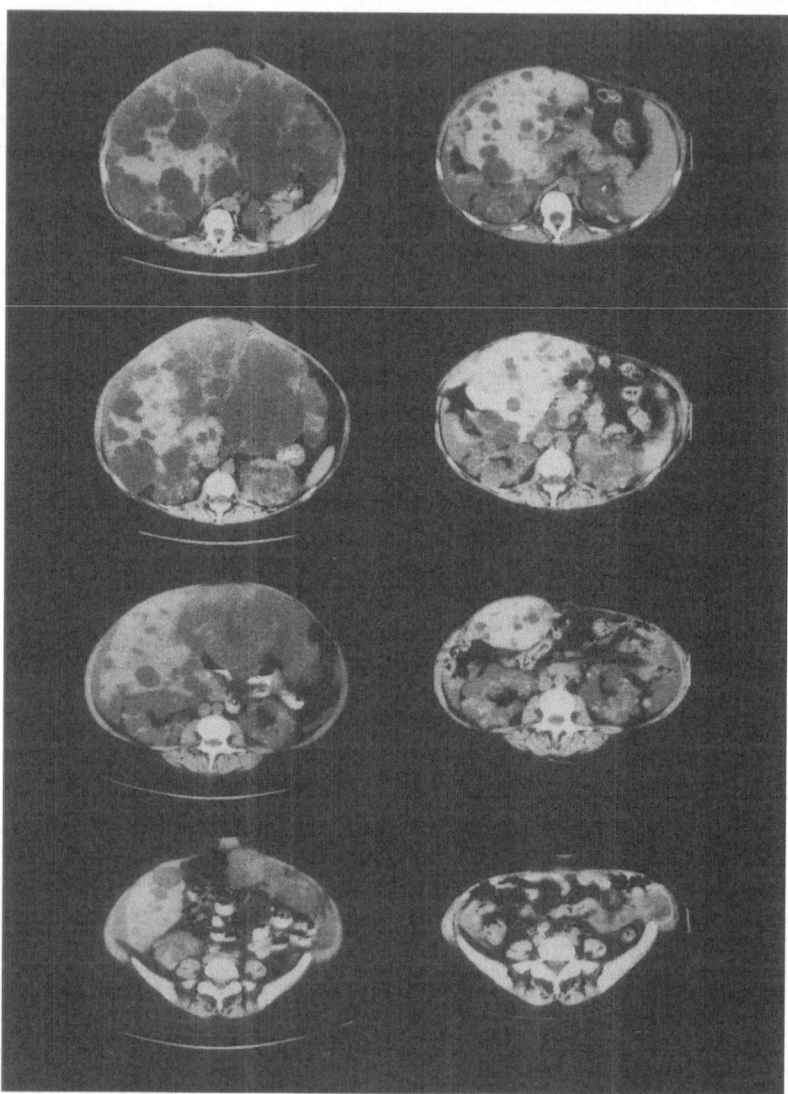

Figure 9.5. Computed tomography before (left panels) and three months after (right panels) a combined fenestration–segmental hepatectomy procedure in a patient with highly symptomatic polycystic liver disease.

of intracranial aneurysms never rupture. Since cerebral angiography has a low but real morbidity and intracranial aneurysm surgery has significant morbidity and mortality, even in the best hands, accurate knowledge of the natural history of unruptured intracranial aneurysms is essential for intelligent treatment decisions. In a recent prospective study of intracranial aneurysms in the general population, the only variable that was found to be of unquestionable value in predicting the risk of rupture was aneurysm size[212]. None of 44 aneurysms smaller than 1 cm in diameter ruptured, whereas 8 of 29 aneurysms 1 cm or more in diameter eventually did. Aneurysmal symptoms other than rupture, such as compression of cranial nerves or other central nervous system structures, distal thromboembolic phenomena, and focal headaches or a change in the character of the headaches, which also predict eventual rupture, correlate with the size of the aneurysm.

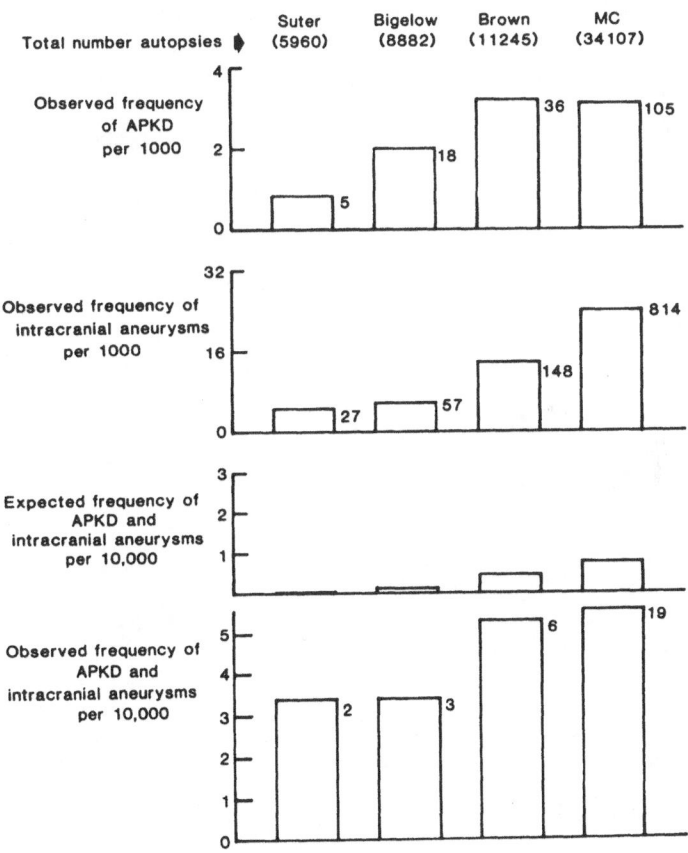

Figure 9.6. Observed and expected frequencies of intracranial aneurysms and polycystic kidney disease in major autopsy series. (Reprinted from Torres *et al.* [196] with permission.)

228

There is no information on the natural history of intracranial aneurysms associated with ADPKD. A decision analysis has been used to assess whether or not patients with ADPKD should undergo routine cerebral angiography for intracranial aneurysms and prophylactic surgery, assuming that the natural history of these aneurysms is not different from the natural history of all intracranial saccular aneurysms[120]. It was found that arteriography should not be carried out routinely because its benefit exceeds one year only if the

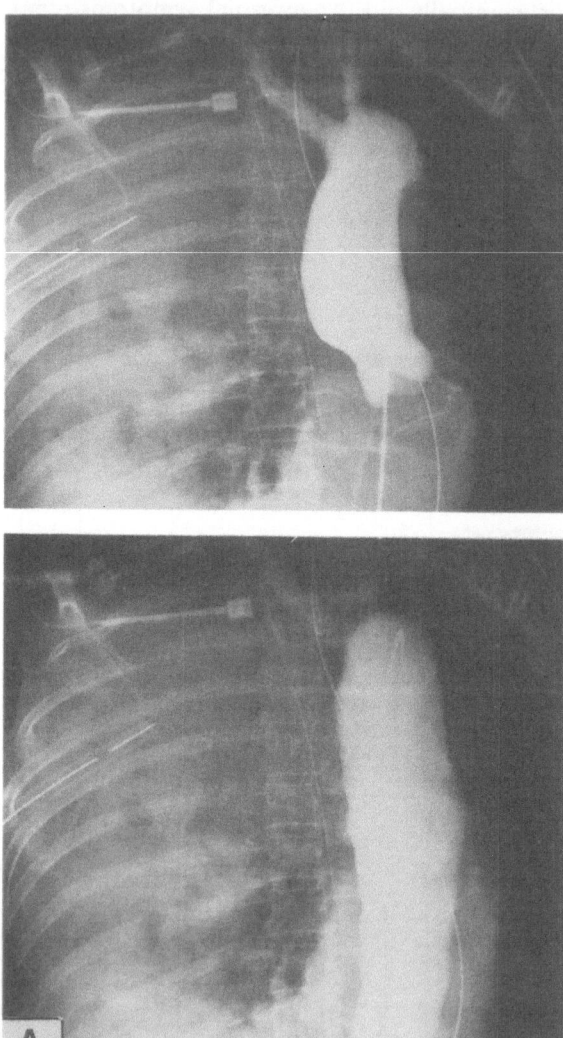

Figure 9.7A. Aortogram demonstrating a dissecting aortic aneurysm in a patient with autosomal dominant polycystic kidney disease.

prevalence of aneurysms exceeds 30%, if the surgical complication rate is 1% or less, and if the patient is under 25 years of age. Therefore, there appears to be little justification to screen for the presence of intracranial aneurysms in asymptomatic patients. Preselection of patients with a high probability of having large intracranial aneurysms by new non-invasive screening techniques might significantly alter this decision tree analysis. The preliminary results of a study using high resolution computed angiotomography and magnetic resonance imaging indicate that routine non-invasive screening of asymptomatic ADPKD patients without a family history of intracranial aneurysms by these techniques has a very low yield[194]. The explanation of the discrepancy between this non-invasive study and the two previously mentioned angiographic studies is not clear. Some authors have reported clustering of intracranial aneurysms in certain families with ADPKD[102,176]. Possibly, screening for intracranial

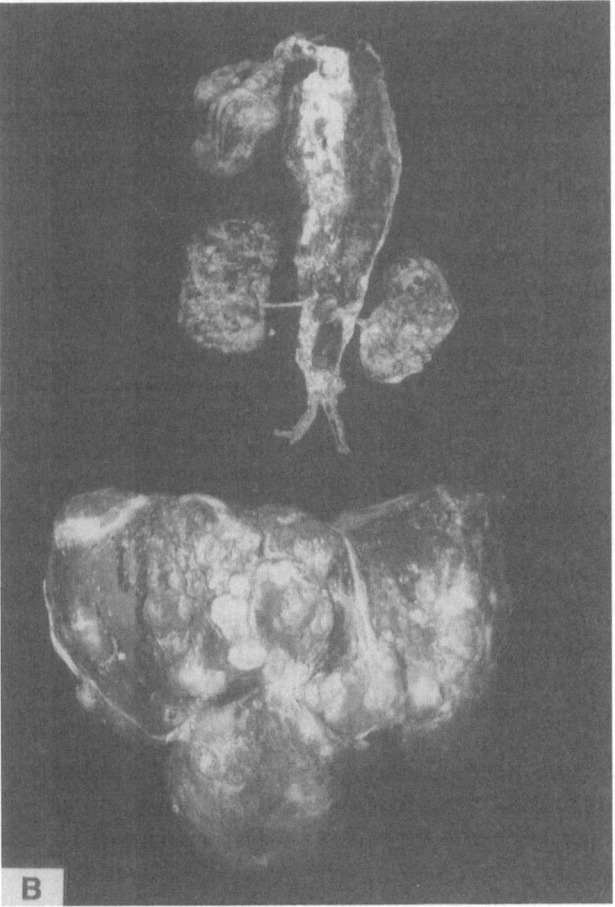

Figure 9.7B. Heart, aorta, polycystic kidneys and polycystic liver of the same patient. (Reprinted from Torres *et al.* [195] with permission.)

aneurysms should be targeted to ADPKD patients with a family history of intracranial aneurysm or subarachnoid hemorrhage.

Surgery is indicated for intracranial aneurysms equal to or greater than 10 mm in diameter[211]. The management of unruptured aneurysms 6–9 mm in diameter is controversial. Aneurysms less than 6 mm in diameter have a low likelihood of rupture and should be restudied yearly. If symptoms develop and/or the aneurysm enlarges, surgery should be considered. The preferred surgical technique involves clipping the aneurysm at its neck. The overall mortality and serious morbidity associated with this procedure for a single unruptured aneurysm is approximately 2–7% when performed by experienced surgeons using the operating microscope. Risk varies with location of the aneurysm, its configuration and the accessibility of its neck to surgical clipping. With multiple aneurysms, the risk is increased for each additional aneurysm. If clipping is successful, it is considered a cure. If clipping of the aneurysm is not possible, other less optimal surgical procedures such as carotid ligation and detachable balloon techniques with or without extracranial to intracranial arterial bypass may be utilized.

4.2.3. Other cardiovascular complications

There have been several case reports of associations of ADPKD and cardio-vascular abnormalities. In a large series, an 18% frequency of cardiovascular abnormalities was found[119]. Dilatation of the aortic root, bicuspid aortic valve, mitral valve prolapse and coarctation of the aorta were the most frequent abnormalities. Valvular and aortic abnormalities have also been found in autopsy series at the Mayo Clinic[196]. Aortic aneurysms or dissections, bicuspid aortic valve and aortic coarctation were observed. Of these, dissecting thoracic aortic aneurysms were the most common (Fig. 9.7). The observed frequency of coexisting polycystic kidney disease and dissecting thoracic aortic aneurysm in these autopsy series was 7.3 times greater than expected from chance association alone. Mitral valve prolapse has been found with increased frequency in these patients in a prospective echocardiographic study[97].

4.2.4. Colon diverticulosis and other associations

The association between ADPKD and colon diverticulosis has been reported by Scheff[177] in a small number of patients. Awareness of this association may be important because these authors also found an increased risk for developing diverticulitis and colonic performation. It has also been suggested that inguinal hernias and congenital skeletal abnormalities may occur with increased frequency in ADPKD patients[69].

4.2.5. Carcinoma in polycystic kidneys

Focal cellular hyperplasia of the tubular epithelium is a common abnormality of ADPKD[10,86]. Whether this constitutes a preneoplastic state is uncertain. Many case reports of ADPKD and renal cell carcinoma have been published, but these do not prove the existence of an association, since chance coexistence of two relatively common disorders can be expected in a considerable number of patients. In many large series of patients, the association of renal cell carcinoma and ADPKD has not been found. Furthermore, development of renal cell carcinoma in polycystic kidney patients on hemodialysis or after renal transplantation has been rarely reported, and it does not appear to be a common problem. The observed frequency of renal cell carcinoma in ADPKD coexisting in the same patient in the Mayo Clinic autopsy series was not higher than expected by chance association alone[196]. The main argument to support the possibility that ADPKD is a premalignant state is the fact that the renal cell carcinoma in many of the reported cases was multicentric or bilateral. When

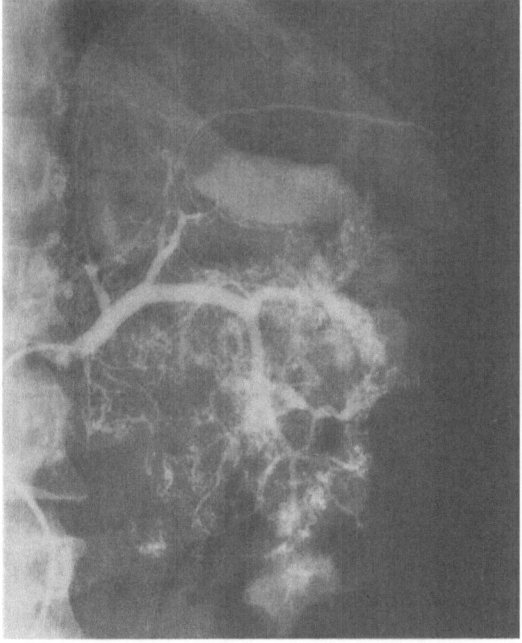

Figure 9.8. Renal cell carcinoma in a patient with autosomal dominant polycystic kidney disease. Hypervascular mass demonstrated by renal arteriography. Polycystic kidney disease had been previously diagnosed. The patient presented with anemia and fever of unknown origin. (Reprinted from Torres *et al.* [195] with permission.)

ADPKD and renal cell carcinoma coexist in the same patient, the diagnosis is challenging. Pain in association with fever, weight loss, anemia, or a striking change in the configuration of the kidney and the presence of mottled calcifications within a renal cyst should raise the suspicion of coexisting renal cell carcinoma. In this situation, renal arteriography is the most helpful diagnostic test (Fig. 9.8).

4.3. Tuberous sclerosis

Tuberous sclerosis is an autosomal dominant disease with high penetrance, extremely variable expression and a high rate of a spontaneous mutation[82,83,104]. It may affect the central nervous system (cortical tubers, subepen-

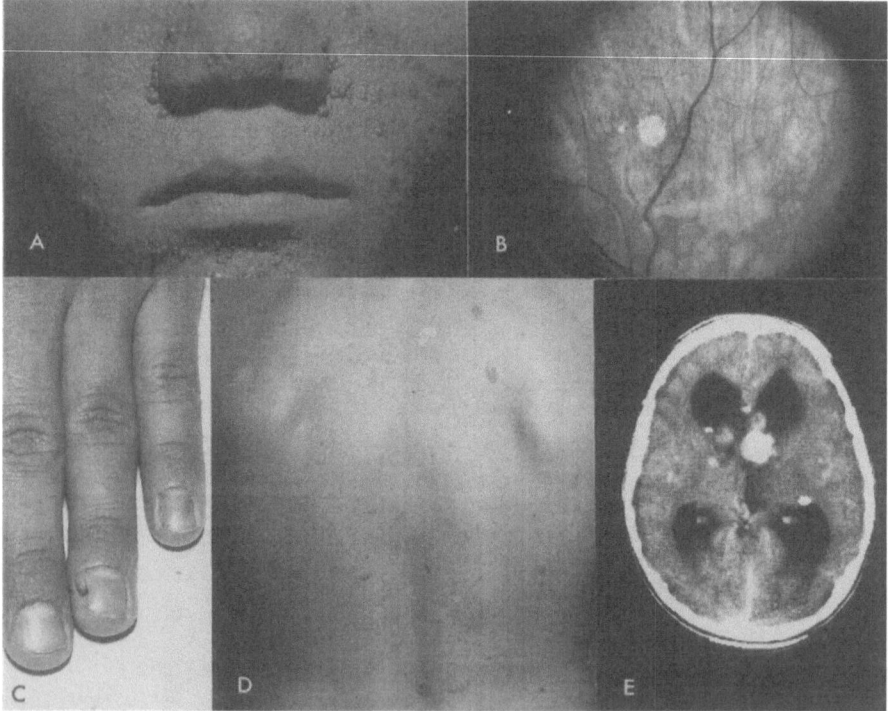

Figure 9.9. Typical lesions of tuberous sclerosis. (A) Adenoma sebaceum. (B) Retinal hamartoma. (C) Subungual fibroma. (D) Hypomelanotic macules and shagreen patch. (E) Computed tomography of the head with contrast: large enhancing subependymal glyoma causing dilatation of the lateral ventricles, multiple calcified subependymal tubers.

cysts), heart (rhabdomyoma) and lungs (Fig. 9.9). Other organs may be involved, but the lesions are usually asymptomatic. Because the clinical features are so variable, minimal diagnostic criteria have been established (Table 9.2).

Table 9.2. Minimal diagnostic criteria of tuberous sclerosis*

One Finding	Two Findings
Facial angiofibroma or periungual fibroma (by biopsy)	Infantile spasms
Cortical tuber, subependymal nodule, or giant cell astrocytoma	Hypomelanotic macules
Multiple retinal hamartomas	Shagreen patch
Combination of renal angiomyolipomas and cysts	Single retinal hamartoma
	Subependymal or cortical calcification (CT scan)
	Bilateral renal tumors (angiomyolipomas or cysts)
	Cardiac rhabdomyoma
	Family history of tuberous sclerosis in a first-degree relative

* According to Gomez et al. [82,83,104]

The majority of patients with tuberous sclerosis seek medical help because of seizures, but the most common findings are the skin lesions. Patients with tuberous sclerosis may have severe diffuse cystic renal disease which, unless associated angiomyolipomas can be demonstrated, is indistinguishable from ADPKD[11,54,112,144,153,188,189]. In order not to misdiagnose these patients as having ADPKD, it is important to recognize the extrarenal manifestations of tuberous sclerosis. When a diagnosis of tuberous sclerosis is considered, the evaluation should include a detailed cutaneous examination with Wood's lamp, ophthalmologic examination with dilatation of the pupils, cranial computed tomography with contrast, and renal ultrasound. Some authors also suggest examination of the teeth for pitted enamel hypoplasia[129] and roentgenograms of the skull, hands and feet to search for bony sclerosis and bone cysts[91].

Several patients with tuberous sclerosis and renal cell carcinomas have been reported[207]. In contrast with patients having renal carcinoma without tuberous sclerosis, there is a female predominance, frequent bilateral involvement and good prognosis following surgery.

4.4. Von Hippel–Lindau disease

Von Hippel–Lindau disease is an autosomal dominant disorder with high penetrance and variable expression[141,150,151]. It most frequently affects the cerebellum, medulla oblongata and spinal cord (hemangioblastomas), retina (angiomatosis), kidney (cysts, hemangiomas, adenomas and carcinomas), pancreas (cysts and, rarely, tumors) and adrenal gland (pheochromocytoma).

Because of the implications for genetic counselling purposes, criteria for a definite diagnosis have been suggested (Table 9.3).

Table 9.3. Diagnostic criteria for von Hippel–Linday disease*

CNS and retinal hemangioblastoma
or
CNS or retinal hemangioblastoma plus one of the following:
Renal, pancreatic, hepatic, or epididymal cysts Pheochromocytoma Renal cancer
or
Definite family history plus
CNS or retinal hemangioblastoma Renal, pancreatic, or epididymal cysts Pheochromocytoma Renal cancer

* From reference 141

The renal lesions of von Hippel–Lindau disease include cysts, hemangiomas, benign adenomas and, most importantly, malignant renal cell carcinomas[128,132]. The cysts are usually multiple and limited in number, and are lined with an epithelium that is often irregularly hyperplastic with mural nodules of clear cell carcinoma. Occasionally, the kidneys may be diffusely cystic, resembling ADPKD, and some of the patients described in the literatures having renal cell carcinoma and ADPKD probably had von Hippel–Lindau disease[67,114]. In autopsy series, nearly one-half of the patients have renal cell carcinomas. In contrast to the general population, they are frequently multicentric and bilateral and there is no male predominance. Recently, a proximal 3p deletion in renal cell carcinoma cells from a patient with von Hippel–Lindau disease was reported[109]. It is possible that the initiation of neoplasia under these circumstances results from the loss of a regulatory mechanism.

In the treatment of renal cell carcinoma in von Hippel–Lindau disease, an effort to spare renal tissue has been recommended since bilateral and multiple lesions are apt to be present or develop subsequently[128,132]. Early diagnosis of the lesions posing a health risk to the patient is essential. Patients diagnosed as having von Hippel–Lindau disease need an annual physical and ophthalmologic examination and a computed tomography of the abdomen[121]. Annual determinations of urinary metanephrines and biannual computed tomography of the head are also reasonable. All first-degree relatives should have physical and ophthalmologic examinations and computed tomography of the head and the abdomen. Any at-risk persons should be rescreened prior to reproduction.

4.5. Orofaciodigital syndrome type I

Orofaciodigital syndrome type I is a rare X-linked dominant disorder with prenatal lethality in males usually diagnosed in childhood[34,50,51,90,140,199]. As many as one-third of female infants with orofaciodigital syndrome type I die in their first year of life. It is characterized by a combination of oral (hyperplastic frenula, cleft tongue, and often cleft palate or lip and malposed teeth), facial (broad nasal root with hypoplasia of nasal alae and malar bone) and digits (brachy, syn, clino, campto, polydactyly). Mental retardation and tremor can be present in up to 30–50% of the patients. The initial report of polycystic kidneys at necropsy in a mother and daughter with this syndrome was considered to be considered to be coincidental[56], but later multiple reports of these associations indicated that cystic kidneys are a manifestation of this syndrome[40,57,95,145,207]. Most of these patients have been adults and often had been previously diagnosed as having ADPKD. Liver cysts are usually absent. Renal failure may ensue at any time during the second through the seventh decade of life.

Since most patients with orofaciodigital syndrome type I come to medical attention in early childhood for surgical repair of the external malformations, their kidney involvement may not be apparent at the time of initial diagnosis. Recognition of this syndrome in the affected individual with renal cystic disease has important genetic implications for the family. The males and the phenotypically normal females are not at risk for kidney disease. Only the female relatives with the clinical findings of orofaciodigital syndrome type I are at risk. Features of this syndrome should be looked for in a family where only females have polycystic kidneys. Conversely, females diagnosed as having orofaciodigital syndrome type I should have renal investigations performed.

References

1. Alpers D. Obstructive jaundice in a patient with polycystic disease (clinicopathologic conference). American Journal of Medicine 1977, 62, 616–626.
2. Alström CH. Alström syndrome. In: Bergsma D, ed., Defects Compendium. New York: Alan R Liss, Inc., 1979, 69–70.
3. Armitage NC and Blumgart LH. Partial resection and fenestration in the treatment of polycystic liver disease. British Journal of Surgery 1984, 71, 242–244.
4. Arnal Monreal FM, Menarguez Palanca J, Arrinda Yeregui JM, et al. Dilataciones quisticas de las vias diliares intrahepatics: enfermedad de Caroli con litiasis masiva

236

intrahepatica y amiloidosis secundaria generalizada. Rev Esp Enferm Apar Dig 1981, 60, 169–174.

5. Avasthi PS, Erickson DG and Gardner KD. Hereditary renal–retinal dysplasia and the medullary cystic disease–nephronophthisis complex. Annals of Internal Mdicine 1976, 157–161.

6. Bean WJ and Rodan BA. Hepatic cysts: treatment with alcohol. American Journal of Roentgenology 1985, 144, 237–234.

7. Bernstein J. A classification of renal cysts. In: Gardner KD, ed., Cystic Diseases of the Kidney. New York: John Wiley and Sons, 1975, 7–30.

8. Bernstein J. Hepatic and renal involvement in malformation syndromes. Mount Sinai Journal of Medicine (New York) 1986, 53, 421–428.

9. Bernstein J. Hepatic involvement in hereditary renal syndromes. Birth Defects: Original Article Series 1987, 23, 115–130.

10. Bernstein J, Evan AP and Gardner KD Jr. Epithelial hyperplasia in human polycystic kidney disease: its role in pathogenesis and risk of neoplasia. Americal Journal of Pathology 1987, 129, 92–101.

11. Bernstein J, Robbins TO and Kissane JM. The renal lesions of tuberous sclerosis. Seminars in Diagnostic Pathology 1986, 3, 97–105.

12. Bernstein J, Stickler GB and Neel IV. Congenital hepatic fibrosis: evolving morphology. Acta Pathologica, Microbiologica et Immunologica Scandinavica 1988, Suppl. 4: 17–26.

13. Biesecker LG, Laxova R and Friedman A. Renal insufficiency in Williams syndrome. American Journal of Medical Genetics 1987, 28, 131–135.

14. Bigelow NH. The association of polycystic kidneys with intracranial aneurysms and other related disorders. American Journal of Medical Sciences 1953, 225, 484–494.

15. Bloom DA and Brosman S. The multicystic kidney. Journal of Urology 1978, 120, 211–215.

16. Bloustein PA. Association of carcinoma with congenital cystic conditions of the liver and bile ducts. American Journal of Gastroenterology 1987, 67, 40–46.

17. Blyth H and Ockenden BG. Polycystic disease of kidneys and liver presenting in childhood. Journal of Medical Genetics 1971, 8, 257–284.

18. Böhm N, Fukuda M, Staudt R and Helwig H. Chondroectodermal dysplasia (Ellis–van Creveld syndrome) with dysplasia of renal medulla and bile ducts. Histopathology 1978, 2, 267–281.

19. Böhm N, Uy J, Kießling M and Lehnert W. Multiple acyl-CoA dehydrogenation deficiency (glutaric aciduria type II), congenital polycystic kidneys, and symmetric warty dysplasia of the cerebral cotex in two newborn brothers. II. Morphology and pathogenesis. European Journal of Pediatrics 1982, 139, 60–65.

20. Boichis H, Passwell J, David R and Miller H. Congenital hepatic fibrosis and nephronophthisis. Quarterly Journal of Medicine 1973, 42, 221–233.

21. Boué J, Chalmers RA, Tracey BM, Watson D, Gray RGF, Keeling JW, King GS, Pettit BR, Lindenbaum RH, Rocchiccioli F and Saudubray J-M. Prenatal diagnosis of dysmorphic neonatal-lethal type II glutaricaciduria. Lancet 1984, 1, 846–847.

22. Brown RAP. Polycystic disease of the kidneys and intracranial aneurysms: the etiology and interrelationship of these conditions: review of recent literature and report of seven cases in which both conditions coexisted. Glasgow Medical Journal 1951, 32, 333–348.

23. Buchta RM, Viseskul C, Gilbert EF, Sarto GE and Opitz JM. Familial bilateral renal agenesis and hereditary renal adysplasia. Zeitschrift für Kinderheilkunde 1973, 115, 111–129.

24. Byrne J and Blanc WA. Malformations and chromosome anomalies in spontaneously aborted fetuses with single umbilical artery. American Journal of Obstetrics 1985, 151, 340–342.

25. Cantani A, Bellioni P, Bamonte G, Salvinelli F and Bamonte MT. Seven hereditary syndromes with pigmentary retinopathy. Clinical Pediatrics (Philadelphia) 1985, 24, 578–583.

26. Carter CO, Evans K and Pescia G. A family study of renal agenesis. Journal of Medical Genetics 1979, 16, 176–188.
27. Chakera TMH. Peripheral dysostosis associated with juvenile nephronophthisis. British Journal of Radiology 1975, 48, 765.
28. Chaudhuri PK, Chaudhuri B, Schuler JJ, et al. Carcinoma associated with congenital cystic dilation of bile ducts. Archives of Surgery 1982, 117, 1349–1351.
29. Churchill DN, Bear JC, Morgan J, Payne RH, McManamon PJ and Gault MH. Prognosis of adult onset polycystic kidney disease re-evaluated. Kidney International 1984, 26, 190–193.
30. Claudy A, Toulon J, Dutoit M, Sabatier J-C and Berthoux F-C. Maladie de darier et polykystose rénale: étude familiale et effets du rétinoide aromatique. Annals Dermatologie Venereologie (Paris) 1981, 108, 675–677.
31. Clermont TJ, Maillard J-N, Benhamou J-P and Fauvert R. Fibrose hépatique congénitale Canadian Medical Association Journal 1967, 97, 1272–1278.
32. Codére F, Brownstein S and Chen MF. Cryptophthalmos syndrome with bilateral renal agenesis. American Journal of Ophthalmology 1981, 91, 734–742.
33. Cohen AH and Hoyer JR. Nephronophthisis: A primary tubular basement membrane defect. Laboratory Investigation 1986, 55, 564–572.
34. Connacher AA, Forsyth CC and Stewart WK. Orofaciodigital syndrome type I association with polycystic kidneys and agenesis of the corpus callosum. Journal of Medical Genetics 1987, 24, 116–122.
35. Contreras CB and Espinoza JS. Discussion clinica y anatomopatologica de enfermos que presentaron un problema diagnostico. Pediatria Santiago 1960, 3, 271.
36. Cryer PE and Kissane JM. Obstructive jaundice in a patient with polycystic disease. Americal Journal of Medicine 1977, 62, 616–626.
37. Curran AS and Curran JP. Associated acral and renal malformations: a new syndrome? Pediatrics 1972, 49, 716–725.
38. Curry CJR, Jensen K, Holland J, Miller L and Hall BD. The Potter sequence: a clinical analysis of 80 cases. Americal Journal of Medical Genetics 1984, 19, 679–702.
39. Datta NS, Wilson GN and Hajra AK. Deficiency of enzymes catalyzing the biosynthesis of glycerol–ether lipids in Zellweger syndrome: a new category of metabolic disease involving the absence of peroxisomes. New England Journal of Medicine 1984, 311m 1080–1083.
40. Dayton MT, Longmire WP and Thompkins RK. A premalignant condition? Americal Journal of Surgery 1983, 145, 41–47.
41. Debakan AS. Hereditary syndrome of congenital retinal blindness (Leber), polycystic kidneys and maldevelopment of the brain. Americal Journal of Ophthalmology 1969, 68, 1029–1037.
42. Del Pino Montes J, Chimpén Ruiz V, Sánchez Garcia P, Pascula González F, Garcia Legido A, Fermoso Garcia J and De Portugal Alvarez J. Medicina Clinica 1983, 81, 595.
43. Delaney VB, Adler S, Bruns FJ, Licinia M, Segal DP and Fraley DS. Autosomal dominant polycystic kidney disease: presentation, complications, and prognosis. Americal Journal of Kidney Diseases 1985, 5, 104–111.
44. DelGuercio E, Greco J, Kim KE et al. Esophageal varices in adult patients with polycystic kidney and liver disease. New England Journal of Medicine 1973, 289, 678–679.
45. De Vos M, Barbier F and Cuvelier C. Congenital hepatic fibrosis. Journal of Hepatology 1988, 6, 222–228.
46. Dieker H and Opitz JM. Associated acral and renal malformations. Birth Defects: Original Article Series 1969, 5, 68–77.
47. Diekman L, Louis C and Schulte-Kemna E. Familiäre nephropathie mit retinitis pigmentosa. Helvetica Paediatrica Acta 1977, 32, 375.
48. Dieterich E and Straub E. Familial juvenil nephronophthisis with hepatic fibrosis and neurocutaneous dysplasia. Helvetica Paediatrica Acta 1980, 35, 261–267.
49. DiMatteo J, Picard R, Vacheron A and Benaid J. Polykstose rénale associée a un

syndrome de Marfan fruste avec dilatation de l'aorte initiale et insuffisance aortique. Bulletins et Mémoires de la Société Médicale des Hôpitaux de Paris 1965, 116, 1665–1673.

50. Doege TC, Thuline HC, Priest JH, Norby DE and Bryant JS. Studies of a family with the oral–facial–digital syndrome. New England Journal of Medicine 1964, 271, 1073–1080.

51. Donnai D, Kerzin-Storrar L and Harris R. Familial orofaciodigital syndrome type I presenting as adult polycystic kidney disease. Journal of Medical Genetics 1987, 24, 84–87.

52. Duplay H, Barillon D, Lebas P, Mattei M, Monnier B, Bauza R and Kermarec J. L'association rein polykystique tumeur du glomus carotidien: origine embryonnaire vasculaire commune? Journal de Urologie Nephrologie 1979, 85, 98–101.

53. Dupond JL, Miguet JP, Carbillet JP, Saint Hiller Y, Perol C and Leconte des Floris R. Polykystose rénale, principale expression de la fibrose hépatique congenitale. Le Nouvelle Presse Médicale 1979, 8, 2885–2888.

54. Durham DS. Tuberous sclerosis mimicking adult polycystic kidney disease. Australian and New Zealand Journal of Medicine 1987, 17, 71–73.

55. Edelman GM. Cell-adhesion molecules: a molecular basis for animal form. Scientific American 1984, 250, 118–129.

56. Emery AEH, Oleesky S and Williams RT. Myotonic dystrophy and polycystic disease of the kidneys. Journal of Medical Genetics 1967, 4, 26–28.

57. Everson GT. Etiology and pathogenesis of PKD characteristics of hepatic cysts. Symposium, Etiology & Pathogenesis of Polycystic Kidney Disease. Sponsored by Baxter and PKF Foundation, Deerfield, IL, 1987.

58. Favre JP, Cayot M, Faivre J, Trigalou D, Klepping C and Viard H. La malade polykystique de foie: á propos de dux cas opérés par fenestration. Revues Francaise Gastroenterologie 1978, 142, 25–30.

59. Ferran JL, Couture A, Veyrac C, Barneon G and Galifer RB. Renal cysts and congenital hemihypertrophy. Annals of Radiology 1981, 25, 136–141.

60. Fillastre JP, Guenel J, Riberi P, Marx P, Whitworth JA and Kunh JM. Senior–Loken syndrome (nephronophthisis and tapeto–retinal degeneration): a study of 8 cases from 5 families. Clinical Nephrology 1976, 5, 14–19.

61. Fitch N and Strolovitz H. Severe renal dysgenesis produced by a dominant gene. American Journal of Diseases in Childhood 1976, 130, 1356–1357.

62. France NE, Crome L and Abraham JM. Pathological features in the De Lange syndrome. Acta Paediatrica Scandinavica 1969, 58, 470–480.

63. Francois J. Syndrome malformatif avec cryptophthalmie. Acta Genetica Medical Gemellol 1969, 18, 18.

64. Fraser FC, Sproule JR and Halal F. Frequency of the branchio–oto–renal (BOR) syndrome in children with profound hearing loss. American Journal of Medical Genetics 1980, 7, 341–349.

65. Friedman A, Bethzhold J, Hong R, Gilbert EF, Viseskul C and Opitz JM. Clinicopathological conference: A three-month-old infant with failure to thrive, hepatomegaly, and neurologic impairment. American Journal of Medical Genetics 1980, 7, 171–176.

66. Friedman WF and Mills LF. The relationship between vitamin D and the craniofacial and dental anomalies of the supravalvular aortic stenosis sydnrome. Pediatrics 1969, 43, 12–18.

67. Frimodt-Møller PC, Nissen HM and Dryreborg U. Polycystic kidneys as the renal lesion in Lindau's disease. Journal of Urology 191981, 125, 868–870.

68. Fryns JP. Chromosomal anomalies and autosomal syndromes. Birth Defects: Original Article Series 1987, 23, 7–32.

69. Gabow PA, Iklé DW, Holmes JH. Polycystic kidney disease: prospective analysis of nonazotemic patients and family members. Annals of Internal Medicine 1984, 101, 238–247.

70. Gaisford W and Bloor K. Congenital polycystic disease of kidneys and liver, portal hypertension – portacaval anastomosis. Proceedings of the Royal Society of Medicine 1968, 61, 304–305.

71. Gang DL and Herrin JT. Infantile polycystic disease of the liver and kidneys. Clinical Nephrology 1986, 25, 28–36.
72. Gardner KD Jr and Evan AP. The nephronophthisis–cystic renal medulla complex. In: Hamburger J, Crosnier J and Grünfeld JP, eds, Nephrology. New York: John Wiley & Sons, 1979, 893–908.
73. Gesundheit N, Dent DL, Fawcett HD et al. Infected liver cyst in a patient with polycystic kidney disease. Western Journal of Medicine 1982, 136, 246–249.
74. Giedion A. Phalangeal cone shaped epiphysis of the hands (PhCSEH) and chronic renal disease – the conorenal syndromes. Pedriatric Radiology 1979, 8, 32–38.
75. Giedion A. Acrodysplasias: peripheral dysostosis, acrodysostosis and Thiemann's disease. Clinical Orthoptics 1976, 114, 107–115.
76. Gilbert E and Opitz J. Renal involvement in genetic–hereditary malformation syndromes. In: Hamburger J, Crosnier J and Grünfeld J-P, eds, Nephrology. New York: John Wiley * Sons, 1979, 909–944.
77. Gilbert EF, Opitz JM, Spranger JW, Langer LO, Wolfson JJ and Visekul C. Chondrodysplasia punctata – rhizomelic form. European Journal of Pediatrics 1976, 123, 89.
78. Gimsing S and Dyrmose J. Branchio–oto–renal dysplasia in three families. Annals of Otology, Rhinology and Laryngology 1986, 95, 421–426.
79. Godel V, Iaina A, Nemet P and Lazar M. Phenotypic variations in renal–retinal dysplasia. Metabolic Pediatric Ophthalmology 1980, 4, 161–163.
80. Godel V, Iaina A, Nemet P and Lazar M. Sector retinitis pigmentosa in juvenile nephronophthisis. British Journal of Ophthalmology 1980, 64, 124–126.
81. Godel V, Blumenthal M and Iaina A. Congenital Leber amaurosis, keratoconus, and mental retardation in familial juvenile nephronophthisis. Journal of Pediatric Ophthalmology Strabismus 1978, 15, 89–91.
82. Gomez MR. Tuberous sclerosis: Part 1. Neurology and Neurosurgery Update Series 1984, 5(35), 2–7.
83. Gomez MR. Tuberous sclerosis: Part 2. Neurology and Neurosurgery Update Series 1984, 5(36), 2–7.
84. Gourdol O, David L, Colon S, Bouvier R, Ayral A, Aguercif M and Francois R. L'Atteinte renale dans le syndrome de Laurence–Moon–Bardet–Biedl. Pediatrie 1984, 39, 175–181.
85. Greene LF, Feinzaig W and Dahlin DC. Multicystic dysplasia of the kidney: with special reference to the contralateral kidney. Journal of Urology 1971, 105, 482–487.
86. Gregoire JR, Torres VE, Holley KE and Farrow GM. Renal epithelial hyperplastic and neoplastic proliferation in autosomal dominant polycystic kidney disease. American Journal of Kidney Diseases 1987, 9, 27–38.
87. Grix A Jr, Curry C and Hall BD. Patterns of multiple malformations in infants of diabetic mothers. Birth Defects: Original Article Series 1982, 18, 55–77.
88. Grünfeld J-P, Albouze G, Jungers P, Landais P, Dana A, Droz D, Moynot A, Lafforgue B, Boursztyn E and Franco D. Liver changes and complications in adult polycystic kidney disease. Advances in Nephrology 1985, 14, 1–20.
89. Halal F, Desgranges M-F, Leduc B, Théorêt and Bettez P. Acro–renal–mandibular syndrome. American Journal of Medical Genetics 1980, 5, 277–284.
90. Harrod MJE, Stokes J, Peede LF and Goldstein JL. Polycystic kidney disease in a patient with oral–facial–digital syndrome – type I. Clinical Genetics 1976, 9m 183–186.
91. Hausser I and Anton-Lamprecht I. Electron microscopy as a means for carrier detection and genetic counselling in families at risk of tuberous sclerosis. Human Genetics 1987, 76, 73–80.
92. Hensinger RN, Lang JE and MacEwen GD. Klippel–Feil syndrome: a constellation of associated anomalies. Journal of Bone and Joint Surgery (America) 1974, 56A, 1246–1253.
93. Herdman RC and Langer LO. The thoracic asphyxiant dystrophy and renal disease. American Journal of Diseases in Childhood 1968, 192–201.
94. Heymans HSA, Oorthuys JWE, Nelck G, Wanders RJA and Schutgens RBH. Rhizomelic

chondrodysplasia punctata: another peroxisomal disorder. New England Journal of Medicine 1985, 313, 187–188.

95. Hoganson G, Berlow S, Gilbert EF, Frerman F, Goodman S and Schweitzer L. Glutaric acidemia type II and flavin-dependent enzymes in morphogenesis. Birth Defects: Original Article Series 1987, 23, 65–74.

96. Hogewind BL, Veltkamp JJ, Polak BCP and van Es LA. Electro-retinal abnormalities in heterozygotes of renal–retinal dysplasia. Acta Medica Scandinavica 1977, 202, 323–326.

97. Hossak KF, Leddy CL, Johnson AM, Schrier RL and Gabow PA: Echocardiographic findings in autosomal dominant polycystic kidney disease. New England Journal of Medicine 1988, 319, 907–912.

98. Howard RJ, Hanson RF and Delaney JP. Jaundice associated with polycystic liver disease. Relief by surgical decompression of the cysts. Archives of Surgery 1976, 111, 816–817.

99. Huguet C, Hcht Y, Ricordeau P and Caroli J. Les énormes polykystoses hépatiques. Medicale Chirurgie Digestif 1973, 2, 227–230.

100. Hunt GM and Whitaker RH. The pattern of congenital renal anomalies associated with neural-tube defects. Dev Med Child Neurol 1987, 29, 91–95.

101. Iglesias CG, Torres VE, Offord KP, Holley KE, Beard CM and Kurland LT. Epidemiology of adult polycystic kidneys disease, Olmsted County, Minnesota: 1935–1980. American Journal of Kidney Diseases 1983, 2, 630–639.

102. Kaehny W, Bell P, Earnest M, Stears J and Gabow P. Family clustering of intracranial aneurysms (ICA) in autosomal dominant polycystic kidney disease (ADPKD). Kidney International 1987, 31, 204 (abstract).

103. Kaehny WD, Manco-Johnson M, Johnson AM, Tangel DJ and Gabow PA. Influence of sex on liver manifestations of autosomal dominant polycystic kidney disease (ADPKD). Kidney International 1988, 33, 196.

104. Kegel MF. Dominant disorders with multiple organ involvement. Dermatology Clinics 1987, 5, 205–219.

105. Kelley RI. Review: The cerebrohepatorenal syndrome of Zellweger, morphologic and metabolic aspects. American Journal of Medical Genetics 1983, 16, 503–517.

106. Kelly CJ and Neilson e.g. Medullary cystic disease: an inherited form of autoimmune interstitial nephritis. American Journal of Kidney Diseases 1987, 10, 389–395.

107. Kerr DNS, Harrison CV, Sherlock S et al. Congenital hepatic fibrosis. Quaterly Journal of Medicine 1961, 30, 91–117.

108. Kieselstein M, Herman G, Wahrman J, Voss R, Gitelson S, Feuchtwanger M and Kadar S. Mucocutaneous pigmentation and intestinal polyposis (Peutz–Jeghers syndrome) in a family of Iraqi Jews with polycystic kidney disease: with a chromosome study. Israle Journal of Medical Sciences 1969, 5, 81–90.

109. King CR, Schimke RN, Arthur T, Davoren B and Collins D. Proximal 3p deletion in renal cell carcinoma cells from a patient with von Hippel–Lindau disease. Cancer Genetics and Cytogenetics 1987, 27, 345–348.

110. Kobayashi Y, Hiki Y, Shigematsu H, Tateno S and Mori K. Renal retinal dysplasia with diffuse glomerular cysts. Nephron 1985, 39, 201–205.

111. Kocoshis SA, Riley CA, Burrell M et al. Cholangitis in a child due to biliary anomalies. Digestive Disease Science 1980, 25, 59–65.

112. Kristal C, Berant M and Alon U. Polycystic kidneys as the presenting feature of tuberous sclerosis. Helvetica Paediatrica Acta 1987, 42, 29–33.

113. Krous HF and Wenzl JE. Familial renal cystic dysplasia associated with maternal diabetes mellitus. Southern Medical Journal 1980, 73, 85–86.

114. Lamiell JM, Stor RA and Hsia YE. von Hippel–Lindau disease simulating polycystic kidney disease. Urology 1980, 15, 287–290.

115. Lanson SZ, Frieden JH and Bierman HR. Polycystic disease of the liver. Journal of the American Medical Asociation 1971, 215, 793–794.

116. Lash JW. Normal embryogenesis and teratogenesis: implications for pathological devel-

opment from experimental embryology. American Journal of Obstetrics and Gynecology 1964, 90, 1193–1207.

117. Lazjuk GI, Lurie IW, Ostrowskaja TI, Kirillova IA, Nedzved MK, Cherstvoy ED and Silyaeva NF. The Wolf–Hirschhorn syndrome. Clinical Genetics 1980, 18, 6–12.

118. Lehnert W, Wendel U, Lindenmaier S and Böhm N. Multiple acyl-CoA dehydrogenation deficiency (glutaric aciduria type II), congenital polycystic kidneys, and symmetric warty dysplasia of the cerebral cortex in two brothers. I. Clinical, metabolical, and biochemical findings. European Journal of Pediatrics 1982, 139, 56–59.

119. Leier CV, Baker PB, Kilman JW and Wooley CF. Cardiovascular abnormalities associated with adult polycystic kidney disease. Annals of Internal Medicine 1984, 100, 683–688.

120. Levey AS, Pauker SG and Kassirer JP. Occult intracranial aneurysms in polycystic kidney disease: when is cerebral arteriography indicated? New England Journal of Medicine 1983, 308, 986–994.

121. Levine E, Collins DL, Horton WA and Schimke RN. CT screening of the abdomen in von Hippel–Lindau disease. American Journal of Roentgenology 1982, 139, 505–510.

122. Lieberman E et al. Infantile polycystic disease of the kidneys and liver: clinical, pathological and radiological correlations and comparison with congenital hepatic fibrosis. Medicine 1971, 50, 277–318.

123. Lin T-Y, Chen C-C and Wang S-M. Treatment of non-parasitic cystic disease of the liver: a new approach to therapy with polycystic liver. Annals of Surgery 1968, 168, 921–927.

124. Linné T, Walkstad I and Zetterström R. Renal involvement in the Laurence–Moon–Biedl syndrome. Acta Paediatrica Scandinavica 1986, 75, 240–244.

125. Lipson M, Waskey J, Rice J, Adomian G, Lachman R, Filly R and Rimoin D. Prenatal diagnosis of asphyxiating thoracic dysplasia. American Journal of Medical Genetics 1984, 18, 273–277.

126. Loh JP, Haller JO, Kassner e.g, Aloni A and Glassberg K. Dominantly-inherited polycystic kidneys in infants: association with hypertrophic pyloric stenosis. Pediatric Radiology 1977, 6, 27–31.

127. Løken AC et al. Hereditary renal dysplasia and blindness. Acta Paediatrica Scandinavica 1961, 50, 177–184.

128. Loughlin KR and Gittes RG. Urological management of patients with von Hippel–Lindau's disease. Journal of Urology 1986, 136, 789–791.

129. Lygidakis NA and Lindenbaum RH. Pitted enamel hypoplasia in tuberous slcerosis patients and first-degree relatives. Clinical Genetics 1987, 32, 216–222.

130. Maillet P, Brette R, Bertrand JL and Tissot E. Trois cas de polykystose hepato–renale. Lyon Médical 1973, 230, 439–442.

131. Mainzer F, Saldino RM, Ozonoff MB and Minagi H. Familial nephropathy associated with retinitis pigmentosa, cerebellar ataxia and skeletal abnormalities. American Journal of Medicine 1970, 49, 556–562.

132. Malek RS, Omess PJ, Benson RC Jr and Zincke H. Renal cell carcinoma in von Hippel–Lindau syndrome. American Journal of Medicine 1987, 82, 236–238.

133. Manes JL, Kissane JM and Valdes AJ. Congenital hepatic fibrosis, liver cell carcinoma and adult polycystic kidneys. Cancer 1977, 39, 2619–2623.

134. Matsumara M, Wada H, Ohwada A and Shinoda T. Unruptured intracranial aneurysms and polycystic kidney disease. Acta Neurochirurgie (Wien) 1986, 79, 94–99.

135. Marsuzaka T, Sakuragawa N, Nakayama H, Sugai K, Kohno Y and Arima M. Cerebro-oculo–hepato–renal syndrome (Arima's syndrome): a distinct clinicopathological entity. Journal of Childhood Neurology 1986, 1, 338–346.

136. Mauseth R, Lieberman E and Heuser ET. Infantile polycystic disease of the kidneys and Ehlers–Danlos syndrome in an 11-year-old patient. Journal of Pediatrics 1977, 90, 81–83.

137. McCarthy LJ, Baggenstoss AH and Logan GB. Congenital hepatic fibrosis. Gastroentology 1965, 49, 27–36.

138. McPherson E, Carey J, Kramer A, Hall JG, Pauli RM, Schimke RN and Tasin MH.

Dominantly inherited renal adysplasia. American Journal of Medical Genetics 1987, 26, 863–872.

139. Melnick M, Hodes ME, Nance WE, Yune H and Sweeney A. Branchio–otorenal dysplasia and branchio–oto dysplasia: two distinct autosomal dominant disorders. Clinical Genetics 1978, 13, 425–442.

140. Méry JP, Simon H, Houitte H, Tanquerel T, Toulet R and Kanger A. A propos de deux observations de maladie polykystique rénale de l'adulte associée au syndrome oral–facial–digital. J Urol Nephrol 1978, 84, 892–893.

141. Michels VV. Von Hippel–Lindau disease. In: Gomez MR, ed, Neurocutaneous Diseases: A Practical Approach. Boston: Butterworths, 1987, 53–66.

142. Milutinovic J, Fialkow PJ, Rudd TG et al. Liver cysts in patients with autosomal dominant polycystic kidney disease. American Journal of Medicine 1980, 68, 741–744.

143. Mitcheson HDm Williams G and Castro JE. Clinical aspects of polycystic disease of the kidneys. British Medical Journal 1977, 1, 1133–1134.

144. Mitnick JS, Bosniak MA, Hilton S, Raghavendra BN, Subramanyam BR and Genieser NB. Cystic renal disease in tuberous sclerosis. Radiology 1983, 147, 85–87.

145. Moore WB, Matthews TJ and Rabinowitz R. Genitourinary anomalies associated with Klippel–Feil syndrome. Journal of Bone and Joint Surgery (America) 1975, 57, 355–357.

146. Moser AE, Singh I, Brown FR III, Solish GI, Kelley RI, Benke PJ and Moser HW. The cerebrohepatorenal (Zellweger) syndrome: increased levels and impaired degradation of very-long-chain fatty acids and their use in prenatal diagnosis. New England Journal of Medicine 1984, 310, 1141–1146.

147. Nagasne N. Successful treatment of Caroli's disease by hepatic resection. Annals of Surgery 1984, 200, 718–723.

148. Nagorney DM, Torres VE, Rakela J and Welch TJ. Surgical anatomy of the liver in adult polycystic kidney disease (APKD). Kidney International 1988, 33, 202 (abstract).

149. Nagorney DM and Torres VE. Unpublished observations.

150. Neumann HPH. Basic criteria for clinical diagnosis and genetic counselling in von Hippel–Lindau syndrome. VASA 1987, 16, 220–226.

151. Neumann HPH. Prognosis of von Hippel–Lindau syndrome. VASA 1987, 16, 309–311.

152. Newsome DA. Retinitis pigmentosa, Usher's syndrome, and other pigmentary retinopathies. In: Newsome DA, ed, Retinal Dystrophies and Degenerations. New York: Raven Press, 1988, 161–194.

153. O'Callaghan TJ, Edwards JA, Tobin M and Mookerjee BK. Tuberous sclerosis with striking renal involvement in a family. Archives of Internal Medicine 1975, 135, 1082–1087.

154. Opitz JM and Gilbert EF. Pathogenetic analysis of congenital anomalies in humans. Pathobiology Annual 1982, 12, 301–349.

155. Opitz JM and Lewin SO. The developmental field concept in pediatric pathology – especially with respect to fibular A/hypoplasia and the DiGeorge anomaly. Birth Defects: Original Article Series 1987, 23, 277–292.

156. Osanondh V and Potter EL. Development of human kidney as shown by microdissection. I. Preparation of tissues with reasons for possible misinterpretations of observations. Archives of Pathology 1963, 76, 271–302.

157. Osanondh V and Potter EL. Pathogenesis of polycystic kidneys: historical survey. Archives of Pathology 1964, 77, 459–512.

158. Paliard P and Partensky C. Traitement par fenestration itérative d'une forme douloureuse, puis cholestatique de polykystose hépatique. Gastroenterol Clin Biol 1980, 4, 854–857.

159. Pathak IG and Williams DI. Multicystic and cystic dysplastic kidneys. British Journal of Urology 1964, 36, 318–331.

160. Pintacuda S, Di Blasi S, Morici G and Amato S. Rene policistico e deficit di alfa$_1$-antitripsina sierica: osservazioni su due gruppi familiari. Minnesota Medicine 1981, 72, 1697–1701.

161. Polak BCP, van Lith FHM, Delleman JW and van Balen TM. Carrier detection in

tapetoretinal degeneration in association with medullary cystic disease. American Journal of Ophthalmology 1983, 95, 487–494.

162. Popovic-Rolovic M, Calic-Perisic G, Bunjevacki G and Negovanovic D. Juvenile nephronophthisis associated with retinal pigmentary dystrophy, cerebellar ataxia, and skeletal abnormalities. Archives of Diseases in Childhood 1976, 51, 801.

163. Price JDE and Pratt-Johnson. Medullary cystic disease with degeneration. Canadian Medical Association Journal 1970, 102, 165–167.

164. Proesmans W, van Damme B and Macken J. Nephronophthisis and tapetoretinal degeneration associated with liver disase. Clinical Nephrology 1975, 3, 160–164.

165. Prouty LA and Myers TL. Oligohydramnios sequence (Potter's syndrome): case clustering in Northeastern Tennessee. Southern Medical Journal 1987, 80, 585–592.

166. Rapola J, Kääriäinen H. Polycystic kidney disease: morphologic diagnosis of recessive and dominant polycystic kidney disease in infancy and childhood. Acat Pathologica, Microbiologica et Immunologica Scandinavica 1988, 96, 68–76.

167. Ratcliffe PJ, Reeders S and Theaker JM. Bleeding esophageal varices and hepatic dysfunction in adult polycystic kidney disease. British Medical Journal 1984, 288, 1330–1331.

168. Rehder H, Weber M, Heyne K and Lituanaia M. Fetal pathology – nonchromosomal. Birth Defects: Original Article Series 1987, 23, 131–151.

169. Resnick JS, Brown DM and Vernier RL. Normal development and experimental models of cystic renal disease. In: Gardner KD, ed, Cystic Diseases of the Kidney. New York: John Wiley & Sons, 1976, 221–241.

170. Ritter R and Siafarikas K. Hemihypertrophy in a boy with renal polycystic disease: varied patterns of presentation of renal polycystic disease in his family. Pediatric Radiology 1976, 5, 98–102.

171. Roberts JBM. Congenital anomalies of the urinary tract and their association with spina bifida. British Journal of Urology 1961, 33, 309–315.

172. Roodhooft AM, Birnholz JC and Holmes LB. Familial nature of congenital absence and severe dysgenesis of both kidneys. New England Journal of Medicine 1984, 310, 1341–1345.

173. Roscher A, Molzer B, Bernheimer H, Stöckler S, Mutz I and Paltauf F. The cerebrohepatorenal (Zellweger) syndrome: an improved method for the biochemical diagnosis and its potential value for prenatal detection. Pediatric Research 1985, 19, 930–933.

174. Rosemberg S, Carneiro PC, Zerbini MCN and Gonzales CH. Brief clinical report: chrondroectodermal dysplasia (Ellis–van Creveld) with anomalies of CNS and urinary tract. American Journal of Medical Genetics 1983, 15, 291–295.

175. Sadler TW. Langman's Medical Embryology, Fifth Edn. Baltimore: Williams & Wilkins, 1985.

176. Saifuddin A and Dathan JRE. Adult polycystic kidney disease and intracranial aneurysms. British Medical Journal 1987, 295, 526.

177. Scheff RT, Zucherman G, Harter H, Delmez J and Koehler R. Diverticular disease in patients with chronic renal failure due to polycystic kidney disease. Annals of Internal Medicine 1980, 92, 202–204.

178. Schinzel A, Savoldelli G, Briner J and Schubiger G. Prenatal sonographic diagnosis of Jeune syndrome. Radiology 1985, 154, 777–778.

179. Schumacher RE, Rocchini AP and Wilson GN. Partial trisomy 2q. Clinical Genetics 1983, 23, 191–194.

180. Scott J, Shousha S, Thomas HC et al. Bile duct carcinoma – a late compliation of congenital hepatic fibrosis. American Journal of Gastroenterology 1980, 73, 113–119.

181. Selgas R, Temes JL, Sobrino JA, Viguer JM, Otero A and Sanchez SL. Enfermedad poliquistica renal del adulto asociada con una forma incompleta de sindrome de Marfan. Med Clin (Barc) 1981, 76, 311–313.

182. Senior B, Friedmann AI and Braudo JL. Juvenile familial nephropathy with tapeto–retinal degeneration. American Journal of Ophthalmology 1961, 52, 625.

183. Senior B. Familial renal–retinal dystrophy. American Journal of Diseases in Childhood 1973, 125, 442–447.

184. Shah KJ. Renal lesions in Jeune's syndrome. British Journal of Radiology 1980, 53, 432–436.

185. Siegelman SS, Zavod R and Hecht H. Neurofibromatosis, polycystic kidneys, and hypernephroma. New York State Journal of Medicine 1971, 71, 2431–2433.

186. Spranger J, Benirschke K, Hall JG, Lenz W, Lowry RB, Opitz JM, Pinsky L, Schwarzacher HG and Smith DW. Errors of morphogenesis: concepts and terms. Journal of Pediatrics 1982, 100, 160–165.

187. Srinivas V, Winsor GM and Dow D. Urologic manifestations of Laurence–Moon–Biedl syndrome. Urology 1983, 581–583.

188. Stapleton BF, Johnson D, Kaplan GW and Griswold W. The cystic renal lesion in tuberous sclerosis. Journal of Pediatrics 1980, 97, 574–579.

189. Stillwell TJ, Gomez MR and Kelalis PP. Renal lesions in tuberous sclerosis. Journal of Urology 1987, 138, 477–481.

190. Summerfield JA, Nagafuchi Y, Sherlock S, Cadafalch J and Scheuer PJ. Hepatobiliary fibropolycystic diseases: a clinical and histologic review of 51 patients. Journal of Hepatology 1986, 2, 141–156.

191. Suter W. Das kongenitale aneurysma der basalen gehirnarterien und cystennieren. Schweiz Medicale Wochenschrift 1949, 79, 471–476.

192. Talwar D and Swaiman KF. Peroxisomal disorders: a review of a recently recognized group of clinical entities. Clinical Pediatrics 1987, 26, 497–504.

193. Tazelaar HD, Payne JA and Patel NS. Congenital hepatic fibrosis and asymptomatic familial adult-type polycystic kidney disease in a 19-year-old woman. Gastroenterology 1984, 86, 757–760.

194. Torres VE, Forbes GS, Wiebers DO, Erickson SB and Smith LH. Value of routine screening for intracranial aneurysms (ICA) in autosomal dominant polycystic kidney disease (ADPKD). Xth International Congress of Nephrology, London, England, 1987, 45 (abstract).

195. Torres VE, Holley KE, Hartman GW and Iglesias CG. Renal cystic disease in the elderly. In: Nuñez JFM and Cameron JS, eds, Renal Function and Disease in the Elderly. London: Butterworths, 1987, 348–399.

196. Torres VE, Holley KE and Gardner KD. Epidemiology. In: Grantham JJ and Gardner KD, eds, Problems in Diagnosis and Management. Kansas City, MD: Kidney Research Foundation, 1985, 49–69.

197. Torres VE. An overview: genetics of renal cystic diseases. In: Spitzer A and Avner E, eds, Topics in Renal Disease. Boston: Martinus Nijhoff Publishers (In press).

198. Trinkl W, Sassaris M and Hunter FM. Nonsurgical treatment for symptomatic liver cyst. American Journal of Gastroenterology 1985, 80, 907–911.

199. Tucker CC, Finley SC, Tucker ES and Finley WH. Oral–facial–digital syndrome, with polycystic kidneys and liver: pathological and cytogenetic studies. Journal of Medical Genetics 1966, 3, 145–147.

200. Turnage RH, Eckhauser FE, Knol JA and Thompson NW. Therapeutic dilemmas in patients with symptomatic polycystic liver disease. American Surgery 1988, 54, 365–372.

201. van Erpecum KJ, Janssens AR, Terpstra JL and Tjon A and Tham RTO. Highly symptomatic adult polycystic disease of the liver. Journal of Hepatology 1987, 5, 109–117.

202. Varma SC, Kaushik SP, Talwar KK and Sharma BK. Association of von Recklinghausen's neurofibromatosis with adult polycystic disase of kidneys and liver. Postgraduate Medicine 1982, 58, 117–118.

203. Verp MS, Amarose AP, Esterly JR and Moawad AH. Mosaic trisomy 7 and renal dysplasia. American Journal of Medical Genetics 1987, 26, 139–143.

204. Wakabayashi T, Fujita S, Ohbora Y et al. Polycystic kidney disease and intracranial aneurysms: early angiographic diagnosis and early operation for the unruptured aneurysm. Journal of Neurosurgery 1983, 58, 488–491.

205. Watchi J-M and Nezelof C. Les maladies polykystiques hepato–renales. Revue Internationale d'Hepatologie 1964, 14, 489–537.
206. Weese-Mayer DE, Smith KM, Reddy JK, Salafsky I and Poznanski AK. Computerized tomography and ultrasound in the diagnosis of cerebro–hepato–renal sydnrome of Zellweger. Pediatric Radiology 1987, 17, 170–172.
207. Weinblatt ME, Kahn E and Kochen J. Renal cell carcinoma in patients with tuberous sclerosis. Pediatrics 1987, 80, 898–903.
208. Welling LW and Welling DJ. Kinetics of cyst development in cystic renal disease. In: Cummings NB and Klahr S, eds, Chronic Renal Disease. New York: Plenum, 1985, 95–104.
209. Whitaker RH and Hunt GM. Incidence and distribution of renal anomalies in patients with neural tube defects. European Urology 1987, 13, 322–323.
210. Whitt JW, Wood BC, Sharma JN and Crouch TT. Adult polycystick kidney disease and lattice corneal dystrophy: occurrence in a single family. Archives of Internal Medicine 1978, 138, 1167–1168.
211. Wiebers DO. Management of unruptured intercranial aneurysms. In: Grantham JJ and Gardner KD, eds, Problems in Diagnosis and Management of Polycystic Kidney Disease. Kansas City: PKR Foundation, 1985, 145–153.
212. Wiebers DO, Whisnant JP and O'Fallon WH. The natural history of unruptured intracranial aneurysms. New England Journal of Medicine 1981, 304, 696–698.
213. Wilcock AR and Emery JL. Deformities of the renal tract in children with meningomyelocele and hydrocephalus, compared with those children showing no such central nerous system deformities. British Journal of Urology 1970, 42, 152–157.
214. Wilson GN, Holmes RG, Custer J, Lipkowitz JL, Stover J, Datta N and Hajra A. Zellweger syndrome: diagnostic assays syndrome delineation, and potential therapy. American Journal of Medical Genetics 1986, 24, 69–82.
215. Witig JH, Burns R and Longmire WP. Jaundice associated with polycystic liver disease. Archives of Surgery 1978, 111, 816–817.
216. Yunis E, Ramírez and Uribe JG. Full trisomy 7 and Potter syndrome. Human Genetics 1980, 54, 13–18.
217. Zerres K, Völpel M-C, Weiß H. Cystic kidneys: genetics, pathologic anatomy, clinical picture, and prenatal diagnosis. Human Genetics 1984, 68, 104–135.

10
Management of Cystic Kidney Disease

W.M. Bennett, L.W. Elzinga and J.M. Barry

Abstract

Management of cystic kidney disease currently is restricted to relief of symptoms and control of complications. There is presently no specific treatment that will reduce cyst formation in patients. Insights gained from basic research should provide a framework on which to base future therapeutic regimens. In this chapter we summarize current therapeutic approaches to the major clinical problems of renal cystic disease, with emphasis on autosomal dominant polycystic kidney disease.

Key words   Hematuria;
Hypertension;
Pain management;
Surgical decompression;
Urinary infection.

1. Infection

1.1. General considerations

Urinary tract infection occurs commonly in patients with cystic kidney diseases. When the renal parenchyma or the cysts themselves are involved, serious consequences such as septicemia, perinephric abscess and loss of renal function may ensue[101]. Most of the information on management of these infections has been obtained in patients with autosomal dominant polycystic kidney disease (ADPKD) and extrapolation to patients with other forms of cystic disease may not be warranted; however, it is likely that the same principles apply.

The vast majority of urinary tract infections associated with renal cystic disease occur in women, as in the general population, and recent urinary tract instrumentation is a risk factor[22,94]. The organisms most often involved in these infections are the enteric Gram-negative bacteria that gain access to the kidney by ascending from the lower urinary tract. However, other infecting organisms, including Gram-positive and anaerobic bacteria, can be present. In some patients with well-documented infections within cysts, urine cultures are persistently negative, making the diagnosis quite difficult. The diagnosis can be further obscured because patients with ADPKD may have flank pain, pyuria and hematuria without infection. It is reasonable to suspect upper tract infection, with possible involvement of cysts, when a patient has persistent fever and flank pain, even if repeated urine cultures are sterile. [67]Gallium and [111]Indium radionuclide scans may help to localize infectious processes. Such studies are helpful if positive, but are often not sensitive enough to exclude cyst infection[31,42].

Instrumentation of the urinary tract should be restricted to only the most pressing of clinical indications – with prophylactic trimethoprim–sulphamethoxazole given before and for 24 hours after the procedure[101]. Asymptomatic bacteriuria should be aggressively eradicated. Although there are no data on the value of long-term antimicrobial prophylaxis in polycystic patients with recurrent lower tract infections, it would appear prudent to institute this measure because of its efficacy in the general population of women with recurrent lower urinary tract infections.

1.2. Antimicrobial drugs

Cyst epithelium is capable of maintaining large gradients of sodium, creatinine and hydrogen ions. These "gradient" cysts are lined with epithelium that demonstrates functional characteristics of distal nephron segments; various molecules, such as lanthanum, undergo transepithelial movement that suggests the presence of tight junctions between adjacent cells[16]. Ultrastructural findings have confirmed that this type of cyst is lined with epithelium of appearance identical to that of cortical collecting ducts[33]. Penetration of such cysts by anionic antibiotics, such as the beta lactams, is poor[68]. Schwab et al. [91] showed that the concentration of clindamycin, with its high pK_a, increases as cyst fluid pH falls, whereas the polar cationic aminoglycoside, gentamicin, has low penetration at all cyst pH values from 5 to 8.

Most cysts are of the "non-gradient type" and are lined with non-specific cells lacking distinctive features of any nephron segment, but some non-gradient cysts are lined with typical proximal tubular cells having villous brush borders[33]. Electrolyte concentrations in non-gradient cysts are typical of a plasma ultrafiltrate. Solute access to these more abundant cysts is probably by diffusion[68]. Although molecules as large as inulin can gain access to cysts, the time course of their appearance within non-gradient cysts is inconsistent with glomerular filtration alone[111].

Beta lactam antibiotics also may gain access to non-gradient cysts by an active organic anion transport pathway, as demonstrated for similar anionic molecules like PAH[68]. However, many non-gradient cysts are lined with epithelium that lacks the capacity to transport organic anions actively[33].

Most therapeutic agents which are water soluble and ionized at physiologic pH will penetrate cyst fluid slowly and irregularly by diffusion, thereby achieving low, steady-state concentrations. Lipophilic agents may, at least theoretically, gain access to cyst fluid of both gradient and non-gradient types[93].

Drugs with a high pK_a accumulate in gradient cysts because of favorable electrochemical gradients. When infected, this type of cyst is particularly difficult to sterilize because water soluble polar drugs, such as beta lactams which are commonly used to treat Gram-negative aerobic bacterial infections, penetrate poorly[7,10,103]. Ionization of these compounds retards their transport across the "tight" epithelium. In addition, the anionic beta lactams have an unfavorable electrical gradient. Table 10.1 summarizes data concerning antibiotic penetration into cyst fluid.

Table 10.1. Antibiotic penetration into cyst fluid

	Gradient cysts	Non-gradient after treatment	*In vitro* efficacy in cyst fluid from patients
Aminoglycosides	–	–[c]	NT
Beta lactams	–	+[a]	NT
Chloramphenicol	+	–	NT
Clindamycin	+	+	NT
Erythromycin	+	+	NT
Fluoroquinolones	+	+	E[b]
Metronidazole	+	+	NT
Trimethoprim–sulphamethoxazole	+	+	E
Vancomycin	+	+	NT

+ Concentration greater than minimum inhibitory concentration (MIC) of likely infecting organism; – Concentration less than MIC of likely infecting organism; NT Not tested; E Increased titre from pretreatment of at least 5-fold; a Some congeners such as ampicillin and cephalosporins achieve adequate levels with prolonged therapy (7–10 days); b Ciprofloxacin more effective than norfloxacin; c Isolated report of adequate concentration with amikacin.

Urinary infections in polycystic patients are often refractory to treatment when renal cysts are infected. Rault[85] has reported treatment failure in this clinical situation despite longterm, specific antibiotics. The nephrectomy specimen contained a sensitive organism identical to that cultured from the original urine. Similarly, in the series of Sweet and Keane, five of eight polycystic patients with symptomatic urinary tract infection developed perinephric abscesses[104]. The abscesses occurred despite prolonged antibiotic therapy directed to organisms known to be sensitive by *in vitro* studies.

The treatment of urinary tract infection in the patient with advanced renal failure may present additional therapeutic problems. Many problems are similar to those in patients with renal failure from other causes. Bacteriologic cure depends on delivery of antibiotic to the site of infection. In patients with marked reduction in glomerular filtration rate, drugs that are filtered, such as the highly polar aminoglycosides, are often ineffective. Gentamicin, when given in doses recommended for patients with severe renal failure, produces urinary drug concentrations lower than the desirable inhibitory concentrations for infecting organisms[9].

Drug delivery into the renal interstitium can also be compromised by chronic renal disease. Trimethoprim-sulphamethoxazole and ampicillin will better treat parenchymal infection in patients with chronic renal failure because of the relative preservation of tubular secretory function[5]. The same considerations also pertain to parenchymal renal infection in renal failure patients with polycystic disease.

Finally, antibiotics may not diffuse well in large cysts with poorly stirred contents. Thus, even if an appropriate drug is identified, prolonged therapy may be necessary even with drugs that are filtered and secreted to assure adequate concentrations in urine, cyst fluid and renal parenchyma. Muther and Bennett[68] obtained fluid from patients with autosomal dominant polycystic disease. Gentamicin, tobramycin, cephapirin and ticarcillin were either undetectable or present in subtherapeutic concentrations.

Elzinga et al.[26] studied cyst fluid obtained by percutaneous aspiration or at surgery from patients having autosomal dominant polycystic disease and receiving trimethoprim–sulphamethoxazole. Cysts were categorized as "non-gradient" or "gradient" by cyst fluid sodium concentration. Mean cyst fluid trimethoprim and sulphamethoxazole concentrations were 15.2 μg/ml and 42.5 μg/ml, respectively. Preferential accumulation of trimethoprim was observed in gradient cysts, exceeding serum levels more than eight-fold. Sulphamethoxazole penetrated both types of cysts to a lesser extent, with concentrations ranging from 10 to 70% of the simultaneous serum. Cyst fluid samples prior to trimethoprim–sulphamethoxazole administration demonstrated no antibacterial activity against *Escherichia coli*, *Proteus mirabilis* and *Streptococcus faecalis*, whereas cyst fluid inhibitory and bactericidal titres following antibiotic administration were 1:32 or greater. These studies indicate the likely effectiveness of trimethoprim–sulphamethoxazole in treating cyst infection.

Clinical experience, although limited, has shown cures in some patients with polycystic disease and refractory urinary tract infections[94]. One failure was associated in a gradient cyst with an amount of sulphamethoxazole inadequate to achieve antibacterial synergism with trimethoprim[95]. Schwab and Weaver[95] recommended withholding trimethoprim–sulphamethoxazole unless the organism was sensitive to trimethoprim alone.

The fluoroquinolones possess favorable antibacterial characteristics against likely pathogens in cyst infections. They also have the property of relatively high lipid solubility, acting as zwitterions at pH 7.4. Elzinga et al. obtained 70 samples of cyst fluid from seven patients who were receiving ciprofloxacin[27]. Ciprofloxacin accumulated in gradient cysts, exceeding serum concentrations by more than four-fold. The mean drug concentration in both types of cysts was 12.7±2 μg/ml, a value well above the minimum inhibitory concentration of the most likely pathogens. Post-treatment cyst fluid, however, demonstrated high bactericidal activity against *E. coli* and *P. mirabilis*, less activity against *Pseudomonas aeruginosa*, *S. faecalis* and Gram-positive cocci.

Similar studies with norfloxacin show adequate concentrations and bactericidal activity only in gradient cysts[8]. Other congeners of this antibiotic class have not been evaluated. In summary, the limited clinical experience with ciprofloxacin has been favorable. Patients with bacteremia and persistent infection refractory to long courses of other antibiotics have been clinically cured within a week of receiving the drug. Recurrence of fever and flank pain can occur unless a full 4–6 week course is given.

Schwab, Bander and Klahr[94] have reported studies of 15 polycystic patients with upper urinary tract infections that were refractory to 5 days of intravenous ampicillin and aminoglycosides. Presumably these patients had pyogenic cyst infections. The authors found a good correlation between the organism cultured from cysts and those grown from blood or urine. Patients developed new discrete areas of palpable tenderness in the affected kidneys. Chloramphenicol in doses of 5 mg/kg/day achieved excellent results within 3–4 days in eight consecutive patients after conventional antibiotic therapy failed[92]. No adverse hematologic consequences were noted. The total treatment course was 14 days. One patient developed a clinical relapse with a chloroamphenicol-resistant organism[27].

Other antibiotics, including doxycycline and tetracycline[93], predicted to accumulate in distal cysts on the basis of hydrophobicity and high pK_a have not been studied clinically or experimentally.

Antibiotic penetration and trapping may be altered by infection, regardless of the functional nature or permeability characteristics of an infected cyst. Amikacin has been found to penetrate non-gradient cysts and sterilize staphylococcal infections because of infection-induced changes in cyst wall permeability to this usually impermeant aminoglycoside[102]. Percutaneous or surgical drainage is usually reserved for patients who fail antibiotic therapy[30]. Recrudescence of fever should prompt a search for calculus, perinephric abscess, or urinary tract obstruction. Nephrectomy may be required when urosepsis is associated with a kidney that does not function because of staghorn calculus or perinephric abscess.

1.3. Treatment of infection in other cystic diseases

In medullary sponge kidney, recurrent calculi and nephrocalcinosis are associated with increased frequency of renal infection. Control of the metabolic factors involved with stone formation, such as elevated urine pH and hypercalciuria, may reduce the frequency of infection. High fluid volumes and suppressive antibiotics may be indicated when symptomatic urinary tract infections recur. In hypercalciuric patients, hyperparathyroidism should be excluded. Thiazide diuretics may be useful to reduce urinary calcium excretion. Renal tubular acidosis should be treated with an appropriate alkali, e.g. approximately 1 mEq/kg/day of sodium bicarbonate or its equivalent.

When infection complicates medullary cystic disease, treatment is often difficult because of renal dysfunction and poor diffusion of antibiotics. Considerations applicable to patients with advanced renal disease are relevant in this situation.

Limited data from patients with acquired renal cystic disease suggest that antibiotic penetration into cysts is similar to that described for ADPKD. No data are available for the treatment of cyst infections in the recessive form of cystic disease in children.

1.4. Treatment guidelines

Theoretical considerations cannot always be equated with effective clinical therapy. In the absence of clinical studies showing efficacy and safety of specific antibiotics in infected patients with cystic renal disease, we have developed the following guidelines:

(1) Consider renal or cyst infection in the differential diagnosis of patients with cystic kidney disease and unexplained fever, gastrointestinal symptoms, flank pain, or generalized constitutional symtoms. A negative urine culture does not exclude cyst infection. Gallium and indium radionuclide scans may be helpful if positive.

(2) Culture urine and treat organisms with antibiotics that are specific for their sensitivity patterns. Consider longterm prophylaxis for recurrent lower tract infections. A 10–14 day course of antibiotics is recommended for lower urinary tract infections. Single dose therapy is not recommended.

(3) When urinary tract instrumentation is necessary, use prophylactic trimethoprim–sulphamethoxazole or a fluoroquinolone.

(4) For upper tract infection with positive blood culture or urine culture, treat for 4–6 weeks with a specific antibiotic based on an *in vitro* sensitivity pattern. If the patient does not improve, presume that antibiotic delivery is poor. Change to a lipophilic antibiotic with efficacy that is either proven or theoretical, and which is based on high pK_a and an antibacterial spectrum against the infecting pathogen. Such drugs include trimethoprim–sulphamethoxazole, chloramphenicol, ciprofloxacin and doxycycline. Consider a search for calculus, upper tract obstruction, or perinephric abscess with gallium or indium scanning and percutaneous, endoscopic or open surgical treatment as necessary.

(5) When an organism cannot be cultured from urine or blood in patients with suspected renal cyst infection, consider diagnostic percutaneous cyst puncture under ultrasound or computed tomography guidance. Therapy should be given with one of the above drugs for 4–6 weeks. If patients

become ill when therapy is discontinued, 6–12 months of low dose therapy may be required. Coverage of Gram-positive organisms with erythromycin or vancomycin and of anaerobic organisms with clindamycin or metronidazole can be used as clinically indicated.

(6) Percutaneous, endoscopic or surgical drainage, or even nephrectomy may be required for antibiotic failures. The possibility of perinephric abscess must be remembered.

(7) Fungal or mycobacterial renal involvement is possible. Medical therapy has a low likelihood of success. Renal fungal infection in the presence of renal insufficiency will not often respond to amphotericin B because worsening renal function prevents delivery of a dose sufficient to eliminate infection.

2. Calculi

The indications for removal of calculi in patients with cystic disease of the kidney include intractable urinary tract infection, urinary tract obstruction and persistent pain[1]. If severe obstruction or sepsis occurs with upper urinary tract calculi, urinary drainage can be provided by retrograde placement of a ureteral catheter or by percutaneous nephrostomy with antibiotic coverage. A nephroscope may be inserted through a nephrostomy tract to remove renal calculi, passing the instruments through renal cysts if necessary (EF Fuchs, personal communication). An ultrasonic probe may be used to fracture large or branched calculi. Extracorporeal shock-wave lithotripsy permits removal of smaller renal stones without direct surgical intervention[112]. An indwelling double-J ureteral stent is usually passed cystoscopically prior to the procedure to assist in the passage of stone fragments and prevent obstruction. Contraindications to the procedure include urinary tract obstruction and active urinary tract infection. Most ureteral calculi will pass spontaneously, especially if they are less than 4 mm in diameter.

Small stones lodged in the ureter may be safely removed endoscopically with stone catheters and ureteroscopy[72]. Proximal ureteral calculi may be removed with percutaneous techniques. Stones associated with sepsis without obstruction are best removed after 10–14 days of organism-specific antibiotics, with absence of fever and leukocytosis at the time of stone manipulation. Rarely, patients who have medullary sponge kidney and multiple, symptomatic calculi will require creation of an ileal ureter[100] or renal autotransplantation with a Boari flap or vesicopyelostomy[79].

3. Hematuria

Hematuria occurs in approximately half the patients with ADPKD[18]. Hematuria from other causes may also occur, e.g. kidney and bladder cancer. If a urinary tract cancer cannot be ruled out in the renal cystic disease patient with recurrent hematuria, antibiotic prophylaxis with trimethoprim–sulphamethoxazole or fluoroquinolone, followed by cystoscopy with cytologic examination and retrograde urography may be necessary. Cystoscopy may demonstrate the origin of gross hematuria, with localization to one kidney. The recognition of renal cell carcinoma in a polycystic kidney may require CT and selective renal arteriography.

Exsanguinating hemorrhage may be treated by segmental renal artery embolization, with continuing hemorrhage requiring nephrectomy. Oral administration of epsilon aminocaproic acid, a competitive blocker of plasminogen, to prevent fibrinolysis may also control hemorrhage[83].

4. Progression of renal failure

4.1. Dietary therapy

Protein-restricted diets have become increasingly popular in treating chronic renal failure, both for symptomatic relief and for retarding progression of renal failure. The pathophysiology of its effect on renal function has been elucidated in animals with chronic renal failure, e.g. the 5/6 nephrectomized rat in which protein loading accelerates renal dysfunction and enhances tubular cystic change[11,50,70]. Protein restriction seems, therefore, to be a reasonable strategy in treating patients with cystic kidney diseases and progressive renal failure.

The optimal timing and details of dietary interventions are not well-studied, with controlled data, for any chronic renal disease, including the cystic diseases. Gretz et al.[38] showed that a diet restricted to 30 g of protein per day slowed the rise in serum creatinine concentrations experienced by patients on an unrestricted diet. Maschio[61] also showed a retarded rate of renal functional deterioration in polycystic patients with modest renal failure fed protein-restricted diets. Uncontrolled studies of protein restriction also show slowed progression to renal failure[28,62,67,88], but other studies, that include polycystic patients with others, have shown little benefit. Critics point out that the reciprocal of serum creatinine may rise because of a drop in muscle mass not an improvement in GFR[56]. Thus, the efficacy of protein restriction in the management of polycystic patients has been questioned. It is nonetheless recommended that protein be moderately restricted (0.8 g/kg/day) in patients with serum creatinine concentrations greater than 2 mg/dl. Care should be taken to provide adequate calories, vitamins and minerals.

A tendency to waste sodium complicates several forms of renal cystic disease. In the subset of patients with ADPKD and an inability to conserve sodium, it is critical to provide enough salt to avoid extracellular volume depletion. Most patients with ADPKD do not waste sodium, however. Martinez-Maldonado[60] showed appropriate sodium conservation in seven patients with relatively preserved glomerular filtration rates on a 10 mmol/day sodium diet. Even patients with advanced renal insufficiency had sodium conserving capability no worse than patients with other types of renal failure.

A defect in urinary concentrating ability may be present at normal glomerular filtration rates[17,82]. It can lead to dehydration unless increased water intake is encouraged during periods thought to be of high insensible loss. Although renal acidification abnormalities have been described in autosomal dominant polycystic kidney disease[82], metabolic acidosis occurs clinically in proportion to other abnormalities of chronic renal failure and should be managed accordingly.

Sodium wasting in medullary cystic disease is clinically prominent, modifying the tendency to hypertension in patients with of chronic renal failure. The clinician will often need to determine the amount of sodium necessary to maintain a normal blood pressure, with specific instructions and counselling from a dietitian to ensure its intake. If oral intake is interrupted for any reason or if diuretics are used indiscriminately, shrinkage of extracellular fluid volume and deterioration of renal function can occur rapidly, requiring prompt intravenous administration of sodium chloride.

Medullary sponge kidney seldom progresses to renal failure. Metabolic acidosis due to type I renal tubular acidosis and hypercalciuria may lead to nephrolithiasis and secondary infection. Attention to hydration and appropriate alkali therapy can minimize these complications.

5. Hypertension

Management of hypertension is critical to maintenance of renal function and avoidance of cardiovascular complications.

Although arterial hypertension occurs in the majority of patients with ADPKD, the pathogenesis is unclear. Primary sodium retention has been suggested[71], but there is no obvious abnormality of the renin–angiotensin system[2]. Infusion of hypertonic saline results in natriuresis above that of healthy control subjects[19]. However, enhanced natriuresis, presumably due to some degree of preexisting volume expansion, occurs in both normotensive and hypertensive patients with ADPKD, casting some doubt on its pathophysiologic significance[19].

Extracellular fluid volume expansion was found in polycystic patients in the absence of an increase in blood pressure[20]. Torres et al. [107] found no difference in plasma concentrations of atrial natriuretic peptide between hypertensive polycystic patients and normotensive controls. While blood pressure correlates positively with kidney size, there are many instances of extremely large kidneys in normotensive individuals.

Thus, the approach to antihypertensive therapy in polycystic disease is empirical. There are no studies, controlled or uncontrolled, comparing various therapeutic regimens. Based on evidence of volume expansion and scattered reports of poor response to angiotensin II antagonists such as saralasin[2], it seems reasonable to assume that the hypertension is volume dependent. The plasma renin activity, albeit normal, may be inappropriately high for the level of volume expansion present.

The most logical therapeutic approach, therefore, is a combination of sodium restriction and diuretics. Reubi reported that hypertension in 50% of his patients with preserved renal function was controlled with diuretics alone[86]. As renal failure progresses, more complicated regimens are required, although there is currently little basis for selection of one drug over another. Converting enzyme inhibitors should probably not be used unless the patient also restricts sodium intake or receives diuretics. Renal function should be closely monitored if converting enzyme inhibitors are used in conjunction with diuretics, since acute renal dysfunction may occur within days to weeks.

Reduction of cyst volume by percutaneous cyst aspiration or surgical marsupialization can ameliorate high blood pressure[6]. The prolonged antihypertensive effect of surgery was emphasized by Yates-Bell[113] and Shangzhi et al. [97], even in patients with severe or malignant hypertension. Our more recent experience suggests that blood pressure improvement is variable and, when it occurs, is usually transient[4]. Hypertension alone cannot be used to justify a surgical approach to ADPKD, particularly when so many safe and effective antihypertensive drugs are now available. Hypertension is an unusual feature of medullary cystic disease and medullary sponge kidney. In fact, if hypertension is present with relative preservation of renal function, another cause of hypertension should be sought. Infantile or autosomal recessive polycystic kidney disease is commonly accompanied by severe hypertension. Most patients respond to salt restriction and the usual types of antihypertensive drugs[36]. It should be remembered that ADPKD can present in early childhood even within the first year of life[15]. The prognosis may not be as poor as had been thought if hypertension is controlled[15,96]. As with hypertensive adults, there are few data on the best therapeutic approach.

6. Management of pain

Abdominal and flank pain are present in the majority of patients, often as the presenting symptom. Pain has a general relationship with cyst size and the weight or volume of the kidneys, but many exceptions exist. Patients with cysts less than 3 cm in diameter may have severe pain, whereas some individuals tolerate massively enlarged cystic kidneys without problems. The precise mechanism by which enlarging cysts cause pain has not been established, but pain and discomfort are thought to be due to stretching of the renal capsule or to traction on the renal pedicle. Although the pain is usually dull and constant,

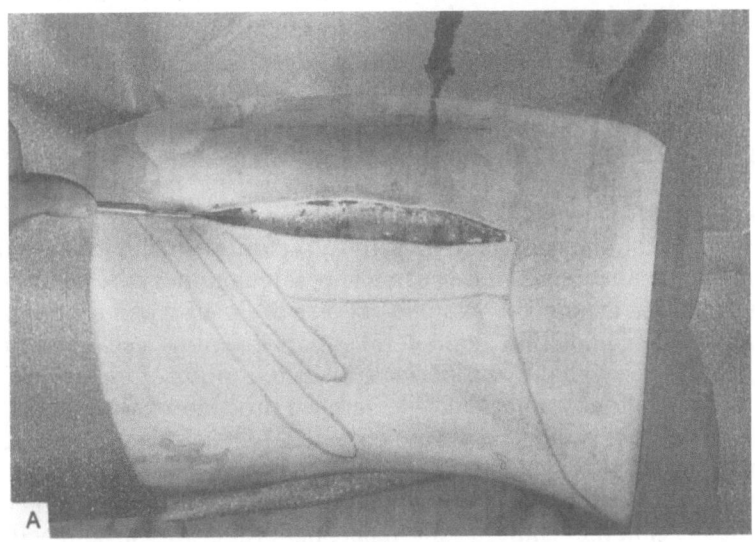

LUMBO-DORSAL FASCIA
SACROSPINALIS M.
QUADRATUS LUMBORUM M.
TRANSVERSALIS FASCIA

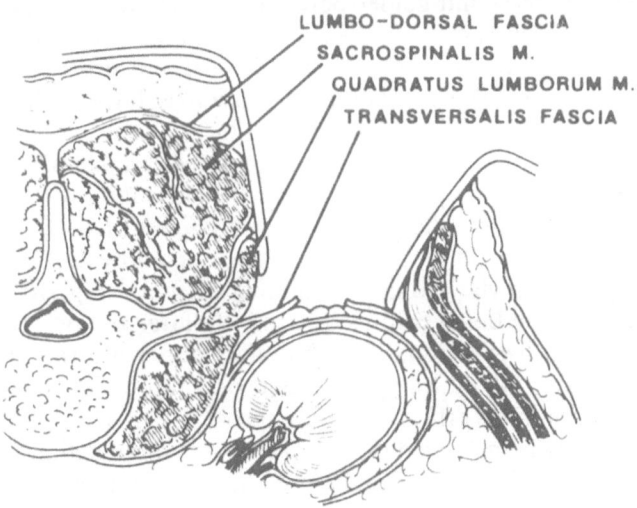

B

Figure 10.1 (A) Posterior surgical approach to kidney. The patient is placed in the lateral decubitus position at an angle of 45° from prone with the table moderately flexed. The incision is made over the belly of sacrospinalis from the proximal portion of the twelfth rib to the iliac crest. (B) The posterior lumbodorsal fascia is incised vertically, the sacrospinalis muscle is retracted medially, and the middle lamella of the lumbodorsal fascia is incised to expose quadratus lumborum, which is retraced medially. The anterior lamella of the lumbodorsal fascia is then incised. The twelfth thoracic and first lumbar nerves must be preserved. The polycystic kidney is exposed within the perirenal fascia. (Reprinted from Journal of Urology[76] with permission.)

localizing to the flank or lateral abdomen, it may be colicky and sharp. The clinician needs to remember that obstruction of the ureter due to a large cyst, a blood clot, a stone, or a neoplasm can produce pain. These complications usually produce an acute exacerbation of pain superimposed on chronic pain. Computed tomography is often helpful in evaluating an exacerbation.

In general, the clinician should be conservative about the prescription of analgesics for chronic renal pain. Single agents, such as acetaminophen, should be prescribed prior to using combination analgesic mixtures or non-steroidal anti-inflammatory drugs because single agents carry a lower risk of causing additional renal damage. Patients with refractory pain should be referred to pain management clinics, because behavioral techniques may be helpful. Narcotics should be avoided, if possible, because of the frequent problems of drug dependence and addiction. Short-term antianxiety drugs can be useful to help patients pass through difficult periods. Despite reports of impressive relief of pain by surgical decompression[87,99], surgical procedures were abandoned 30 years ago because poor results were obtained[12,13,65]. Recently, because of the encouraging long-term pain relief reported by Shangzhi et al. [97], we undertook a reevaluation of cyst decompression in patients with refractory pain requiring narcotics[6]. As in the Chinese experience, pain relief was striking with no loss of renal function. Ultrasound-guided percutaneous aspiration of cyst fluid from three to five of the largest cysts on the affected side was accomplished without complications. Dramatic pain relief was universal, but in some patients was unfortunately transient. The probability of a patient being pain-free 18 months after percutaneous cyst aspiration was 33 ± 17%. Patients with recurrence of pain within 6 months underwent cyst decompression or cyst reduction. Unilateral cyst decompression was performed by vertical lumbotomy[76], since it is one of the least painful approaches to the kidney (Fig. 10.1A–B). The surgeon manually mobilized the kidney as cysts were decompressed. Bilateral cyst reduction surgery was via midline abdominal incision (Fig. 10.2A–D). The probability of a patient being pain-free 18 months after an operation was 81 ± 12%. There was no loss of renal function after either aspiration or surgery. Further experience with cyst aspiration and decompression surgery has not demonstrated diminished efficacy of this approach (Fig. 10.3).

Pain relief may be achieved by bilateral renal embolization[55]. Reduction of cyst size in simple renal cysts can be obtained by percutaneous installation of iophendylate or alcohol after aspiration[3,41]. To the best of our knowledge, this approach has not been studied in the polycystic kidney diseases. Symptomatic relief should be at least as good as with aspiration alone. Theoretically, nerve blocks and even renal denervation could be attempted.

7. Preservation of renal function by cyst reduction surgery

Relief of symptoms by cyst decompression was first reported by Rovsing in

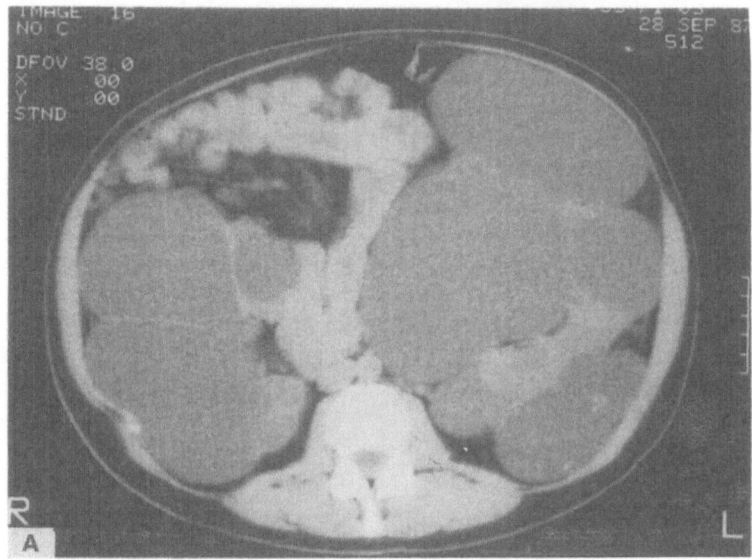

Figure 10.2A CT scan of 46-year old woman with massive polycystic kidney disease and disabling abdominal pain.

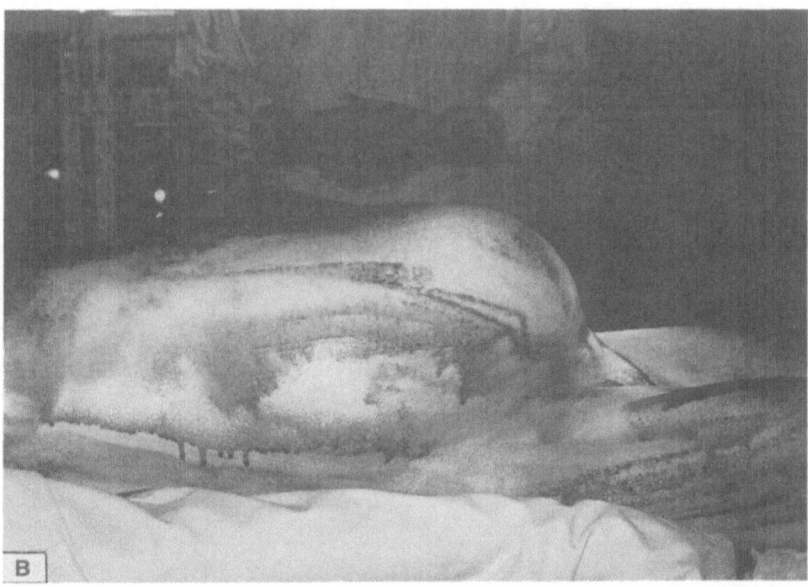

Figure 10.2B Abdominal distortion prior to cyst marsupialization via vertical midline abdominal incision.

260

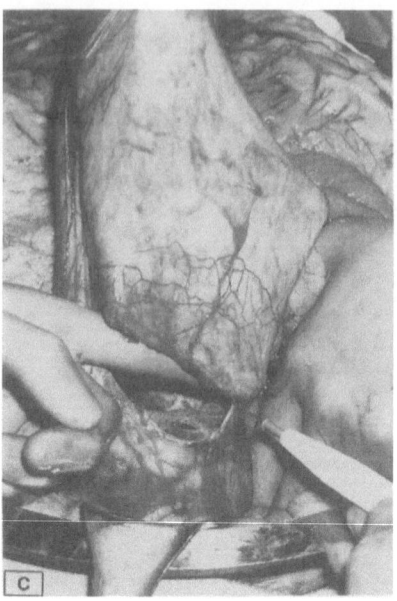

Figure 10.2C Marsupialization of cysts with electrocautery eliminates the need for whip-stitching the edges.

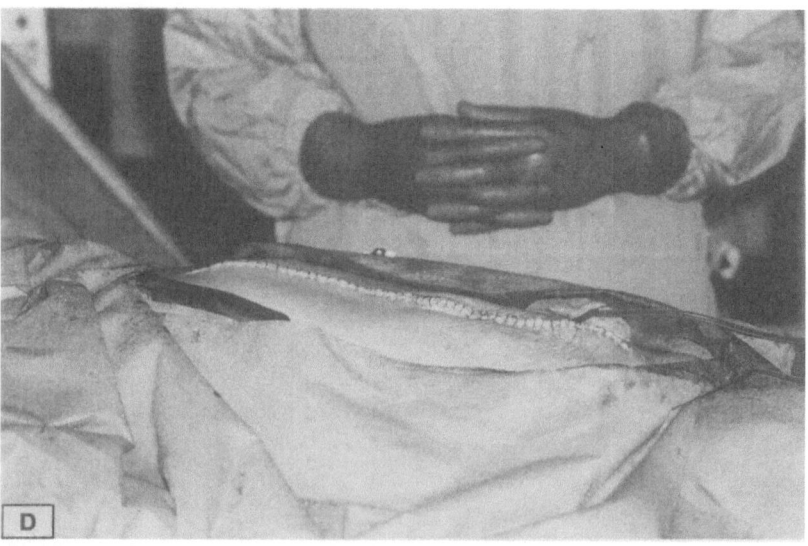

Figure 10.2D Immediate post-operative result. Abdominal girth was decreased from 114 cm to 88 cm and pain was relieved.

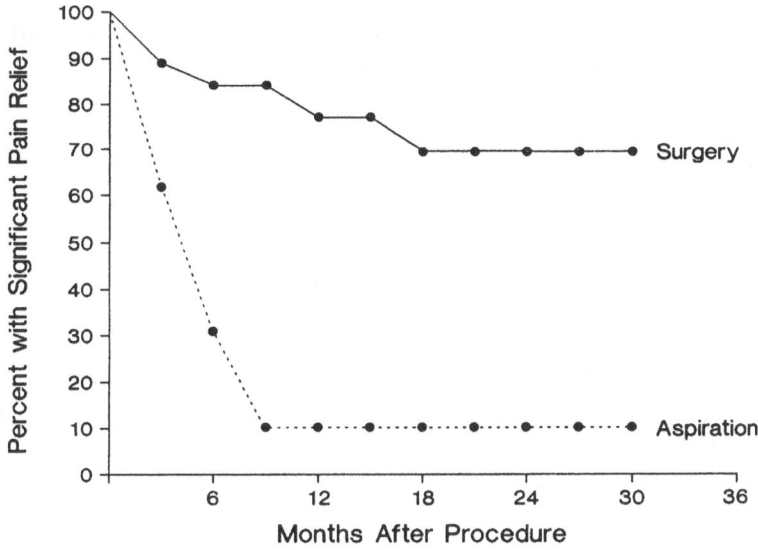

Figure 10.3. Pain relief following cyst reduction in patients with autosomal dominant polycystic kidney disease. There were 11 patients treated by percutaneous needle aspiration and 19 patients treated by surgical renal cyst marsupialization. Maximum follow-up was 6½ years.

1911[87]. Emptying of cysts by needle puncture or actual removal of cyst walls, allowing drainage of fluid into the abdomen, was abandoned in the 1960's primarily because of the report by Bricker and Patton about two patients who subsequently suffered decreased glomerular filtration rate[12,81]. One of the patients actually had a transient improvement in renal function, and the rate of renal functional decline prior to surgery was not specified. The authors argued that cyst reduction surgery should be avoided because of the loss of functioning cystic nephrons. On theoretical grounds, the loss of even several hundred cystic nephrons should make little difference to whole kidney function, since each adult kidney has approximately 1 million nephrons and only 2–10% are cystic[99,109].

The other negative report regarding surgery came in 1963 from Milam *et al.* [65], who showed a post-operative loss of function even in non-operated kidneys.

In fact, however, most of the literature on the effects of cyst reduction surgery showed little adverse and many favorable outcomes on renal function[6,8,12,14,58,64,65,81,87,97,113] (Table 10.2). This experience is remarkable, because most of the surgery was done prior to the availability of dialysis and modern antibiotics. Nearly all the patients who died following surgical decompression had advanced preoperative renal failure or post-operative infections. In the report of Simon and Thompson in 1955[99], for example, survival for 8–21 years was achieved in four patients who had unilateral nephrectomy of a non-functional kidney and cyst reduction on the opposite side. This surgery was associated with prolonged survival despite extensive nephron removal, far greater in extent than in the patients reported by Bricker and Patton.

Our recent experience with cyst reduction aspiration or surgery in patients with refractory pain has revealed no deleterious effects on renal function[6] (Fig. 10.4). Thus the reports (since 1966) have shown no operative mortality in 63 patients and no loss of renal function due to the surgery *per se* [6,97]. It is difficult to determine if any intervention changes the course of renal disease in a particular patient. The anatomic studies of Grantham *et al.* [34] show that cysts are larger, but not more numerous, in azotemic patients, suggesting that renal failure develops because of progressive cyst enlargement that compresses and compromises non-cystic nephrons.

Franz and Reubi[28] have shown direct correlations among cyst size, the number of large renal cysts and serum creatinine concentrations. This observation is compatible with attempts at cyst volume reduction to preserve renal function. Carefully designed prospective studies are needed to demonstrate the efficacy of these approaches, because the progression of renal disease is so variable among individual patients[92]. We have begun such studies on patients with progressively declining renal function and serum creatinine values between 2–5 mg/dl, because these are the patients expected to experience the most rapid declines according to both the model of Franz and Reubi[28] and the linear declines in renal function observed by Delaney *et al.* [22]. Unilateral aspiration or surgery is accompanied by follow-up, split non-invasive renal function studies using the non-operated kidney as a control. At present, surgery

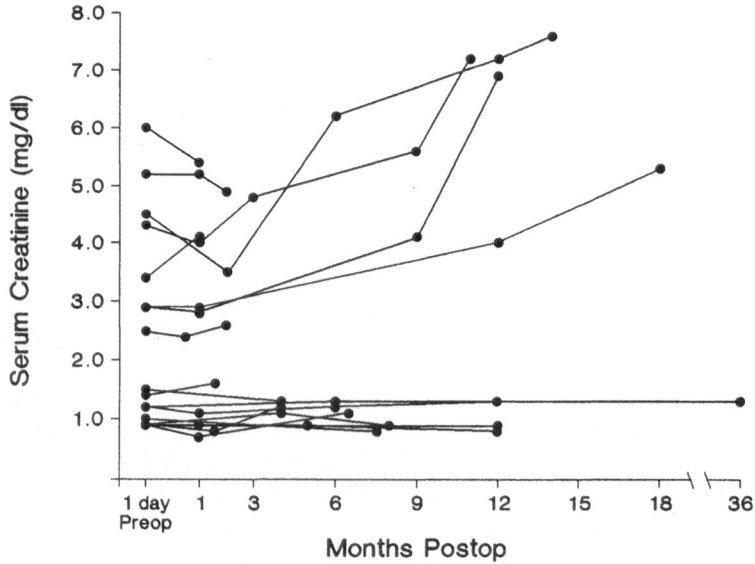

Figure 10.4. Influence of cyst reduction surgery on renal function in patients with autosomal dominant polycystic kidney disease.

Table 10.2. Effect of surgical cyst decompression on renal function

Author	Ref	Year	No. of patients	Peri-operative mortality (%)	Results	Comment
Rovsing	(87)	1911	3	0	"Improved kidney function"; no data given	–
Lund	(58)	1914	4	0	Preservation of function for up to 5 y; no data	Indicated only in "non-uremic patient"
Meltzer	(64)	1929	31	not discernable probably minimal	"Prognosis more hopeful"; no function data given	Based on a questionnaire sent to American Urological Association members
Cahill and Fish	(14)	1941	23	9	Improved kidney function; little data given	74% longterm survivors (1–16 y)
Dodson	(23)	1947	6	33	Improves PSP excretion at 2 y follow-up	Deaths due to renal failure in azotemic patients with infection also pre-existing
Kohler	(51)	1947	3	0	"Improved function"; no data presented	Injected a sclerosing solution into emptied cysts
Mayers	(63)	1948	2	0	"Marked improvement" no function data given	Injected a quinine hydrochloride solution into emptied cysts
Nielsen	(74)	1950	1	0	Longterm survival	Kidney infected pre-operatively; 50% glucose injected into emptied cysts
Newman	(73)	1950	10	0	Mean BUN 35 mg/dl before and 32 mg/dl 3 months after	Operation of little help when BUN >70 mg/dl
Buck et al.	(13)	1951	6	33[a]	Improved intravenous pyelograms. Survival of 13 y and 7 y in 2; lost to to follow-up	Deaths in patients with pre-existing renal failure

Table 10.2. Effect of surgical cyst decompression on renal function (continued)

Author	Ref	Year	No. of patients	Peri-operative mortality (%)	Results	Comment
Higgins	(39)	1952	8	0	Improved renal function; no data given	Warned to not operate with BUN >40 mg/dl
Simon and Thompson	(99)	1955	62	3[a]	5 year survival 78% vs 50% in 230 non-surgical patients over same time period (1925–1944); uniphrectomy of non-functional kidney and cyst puncture at surgery followed by survival of >8, >12, >17 and 21 y in the 4 patients who had both procedures[b]	Both deaths in patients with pre-operative azotemia
Patton and Bricker	(81)	1954	2	0	GFR decreased from 86 to 80 ml/min at 2 month follow-up and from 67 to 46 in the other patient at 1 month GFR decreased over the next 10 months from 80 ml/min to 65 ml/min in the first patient, and increased from 46 ml/min to 49 ml/min over 11 months in the other	No data on rate of renal function decline preoperatively
Bricker and Patton	(12)	1957	2[c]	0		
Yates-Bell	(113)	1957	18[a]	11	Transient decrease in function (unspecified) then "delay of deterioration"; survival of patients with mean pre-operative BUN of 69 mg/dl was a mean of 5.9 y (1–23)	1 death in patient with pre-operative BUN of 146 mg/dl, the other from bleeding, after a biopsy of cystic liver – pre-operative BUN 112 mg/dl
Dalgaard	(18)	1957	54	13	No actual function given, but fatality rate diminished compared to non-operated patients observed concurrently	Cautioned about operating on patients with advanced uremia

Table 10.2. Effect of surgical cyst decompression on renal function (continued)

Author	Ref	Year	n	%	Findings	Notes
Goldstein and Goldstein	(32)	1960	38	31[d]	Survival >4.9 y in operated patients operated patients versus >2.5 y in 19 non-operated controls	13 operated patients lived >5 y, 7>10 y and 2 >15 y; longest non-operated survivor, 9 y
Milam et al.	(65)	1963	9	0	Unilateral surgery performed; operated side had decreased GFR in 8/9 patients (x=41%) while non-operated decreased in 1/9 (x=35%; follow-up 3–40 months)	Operated kidneys frankly infected; no pre-operative rate of renal function measured under anaesthesia
Lue et al.	(57)	1966	27	30*	In 7 patients with normal BUN, 5 improved; 6 patients BUN <80, 4 improved; 14 patients BUN >80, 7 improved	All deaths in patients with pre-operative BUN greater than 80 mg/dl
Shangzhi et al.	(97)	1980	52	0	2 patients with BUN >60 mg% progressed to ESRD 33 patients BUN 17–30 with hypertension, 11 have BUN <17, 20 stable and 2 progressed over 5–14 y; 17 patients with BUN <17, 13 stable, 3 between 17–30 and 1>60 mg/dl over 3–20 y	Impressive blood pressure improvement
Bennett et al.	(6)	1987	11	0	Creatinine clearance and/or GFR stable over 6 months to 5 y	
Total			369	9.5	18 or 21 reports are "positive regarding some potential benefit; 3 reports involving 11 patients are negative"	

a No dialysis for supportive care; b Alive at time of report; c Same patients as 1954 report by same authors; d Mortality within 1 year of surgery. All died of advanced uremia which was present preoperatively.

for the purpose of preservation of function should be undertaken only as part of an investigative study.

8. Special considerations for management of endstage renal failure in patients with cystic kidney disease

Progression to endstage renal failure is a common outcome. Both chronic dialysis and renal transplantation are successful in most cases, and selection of the precise modality of treatment is highly dependent on individual patient factors, such as the extent of extrarenal cardiovascular disease, presence of active infection and suitability for immunosuppressive treatment. Polycystic kidney disease accounts for about 5% of renal diseases treated by renal transplantation. The graft survival rate is about 5% lower than the rates in patients with glomerulonephritis or pyelonephritis[105], probably because polycystic patients are older at the time of grafting. The indications for removal of polycystic kidneys prior to renal transplantation are the following: pyelonephritis, renal cystitis, hematuria requiring repeated blood transfusions and kidneys so large that they cause inferior vena caval obstruction or preclude placement of a renal allograft in the true pelvis.

Bilateral nephrectomies are usually performed via a transperitoneal midline approach. Care must be taken not to remove the adrenal glands which may adhere to the upper poles of the kidneys. The distal third of each ureter is left *in situ* to allow for reconstruction of the kidney transplant's urinary tract as a primary procedure, or for revision of ureteral obstruction as a secondary procedure. Unilateral nephrectomies are performed through either the transperitoneal or the flank approach.

In the experience of the Cleveland Clinic treating 56 patients with ADPKD there were no complications from the native kidneys in the 29 patients whose kidneys remained *in situ* [77]. Thaysen and Thomsen[106] reported an actual decrease in kidney size based on serial computed tomograms in patients treated with either dialysis or transplant for endstage polycystic kidney disease.

The standard criteria for a living related renal donor are employed with the addition of a renal ultrasonography or computed tomography to ascertain that polycystic kidney disease is not present in the donor. When a cadaver kidney transplant is necessary, a kidney from a cytomegalovirus seropositive donor for a cytomegalovirus seronegative recipient is not recommended because, in our experience, the older, high-risk, highly immunosuppressed patient does not tolerate post-transplant cytomegalovirus infections as well as does the younger, good-risk recipient.

Because patients with endstage ADPKD are usually in their fifth and sixth decades, pelvic arteriosclerosis may provide a challenge to the transplanting surgeon. In our series, fewer than one-third of these patients had the standard end-to-end renal artery to internal iliac artery anastomosis, and a side-to-end anastomosis to the renal artery was usually necessary.

Pretransplant evaluation of the lower urinary tract of the older man may reveal bladder outlet obstruction because of prostatic hypertrophy. It is best managed with a pretransplant transurethral prostatectomy or by transurethral incision of the prostate[80] to avoid urinary retention after renal transplantation. If the patient is anuric, a suprapubic catheter is placed at the time of bladder outlet surgery to allow the patient to fill his urinary bladder and to void 3–4 times per day during the 6 weeks of healing to prevent occlusion of the prostatic fossa prior to its natural reepithelialization.

Some clinics include routine screening for coronary heart disease in older, high-risk patients, and correct any surgically remediable lesions, even in asymptomatic patients[77]. They also recommend screening of patients for diverticular disease of the colon and resection of involved segments prior to elective renal transplantation. Although this practice is based on the known high prevalence of diverticular disease in patients with ADPKD[21,90], this prophylactic surgery has not achieved a widespread acceptance, and we reserve anterior colon resection for patients with documented prior diverticulitis.

In individual patients, the sheer bulk of cystic kidneys and liver may contribute to poor nutrition. However, the presence of large cystic kidneys *per se* does not preclude dialysis modalities, including continuous ambulatory peritoneal dialysis[47]. Dialysis-induced hypotension caused by massive kidneys obstructing the inferior vena cava has been reported[84]. Nephrectomy or cyst reduction surgery should be considered in unusual cases where morbidity is caused by cyst size alone.

Hemodialysis patients with ADPKD may have problems maintaining vascular access because of relatively high hematocrits and blood viscosity. Primary or secondary polycythemia and dialysis-induced hypotension may develop and further aggravate this tendency[48]. Periodic phlebotomy and occasionally bilateral nephrectomy may be required. Recombinant erythropoietin therapy should be used with caution in hemodialysis patients with cystic disease.

In children with endstage dominant or recessive disease, management should be undertaken by pediatric nephrologists. Despite the risk of progressive liver disease in patients with recessive disease, many patients are successfully rehabilitated.

Patients with endstage medullary cystic disease tend to do well on dialysis because of good urinary output and the absence of hypertension.

In patients who are candidates for immunosuppression, the question of preexisting neoplasia in polycystic kidneys may be clinically relevant. Gregoire *et al.* [37] found 24% of patients with ADPKD to have renal neoplasms, although none had been diagnosed clinically. Neoplasms were much more common in older and male patients.

As a practical matter, patients with polycystic kidney disease should be considered at risk for development of neoplastic transformation. Gross hematuria, progressive constitutional symptoms and increased renal size should prompt the exclusion of a neoplasm. We and others have found computed tomography useful as a diagnostic modality[53]. Prior to acceptance for renal transplantation, this examination is routinely performed. The finding of a solid mass or high density cyst should prompt a diagnostic search with magnetic resonance imaging or arteriography for a neoplasm[40]. Bilateral nephrectomy should be performed if neoplasia is found, since these tumors are bilateral in a high percentage of cases. Similar symptoms in dialysis patients with cystic disease should also prompt a diagnostic workup to exclude neoplasm.

9. Pregnancy and fertility in patients with polycystic kidney disease

Patients with ADPKD frequently reach childbearing age without knowledge of their disease or with minimal symptomatology. Milutinovic *et al.* [66] showed a similar prevalence of spontaneous abortion, stillbirth and urinary infection between polycystic women and unaffected women from families at risk. Pregnancy did not seem to have an adverse effect on the course of polycystic disease, because women with greater than three pregnancies had renal function similar to that in aged-matched women with fewer pregnancies. Hypertension in pregnancy was common in affected patients, and thus the prospective mother needs careful prenatal care to avoid fetal complications associated with hypertension. As expected, patients with severe hypertension, proteinuria and renal insufficiency prior to pregnancy had an excessive fetal wastage and higher maternal morbidity[78]. The size of fetal polycystic kidneys occasionally causes dystocia.

10. Intracranial aneurysms

The management of intracranial aneurysms associated with polycystic disease is of great importance, since rupture confers a grim prognosis on the patient[75]. Most authors agree that the presence of an unruptured aneurysm in a patient with headache, subarachnoid hemorrhage or cranial nerve paralysis should lead to elective surgical repair. In the general population, rupture of saccular aneurysms relates to their size. Those less than 1 cm in diameter virtually never ruptured, whereas those greater than 1 cm in diameter had a rupture rate of 27% in the 8 year study by Wiebers *et al.* [110].

Asymptomatic patients at risk or known to have small aneurysms present a therapeutic dilemma, particularly when they are considered for endstage renal disease management by hemodialysis with its attendant anticoagulation or renal transplantation with immunosuppression. Wakabayashi[108] and Ishibashi *et al.* [44] both found the prevalence of aneurysms to be around one-third, commonly without hypertension. Although hypertension may not cause the aneurysms, elevated blood pressure may increase the chances of rupture. Recent information has suggested a family clustering of aneurysms[49,89]. In the absence of data confirming that a negative angiogram precludes future development of aneurysm, we have limited our investigation of asymptomatic patients to those considered at highest risk, namely those with family histories of aneurysm or subarachnoid hemorrhage. This is particularly important for patients about to embark on chronic hemodialysis or renal transplantation.

Using decision analysis, Levey et al.[52] concluded that the benefit of routine cerebral arteriography does not exceed its risk to survival, except in certain selected patients. The analysis was based on a set of assumptions concerning the risk of surgical complications and the prevalence of aneurysm. The benefit for patients under 25 years of age exceeds a 1-year survival gain only if aneurysm prevalence is greater than 30%. Although smaller studies have shown prevalence figures greater than 30%[44,108], family clustering and much larger populations need to be considered before new recommendations can be made. Evolution of new non-invasive imaging techniques may change the screening of asymptomatic patients at risk for this serious complication.

11. Acquired cystic disease

Since the original report of Dunnill et al. in 1977[24], it has been recognized that approximately one-third of all patients receiving dialysis treatment for chronic renal disease develop cysts in their retained native kidneys, regardless of the etiology of renal failure[35,69]. In most patients this condition is asymptomatic; however, some patients develop hematuria, flank pain, flank masses and even retroperitoneal hemorrhages. The symptoms may be precipitated or aggravated by heparin used in dialysis. Despite a lack of conclusive evidence, it has been our policy to evaluate such patients for acquired cystic disease and associated neoplasm. Another clue to the presence of acquired cystic disease is a spontaneous rise in hemoglobin concentrations or hematocrits from previously stable values.

The most serious complication of acquired cystic disease is malignant transformation. Although intracystic renal adenomas and adenocarcinomas may occur in up to 25% of these patients, metastatic spread is unusual, occurring in less than 5%[25,29,43,45]. Largely because of the risk of neoplasia, we screen all patients under consideration for transplantation and those patients who have been maintained on chronic dialysis for at least 2 years. Computed tomography provides better resolution and diagnostic information than does ultrasonography. Using computed tomography, Ishikawa et al.[46] prospectively followed 96 patients on longterm hemodialysis and showed an increase in kidney size beginning after 3 years of treatment. Almost four-fifths of patients had multiple cysts. Some patients with metastatic adenocarcinomas have been reported[54,59]. Solid masses or complex cysts discovered by such screening should be evaluated further. Retroperitoneal lymphadenopathy on computed tomography scan may be a sign of malignancy[98].

Prior to renal transplantation, kidneys containing suspicious changes should be removed because the risk of neoplasia increases with immunosuppression. Although non-neoplastic cystic change in native kidneys may regress with resumption of normal renal function by transplantation[46], the natural history of neoplasms arising in kidneys with acquired cystic disease is unclear. Thus, it has been our feeling that they must be regarded as potential life-threatening malignancies until evidence to the contrary is available.

References

1. Amar AD, Das S and Egen RM. Management of urinary calculus disease in patients with renal cysts: Review of 12 years of experience in 18 patients. Journal of Urology 1981, 125, 153–156.
2. Anderson RJ, Miller PD, Linas SL, Katz FH and Holmes JH. Role of renin–angiotensin systm in hypertension of polycystic kidney disease. Mineral and Electrolyte Metabolism 1979, 2, 137–141.
3. Ban WJ. Renal cysts: treatment and alcohol. Radiology 1981, 138, 329–331.
4. Bennett WM, Barry J, Elzinga L, Golper T and Torres V. Renal functional and symptomatic responses to reducing cyst volume in patients with autosomal dominant polycystic kidney disease. Kidney International 1988, 33, 181.
5. Bennett WM and Craven R. Ampicillin and trimethoprim–sulfamethoxazole disease. Journal of the American Medical Association 1976, 236, 946–950.
6. Bennett WM, Elzinga L, Golper TA and Barry JM. Reduction of cyst volume for symptomatic management of autosomal dominant polycystic kidney disease. Journal of Urology 1987, 137, 620–622.
7. Bennett WM, Elzinga L, Pulliam JP, Rashad AL and Barry JM. Cyst fluid antibiotic concentrations in autosomal dominant polycystic kidney disease. American Journal of Kidney Diseases 1985, 6, 400–404.
8. Bennett WM, Golper TA and Elzinga L. Fluoroquinolones in patients with polycystic kidney disease. Kidney International 1989, 35, 738.
9. Bennett WM, Hartnett M, Craven R, Gilbert D and Porter GA. Gentamicin concentrations in blood, urine and tissue of patients with end-stage renal disease. Journal of Laboratory and Clinical Medicine 1977, 90, 389–393.
10. Bonadio M, Marino O, Catania B and Giannotti P. Slow penetration of piperacillin into renal cysts. Proceedings of the Internation Congress of Nephrology 1984, 9m 73A.
11. Brenner BM. Hemodynamically mediated glomerular injury and the progressive nature of renal disease. Kidney International 1983, 23, 647–655.
12. Bricker NS and Patton JF. Renal function studies in polycystic disease of the kidney with observations on the effect of surgical decompression. New England Journal of Medicine 1957, 256, 212–214.
13. Buck FN, Bunts RC and Dodson AI. Preservation of renal function in polycystic disease. Journal of Urology 1951, 66, 46–53.
14. Cahill GF and Fish GW. Surgical aspects of polycystic disease. Transactions of the American Society for Genitourinary Srugery 1941, 34, 81–87.
15. Cole BR, Conley SB and Stapleton FB. Polycystic kidney disease in the first year of life. Journal of Pediatrics 1987, 111, 693–699.
16. Cuppage FE, Huseman RA and Chapman A. Ultrastructure and function of cysts from human adult polycystic kidneys. Kidney International 1980, 17, 372–381.

17. D'Angelo A, Mioni G, Ossi E, Lupo A, Valvo E and Maschio G. Alterations in renal tubular sodium and water transport in polycystic kidney disease. Clinical Nephrology 1975, 3, 99–105.
18. Dalgaard OZ. Bilateral polycystic disease of the kidneys: A follow-up study of 284 patients and their familieis. Acta Medica Scandinavica 1957, 158 (Suppl. 328), 1–255.
19. Danielsen H, Nielsen AH, Pedersen EB, Herlevsen P, Kornerup HJ and Posborg V. Exaggerated natriuresis in adult polycystic kidney disease. Acta Medica Scandinavica 1986, 219, 59–66.
20. Danielsen H, Pedersen EB, Nielsen AH, Herlevsen P, Kornerup HJ and Posborg V. Expansion of extracellular volume in early polycystic kidney disease. Acta Medica Scandinavica 1986, 219, 399–405.
21. DeBono DP and Evans DB. The management of polycystic kidney disease with special reference to dialysis and transplantation. Quarterly Journal of Medicine 1977, 46, 353–363.
22. Delaney VB, Adler S and Bruns FJ. Autosomal dominant polycystic kidney disease: presentation, complications and prognosis. American Journal of Kidney Diseases 1985, 5, 104–111.
23. Dodson AI. The surgical treatment of polycystic disease of the kidney: case reports. Journal of Urology 1947, 57, 209–212.
24. Dunnill MS, Millard PR and Oliver D. Acquired cystic disease of the kidneys: a hazard of long term intermittent maintenance hemodialysis. Journal of Clinical Pathology 1977, 30, 868–877.
25. Dunnill MS. Acquired cystic disease. In: Grantham JJ and Gaardner KD, eds, Problems in Diagnosis and Management of Polycystic Kidney Disease. Kansas City: Intercollegiate Press, 1985, 211–223.
26. Elzinga L, Golper TA, Rashad A, Carr M and Bennett W. Trimethoprim–sulfamethoxazole activity in cyst fluid from autosomal dominant polycystic kidneys. Kidney International 1987, 32, 884–888.
27. Elzinga LW, Golper TA, Rashad AL, Carr ME and Bennett WM. Ciprofloxacin activity in cyst fluid from polycystic kidneys. Antimicrobial Agents and Chemotherapeutics (In press).
28. Franz KA and Reubi FC. Rate of functional deterioration in polycystic kidney disease. Kidney International 1983, 23, 526–529.
29. Gasrdner KD and Evan AP. Cystic kidneys: an enigma evolves. American Journal of Kidney Diseases 1984, 3, 403–413.
30. Gerzof SG and Gale ME. Computed tomography and ultrasonography for diagnosis and treatment of renal and retroperitoneal abscesses. Urology Clinics of North America 1982, 9, 185–193.
31. Gilbert BR, Cerqueira MD, Eary JF, Simmons MC, Nabi HA and Nelp WB. Indium-111 white blood cell scan for infectious complications of polycystic renal disease. Journal of Nuclear Medicine 1985, 26, 1283–1286.
32. Goldstein AE and Goldstein RB. Polycystic renal disease: an analysis of operative and non-operative cases. Journal of Urology 1960, 84, 268–272.
33. Grantham JL and Evan AE. Cyst formation and growth in autosomal dominant polycystic kidney disease. Kidney International 1987, 31, 1145–1152.
34. Grantham JJ, Geiser JL and Evan AP. Cyst formation and growth in autosomal dominant polycystic kidney disease. Kidney International 1987, 31, 1145–1152.
35. Grantham JJ and Levine E. Acquired cystic disease: replacing one kidney disease with another. Kidney International 1985, 28, 99–105.
36. Grantham JJ and Slusher S. Management of renal cystic disorders. In: Suki WN and Massry SG, eds, Therapy of Renal Disease and Related Disorders. The Hague: Martinus Nijhoff, 1985, 383–404.
37. Gregoire JR, Torres VE, Holley KE and Farrow GM. Renal epithelial hyperplastic and neoplastic proliferation in autosomal dominant polycystic disease. American Journal of Kidney Diseases 1987, 9, 27–38.

38. Gretz N, Korb E and Strauch M. Low protein diet supplemented by keto acids in chronic renal failure: a prospective controlled study. Kidney International 1983, 24 (Suppl. 16), S263–S267.
39. Higgins CC. Bilateral polycystic kidney disease: review of 94 cases. Archives of Surgery 1952, 65, 318–329.
40. Hilpert P, Friedman AC, Radecki PD, Caroline DF, Fishman EK, Meziane MA, Mitchell DG and Kressel HY. MRI of hemorrhagic renal cysts in polycystic kidney disease. American Journal of Radiology 1986, 146, 1167–1172.
41. Hirsch M and Blinder G. Combined percutaneous diagnostic puncture and management of renal custs. Israel Journal of Medical Sciences 1982, 18, 609–613.
42. Hopkins GB, Hall RI and Mende CW. Gallium-67 scintigraphy for the diagnosis and localization of perinephric abscesses. Journal of Urology 1976, 115, 126–128.
43. Hughson MD, Buchwald D and Fox M. Renal neoplasia and acquired cystic kidney disease in patients receiving long term dialysis.Archives of Pathology and Laboratory Meidicine 1986, 110, 592–601.
44. Ishibashi A. Renal imagings in the diagnosis of polycystic kidney disease.Japanese Journal of Nephrology 1981, 23, 1003–1005.
45. Ishikawa I, Saito Y, Onouchi Z, Kitada H, Suzuki S, Kurihara S, Yuri T, Kitada H and Shinoda A. Development of acquired cystic disease and adenocarcinoma of the kidney in glomerulonephritic chronic hemodialysis patients. Clinical Nephrology 1980, 14, 1–6.
46. Ishikawa I, Yuri T, Kitada H and Shinoda A. Regression of acquired cystic disease of the kidney after successful renal transplantation. American Journal of Nephrology 1983, 3, 310–314.
47. Io Y, Singh S and Pollak VE. Efficacy of dialysis treatment. In: Grantham JJ and Gardner KD, eds, Problems in Diagnosis and Management of Plycystic Kidney Disease. Kansas City: Intercollegiate Press, 1985, 160–168.
48. Jermanovich NB. Polycystic kidney disease and polycythemia vera. Archives of Internal Medicine 1983, 143, 1822–1823.
49. Kachney W, Bell P, Earnest M, Stears J and Gabow P. Familial clustering of intracranial aneurysms in autosomal dominant polycystic kidney disease. Kidney International 1987, 31, 204.
50. Kenner CH, Evan AP, Blomgren P, Aronoff GR and Luft FC. Effect of protein intake on renal structure and function in partially nephrectomized rats. Kidney International 1985, 27, 739–750.
51. Kohler B. Surgical treatment of the polycystic kidney. Acta Chirurgie Scandinavica 1947, 96, 283–295.
52. Levey AS, Pauker SG and Kassirer JP. Occult Intracranial aneurysms in polycystic kidney disease. New England Journal of Medicine 1983, 308, 986–994.
53. Levine E and Grantham JJ. High-density renal cysts in autosomal dominant polycystic kidney disease demonstrated by CT. Radiology 1985, 154, 477–482.
54. Levine E, Grantham JJ, Slusher SL, Greathouse JL and Krohn BP. CT of acquired cystic kidney disease and renal tumors in long term dialysis patients. American Journal of Roentgenology 1984, 142, 125–131.
55. Lowance DC, Estes R and Underwood F. Selected embolization of polycystic kidneys to modulate polycythemia, pain and renal size. Proceedings of the International Congress of Nephrology 1984, 9, 106A.
56. Lucas PA, Meadows JH, Roberts DE and Coles GA. The risks and benefits of a low protein–essential amino acid–keto diet. Kidney International 1986, 29, 995–1003.
57. Lue Y, Anderson E and Harrison JH. The surgical management of polycystic renal disease. Surg Gynecol Obstet 1966, 45–49.
58. Lund FB. Rovsing's operation for congenital cystic kidney. Journal of the American Medical Association 1914, 63, 1083–1086.
59. MacDougall M, Welling LW and Weigman TB. Renal adenocarcinoma and acquired

cystic disease in chronic hemodialysis patients. American Journal of Kidney Diseases 1987, 9, 166–171.

60. Martinez-Maldonado M, Yium JJ, Suki WN and Eknoyan G. Electrolyte excretion in polycystic kidney disease: inter-relationship between sodium, calcium, magnesium and phosphate. Journal of Laboratory and Clinical Medicine 1977, 90, 1066–1075.

61. Maschio G, Oldrizzi L, Rugill C, Valvo E, Lupo A, Tessitore N, Loschiavo C, Fabris A, Gammaro L and Panzetta GO. Dietary Management. In: Grantham JJ and Gardner KD, eds, Problems in Diagnosis and Management of Polycystic Kidney Disease. Kansas City: Intercollegiate Press, 1985, 87–92.

62. Maschio G, Oldrizzi L, Tessitore N, D'Angelo A, Valvo E, Lupo A, Loschiavo C, Fabris A, Gammaro L, Rugiu C and Panzetta G. Effects of dietary protein and phosphorus restriction on the progression of early renal failure. Kidney International 1982, 22, 371–376.

63. Mayers MM. Polycystic kidney disease. Journal of Urology 1948, 59, 471–476.

64. Meltzer M. Surgery for polycystic kidney disease. American Journal of Surgery 1929, 7, 420–423.

65. Milam JH, Magee JH and Bunts RC. Evaluation of surgical decompression of polycystic kidneys by differential renal clearance. Journal of Urology 1963, 90, 144–149.

66. Milutinovic J, Fialkow PJ, Agodoa LY, Phillips LA and Bryant JI. Fertility and pregnancy complications in women with autosomal dominant polycystic disease. Obstetrics and Gynecology 1983, 61, 566–570.

67. Mitch WE, Walser M, Buffington GA and Lemann J. A simple method of estimating progression of chronic renal failure. Lancet 1976, 2, 1325–1328.

68. Muther RS and Bennett WM. Cyst fluid antibiotic concentrations in polycystic kidney disease: difference between proximal and distal cysts. Kidney International 1980, 20, 519–522.

69. Narasimhan N, Golper T, Wolfson M, Rahatzahad M and Bennett WM. Clinical characteristics and diagnostic considerations in acquired renal cystic disease. Kidney International 1986, 30, 748–752.

70. Narasimhan N, Golper TA, Wolfson M and Bennett WM. Discrepancy between histology and function in the high protein fed remnant model. American Journal of Kidney Diseases 1985, 6, A13.

71. Nash MD. Hypertension in polycystic kidney disease without renal failure. Archives of Internal Medicine 1977, 137, 1571–1575.

72. Netto NR Jr, Lemos GC and Claro JFA. Methodology for endoscopic treatment of ureteral calculi. Journal of Urology 1986, 135, 909–911.

73. Newman HR. Congenital polycystic kidney disease. American Journal of Surgery 1950, 80, 410–418.

74. Nielsen SS. Infected cystic kidney. Nordic Medicine 1950, 44, 1145–1146.

75. Nishioka H, Torner JG, Graf CJ, Kassell NF, Sahs AL and Goettler LC. Cooperative study of intercranial aneurysms and subarachnoid hemorrhage: A long term prognostic study. II. Ruptured intercranial aneurysms managed conservatively. Archives of Neurology 1984, 41, 1142–1146.

76. Novick AC. Posterior surgical approach to the kidney and ureter. Journal of Urology 1980, 124, 129–195.

77. Novick AC and Ho-Hsieh H. Renal transplantation. In: Grantham JJ and Gardner KD, eds, Problems in Diagnosis and Management of Polycystic Kidney Disease. Kansas City: Intercollegiate Press, 1985, 172–179.

78. Oken DE. Chronic renal diseases and pregnancy: a review. American Journal of Obstetrics and Gynecology 1966, 94, 1023–1043.

79. Olsson CA and Idelson B. Renal autotransplantation for recurrent renal colic. Journal of Urology 1980, 193, 467–474.

80. Orandi A. Transurethral incision of prostate compared with transurethral resection of prostate in 132 matching cases. Journal of Urology 1987, 138, 810–815.

81. Patton JF and Bricker NS. Renal function studies in polycystic disease of the kidney: A preliminary report. Journal of Urology 1954.

82. Preuss H, Geoly K, Johnson M, Chester A, Kliger A and Schreiner G. Tubular function in adult polycystic kidney disease. Nephron 1979, 24, 198–204.

83. Rao KV. Use of epsilon aminocaproic acid in protracted bleeding from polycystic kidneys: A case report. Journal of Urology 1986, 136, 887–888.

84. Raulerson JD, Juncos LI, Fuller TJ and Cade R. Obstruction of the inferior vena cava complicating hemodialysis in polycystic kidney disease. Southern Medical Journal 1979, 72, 1389–1392.

85. Rault R. Symptomatic urinary infections in patients on maintenance hemodialysis. Nephron 1984, 37, 82–84.

86. Reubi FC. Hypertension. In: Grantham JJ and Gardner KD, eds, Problems in Diagnosis and Management of Polycystic Kidney Disease. Kansas City: Intercollegiate Press, 1985, 121–128.

87. Rovsing T. Treatment of multiocular renal cyst with multiple punctures. Hospitalstid 1911, 4, 105.

88. Rutherford WE, Blondin J, Miller JP, Greenwalt AS and Vavra JD. Chronic progressive renal disease: rate of change of serum creatinine. Kidney International 1977, 11, 62–70.

89. Saifuddin A and Dathan JR. Adult polycystic kidney disease and intracranial aneurysms. British Medical Journal 1987, 295, 526.

90. Scheff RT, Zuckerman G, Harter H, Delmez J and Koehler R. Diverticular disease in patients with chronic renal failure due o polycystic kidney disease. Annals of Internal Medicine 1980, 92, 202–204.

91. Schwab S, Hinthorn D, Diederich D, Cuppage F and Grantham JJ. pH-dependent accumulation of clindamycin in a polycystic kidney. American Journal of Kidney Diseases 1983, 3, 63–66.

92. Schwab SJ. Efficacy of chloramphenicol in refractory cyst infections in autosomal dominant polycystic kidney disease. American Journal of Kidney Diseases 1985, 5, 258–261.

93. Schwab SJ. Experience with chloramphenicol in refractory renal infection. In: Grantham JJ and Gardner KD, eds, Problems in Diagnosis and Management of Polycystic Kidney Disease. Kansas City: Intercollegiate Press, 1985, 105–110.

94. Schwab SJ, Bander SJ and Klahr S. Renal infection in autosomal dominant polycystic kidney disease. American Journal of Medicine 1987, 82, 714–718.

95. Schwab SJ and Weaver ME. Penetration of autosomal dominant polycystic kidney disease. American Journal of Kidney Diseases 1986, 7, 434–438.

96. Sedman A, Bell P, Manco-Johnson M, et al. Autosomal dominant polycystic kidney diseases in childhood: a longitudinal study. Kidney International 1987, 31, 1000–1005.

97. Shangzhi H, Shiyuan A, Henning J, Rong Y and Yufeng C. Cyst decapitating decompression operation in polycystic kidneys. Chinese Medical Journal 1980, 93, 773–778.

98. Siegel SC, Sandler MA, Alper MB and Pearlberg JL. CT of renal carcinoma in patients on chronic hemodialysis. American Journal of Radiology 1988, 150, 583–585.

99. Simon HB and Thompson GJ. Congenital renal polycystic disease. Journal of the American Medical Association 1955, 159, 657–662.

100. Skinner DG and Goodwin WE. Indications for the use of intestinal segments in management of nephrocalcinosis. Journal of Urology 1975, 112, 436–442.

101. Sklar AH, Caruana RJ, Lammers JE and Strauser GD. Renal infections in patients with adult polycystic kidney disease. American Journal of Kidney Diseases 1987, 10, 81–88.

102. Spiegal D and Molitoris BA. The role of percutaneous cyst aspiration in the management of polycystic kidney disease patients with cyst infections. Clinical Research 1986, 34, 85A.

103. Stout RL, Watson AJ and Whelton A. Azthreonam concentrations in severely diseased human and healthy canine kidneys: therapeutic implications. Proceedings of the International Congress on Nephrology 1987, 10, 133A.

104. Sweet R and Keane WF. Perinephric abscess in patients with polycystic kidney disease undergoing chronic hemodialysis. Nephron 1979, 23, 237–240.

105. Terashita GY and Cook DJ. Original disease of the recipient. In: Terasaki PI ed, Clinical Transplants – 1987, Chapt. 36. Los Angeles: UCLA Tissue Typing Laboratory, 1987, 373–379.
106. Thaysen JH and Thomsen HS. Involution of polycystic kidneys during replacement therapy of terminal renal failure. Acta Medica Scandinavica 1982, 212, 389–394.
107. Torres VE, Wilson DM, Offord KP, Burnett JC and Romero JC. Natriuretic response to volume expansion in adult polycystic kidney disease with normal renal function. Proceedings of the American Society of Nephrology 1987, 10, 64A.
108. Wakabayashi T, Fujita S, Ohbora Y, Suyama T, Tamaki N and Matsumoto S. Polycystic kidney disease and intracranial aneurysms. Journal of Neurosurgery 1983, 58, 488–491.
109. Welling LW and Grantham JJ. Cystic and developmental diseases of the kidney. In: Brenner BM and Rector FC, eds, The Kidney. Philadelphia: W.B. Saunders, 1986, 1346.
110. Wiebers DO, Whisnant JP and O'Fallon WM. The natural history of unruptured intracranial aneurysms. New England Journal of Medicine 1981, 304, 696–726.
111. Wikre C and Bennett WM. Renal cyst epithelial transport in non-uremic polycystic kidney disease. Kidney International 1983, 23, 514–518.
112. Winfield HN, Clayman RV, Chaussy CG, Weyman PJ, Fuchs GJ and Lupu AN. Monotherapy of staghorn renal calculi: A comparative study between percutaneous nephrolithotomy and extracorporeal shock wave lithotripsy. Journal of Urology 1988, 139, 895–899.
113. Yates-Bell JG. Rovsing's operation for polycystic kidney. Lancet 1987, 1, 125.

11
Ethical Issues and Cystic Kidneys

W. B. Weil Jr

Abstract

Ethical problems arise in patients with renal cystic disease much as they do in any medical condition; however, these patients do present special circumstances that add particular significance to specific issues. The conflict between autonomy and paternalism in the care of cystic diseases is evident when considering the type and location of treatment and in managing the dialysis patient whose behavior interferes seriously with operation of the dialysis unit. Voluntary vs. mandatory testing for non-curable disease raises similar issues for all patients. These issues have particular sensitivity when they apply to such conditions as ADPKD, Huntington disease or AIDS. Maintaining patient confidentiality is a long-held value that is challenged when a patient with known ADPKD refuses to inform the partner in planning for children. The physician's need to cause no harm may lead to a need to inform the partner without the patient's consent, an act that would be difficult for most physicians. Allocation of scarce or expensive resources is a problem that arises in many areas, but becomes especially difficult in the search for principles that will not unfairly discriminate against potential transplant recipients over a range of ages, incomes, education and future potential. Thus, although renal cystic diseases do not generate any unique class of ethical problems, they do provide some complex and special examples of problems that may be encountered with many other diseases.

Key words   Allocation of resources;
Beneficent deception;
Justice;
Paternalism;
Personal autonomy;
Truth telling.

Abbreviations

ADPKD   Autosomal dominant polycystic kidney disease;
DNR   Do not resuscitate.

1. Introduction

As with almost any illness state, ethical issues abound in the care of persons with cystic kidney diseases. Because the range of ethical issues is so broad and at the same time has a large degree of universality, the ethical problems discussed in this chapter will focus on ADPKD as the prototypical problem. Where appropriate, problems posed by other cystic kidney diseases will be discussed.

Before examining specific ethical problems it is helpful to review some of the characteristics of ethical issues in the medical context. Ethical problems are often couched in the form of a question: What *should* be done in these circumstances? Decisions are based on moral values such as truth telling and not doing harm. When there is only one moral value involved, there is little question about what ought to or should be done: one should tell the truth, one should not produce harm, etc. Ethical problems arise when moral values or interests are in conflict. For example, if one were to tell someone the truth about his/her dismal prognosis at a time that that person were in a critical condition and might not recover, one might generate such a negative state of mind as to impair recovery. Thus, truth telling and not doing harm could be in conflict. How we resolve such a problem will depend to some extent on the specific circumstances, and, to some extent, on how we ourselves evaluate the relative moral weight of each principle, which in turn depends on our own values. However, in many such circumstances, cogent moral discussion has already taken place, and we can use such information in arriving at our own decision.

2. Common ethical conflicts

2.1 Autonomy and paternalism

Most of the ethical problems that arise in medical care in general will also arise in the care of patients with renal cystic disease. Some of these, such as discontinuing life support, including termination of dialysis, upon request of a patient or the patient's surrogate and the issues related to DNR orders, have been discussed at great length in the current literature[20,25,26,29,30,32]. The problems of AIDS have also been discussed in a wide variety of contexts[12]. Because the patient with renal cystic disease in general does not raise new or different issues in these areas, they will not be further discussed in this chapter. Failure to consider these issues at greater length does not imply that they are of any less significance in patients with cystic diseases, but only that they have been well-considered in other publications.

Issues chosen for discussion include patient autonomy, informed consent, disclosure of confidential information and allocation of limited resources.

The most prominent ethical conflict at present lies between personal autonomy and professional paternalism (parentalism). It is being increasingly recognized in contemporary medical care that mature individuals should have the right to determine their own life courses as long as such decisions do not interfere with the interests of other persons (autonomy). The converse of this is that the physician or other health care provider is more knowledgeable than the patient about the patient's illness, and that the physician is in a better position to make decisions about health care than is the patient (paternalism). In practice, "medical paternalism" has been the dominant mode of physician–patient interaction for many centuries. Only in the past few decades has recognition of the patient's prerogatives in decision-making become apparent[31]. Even today, however, the vast majority of decisions regarding diagnostic tests and therapeutic interventions remain physician-determined. Most laboratory procedures are ordered without much discussion with the patient, and many treatments – especially minor ones – are established by the physician. Nevertheless, when either diagnostic or therapeutic procedures could seriously affect the patient or could conflict with the patient's values or interests, it is a prudent physician who involves the patient in the decision-making process. This respect for the patient as an individual represents the recognition of the patient's personal autonomy.

For an individual to exercise his/her autonomy, several conditions must be met. The patient, first of all, must be capable of understanding the information provided. That information should include the proposed procedure and its risks and benefits, and all reasonable alternative procedures and their attendant risks and benefits, including the option of foregoing the procedure entirely. The information must be provided in terms the patient can understand, and it should include all that any reasonable patient would wish to know plus any information this specific patient wants to know.

The second requirement for the exercise of personal autonomy is that the patient be capable of evaluating the options available in terms of his/her own value system and of making a decision based on this evaluation[18]. If the patient is incapable of carrying out these functions, information needs to be provided to the appropriate proxy, who then may be empowered to carry out the decision-making process. If there is doubt about the capability of the patient to carry out the appropriate functions, competence may need to be ascertained by the judicial system, and a court-appointed guardian assigned. Except in a true emergency, it is not the physician's prerogative to assume these functions.

Expression of the patient's autonomy occurs by the process of informed consent. By its definition, informed consent requires that the patient (or his/her proxy/surrogate) is fully informed and provides the consent without undue influence or coercion by others. Thus the third condition is that the informed consent be made voluntarily.

The right of the patient to be autonomous implies an obligation by the physician to respect the patient's decision regardless of whether the decision coincides with the physician's views. A special problem in autonomy occurs with the non-compliant patient, and a major problem is the impact of non-compliance on the autonomy of others[5].

2.2 *Truth telling and benevolent deception*

Truth telling and benevolent deception are another pair of often conflicting values. Telling the truth to a patient is a value based on our respect for the patient as a person and on the concept that a medical care relationship is a fiduciary one, i.e. a relationship based on mutual trust and respect. The physician generally expects the patient to tell the truth, and the patient, if he/she is to continue to trust the physician, expects the truth in return. Most commonly, telling the truth does not harm; thus, beneficence and non-maleficence are associated with honesty. There are occasions, however, when a physician believes that honesty could be harmful, and therefore truth-telling is in conflict with non-maleficence. Under such circumstances, the physician might engage in what has been termed "benevolent deception" or "therapeutic privilege"[27]. The danger inherent in this practice is that truth telling may not be harmful, but is avoided because it is unpleasant for the physician[14], because it may reveal an error in care, or because it may lead the patient to make a decision contrary to what the physician believes to be "correct". As a result of these considerations, several constraints on benevolent deception have evolved. One such constraint is that benevolent deception should not be used to insure that a patient will accept a procedure he/she might otherwise refuse. Benevolent deception cannot be applied to any research proposal or as the basis for non-disclosure of a DNR order. It cannot be invoked when informing a proxy or surrogate for the patient. It should not be used to withhold a diagnosis from a patient and should be considered only when the harm of truthful disclosure clearly outweighs the benefits of such disclosure.

2.3 *Allocation of resources and distributive justice*

The third ethical dilemma arises in the allocation of resources. The conflict occurs when the principle of justice, or equal treatment for all individuals of a group, must be modified because there are not enough resources to treat everyone equally. Under such circumstances, allocation decisions must be made that provide greater access to treatment for one subgroup of patients over another. Criteria commonly used for such allocation decisions have included preferences for those most ill, those most likely to benefit from the treatment, those who have waited longest, and those with the resources to meet the costs of the treatment. Each of these allocation principles has advantages and disadvantages. The greatest danger that can arise from any failure to treat everyone equally is that the allocation will directly or indirectly discriminate against patients on the basis of what many would consider as irrelevant criteria, such as sex, race, life-style or educational attainment.

2.4 Confidentiality and disclosure

The fourth ethical dilemma involves the limits of confidentiality because of potential harm to others. "Confidentiality refers to the boundaries surrounding shared secrets and to the process of guarding these boundaries"[2]. The principles supporting the concept of confidentiality include respect for personal autonomy, respect for the secrets of patients, obligations to uphold an explicit or implicit promise of non-disclosure, and expectations of non-disclosure to enhance the therapeutic relationship. Nevertheless, limits on confidentiality occur when maintaining information as confidential will bring harm to others. As stated by Sissela Bok[2], "Once professionals undertake to receive and even probe for information threatening to others, they can no longer ignore those others, out of concern for their patients or for society. The *prima facie* premises supporting confidentiality are overridden at such times". However, she goes on to state "the doctor is therefore free to speak, but with certain limitations: he must reveal only so much of the secret as is necessary to avert harm and only to the person threatened, who has a right to this information...".

An excellent general reference to these four ethical problems and related issues is the multivolume publication of the *President's Commission for the Study of Ethical Problems in Medicine and Biomedical and Behavioral Research*[21].

3. Problems specific to cystic disease

With this general background in basic ethical principles and the ways in which they may conflict, the problems arising in consideration of cystic disease of the kidney will be examined under three headings: testing, disclosure, and treatment.

3.1 Issues related to testing

In the testing for any medical condition, the primary issue is patient autonomy. Testing for cystic conditions of the kidney is no exception. In general, testing can be described as either voluntary or mandatory. Mandatory testing may occur for two reasons: (1) to assure appropriate medical care for those unable to provide consent for themselves; this could occur if there were a possibility that the person had a condition both remedial and seriously threatening to health (e.g. thyroid and PKU testing of newborn infants); (2) if there were a serious threat to the public health, and such a threat could be prevented by detection of persons with the condition; mandatory testing for syphilis prior to marriage was predicated on this basis, but has been shown to be relatively ineffective and has been abandoned in many jurisdictions. The latter basis for mandatory testing is controversial because it depends on the perceived seriousness of the threat to the public health, and even more on the perceived ability to protect against that threat by knowledge of the carriers of the condition. These perceptions of benefit must be weighed against the potential burdens generated by the invasion of privacy imposed by any mandatory procedure[1,13]. At the present time there does not appear to be any aspect of cystic kidney diseases that would warrant the invoking of mandatory testing[9].

One might propose that, in a family with a known heritable condition, e.g. ADPKD, adults should mandatorily be tested before they have children to prevent the condition in their offspring. Alternatively, that if a child were conceived, the fetus be tested to prevent the birth of an affected child[22,33]. The problem with these suggestions is that such testing, either of parents or fetus, while it might have value to the unborn child, would not result in a physician's being able to treat the child, nor would the results of the testing seriously affect the public health.

Thus, in testing for cystic diseases of the kidney, there has been no basis yet established for mandatory testing. That is not to say that all such testing is purely voluntary. If one were a member of a family with ADPKD and chose not to be tested, it would be well within one's individual rights to forego such a test[17]. If, however, one were married and contemplating having children, one's spouse would have a strong moral argument in trying to persuade one to be tested. Thus pressure from one's spouse or other family members could lead to a less than purely voluntary decision[24]. Such coercion is less problematic for a standard procedure than a research study.

In both the issue of standard testing and the issue of research, but especially in the latter circumstance, it is incumbent on the physician to ascertain that the patient's informed consent is voluntary, and that full disclosure of the risks and benefits includes the information that the physician will undertake the proposed studies only if the patient truly volunteers for them. If this is not the case, it might prove helpful to invite discussion of the situation more fully with the patient and other involved family members. Under such circumstances, it would be important to emphasize that respect for another person is incumbent upon allowing individuals to base such decisions on their own volition. In addition, one might well add that the procedure can be carried out only if the individual freely consents after being fully informed.

Other circumstances in which the voluntary nature of informed consent may be questionable occur when testing is required for employment or for insurance purposes. It is quite conceivable that knowledge of an individual's family history of ADPKD would influence a potential employer or insurer in considering him/her for longterm employment or for health or life insurance coverage. If the person were unwilling to be tested, he/she could forego the position or the insurance, but that might not be a practical consideration. Again, such a voluntary informed consent is not truly voluntary in the truest sense of the term. In this case, the issue of disclosure becomes involved and is discussed later in this chapter.

It should be apparent that counselling services may be an important adjunct to the actual testing procedure. Such counselling should occur both prior to any testing and again at the time that results of the tests become known, whether they are positive or negative. Although the physician may feel competent to carry out the counselling, there are advantages to using someone who is trained in the field of psychology or social work. In addition, the use of someone other than the physician provides the benefit of impartiality and the avoidance of any semblance of bias or conflict of interest.

However, the avoidance of bias is likely only if the counsellor is not a member of the physician's "team". If the counsellor were associated with the physician's group, he/she may be put in the position of being a "double agent". The team member under such circumstances has a loyalty to the group and may see his/her role as supporting the group's goals. If one of the group's goals were to carry out a study of persons with cystic disease, the counsellor could have difficulty reconciling the conflicting roles of being a good group member and of supporting the patient's decision if he/she were reluctant to undergo the study. The obvious way out of this dilemma is either to utilize an independent counsellor, or to have as an explicit group goal the preservation of patient autonomy[15].

Prenatal testing, as mentioned previously, is just becoming available and almost certainly will be widely used in the near future. Parents may request such testing with the possibility of aborting an affected fetus. While the parents are fully entitled to consider and to undertake an abortion, there are ethical issues that distinguish abortion for terminating the pregnant state from abortion for a specific disability[16]. People who are are active in disability issues are often staunch advocates of the right to choose abortion to achieve a non-pregnant state, but are opposed to abortion for a specific disability. They make the point that the latter type of abortion indicates the undesirability of individuals with that disability and thereby devalues such persons in the public image. In a discussion of such an issue relative to Huntington disease, Woody Guthrie's widow is quoted as asking, "Would the world be better off if Woody Guthrie had not been born?"

It seems clear that the testing of children, especially for ADPKD, should be done only for a specific indication, e.g. to determine the pattern of inheritance, among siblings of a child with cystic kidneys, for purposes of genetic counselling. Testing should otherwise be deferred until the child is old enough to make his/her own decision. Since there is currently nothing that can be done to alter the course of the disease, and since it rarely becomes clinically manifest in childhood, there is no reason to abrogate the child's autonomy and to make a decision for testing prior to the child's maturity.

In summary, testing for cystic disease of the kidney should be a voluntary, autonomous undertaking, and should usually be accompanied by pre- and post-testing counselling, especially if there appears to be any ambivalence in the individual to be tested.

3.2 Disclosure and confidentiality

The second major ethical area in the care of individuals with renal cystic disease is that of disclosure and its relation to the principle of confidentiality. In many situations the individual involved will have no problem, as he or she may wish to disclose the test results and the consequences of being at risk to those directly affected by his or her condition. When such disclosure is voluntary it presents no ethical problems. However, to one extent or another, anyone who may be at risk for cystic diseases may wish to limit either the disclosure of risk status or the results of a positive test. Under such circumstances there may be a conflict between the traditional confidentiality of the doctor–patient relationship and the responsibility of the physician not to harm (non-maleficence)[2,13,24].

The best way to avoid the conflict between confidentiality and disclosure is to discuss the matter prior to the time any testing or diagnostic procedures are undertaken. In such a discussion the physician can ascertain the patient's views on disclosure to a sexual partner, to children, to insurance companies and to employers. The physician can also make certain that the patient understands the physician's position on these matters. This will allow the patient to make an informed consent knowing in advance the implications of testing as well as the more standard risk/benefit analysis.

What should govern the physician's behavior in matters of disclosure? There are some who believe that the issue of confidentiality is so significant that it should not be violated under any circumstances. Nevertheless, as important as confidentiality is to the maintenance of trust in the professional relationship and to the respect owed to the person who has shared information, there are limits imposed by the principle of not producing harm. The individual with the condition may create harm by withholding such information. Under such circumstances, one might reasonably consider that such a person has forfeited the right to confidentiality. Alternatively the physician may reveal the information, to avoid creating harm, to others because of respect for their status as persons who deserve protection from harm. In either case, the physician should inform the patient that the physician plans to reveal the findings unless the patient chooses to do so.

Breaking confidentiality to avoid serious harm usually arises in situations when one member of a couple refuses to inform the partner of his or her condition. This becomes more compelling when the couple contemplates having children. Each partner has what may be termed procreative rights, which include the knowledge about known serious genetic risks or the chance that an offspring will acquire a serious congenital illness from an affected partner. If one withholds such information, serious harm may occur to the child to be born, and the procreative rights of the partner are thus violated. Under such circumstances a physician may choose to request that the individual inform the partner. If the person refuses to do so, the physician may state that the physician will feel compelled to make such information known to the partner. As mentioned before in Section 2.1, the right to be autonomous does not include the right to make decisions that interfere with the autonomy of another person.

Any action to disclose information without the patient's consent should not be undertaken casually. The necessity to reveal information without consent must be premised on averting serious harm to another individual. Thus, there would be no cause to provide information to parents or other relatives, to employers, or to insurance companies. However, if the patient has given consent to employers or insurance companies to obtain medical information, one cannot refuse to reveal whatever information is appropriate to that inquiry. If the patient has not provided consent for release of information, then any request for information is appropriately refused, unless it is the patient's partner. Although some harm to others may result from such a refusal, that harm is not of sufficient magnitude to harm the privacy of the patient.

There remains the issue of telling children in at-risk families of their being at risk for any of the heritable problems. There are two kinds of situations in which this issue could arise. The more likely event would occur if one of the child's parents requires treatment for renal failure and the child asks "what is wrong with daddy/mommy?" and then follows with "could that happen to me?"The other situation would occur if the child is unaware of renal disease in a parent, but the parents feel either an obligation to tell the child or to keep such information secret. If the child is truly unaware of renal disease in the family (parenthetically, that is not as common as many parents believe), then there is no need to inform the child prior to adolescence. Sometime between the onset of adolescence and the age when the child becomes independent, it is ethically imperative that the child be told of his/her potential risk for renal disease. Ideally the time chosen to reveal this information is when the child can handle it with some degree of emotional stability, comprehension and the capacity to take whatever action he/she deems appropriate. Should the parents refuse to provide their child with such information, even at maturity, the physician may need to intervene to prevent a harm greater than that of overriding parental discretion and privacy[7,9,10].

The more difficult problem occurs when the child asks about the likelihood of having the same disease as a parent already seriously ill with cystic disease. Telling the child the truth, at some level or another, is clearly the best solution for the longterm. The amount of detail and the degree of explanation should obviously vary with the age and development of the child. In such circumstances the answer can begin with "yes, that is a possibility". What follows after that will depend on what the child responds. For the young child, that is all that may be asked. If the child is older, the child may follow with additional questions, each of which needs to be answered as truthfully, but as simply as possible.

In every case, however, there are two issues that the parent should volunteer. First, the parent should make it clear that additional questions can be asked at any time. Second, the parent needs to reassure the child of any age that, even if he or she were to have such a condition, it would not present a problem until the child has grown up. Further, it needs to be added that in any case the child will be entirely normal as a child, can go to school, ride a bike, play as hard as wanted, and do all the things that any child would be allowed to do. This kind of reassurance is especially important for young children, because their sense of time, especially long time periods, is poorly developed.

In summary, confidentiality in the doctor–patient relationship is a value of great importance. As with many moral principles, this one is not absolute; there usually is some other principle that may be in conflict, and the decision then rests on which value in the specific circumstances carries the greater moral weight. In the case of harm to another individual, if that harm is sufficiently grave and is avoidable, the moral value of not harming another may outweigh the harm in breaking the confidential relationship.

3.3 Treatment and allocation of resources

Of the ethical issues relative to renal disease in general, the one that has received the most scrutiny and review is that related to the allocation of resources to persons with chronic renal failure.

Prior to the passage of the USA Federal legislation in 1973 that provides payment for the care of persons with endstage renal disease, the most controversial problem was the determination of which patients should have access to dialysis and transplantation. Various strategies were utilized to determine which lives were worth saving. Criteria often had a social value factor, and thus created a tendency to discriminate against the poor, the less well-educated, those with decreased mental capacity, and the aged[4]. With the advent of a payment mechanism for virtually all persons in need of dialysis, the situation has changed radically. There were close to 100,000 persons undergoing dialysis in 1988. The endstage renal disease program, including dialysis and transplantation, had in 1988 a US Federal price tag of about 2.5 billion dollars, that is, a direct cost to the Federal government of at least $25,000 per patient per year. The actual cost to society was greatly in excess of this amount.

The national concern for reduction in the Federal budget across all categories has raised the issue of limiting the cost of the endstage renal disease program. The ethical problems inherent in such discussions include those relating to the type of therapy to be employed and those related to the selection of patients for any type of therapy. Numerous proposals have been advanced to accomplish this goal. For example, it has been estimated that up to 30% of

patients undergoing dialysis are either not benefited or only minimally benefited by such treatment, and their identification would not be too difficult.
Another proposal has been to further alter the reimbursement system, which
currently favors in-center dialysis over home dialysis, hemodialysis over peritoneal dialysis, and any form of dialysis over transplantation. In each case, the
physician–center reimbursement system favors the more costly alternative over
the socially less costly one. In addition, several analyses have shown the socially
less costly alternative to yield improved patient outcomes. With the current
cost of immunosuppressive therapy, the cost advantage of transplantation over
dialysis may not be as great as originally perceived, but the improved patient
outcome would still favor transplantation over any form of dialysis. Similarly,
home dialysis is associated with better outcomes for the patient than is in-center
dialysis[8].

Costs are determined by type of dialysis, location of dialysis and choice of
transplantation versus dialysis. The differences in reimbursement for the various procedures, while to some extent based on differences of time and effort
involved, have favored the more expensive alternative in each case. By itself
this is more a problem in economic policy than of ethical issues. The ethical
problem arises in the analysis of risk and benefit to the patient. If, as some
suspect, the risk–benefit ratio from the patient's perspective were more favorable for the lower cost alternative in each case, then favoring the procedures
with the poorer risk–benefit ratio would represent a conflict of interest for the
physician[3]. Furthermore, the favored choice of alternatives, despite the conflict
of interest, would appear to favor the financial interests of the physician over
the medical interests of the patients. Such a balance of interests would clearly
pose difficulty for the principle of beneficence. Data from a broadly based,
longterm outcome management analysis would be of great assistance in resol-
ving such issues. Should such an analysis confirm the suspicion that the lower
cost alternatives are associated with better patient outcomes, a major financial
rearrangement would be called for. Although such financial restructuring
might have to be carefully staged to avoid a serious disruption of the entire
endstage renal care program, it is certainly conceivable that it could be accomplished if warranted.

Conversely, should the outcome analysis favor the more expensive forms
of therapy, there would be less of an ethical basis for major alterations in the
reimbursement patterns. The ethical basis for change under these conditions,
as well as under the former premises, would relate to the cost–benefit values
of this program versus the cost–benefit of other programs that may save lives
and improve health and well-being. Such programs would include increased
prevention efforts and increased research on methods to circumvent the development of endstage illness.

On the other hand, several commentators have suggested that making all
of the changes in reimbursement that have been recommended would result
in only a short period of cost reduction. Costs inevitably would again rise unless

a ceiling were imposed, and a major rethinking of the problem would then become necessary[19].

The other issue of limiting access to therapy for certain patients is more complex. Basically it amounts to setting priorities as to the order in which patients are served, recognizing that individuals with the lowest priorities may never be served before death intervenes.

The ethical issue that is violated when such allocation decisions occur is the principle of justice or equity, which holds that persons in comparable circumstances should be treated comparably. When resources are plentiful there is a clear moral mandate to provide the same resources to everyone who needs them. In a somewhat limited fashion that has been the principle guiding endstage renal disease care in the United States for the past 15 years. However, even within this equity-driven system, some degree of priority or allocation has been taking place. When resources are limited, one alternative to allocation is to provide a fraction of needed resources to everyone in need. However in endstage renal disease, such an approach could be devastating if, as is likely, partial treatment would be equivalent therapeutically to no treatment. Under such circumstances, no one would be saved and all would die. Thus, some kind of allocation is necessary.

Allocation algorithms are found throughout the transplantation field – more so in the transplanting of hearts and livers than of kidneys, but even in the renal field such practices exist. The most important ethical problem with any allocation or priority-setting system is that it not be intentionally or unintentionally biased to favor or discriminate against individuals for medically irrelevant reasons. A policy that excluded one sex or racial group or geographic area would be unethical on this basis. The unofficial selection process in the British National Health Service, which treats about half as many persons as does the American program, is an example of such a system[6,23].

The priority criteria that have been found to be morally acceptable in various settings have included:

(1)　length of waiting time – a principle of first come, first served;
(2)　urgency – a policy that treats those most in danger of dying before undertaking care for those with a less immediate threat of death;
(3)　benefit – a complex system that gives priority to those most likely to benefit from the procedure;
(4)　technical factors – a system that recognizes the need to give small organs to small people and large organs to large people, or, when time is short, to select a person that is readily available ahead of one that would take more time to appear.

Each of these priority criteria has both positive and negative ethical values. One approach to minimizing the negative aspects and maximizing the positive elements in each criterion has been to combine them in some sort of weighted system that yields a combined "priority score". This approach used by the

Pittsburgh group, was published in 1987[28]. Although currently being applied in the field of transplantation, such a system should be applicable to dialysis if serious curtailment of that program becomes a reality. Whenever a systematic selection process is adopted for any procedure, outcome data must be accumulated for periodic retrospective review. Such a review process is necessary to determine if some unexpected bias in selection has occurred, a bias that discriminates against one group of patients for factors that are irrelevant to the process and consequently unjust or unethical.

3.4 Prevention

Currently there are no known primary prevention methods for cystic conditions of the kidney[11]. However, two potential approaches that have considerable ethical implications deserve mention. The first of these is gene therapy. Assuming that a specific gene will be identified, there would be two approaches possible for modifying the abnormal gene. One of these would be to modify or replace the gene in the somatic cell line. The other approach would be to attempt such changes in the germ cell line. Should somatic cell gene therapy prove feasible, there would be few ethical issues involved in proceeding with such an approach on an experimental basis. The major problems would be those concerned with research on a fetus or child. At the present time the approval process is a complex one, but approval should be ultimately obtainable because the research is orientated at directly benefitting that specific fetus or child. Germ cell line research is much more problematic because of the potential for multigenerational effects – harmful as well as beneficial. Under such circumstances there is a general negative attitude toward any research that would directly impact on the germ cell line.

Another alternative more feasible at the present time is the use of donated ova or sperm depending on which parent is affected. While there exist numerous concerns about the use of donor gametes, the use of donor sperm has a long history in the field of alternative reproductive practices. Although ovum donation is relatively recent, there is little from an ethical perspective to distinguish it from sperm donation. Other reproductive practices that could be considered would be embryo donation or surrogate pregnancy, but neither of these approaches offers any advantage over gamete donation and the ethical and social problems would be far greater.

Thus, cystic disease of the kidney presents the clinician with a wide variety of ethical issues. The most prominent issues are those involving personal autonomy and its conflict with medical paternalism, confidentiality and the principle of not allowing harm to come to others, problems in the allocation of limited resources, and prevention of the genetically determined conditions by alternative modes of reproduction or selective abortion.

290

References

1. Barry M, Cleary P and Fineberg H. Screening for HIV infection: risks, benefits, and the burden of proof. Law, Medicine and Health Care 1986, 14, 259–267.
2. Bok S. The limits of confidentiality. Hastings Center Report 1983 (February), 13, 24–31.
3. Bovbjerg R, Held P and Diamond L. Provider–patient relations and treatment choice in the era of fiscal incentives: the case of end-stage renal disease program. Milbank Quarterly 1987, 65, 177–202.
4. Caplan A. Kidneys, ethics, and politics: policy lessons of the ESRD experience. Journal of Health Politics, Policy and Law 1981, 6, 488–503.
5. Conrad P. The noncompliant patient in the search of autonomy. Hastings Center Report 1987 (August), 17, 15–17.
6. Challah S, Wing A, Bauer R, Morris R and Schroeder S. Negative selection of patients for dialysis and transplantation in the United Kingdom. British Medical Journal 1984, 288, 1119–1122.
7. Dubler N. My Husband Won't Tell the Children. Hastings Center Report 1984 (August), 17, 15–17.
8. Evans R, Mannine D, Garrison L, Hart G, Blagg C, Gutman R, Hull A and Lowrie E. The quality of life of patients with end-stage renal disease. New England Journal of Medicine 1985, 312, 553–559.
9. Gabow P, Grantham J, Childress J, Cole B, Gardner K, Bennett W, Kimberling W, Reeders S and Conneally P. Gene testing in autosomal dominant polycystic kidney disease. National Kidney Foundation
10. Gaylin W. The competence of children: no longer all or none. Hastings Center Report 1982 (April), 12, 33–38.
11. Goodman L and Goodman M. Prevention – how misuse of a concept undercuts its worth. Hastings Center Report 1986 (April), 16, 26–38.
12. Gostin L and Curran W, eds., AIDS Science and Epidemiology. Law, Medicine and Health Care 1986, 14.
13. Gostin L and Curran W. AIDS screening, confidentiality and the duty to warn. American Journal of Public Health 1987, 77, 361–365.
14. Katz J. Why doctors don't disclose uncertainty. Hastings Center Report 1984 (February), 14, 35–44.
15. Mackilin R. Ethical issues in treatment of patients with end-stage renal disease. Social Work Health Care 1984, 9, 11–20.
16. Mathieu D. Respecting liberty and preventing harm: Limits of state intervention in prenatal choice. Harvard Journal Law Public Policy, 8, 19–55.
17. Meissen G, Myers R, Mastromauro C, Koroshetz W, Klinger K, Farrer L Watkins P, Gusella J Bird E and Martin J. Predictive testing for Huntington's Disease with use of a linked DNA marker. New England Journal of Medicine 1988, 318, 535–542.
18. Miller B. Autonomy and the refusal of lifesaving treatment. Hastings Center Report 1981 (August), 11, 22–15.
19. Moskop J. The moral limits to federal funding for kidney disease. Hastings Center Report 1987 (April), 17, 11–15.
20. Nolan K. In death's shadow: the meanings of withholding resuscitation. Hastings Center Report 1987 (October/November), 17, 9–14.
21. President's Commission for the Study of Ethical Problems in Medicine and Biomedical and Behavioral Research. Summing Up – The Ethical and Legal Problems in Medicine and Biomedical and Behavioral Research 1983 (March).
22. Reeders S, Gal A, Propping P, Waldherr R, Davies K, Zerres K, Hogenkamp T, Schmidt W, Dolata M and Weatherall D. Prenatal diagnosis of autosomal dominant polycystic kidney disease with a DNA probe. Lancet 1986, 6–7.
23. Rennie D, Rettig R and Wing A. Limited resources and the treatment of end-stage renal

failure in Britain and the United States. Quarterly Journal of Medicine 1985, New Series 56, 321–336.

24. Rosenfeld A. At risk for Huntington's Disease: who should know what and when? Hastings Center Report 1984 (June), 14, 5–8.

25. Ruark J and Raffin T, Stanford University Medical Center Committee on Ethics. Initiating and withdrawing life support: principles and practice in adult medicine. New England Journal of Medicine 1988, 318, 25–30.

26. Schneiderman L. Sounding board – ethical decisions in discontinuing mechanical ventilation. New England Journal of Medicine 1988, 318, 984–988.

27. Somerville M. Therapeutic privilege: variation on the theme of informed consent. Law, Medicine and Health Care 1984, 12, 4–12.

28. Starzl T, Hakala T, Tzakis A, Gordon R, Stieber A, Makowka L, Klimosi J and Bahnson H. A multifactorial system for equitable selection of cadaver kidney recipients. Journal of the American Medical Association 1987, 257, 3073–3075.

29. Tomlinson T and Brody H. Sounding board – ethics and communication in do-not-resuscitate orders. New England Journal of Medicine 1988, 318, 43–46.

30. Viederman M. Saying "No" to hemodialysis: should a minor's decision be respected? Hastings Center Report 1974 (September), 14, 8–10.

31. Weil W. Problems related to personal autonomy and informed consent. Delaware Medical Journal 1987, 59, 189–203.

32. Younger S. DNR orders: no longer secret, but still a problem. Hastings Center Report 1987 (February), 17, 24–33.

33. Zerres K, Hansmann R and Gembruch U. Autosomal recessive polycystic kidney disease – problems of prenatal diagnosis. Prenatal Diagnosis 1988, 8, 215–229.

Section 4

12
Autosomal Dominant Polycystic Kidney Disease

P. A. Gabow

Abstract

Autosomal dominant polycystic kidney disease (ADPKD) is a hereditary disease occurring in 1 in 200 to 1 in 1,000 individuals. ADPKD is characterized by cystic lesions in the kidneys and often by structural abnormalities in the gastrointestinal tract and cardiovascular system. The pathogenesis of the disorder appears to involve both cellular proliferation and altered extracellular matrix synthesis. Diagnosis can be established most readily by the sonographic demonstration of renal cysts or by gene linkage analysis. Renal manifestations of ADPKD include hypertension, infection, nephrolithiasis and malignancy. The prominent extrarenal manifestations include hepatic cysts, mitral valve prolapse and intracranial aneurysms. Although only 2% of nephrons appear to be involved in cyst formation, the renal function often slowly deteriorates. Presently, there is a 52% probability of an ADPKD subject's being alive without renal replacement therapy at age 73. ADPKD patients with endstage renal disease respond to renal replacement therapy as well as other patient groups.

Key words   Autosomal dominant polycystic kidney disease;
                      Intracranial aneurysms;
                      Mitral valve prolapse;
                      Polycystic liver disease.

1. Introduction

Autosomal dominant polycystic kidney disease (ADPKD) came to the attention of the medical community through autopsy observation of large kidneys replaced by cysts. The kidneys can be of gargantuan proportions, weighing 7–8 kg and measuring 40 × 25 × 20 cm. Hence the name focused on the renal abnormality, and the disorder was considered to be solely a kidney disease. The early reports of ADPKD culminated in the classic treatise by Dalgaard in 1957[33]. The thesis detailed the clinical features in advanced disease and documented the natural history of the disorder as it unfolded in the preantibiotic, preantihypertensive era. For the next several decades ADPKD received little attention from the medical community. However, in recent years there has been a flurry of investigative activity with identification of the chromosome carrying a putative gene[146], with description of the early phases of the disorder[59], and with broadening of the concept of the disorder into that of a systemic disease. This new knowledge and the application of modern investigative techniques are likely to result in this disorder becoming one of the first kidney diseases to be understood completely from the gene to the gene product to the pathogenesis of the clinical abnormalities.

2. Definition and pathogenesis

We define ADPKD as a systemic, dominant hereditary disorder producing cysts in the kidneys and structural abnormalities in the gastrointestinal tract and the cardiovascular system.

Several pathogenetic mechanisms have been considered to be operative in ADPKD (Table 12.1) and are discussed in more detail in Chapter 5 of this volume.

Table 12.1 Pathogenesis of ADPKD

(1)	Failure of union of embryonic kidney segments
(2)	Abnormal cell growth
(3)	Intratubular obstruction
(4)	Abnormal extracellular matrix
(5)	White cell alteration of the tubular microenvironment

ADPKD was initially thought to be a congenital non-union of portions of the embryonic kidney, resulting in blind sacs or cysts. Microdissection studies, which demonstrated tubular continuity with the cysts, rendered this hypothesis untenable[8,138,141]. Another early hypothesis ascribed ADPKD to neoplasia. After decades of no interest in this concept, evidence supporting altered growth is again gaining credance[46,47,78]. It is possible that the altered growth observed is a non-specific response to renal injury, particularly since polyp formation is also observed in the remnant kidney model[98] or a result of response to altered extracellular matrix. The micropolyps in ADPKD have been envisioned to develop in a critical position in tubular lumens, producing obstruction and an antegrade increase in intraluminal pressure with cyst formation[47]. However, epithelial hyperplasia more likely contributes directly to cyst formation. Calculations relating cyst size, epithelial cell number and cell size demonstrate that cell proliferation must occur for any cyst to form[76]. Moreover, tissue culture of ADPKD cyst epithelium has demonstrated accelerated growth in some studies[182].

Although altered cell growth appears to be a critical aspect of cyst formation in the kidney, and presumably in the liver, it does not provide as ready an explanation for non-cystic extrarenal manifestations. These extrarenal manifestations are most consistent with a derangement of extracellular matrix. Moreover, there are experimental data lending support to this interpretation[22,73,124,182]. The hypotheses of altered growth and abnormal extracellular matrix are not necessarily mutually exclusive, since growth and matrix properties are intimately related aspects of cell proliferation and differentiation[100].

Given the fluid-filled nature of a cyst, accumulation of fluid is critical to cyst development. The importance of this aspect of cyst formation remains to be completely examined.

Environmental influences have been implicated in the pathogenetic mechanisms of experimental cystic disease, particularly in relation to chemical cystogens[24,31,35,39,45,46,48,64,67,70,140,172]. No such association has been made in human cystic disease.

Given the ultimate genetic nature of the disease, one must explain why only some portions of some nephrons are involved in cyst formation. This could be compatible with modulation of gene expression by local factors. In this regard, Gardner et al.[64,65] have demonstrated that experimental renal cyst formation is substantially influenced by exposure to bacteria and endotoxins.

Currently no one hypothesis provides a comprehensive explanation of all aspects of the disorder. Multiple interrelated factors are likely to be involved in producing the varied phenotypic manifestations of ADPKD.

3. Inheritance and epidemiology

The early descriptions of polycystic kidney disease revealed a biphasic distribution of the age of presentation, with peak incidences in both the first and fourth to fifth decades. Application of the principles of Mendelian genetics to the observed family pedigrees suggested that the childhood form commonly followed autosomal recessive transmission and the adult form followed autosomal dominant inheritance. The nomenclature used for these principal varieties of renal cystic disease came to reflect the age of presentation rather than the genetics, that is, "infantile" and "adult" polycystic kidney disease. As a consequence of this terminology, polycystic kidney disease in childhood tended to be regarded as autosomal recessive, but the recognition of dominant disease in children[7,10,12,17,27,29,44,50,55,79,96,97,115,117,118,122,143,145,149,150,162,164,168,178, 183,185] mandates a terminology based on inheritance as well as other clinical characteristics.

ADPKD has been assumed to represent one genetic disorder. However, current data suggest that more than one gene may be responsible. In 1985, Reeders et al.[146] applied gene linkage techniques to ADPKD, using a highly polymorphic DNA probe for the alpha-hemoglobin region on the short arm of chromosome 16. It was determined that PKD-1 gene was relatively near this marking probe and on chromosome 16. However, the PKD-1 gene itself was not identified. In 1988, Kimberling et al.[99] demonstrated non-linkage to the chromosome 16 markers in several generations of a large family, thus indicating the presence of a second PKD gene. The chromosome bearing the PKD-2 gene remains to be identified. Present information suggests that the majority of ADPKD is due to the PKD-1 gene on chromosome 16[99].

Regardless of which PKD gene is responsible for ADPKD in a given family, each affected person has the PKD gene on one of a pair of autosomal chromosomes. Thus, each offspring of an affected parent has a 50% chance of inheriting the PKD gene and the disorder. ADPKD occurs with equal frequency and penetrance in males and females[33]. Dalgaard[33] has suggested a 90% penetrance of the gene, defined as the occurrence of renal cysts, by age 90.

Some cases of ADPKD occur as a result of spontaneous mutation because both parents are unaffected. Only about 60% of affected individuals provide a positive family history of ADPKD[33,90]. However, testing of parents with appropriate imaging modalities generally reveals that one parent is affected, albeit asymptomatic. Thus, it would appear that the spontaneous mutation rate is under 10%.

ADPKD has been described throughout the world and among all ethnic groups. However, there are fewer reported cases within black populations[42,151,170,175]. The prevalence of ADPKD in Europe and the United States is between one in 200 and one in 1000, making it more common than sickle cell disease, cystic fibrosis and Huntington disease[33,34,86,90]. The age- and sex-adjusted incidence rate in the United States is 1.38 in 100,000[90,175]. If those individuals who are diagnosed at autopsy are included, the incidence almost doubles, emphasizing both the paucity of symptomatology and low index of clinical suspicion in oligosymptomatic individuals[90,175].

4. Methods of diagnosis

The methods of diagnosis include clinical, routine laboratory studies, radiographic studies and gene linkage analysis (Table 12.2).

Table 12.2 Methods of diagnosis of ADPKD

(1)	Family history
(2)	Routine history and physical examination
(3)	Routine laboratory data
(4)	Renal concentrating test
(5)	Imaging studies
	Excretory urography
	Isotope scanning
	Arteriography
	Ultrasonography
	Computed axial tomography
	Magnetic resonance imaging
(6)	Gene linkage analysis

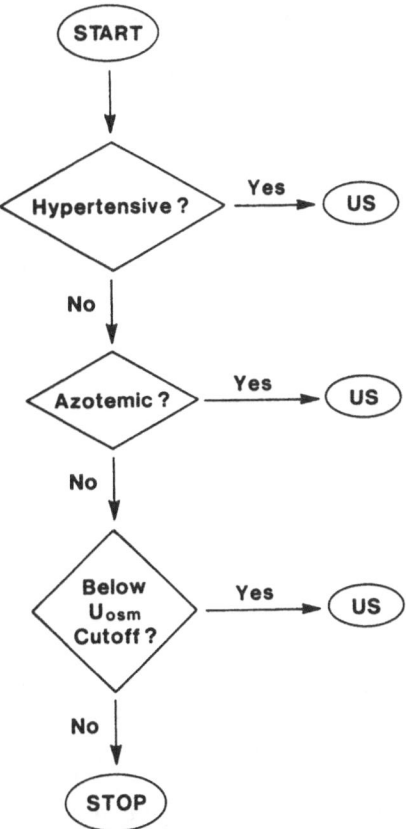

Figure 12.1 An algorithm developed from a population of 56 ADPKD and 79 non-ADPKD subjects. The decision points are diamonds. US represents ultrasound of the kidneys. The U_{osm} cutoff is the minimal value for maximal U_{osm} derived from a formula which minimizes false negatives.

As discussed above, family history is positive in only 60% of cases[33,90]. Moreover, a positive family history only conveys a 50% risk and, therefore, cannot establish the diagnosis. Routine history and physical examination do not yield sufficiently sensitive or specific data to identify true gene carriers, since there is considerable overlap in signs and symptoms between affected and unaffected family members[59] (Table 12.3).

Similarly, normal routine laboratory data, including tests of renal function, do not eliminate the possibility of ADPKD, as renal functional impairment is a relatively late manifestation of the disease[59]. Although abnormal renal function in an at-risk individual warrants evaluation for ADPKD, it does not establish ADPKD as the definitive cause of renal impairment without further study.

Table 12.3 Comparison of signs and symptoms in affected and unaffected family members[*]

Symptoms	Unaffected (% of 250)	Affected (% of 164)
Bloating	0.0	1.3
Abdominal mass	0.0	1.3
Abdominal distention	0.0	3.8
Urinary frequency	3.1	5.5
Peripheral edema	4.3	5.5
Dysuria	5.9	7.9
Nocturia	5.9	7.9
Nausea	0.4	4.9[a]
Headache	3.1	18.9[a]
Hematuria	8.3	31.1[a]
Flank and back pain	20.5	61.0[a]
Systolic murmur	4.9	10.5[a]
Peripheral edema	3.3	9.3[a]
Abdominal tenderness	7.6[a]	19.1[a]
Palpable liver	6.4[a]	27.2[a]
Palpable kidney	4.4[a]	51.6[a]
Abnormal funduscopic findings	6.0[a]	22.2[a]

[a]Statistically significant p < 0.05
[*]From: Gabow PA, Ikle DW and Holmes JH[59] (with permission).

Impaired renal concentrating ability occurs early in ADPKD[32,60,120,144]. Its presence is sufficiently predictable to establish its usefulness as a screening test in subjects at risk[60]. Impaired concentrating ability warrants further evaluation by ultrasonography[60]. If concentrating ability is coupled with blood pressure determination and serum creatinine measurement, an algorithm can be developed with a predictive value for a normal result of 93% (Fig. 12.1)[60]. With this inexpensive office-based screening, only 2–3% of true positives will be missed, and 20–30% of negative family members will not require ultrasonography[60].

Prior to the demonstration of the PKD-1 gene on chromosome 16, an affected individual could be identified with certainty only after the detection of renal cysts by one of the imaging modalities (Table 12.2). Ultrasonography is the preferred modality. It is sensitive, detecting cysts of 2–5 mm or more in diameter. It requires no contrast or radiation exposure, and it can be performed with ease in young children and pregnant women. It has been stated that ultrasonography will be positive in 86% of ADPKD subjects by age 30 years[9]. The typical ultrasonographic appearance is renal enlargement with multiple cysts distributed throughout the parenchyma. However, as many as 18% of ADPKD subjects have normal sized kidneys[59]. Despite a lack of agreement on how many cysts actually constitute polycystic kidney disease, most radiologists and clinicians require multiple cysts and bilateral involvement. Completely reliable interpretation of a normal or minimally abnormal renal ultrasonogram at a given age awaits the systematic correlation of gene status with serial

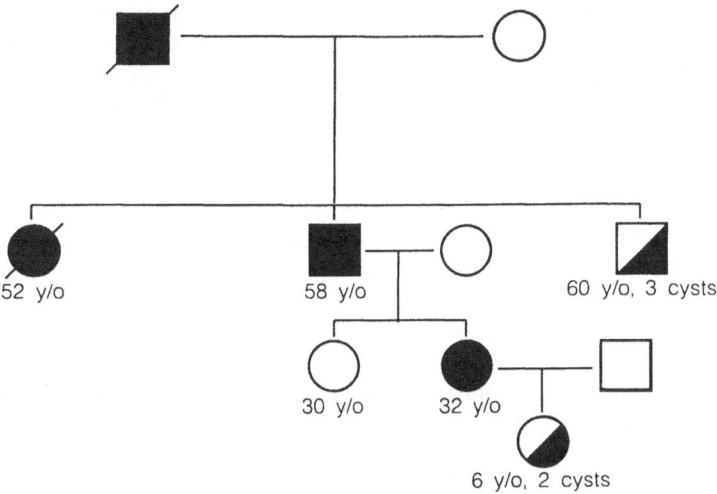

Figure 12.2. This is a pedigree of a four generation ADPKD family. Solid symbols indicate subjects with definite ADPKD. Half shaded symbols represent individuals who are suspicious for ADPKD. Lined symbols indicate deceased persons. One male in the second generation has only three cysts and may be normal. However, the child in the fourth generation with two cysts is likely to be affected.

ultrasonography studies. Moreover, ultrasonography can yield both false positive and false negative tests. Medullary pyramids have been interpreted as cysts in children[162]. Enhanced computed tomography (CT) scan appears to yield the diagnosis in 6–10% of subjects who have normal ultrasonography[91,108,112] (Table 12.2). This small increment in sensitivity does not warrant utilization of CT scan for routine screening because of its radiation and contrast exposure and the difficulty of performing the study in children. CT should be reserved for subjects in whom the level of clinical suspicion is high despite normal ultrasonography, and for those individuals in whom renal complications of ADPKD are suspected. Although renal cysts can be identified by MRI without either contrast or radiation exposure, preliminary information suggests it offers no advantage over, and greater expense, than ultrasonography[88,109].

The differential diagnosis of familial cystic disease includes tuberous sclerosis. This disorder is also an autosomal dominant trait. Although the classic renal abnormality is angiomyolipoma, isolated cystic disease has occurred[41,169]. Thus, any new patient, particularly with a history of seizure disorder, should have a skin examination for shagreen patches, ash leaf spots, adenoma sebaceum and subungual fibroma, and an ophthalmologic examination for retinal lesions. CT examination for cerebral abnormalities is indicated when doubt persists. The presence of the extrarenal manifestations of ADPKD militates against tuberous sclerosis.

Simple renal cysts remain in the differential diagnosis, because cysts are few and renal size may be normal early in the course of ADPKD. Patient age is, of course, a strong consideration, because simple cysts increase in number and frequency with age, and it has been estimated that one-half of individuals past the age of 50 years have at least one renal cyst[81]. Simple cysts do occur in children[2,71,103,128,166], but the condition remains rare in youngsters. In fact, 70% of children at risk for ADPKD and having unilateral renal cysts or fewer than five cysts proceed to develop ADPKD[162]. The significance of this observation is demonstrated by the pedigree shown in Fig. 12.2. Thus, the diagnosis of multiple, simple cysts is more tenable when three renal cysts are found in a 60-year-old at-risk individual than when two cysts are found in a 6-year-old at risk.

In young children and fetuses there is difficulty distinguishing ARPKD from ADPKD. The single best criterion is the status of the parents (Table 12.4). Parents of children with renal cysts must undergo ultrasonography for the child's condition to be evaluated.

Table 12.4 Patterns of ADPKD in childhood[*]

Patient age (years)	6
Mother's age (years)	31
Mother's status	normal sized kidneys, single renal cyst
Father's status	unaffected
Maternal grandparents' status	grandfather-age 56, single renal cyst
Paternal grandparents' status	unknown
Siblings' status	12 y/o brother – nl 10 y/o brother – increased kidney size, hyperechogenic 8 y/o brother – nl 3 y/o sister – increased kidney size, liver hyperechogenic
Patient's renal ultrasonogram	increased kidney size and echogenicity
Patient's renal function	normal
Patient's hepatic function	normal
Extrarenal abnormalities	two liver cysts

[*]Gabow PA[56] (with permission)

History and physical examination of the parents are insufficient. In one study, 38% of the parents of children with ADPKD were unaware that they had ADPKD[143]. The ultrasonographic appearances of ARPKD and ADPKD are not sufficiently different to permit definite diagnosis[143]. Similar confusion can occur with excretory urography. In one study only one of six children was correctly diagnosed as ADPKD by the radiographic appearance of the kidneys[29]. Liver biopsy more often shows hepatic fibrosis in ARPKD than in

ADPKD[113], but hepatic portal enlargement and biliary abnormalities occur in some infants with renal cystic disease of clearly dominant type. In addition, sonographically demonstrable hepatic cysts occur in both ADPKD and ARPKD. Resolution of the diagnosis in individual cases with uncertain family histories may require long-term follow-up.

Gene linkage analysis can now provide a diagnosis prior to the development of renal cysts in some asymptomatic at-risk individuals (see Chapter 6). Prenatal diagnosis can also be performed via amniocentesis[147]. Since the gene itself has not yet been identified, the status of an individual requires testing of other family members and the presence of at least two affected individuals who will supply blood samples (see Chapter 6). The linkage analysis utilizes highly polymorphic probes, and it is likely that the affected and the unaffected parent will be genetically different. The type travelling with the PKD-1 is thus likely to be identified. A lack of linkage may mean that the abnormality resides elsewhere than in PKD-1. If gene linkage analysis can be employed in a particular family, gene status can be established with greater than 99% accuracy by the use of flanking probes[20]. Each offspring would have to assume, without linkage analysis, a 50% chance of having the gene. The odds change to 95% and 5% when linkage analysis is employed (Fig. 12.3).

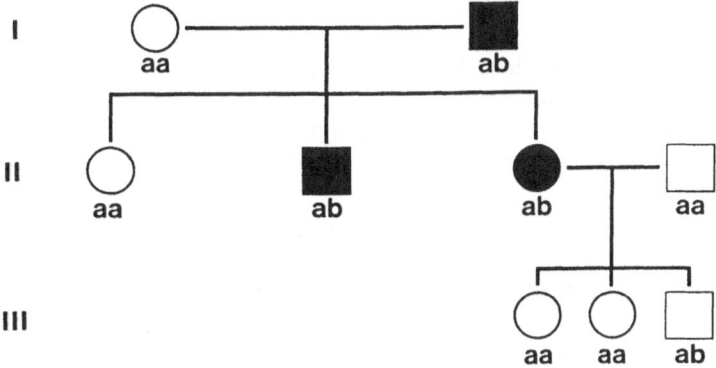

Figure 12.3 This is a pedigree of a three generation family with ADPKD. The closed symbols represent known affected subjects; the open symbols in generations I and II are unaffected subjects. The family was studied using gene linkage analysis and the linkage types are displayed under each symbol. In generations I and II ADPKD is occurring with the b type. Thus, ADPKD is segregating with the b type. Therefore, in the III generation the two females have < 5% chance of having ADPKD and the male has a 95% chance of having the ADPKD gene.

Should linkage analysis then become the preferred method of diagnosing ADPKD? The answer is dependent upon the clinical issue to be addressed. An individual sees a physician either for the evaluation of symptoms and signs that suggest ADPKD or for evaluation of increased risk of ADPKD.

In the first instance, an individual should undergo ultrasonography. A characteristic positive ultrasonogram establishes the gene status with almost 100% assurance and informs the clinician about the severity of the renal abnormality and perhaps about the involvement of other organs.

In the second instance, an asymptomatic subject can be evaluated in one of three ways: a test of renal concentrating ability, ultrasonography, or gene linkage analysis. The choice is dictated by cost, ease of performance, family structure, diagnostic precision desired and structural information required. The renal concentrating test is the least expensive, least difficult and least precise. Gene linkage analysis is the most expensive, most difficult and most precise prior to the development of renal cysts. Ultrasonography is intermediate in cost and ease of performance. It is less sensitive than gene linkage, particularly in younger individuals who may not have developed cysts. It is the only modality to provide data on severity. In a young transplant donor (less than 30 years of age) or in an individual whose family planning is to be absolutely dictated by gene status, gene linkage analysis would appear to provide the most definitive diagnostic test. Linkage analysis will not ascertain whether an unknown cystic disease is ADPKD, a task for which identification of the ADPKD gene is necessary.

Although this array for diagnostic possibilities exists, which at-risk individuals should be screened? Every at-risk adult should be informed of the status and the availability of testing of patient, offspring and unborn fetus. The patient should also be apprised of the impact of a positive diagnosis on insurability, and perhaps employability. If patient care is to be altered by a definitive diagnosis, diagnostic testing is clearly indicated. Non-clinically directed, random screening without appropriate counselling should be avoided in both adults and children, and early diagnosis of completely asymptomatic youngsters may not be helpful.

5. Clinical manifestations

Autosomal dominant disorders are in general characterized by variability in age of onset and in phenotypic expression[173]. ADPKD is no exception. Variability may reflect the influence of environmental factors, the influence of the non-ADPKD allele on the chromosome inherited from the unaffected parent, and the overall genetic background of the individual. The possible involvement of these factors will be discussed as they apply in the various clinical settings.

5.1 Age of onset

ADPKD is an inherited disorder. It begins at conception. Its clinical age of onset is defined by the age at which symptoms appear or cysts can be found. These ages differ, depending upon the circumstances of inquiry. For example, symptomatic subjects are older than asymptomatic subjects (38.1±1.4 vs. 27.3±2.1 years)[59]. If, however, familial occurrence prompts a diagnostic search, a younger age of onset will be identified. Age at onset is also influenced by the technique used for screening: physical examination vs. ultrasonography, for example. The latter is obviously far more sensitive in demonstrating cysts. Diagnosis of renal cysts by ultrasonography can range from 22 weeks of gestational age to 80 years[33,143].

The extent to which age of onset is or can be influenced is debatable. Although no modulating external environmental influences have been described in humans, exposure to bacteria and bacterial toxins has been demonstrated to be a critical influence in experimental cystic disease[65,66,70]. Sedman *et al.*[162] have reported that individuals with childhood presentation of ADPKD were more likely to have an affected father than an affected mother, but other reports have not demonstrated this difference[93]. However, there is some precedent in that the gender of affected parents affects age of onset in offspring with Huntington disease[18].

5.2 Symptoms and signs

The clinical manifestations of ADPKD are influenced by the age of the subject. The early literature detailing ADPKD in childhood describes a severe disease.

Table 12.5 Signs and symptoms in children at presentation[*]

SADPKD ADPKD	Unaffected $n = 103$ %	Suspicious[a] $n = 28$ %	Affected $n = 23$ %
Abdominal or flank pain	11	7	22
Headaches	8	7	13
Urinary tract infections	6	21	13
Gross hematuria	3	4	26[b]
Proteinuria	1	0	9
Hypertension (by history)	5	7	22[b]
Palpable abdominal mass	0	0	22[c]
Hernias	1	4	22[b]

[a]unilateral, <5 cysts total.
[b]$p < 0.005$, vs unaffected.
[c]$p < 0.05$, vs unaffected or suspicious.
[*]From: Sedman A, Bell P, Manco-Johnson M, Schrier R, Warady BA, Heard EO, Butler-Simon N and Gabow p[162] (with permission).

Recent studies undoubtedly present a more accurate description of the range of findings in childhood ADPKD[29,162]. Thirty percent of children come to medical attention because of clinical symptoms[162]. However, 74% of ADPKD children actually have symptoms, when questioned specifically[162]. The symptoms and signs include abdominal masses, hematuria, proteinuria and hypertension[29,93,143,162] (Table 12.5).

Hypertension, defined as a blood pressure above the 95% confidence limits for age, was reported in 20% of the children[29,162]. The urinalysis is often mildly abnormal: 14% have at least 1+ or greater proteinuria, 19% have 1 or more RBC/hpf, and 45% have 1 or more WBC/hpf[29,162]. However, only 5–10% of children have severe abnormalities, such as + 2 or greater proteinuria, more than 5 RBC/hpf, or more than 5 WBC/hpf. Only 13% of children in Sedman's study had abnormal renal function at the time of presentation[162].

Extrarenal manifestations have not been evaluated systematically, but appear to be unusual in children with ADPKD.

Pain is clearly the most common clinical symptom of ADPKD in adults (Table 12.6).

Table 12.6 Symptoms of ADPKD*

	Numbers	Range in reports	Mean percentage
Flank pain	601/1194	(19–78%)	50
Abdominal pain	114/185	(60–75%)	62
Hematuria	555/1534	(13–57%)	35
Headache	87/317	(15–50%)	27
Gastrointestinal complaints	114/776	–	15
Nocturia	32/233	–	14
Colicky pain	127/993	–	13
Dysuria	20/223	–	9
Frequency	20/223	–	9
Polyuria	5/59	–	8

*The chart is compiled from available data in series by Braasch, Dalgaard, Delaney, Gabow, Higgins, Iglesias, Milutinovic, Oppenheimer, Simon and Ward. The denominator refers to the total patient population in the series mentioning the symptom.
From: Grantham JJ and Gabow PA[75] (with permission).

Women appear to have more abdominal pain than men[33]. The pain can vary from intermittent to constant and from dull aching to severe disabling pain. Many patients require regular use of analgesics. Patients with recurring pain are more likely to have more renal cysts that exceed 3 cm in size when compared to patients without pain[83]. This may explain why pain is relieved in some patients by surgical unroofing and decompression of cysts[14,53,165]. Sudden increase in severity of pain or change in quality of pain deserve attention. Renal infection, bleeding, cyst infection or rupture, stone, or renal malignancy should be considered.

Thirty to 50% of adult subjects with ADPKD experience hematuria at some time prior to diagnosis[19,33,37,90,125,167,179]. Gross hematuria often prompts a patient to seek medical advice. Although episodes of gross hematuria can occur with strenuous physical activity and abdominal or flank trauma, the role of these events in the provocation of gross hematuria has not been systematically examined. Hematuria does appear to occur more commonly in subjects with large kidneys or hypertension[59]. Episodes of gross hematuria may last from days to weeks. Patients should be treated with bed rest, hydration and analgesics. Hospitalization or transfusion is rarely required. There are no guidelines defining which individuals with gross hematuria should undergo further investigation, but causes other than ADPKD should be considered when bleeding continues beyond one week or when bleeding first develops in patients older than 50 years. Although gross hematuria may be accompanied by clots and colicky pain, stones also need to be considered.

Polyuria is a complaint listed by approximately 8% of ADPKD patients[19,33,59,90,125]. This may not differ from the frequency in control subjects[60]. Although a decrease in renal concentrating ability is an early manifestation of ADPKD, it usually is mild and unlikely to result in substantial polyuria. The mean normal urinary osmolality in 87 subjects with ADPKD and normal renal function was 680 ± 14 mosm/kg H_2O, compared with 812 ± 13 mosm/kg in 106 unaffected family members[60]. The usual obligate osmolar excretion/24 h is 600 mosm. Thus, roughly 20% more urine, or approximately one litre, would be required by affected subjects to remove their osmotic load in the face of this reduced renal concentrating ability.

Gastrointestinal complaints of nausea, vomiting and diarrhea are less common than the renal symptoms, but can pose significant problems for occasional patients[59]. The mechanism of these symptoms is not known.

Twenty-one percent of ADPKD subject have a precordial systolic murmur and 14% have a click, compared with 9% and 5%, respectively, of random control subjects[87]. The presence of murmur cannot be related to hypertension; it most likely is due to mitral valve prolapse.

Headaches, often severe and recurring, are a common occurrence unrelated to hypertension[59,86]. Although chronic headaches may be caused by berry aneurysms in the general population, this relationship has not been examined in ADPKD[36]. Headaches often contribute to the chronic use of analgesics by these patients.

Palpable hepatomegaly occurs in 30% and palpably enlarged kidneys in 50–94% of non-azotemic adult ADPKD subjects[19,33,59]. Hernias are more common in ADPKD patients and should be evaluated in the initial physical examination[59,162].

Hypertension occurs in approximately 60% of non-azotemic patients[59,131,148,176]. Braasch and Schacht[19] first suggested that the mechanism of hypertension was not simply endstage renal disease. They noted a 71% incidence of hypertension in a group of ADPKD subjects, compared with a 26% incidence in a group of age- and sex- matched subjects with chronic pyelonephritis[19]. Among ADPKD subjects with normal renal function, those with hypertension have significantly larger kidneys than those with normotension[58]. This relationship between cystic deformity of the kidneys and hypertension is further emphasized by the significant improvement in blood pressure that occurs after extensive surgical unroofing of renal cysts[14,53]. Structural severity could relate to hypertension through the renin–angiotensin system (activated by attenuation of vessels around cysts and relative renal ischemia) or through impaired sodium excretion secondary to tubular abnormality.

There are conflicting data regarding sodium balance and intravascular volume[11,32,131,176]. D'Angelo[32] reported impaired renal sodium excretion in response to an acute sodium load in non-azotemic ADPKD subjects. Nash[131] found most non-azotemic subjects become normotensive on a diet containing 10 mEq sodium per day. Valvo et al.[176] found an increased plasma volume in hypertensive compared to normotensive ADPKD subjects; however, some of the hypertensive subjects had advanced renal failure[176]. Bell et al.[11] found no effect of sodium intake and plasma volume on blood pressure in ADPKD patients. Although plasma renin activity and aldosterone measurements were not different in hypertensive and normotensive subjects, the renin response to captopril was significantly greater in hypertensive patients, suggesting some element of renal ischemia, even though the blood pressure response was not different. This lack of blood pressure response is similar to the failure of saralasin infusion in hypertensive patients with ADPKD compared with hypertensive patients with renal artery stenosis[6]. However, immunohistochemical studies of renin in the kidney have shown more than normal juxtaglomerular and vascular renin granularity in ADPKD kidneys, supporting a role for renin in the hypertension of ADPKD[72]. Despite these data to implicate the renin–angiotensin system, the mechanism of hypertension in the disorder awaits further study.

5.3 Laboratory data

Early in the course of the disease, all routine laboratory data including complete blood count, serum electrolytes, blood urea nitrogen, serum creatinine and liver function enzyme values are normal[59]. Although ADPKD patients undergoing hemodialysis may have higher mean hematocrits than non-ADPKD hemodialysis patients, polycythemia is a rare occurrence[25,26,52,59]. Liver function tests are virtually always normal, even though hepatic cyst formation is common (see below)[51,59,127,137].

Hyperuricemia and gout have been thought to be increased in frequency in ADPKD, but the examination of a large number of non-azotemic patients has demonstrated that more important factors are sex, hypertension and renal function[95].

A majority of adults with ADPKD have a mildly abnormal urinalysis[19,33,59,136,167,179]. Pyuria is a common finding, but it does not necessarily indicate urinary tract infection[19,33,59,136,167,179]. Urine cultures are necessary to establish the diagnosis of active infection. Milutinovic[125] found low grade pyuria in 46% of females and 33% of males, but positive urine cultures in only 7%.

Twenty-four hour protein excretion is less than 1 g in most patients[144], but some examples of nephrotic range proteinuria have been reported[1]. Severe proteinuria and early onset of renal failure suggest the possibility of a superimposed abnormality[1].

5.4 Renal pathology

Renal cysts are epithelial-lined cavities distributed throughout the renal parenchyma. The cysts contain fluid that varies in appearance from clear to hemorrhagic. The cysts are more or less uniformly distributed throughout the parenchyma. Even in far advanced disease, with little apparently normal tissue, histopathologic examination shows renal parenchyma interspersed among cysts. Dissection of a kidney from a non- azotemic individual suggests that less than 2% of the total nephrons are involved[76]. Some microdissection studies have shown cysts to be tubular outpouchings distributed along the nephrons from the glomerulus to the collecting duct[84,107,138,141]. Recent electron microscopic studies fail to demonstrate tubular orifices in large cysts, suggesting a secondary loss of continuity[76]. Mathematical calculations relating single nephron glomerular filtration rate to cyst fluid volume and information on cyst epithelial transport support a conclusion that fluid accumulation depends significantly upon active secretion rather than just passive filling from glomerular filtration[74,76,130,157].

The epithelial linings of a majority of cysts lack morphologic characteristics of specific renal tubular segments[76]. Nonetheless, cyst puncture data reveals epithelial function characteristic of specific tubular segments. Some cysts contain fluids with high sodium concentrations or high pH values as in proximal tubules. Other cyst fluids have low sodium concentrations and low pH values as in distal tubules[62,74,89].

It is not clear whether all of the cysts that develop throughout life are present in microscopic size at birth, simply increasing in size with age, or whether cyst number actually increases. Clinically, it appears that both cyst number and size increase over time[59,86]. Children have normal or only moderately enlarged kidneys that manifest occasional small cysts[162]. The endstage kidney in the adult is large and seemingly replaced by cysts. Although a predominant cyst size can be determined in many instances of advanced disease, there is great variability. In general, but not invariably, cyst number, cyst size and renal size increase concordantly in both kidneys[59]. Discrepancies in kidney sizes should raise the question of a superimposed process.

5.5 Renal infection

Urinary tract infections in ADPKD include cystitis, pyelonephritis, cyst infection and perinephric abscess[159,171]. Cystitis is differentiated from upper tract disease by the usual clinical criteria, with fever, leukocytosis and flank pain suggesting upper tract infection. Risk factors include previous instrumentation of the urinary tract[37] and female sex[159]. The differentiation of pyelonephritis from cyst infection is less clear. The presence of white cell casts and the prompt response to the standard antibiotic therapy for urinary tract infection are more compatible with pyelonephritis than with cyst infection[159].

Most antibiotics used in treating routine urinary tract infections fail to penetrate renal cysts[13,130,158,161] (Table 12.7); hence failure of the patient to defervesce promptly can be taken as evidence of infection within a cyst rather than within the renal parenchyma.

Lipophilic antibiotics have the best cyst penetration. Cyst puncture studies have demonstrated therapeutic antibiotic levels in cyst fluid for trimethoprim–sulphamethoxazole, chloramphenicol and ciprofloxacin, and inadequate levels for ampicillin and aminoglycosides[13,43,130,157-161].

Table 12.7 Antibiotic concentration in cysts of proximal and distal origin*

Antibiotic		Serum conc. (μg/ml)	Cyst fluid (μg/ml)	
			Proximal	Distal
Gentamicin		2.3–3.8	1.04–1.3	0–0.07
Tobramycin		3.7	0	0
Cephapirin		46.0	8.1	38
Ticarcillin		400	135	0
Ampicillin		179	0.4	—
Clindamycin		3.9	9.2	34
Trimethoprim–sulpha	T	7.7	16.1	228
	S	75.3	94.7	9.7

*From: Grantham JJ, Gabow PA[75] (with permission).

Patients with presumed upper tract disease and failure to respond to standard antibiotic regimens within 72 hours should be switched to one of the antibiotics that are known to penetrate cysts. Positive blood cultures slightly favor cyst infection; 93% of individuals with cyst infection have positive blood cultures compared to to 45% with interstitial infections[159]. The organisms causing cyst infection include *Escherichia coli, Proteus vulgaris, Staphylococcus albus or aureus, Streptococcus faecalis* and anaerobic organisms[13].

Localization of an infected cyst or cysts by imaging techniques, including ultrasonagraphy, CT, magnetic resonance imaging and gallium scan often yields unreliable results[159]. There are insufficient data to assess indium-tagged white blood cells. If antibiotics with adequate cyst penetration are utilized there should be very few indications for treating renal infection by surgery.

5.6 Nephrolithiasis and intrarenal calcification.

Nephrolithiasis occurs in approximately 20% of patients, and should be considered in a patient who has increased pain, colicky pain or gross hematuria[5,37,125,163,174]. CT appears to be the best imaging modality for stone identification[112]. The frequency of nephrolithiasis is similar in men and women[174]. The mean age of presentation of symptomatic nephrolithiasis is 39 ± 14 years[174].Uric acid (57%) and calcium (76%) are the most common components of the stones[174]. Potentially relevant metabolic abnormalities have been identified. In ADPKD patients who had normal renal function and were not taking diuretics, Torres *et al.* found 64% with hypocitric aciduria, 20% with hyperoxaluria, 17% with hyperuricemia and 13% with hyperuricosuria[174]. First morning urines had lower pH values[174].

In addition to nephrolithiasis, calcification occurs within cyst walls. It may result from previous bleeding into cysts.

5.7 Renal malignancy.

Hypernephroma and benign renal adenoma have been reported in ADPKD. Autopsy examination of 84 kidneys from 87 ADPKD patients at the Mayo Clinic revealed renal neoplasms in 24%[78]. One patient had bilateral low-grade clear cell carcinoma and another a transitional cell tumor. The remaining tumors were only microscopic adenomas[78]. This study did not demonstrate an increased frequency of renal cell carcinoma in ADPKD[78]. However, calculations by Bernstein *et al.*[15] support the association.

The diagnosis of hypernephroma can be difficult in the setting of ADPKD because of preexisting anatomical distortion, hematuria and pain. A change in the pattern of pain or hematuria, or weight loss, fever, increased sedimentation rate, abnormal liver function tests, anemia disproportionate to renal function and erythrocytosis should raise the possibility of renal malignancy. The preferred diagnostic tests are CT and, if necessary, renal arteriogram. Disproportionate size of one kidney, suggesting a unilateral mass, is not common but also may be caused by malignancy. Bilateral hypernephromas occur[63,132]. They appear to be more common in ADPKD than in the general population[63]. The increased frequency of neoplasia may relate to altered cell growth in the pathogenesis of ADPKD[15].

6. Extrarenal manifestations of ADPKD

We consider ADPKD to be a systemic disorder in which the phenotypic manifestations of the abnormal gene span an array of organ systems (Table 12.8).

Not every affected individual manifests all of the possible aspects. The assumption that every genetically affected individual will express renal cysts is based on the fact that renal cysts rather than gene identification has been the *sine qua non* of the diagnosis. We have observed individuals in ADPKD families who have no renal cysts but have other organ system manifestations, such as hepatic cysts or mitral valve prolapse[59,87]. If these individuals prove to be gene carriers, our notions of phenotypic presentation will be altered.

Table 12.8 Organ system involvement in ADPKD*

Genitourinary system
Renal cysts
Gastrointestinal tract
Hepatic cysts
Pancreatic cysts (rare)
Colonic diverticulae
Cardiovascular system
Cardiac valvular abnormalities
Berry aneurysm
Thoracic aortic aneurysm
Musculoskeletal
Inguinal hernias

*From: Gabow PA[56] (with permission)

Both interfamilial and intrafamilial variability occur in the extrarenal manifestations of ADPKD. Interfamily variability is best exemplified by apparent differences in the occurrence of berry aneurysms, which may reflect genetic heterogeneity or environmental influences. Intrafamily variability is illustrated by differing manifestations and severities of structural defects despite similar ages (Table 12.9). Such intrafamilial variability may reflect the influence of the non-ADPKD allele, of other genes, or of environmental factors.

Table 12.9 Intrafamily variability in ADPKD[*]

Subject	PP	KP	GP
Sex	F	M	M
Age	34	30	33
Hypertension	–	+	+
Renal size	1142 cm^3	1243 cm^3	580 cm^3
MVP	+	+	+
Hepatic cysts	+	–	–
Ovarian cysts	+	N/A	N/A
Uterine prolapse	+	N/A	N/A

[*]From: Gabow PA and Schrier RW[61] (with permission).

6.1 Gastrointestinal manifestations

Hepatic cysts are the most common extrarenal manifestation of ADPKD, found in as many as two-thirds of patients[59,80,91,127]. Since not every individual with renal cysts manifests hepatic cysts, there must be factors that modulate the ADPKD gene's hepatic expression, but do not affect the gene's renal expression. Age, severity of the renal structural lesion, degree of renal functional impairment, gender and pregnancy influence the presence, number and size of hepatic cysts[49,57,59,80,127]. Cyst development can cause enormous hepatic enlargement, generally with preservation of hepatic function and maintenance of hepatic cell mass[49].

Some, but not all, studies demonstrate an increased frequency of diverticular disease in ADPKD[104,155] and others report colonic perforation[68,69,114]. These manifestations are compatible with the hypothesis that a disordered extracellular matrix yields an abnormal intestinal wall[3].

6.2 Cardiac manifestations

Individuals with ADPKD suffer a 25% incidence of atypical chest pain and a 40% frequency of palpitations, significantly more than reported by their unaffected family members[87]. Physical examination reveals regurgitant cardiac murmurs in 21% of patients and a mitral click in 14%[87]. These findings are suggestive of frequent mitral valve prolapse in ADPKD. A prospective study of ADPKD subjects by echocardiography and doppler examination has confirmed a 26% frequency of mitral valve prolapse compared with a 2% frequency in 100 random control subjects[87]. In addition ADPKD subjects demonstrated an increased frequency of aortic valve and tricuspid valve incompetence.

There are potential short–and longterm clinical implications of mitral valve prolapse in ADPKD patients relating to the question of antibiotic prophylaxis, the occurrence of cardiac arrhythmia, cerebral embolism and sudden death[40].

Mitral valve prolapse is considered by some to represent a disorder of collagen matrix[30]. The association of mitral valve prolapse with ADPKD can be cited in support of the hypothesis that ADPKD is a disorder affecting extracellular matrix.

6.3 Vascular manifestations

The association of berry aneurysms and ADPKD has been noted by numerous investigators since the early 1900's. Its reported frequency ranges from 10 to 40%[16,21][33,38,90,121,142,175,177]. Variation may reflect the ethnic backgrounds of the groups studied, the diagnostic methods utilized, or the families studied. A prospective study of 17 Japanese ADPKD subjects from ten families revealed a 41% incidence of berry aneurysms[177]. Nine percent of ADPKD subjects die from ruptured berry aneurysms[34,82]. If 50% of berry aneurysms rupture, this would suggest a frequency of 18% among persons with ADPKD.

The role of hypertension in berry aneurysms rupture has been debated. The hypertension of ADPKD may modify the rate of rupture that is observed in the general population[36,180]. Certain families with ADPKD may have a greater frequency of berry aneurysms than do other ADPKD families[94]. Inter-family variability is compatible with genetic heterogeneity. Thus, one PKD gene could be associated with berry aneurysm and another not.

Despite the considerable range of reported frequencies, it is clear that the frequency of aneurysm rupture in ADPKD is substantially above that reported in the general population[129]. This raises questions of who with ADPKD should be studied and what is the diagnostic modality of choice. Clearly any individual with symptoms suggestive of aneurysm rupture (sudden onset of a severe headache different from previous headaches, nerve paresis, signs of meningeal irritation) should be examined. The more difficult clinical question is which, if any, *asymptomatic* subjects should be examined.

Decision analysis strategies suggest that routine screening is not indicated[110]. The possibility of family clustering and specific circumstances, such as a subject's work or avocation,were not considered in this study. Given current data, it seems reasonable to advise screening for those ADPKD subjects who have a family history of berry aneurysm, or who perform activities in which sudden loss of consciousness would endanger the lives of others.

The pathogenesis of berry aneurysm has not been examined in ADPKD. There is no unanimity of opinion, and some information suggests an abnormality of the internal elastic membrane in all aneurysm formation[129]. This defect would be compatible with altered extracellular matrix formation, and would support the hypothesis that such a defect plays a role in the pathogenesis of ADPKD.

7. Natural history and treatment

The natural history of ADPKD equates approximately to the progression of renal cysts. As recognition of manifestations broadens, more attention may need to be paid to the natural history of gastrointestinal and cardiovascular aspects.

The natural histories of the renal abnormalities in adults and children require separate discussions. Initial descriptions of childhood presentation largely suggested that renal disease usually progressed to endstage renal disease or death early in life[12,44,145,164]. Recent data indicate a substantially better prognosis[29,162]. Only 27% of the 18 children with ADPKD that were followed for 7.6 years by Sedman et al.[162] suffered disease progression, that is, developed hypertension or worsening renal function. In that time-span only three children progressed to endstage renal disease. Moreover, Cole et al. has shown relative stability of renal function over a 31.9±15 month follow-up in children who present in the first year of life[29].

Overall, ADPKD is a slowly progressive renal disease that rarely results in endstage renal disease prior to the fourth or fifth decade of life. Early data suggested that endstage renal disease occurred at age 50, approximately ten years after the onset of symptoms[33,86]. Only 58% of women and 53% of men were alive two and one-half years after palpable renal enlargement occurred[33].

A more optimistic outlook appears to be emerging. Data from the Mayo Clinic reveals a better kidney and patient survival in the decades between 1956 and 1980 than between 1935 and 1955 (kidney survival 92% versus 48%; patient survival 80% versus 40%)[90]. Churchill et al.[28] have found a 77% probability that ADPKD patients will be alive without the need for renal replacement therapy at age 50, a 57% probability by age 58 and a 52% probability by age 73.

There are several factors that might affect the rate of disease progression. They include family grouping, cyst growth and development, hypertension and urinary tract infection. Dalgaard[33] found that time from development to endstage renal disease was similar within families. There are many exceptions to this "rule of thumb". It is possible that prior to the availability of antihypertensive and antibiotic therapies there was less variability within families than seems now to occur.

There appears to be a relationship, albeit not perfect, between cyst growth and the progression of renal disease[59,86,106]. Patients with larger kidneys and larger cysts have higher serum creatinine concentrations even among individuals with concentrations less than 3.0 mg/dl[59]. This observation may relate to compression of surrounding parenchyma by larger cysts[54]. Compression of adjacent tissue by cysts is observed in kidneys from ADPKD subjects[76].

One recent study in rats suggests that the decline in renal function in cystic kidneys is predominantly the result of tubular rather than glomerular involvement[23].

Not all investigators have demonstrated a negative influence of hypertension on the preservation of renal function in ADPKD. Data suggest poorer kidney and patient survivals in subjects who were hypertensive at the time of diagnosis[54,90,167]. While conclusive data are lacking for ADPKD, it seems prudent to vigorously control blood pressure. There are insufficient data from large numbers of patients with documented urinary tract infections to define the role of recurrent parenchymal or cyst infection on the course of ADPKD. Avoidance of urinary tract instrumentation and prompt treatment of urinary tract infections appear to be appropriate management.

Given the extent of their use by some ADPKD patients, analgesics could conceivably play a role in disease progression. Patients should be cautioned regarding the excessive use of analgesics in general. Potential nephrotoxic analgesics should be used with caution.

Current data suggest that pregnancy in ADPKD does not have an adverse effect on renal function[126,134,152]. However, new onset hypertension during pregnancy is more common in women with ADPKD than in at-risk, unaffected subjects[126].

The role of dietary protein restriction in ADPKD remains to be defined. One study of protein and phosphate restriction in 17 ADPKD subjects suggested that renal deterioration slowed over a follow-up period of 41–44 months[135].

Surgical unroofing of renal cysts did not worsen renal function in 11 patients. It remains to be determined if this form of intervention can actually preserve renal function[14].

Counselling of patient and family is a critically important aspect of management[156]. To date there is no disease-specific therapy. However, as more data implicate accelerated cell growth and cyst secretion, therapies aimed at these mechanisms can be explored. Lacking specific therapy, clinicians must apply principles that are involved in treating other renal diseases. When individuals with ADPKD reach endstage renal disease, they are candidates for renal replacement therapy. ADPKD patients account for 10–12% of the chronic hemodialysis population. Their survival on hemodialysis is the same as that of other non-diabetic patients[85,92,102,111]. There are fewer data on peritoneal dialysis in ADPKD, but it appears feasible in some patients[102].

One patient has been reported to develop an infected hepatic cyst shortly after initiation of peritoneal dialysis, suggesting increased risk of infection with this therapy[116]. However, the same risk of infection appears to occur with hemodialysis as well. Grünfeld et al.[80] have detailed a 3% frequency of serious hepatic infection in the ADPKD population on hemodialysis. In addition, Scheff et al.[155] reported four intra-abdominal abscesses in 12 ADPKD hemodialysis patients with diverticular disease compared to a zero occurrence among non-ADPKD patients. One study did demonstrate greater frequency of death from bacterial sepsis in ADPKD, suggesting that longer survival through renal replacement therapy allows extrarenal manifestations of the disease to become more prominent and to be a greater source of morbidity and mortality.

Most data indicate that ADPKD patients have kidney and patient survival rates with transplantation that are equivalent to those of non-diabetic patients[4,77,119,123,139,153,154,181,184]. There is variability from center to center regarding criteria for removal of native kidneys prior to transplantation. However, there is general agreement that kidneys should be removed in individuals with recurrent renal infection, recurrent severe hematuria, intractable pain, renal neoplasm and kidney-dependent hypertension[77,133,155].

Sanfilippo et al.[154] noted a decreased patient survival at one and two years post-transplant in ADPKD patients with graft failure and bilateral nephrectomy as compared to patients with unilateral nephrectomy or retention of both kidneys. Some centers also recommend barium enema examination for diverticular disease and surgical removal of severely affected colon segments prior to transplantation. The use of a living related donor in ADPKD raises the question of which methods are appropriate to screen such a donor. Certainly an ultrasonogram is an appropriate screening examination. However, a normal ultrasonogram in a young donor is not sufficient. CT scan with contrast improves the diagnostic precision. Given its availability, gene linkage analysis is probably indicated if the family is genetically informative, and if the donor is young or has extrarenal manifestations that suggest ADPKD.

ADPKD is emerging as a clinically important systemic disease whose pathogenesis is being rapidly unravelled, whose clinical dimensions are broadening, and whose therapy may be soon radically altered by techniques aimed at reducing cyst growth.

References

1. Ackerman GL. Nephrotic syndrome in polycystic renal disease. Journal of Urology 1971, 105, 7–9.
2. Ahmed S. Simple renal cysts in childhood. British Journal Urology 1972, 44, 71–75.
3. Almay TP and Howell DA. Diverticular disease of the colon. New England Journal of Medicine 1980, 302, 324–331.
4. Amamoo DG, Woods JE and Anderson CF. Renal transplantation in end stage polycystic renal disease. Journal of Urology 1974, 112, 443–444.
5. Amar AE, DAS S and Egan RM. Management of urinary calculous disease in patients with renal cysts: Review of 12 years of experience in 18 patients. Journal of Urology 1981, 125, 153–156.
6. Anderson RJ, Miller PD, Linas SL, Katz FH and Holmes JH. Role of the renin–angiotensin system in hypertension of polycystic kidney disease. Mineral and Electrolyte Metabolism 1979, 2, 137–141.
7. Anton P and Abramowsky CR. Adult polycystic renal disease presenting in infancy: a report emphasizing the bilateral involvement. Journal of Urology 1982, 128, 1290–1291.
8. Baert L. Hereditary polycystic kidney disease (adult form): A microdissection study of two cases at an early state of the disease. Kidney International 1978, 13, 519–525.
9. Bear JC, McManamon P, Morgan J, Payne RH, Lewis H, Gault MH and Churchill DN. Age at clinical onset and at ultrasonographic detection of adult polycystic kidney disease: Data for genetic counselling. American Journal of Medical Genetics 1984, 18, 45–53.
10. Begleiter ML, Smith TH and Harris DJ. Letter: Ultrasound for genetic counselling in polycystic kidney disease. Lancet 1977, 2, 1073–1074.

11. Bell PE, Hossack KF, Gabow PA, Durr JA, Johnson AM and Schrier RW. Hypertension in autosomal dominant polycystic kidney disease. Kidney International, 1988, 34, 683–690.

12. Bengtsson U, Hedman L and Svalander C. Adult type of polycystic kidney disease in a new-born child. Acta Medica Scandinavica 1975, 197, 447–450.

13. Bennett WE. General features of autosomal dominant polycystic kidney disease: Evaluation and management of renal infection. In: Grantham JJ, Gardner KD Jr, eds, Problems in Diagnosis and Management of Polycystic Kidney Disease. Kansas City: PKR Foundation, 1985, 98–105.

14. Bennett WM, Elzinga L, Golper TA and Barry JM. Reduction of cyst volume for symptomatic management of autosomal dominant polycystic kidney disease. Journal of Urology 1987, 137, 620–622.

15. Bernstein J, Evan AP and Gardner KD Jr. Epithelial hyperplasia in human polycystic kidney diseases: Its role in pathogenesis and risk of neoplasia. American Journal of Pathology 1987, 129, 92–101.

16. Bigelow NH. The association of polycystic kidneys with intracranial aneurysms and other related disorders. American Journal of Medicine Sci 1953, 225, 485–494.

17. Blyth H and Ockenden B. Polycystic disease of kidneys and liver presenting in childhood. Journal of Medical Genetics 1971, 8, 257–284.

18. Boehnke M, Conneally PM and Lange K. Two models for a maternal factor inheritance of Huntington disease. American Journal of Human Genetics 1983, 35, 845–860.

19. Braasch WF and Schacht FW. Pathological and clinical data concerning polycystic kidney. Surgery and Gynecological Obstetrics 1933, 57, 467–475.

20. Breuning MH, Brunner H, Saris JJ, van Ommen GJB, Reeders ST, Ijdo JW, Verwest A and Pearson PL. Improved early diagnosis of adult polycystic kidney disease with flanking DNA markers. Lancet 1987, 2, 1359–1361.

21. Brown RAP. Polycystic disease of the kidneys and intracranial aneurysms. The etiology and interrelationship of these conditions: Review of recent literature and report of seven cases in which both conditions coexisted. Glasgow Medical Journal 1951, 32, 333–348.

22. Butkowski RJ, Carone FA, Grantham JJ and Hudson BG. Tubular basement membrane changes in 2–amino–4, 5–diphenylthiazole–induced polycystic disease. Kidney International 1985, 28, 744–751.

23. Carone FA. Functional changes in polycystic kidney disease are tubulo–interstitial in origin. Seminars in Nephrology 1988, 8, 89–93.

24. Carone FA, Rowland RG, Perlman SG and Ganote CE. The pathogenesis of drug-induced renal cystic disease. Kidney International 1974, 5, 411–421.

25. Chandra M, Miller ME, Garcia JF, Mossey RT and McVicar M. Serum immunoreactive erythropoietin levels in patients with polycystic kidney disease as compared with other hemodialysis patients. Nephron 1985, 39, 26–29.

26. Chester AC, Argy WP Jr, Rakowski TA and Schreiner GE. Polycystic kidney disease and chronic hemodialysis. Clinical Nephrology 1978, 10, 129–133.

27. Chevalier RL, Garland TA and Buschi AJ. The neonate with adult- type autosomal dominant polycystic kidney disease. International Journal of Pediatric Nephrology 1981, 2, 73–77.

28. Churchill DN, Bear JC, Morgan J Payne RH, McManamon PJ and Gault MH. Prognosis of adult onset polycystic kidney disease re-evaluated. Kidney International 1984, 26, 190–193.

29. Cole BR, Conley SB and Stapleton FB. Polycystic kidney disease in the first year of life. Journal of Pediatrics 1987, 111, 693–699.

30. Cole WG, Chan D, Hickey AJ and Wilken EL. Collagen composition of normal and myxomatous human mitral heart valves. Biochemical Journal 1984, 219, 451–460.

31. Crocker JFS, Brown DM, Borch RF and Vernier RL. Renal cystic disease induced in newborn rats by diphenylamine derivatives. American Journal Pathology 1972, 66, 343–350.

32. D'Angelo A, Mioni G, Ossi E, Lupo A, Valvo E and Maschio G. Alterations in renal

tubular sodium and water transport in polycystic kidney disease. Clinical Nephrology 1975, 3, 99–105.

33. Dalgaard OZ. Bilateral polycystic disease of the kidneys: A follow- up of two hundred and eighty-four patients and their families. Acta Medica Scandanavica 1957, 158, 326–329.

34. Danovitch GM. Clinical features and pathophysiology of polycystic kidney disease in man. In: Gardner KD Jr, eds., Cystic Diseases of the Kidney. New York: Wiley, 1976, 125–150.

35. Darmady EM, Offer J and Woodhouse MA. Comparison of experimental and human polycystic disease: Thoughts on etiology. Nephron 1965, 4, 254–255.

36. De la Monte S, Moore GH Monk MA and Hutchins GM. Risk factors for the development and rupture of intracranial berry aneurysms. American Journal of Medicine 1985, 78, 957–964.

37. Delaney VB, Adler S, Bruns FJ, Licinia M, Segel DP and Fraley DS. Autosomal dominant polycystic kidney disease: Presentation, complications, and prognosis. American Journal Kidney Diseases 1985, 5, 104–111.

38. Ditlefsen EML and Tonjum AM. Intracranial aneurysms and polycystic kidneys. Acta Medica Scandanavica 1960, 168, 51–54.

39. Dobyan DC, Hill D, Lewis T and Bulger RE. Cyst formation in rat kidney induced by cisplatinum administration. Laboratory Investigation 1981, 45, 260–268.

40. Duren DR, Becker AE and Dunning AJ. Long-term follow-up of idiopathic mitral valve prolapse in 300 patients: A prospective study. JACC 1988, 11, 42–47.

41. Durham DS. Tuberous sclerosis mimicking adult polycystic kidney disease. Australi and New Zealand Journal of Medicine 1987, 17, 71–73.

42. Eggers PW, Connerton R and McMullan M. The Medicare experience with end-stage renal disease: Trends in incidence, prevalence, and survival. Health Care Financing Review 1984, 5, 69–88.

43. Elzinga L, Rashad A, Golper TA and Bennett WM. Antibiotic activity in cyst fluid of patients with cystic kidney disease (CKD). Abstract: Tenth International Congress of Nephrology, 1987.

44. Eulderink F and Hogewind BL. Renal cysts in premature children. Archives of Pathology and Laboratory Medicine 1978, 102, 592–595.

45. Evan AP and Gardner KD Jr. Comparison of human polycystic and medullary cystic kidney disease with diphenylamine–induced cystic disease. Laboratory Investigation 1976, 35, 93–101.

46. Evan AP and Gardner KD Jr. Nephron obstruction in nordihydroguaiaretic acid-induced renal cystic disease. Kidney International 1979, 15, 7–19.

47. Evan AP, Gardner KD Jr and Bernstein J. Polypoid and papillary epithelial hyperplasia: A potential cause of ductal obstruction in adult polycystic disease. Kidney International 1979, 16, 743–750.

48. Evan AP, Hong SK, Gardner KD Jr, Park YS and Itagaki R. Evolution of the collecting tubular lesion in diphenylamine–induced renal disease. Laboratory Investigation 1978, 38, 242–252.

49. Everson GT, Scherzinger A, Leff N, Reichen J, Lezotte D Manco-Johnson M, and Gabow P,. Polycystic liver disease: Quantitation of parenchymal and cyst volumes from CT images and clinical correlates of hepatic cysts. Hepatology 1988, 8, 1627–1634.

50. Fellows RA, Leonidas JC and Beatty EC. Radiologic features of "adult type" polycystic kidney disease in the neonate. Pediatric Radiology 1976, 4, 87–92.

51. Fisher J, Mekhjian H, Pritchett ELC and Charms LS. Polycystic liver disease: Studies in the mechanism of cyst fluid formation: A case report. Gastroenterology 1974, 66, 423–428.

52. Forssell J. Nephrogenous polycythemia. Acta Medica Scandanavica 1958, CLXI, 169–179.

53. Frang D, Czvalinga I and Polyak L. A new approach to the treatment of polycystic kidneys. International Urology and Nephrology 1988, 20, 13–21.

54. Franz KA and Reubi FC. Rate of functional deterioration in polycystic kidney disease. Kidney International 1983, 23, 526–529.

320

55. Fryns JP and Van Den Berghe H. Letter: "Adult" form of polycystic kidney disease in neonates. Clinical Genetics 1978, 15, 205–206.
56. Gabow PA. Epidemiology of autosomal dominant polycystic kidney disease: Implications for genetic counselling. In: Spitzer A and Avner E, eds., Topics in Renal Medicine: The Genetics of Hereditary Nephropathies. Boston: Martinus Nijhoff, 1988. (In Press).
57. Gabow PA, Everson GT, Kaehny WD, Johnson AM and Schrier RW. Clinical characteristics and determinants of hepatic cysts in autosomal dominant polycystic kidney disease. Kidney International (Abstr), 1988, 33, 196.
58. Gabow PA, Heard E, Pretorius D, Duley I, Bell P, Kaehny W and Schrier RW. Relationship between renal structure and hypertension in autosomal dominant polycystic kidney disease (ADPKD). American Society of Nephrology 1986, 19, 140A.
59. Gabow PA, Ikle DW and Holmes JH. Polycystic kidney disease: Prospective analysis of nonazotemic patients and family members. Annals of Internal Medicine 1984, 101, 238–247.
60. Gabow PA, Kaehny WD, Johnson AM, Duley IT, Manco-Johnson M, Lezotte DC and Schrier RW. The clinical utility of renal concentrating capacity in polycystic kidney disease. Kidney International 1988. American Journal of Kidney Diseases 1987, 9, 27–38.
61. Gabow PA and Schrier RW. Physiopathologie de la polykystose renale de l'adulte. Flammarion Medecine-Sciences – Actualites Nephrologiques 1988, 25–38.
62. Gardner KD. Composition of fluid in twelve cysts of a polycystic kidney. New England Journal of Medicine 1969, 281, 985–988.
63. Gardner KD Jr and Evan AP. Cystic kidneys: An enigma evolves. American Journal of Kidney Diseases 1984, 3, 403–413.
64. Gardner KD Jr and Evan AP. Renal cystic disease induced by diphenylthiazole. Kidney International 1983, 24, 43–52.
65. Gardner KD Jr, Evan AP and Reed WP. Accelerated cyst development in deconditioned germfree rats. Kidney International 1986, 29, 1116–1123.
66. Gardner KD Jr, Reed WP, Evan AP, Zedalis Journal Hylarides MD and Leon AA. Endotoxin provocation of experimental renal cystic disease. Kidney International 1987, 32, 329–334.
67. Gardner KD Jr, Solomon S, Fitzgerrel WW and Evan AP. Function and structure in the diphenylamine-exposed kidney. Journal of Clinical Investigation 1976, 57, 796–806.
68. Ghose MK, Sampliner JE, Cohn P and Roza O. Spontaneous colonic perforation: A complication in a hemodialysis patient. Journal of the American Medical Association 1970, 214, 145.
69. Goldman R. Colon perforation in polycystic kidney disease. Journal of the American Medical Association 1975, 233, 137.
70. Goodman T, Grice HC, Becking GC and Salem FA. A cystic nephropathy induced by nordihydroguaiaretic acid in the rat. Laboratory Investigation 1970, 23, 93–107.
71. Gordon RL, Pollack HM, Popky GL and Duckett JW Jr. Simple serous cysts of the kidney in children. Pediatric Radiology 1979, 131, 357–361.
72. Graham PC and Lindop GBM. The anatomy of the renin–secreting cell in adult polycystic kidney disease. Kidney International 1988, 33, 1084–1090.
73. Granot Y, Van Putten V, Summer S, Granot H, Gabow P and Schrier R. The Biosynthesis of intra– and extracellular proteins by cultured human polycystic kidney (HPKD) cells. Abstract: Western Association of Physicians, 1988.
74. Grantham JJ. Polycystic kidney disease: A predominance of giant nephrons. American Journal of Physiology 1983, 244, F3–F10.
75. Grantham JJ and Gabow PA. Polycystic kidney disease. In: Schrier RW and Gottschalk CW, eds, Diseases of the Kidney. Boston: Little, Brown and Company, 1988, 583–615.
76. Grantham JJ, Geiser JL and Evan AP. Cyst formation and growth in autosomal dominant polycystic kidney disease. Kidney International 1987, 31, 1145–1152.
77. Grantham JJ and Slusher SL. Management of renal cystic disorders. In: Suki WN and

Massry SG, eds, Therapy of Renal Diseases and Related Disorders. Boston: Martinus Nijhoff, 1984, 383–404.

78. Gregoire JR, Torres VE, Holley KE and Farrow GM. Renal epithelial hyperplastic and neoplastic proliferation in autosomal dominant polycystic kidney disease.

79. Grossman H, Winchester PH and Chisari FV. Roentgenographic classification of renal cystic disease. American Journal of Roentgenology 1968, 104, 319–331.

80. Grünfeld JP, Albouze G, Jungers P, Landais P, Dana A, Droz D, Moynot A, Lafforgue B, Boursztyn E and Franco D. Liver changes and complications in adult polycystic kidney disease In: Bach JF, Crosnier J, Funck-Bretano JL and Grünfeld JP, eds, Advances in Nephrology. Chicago: Year Book Medical Publishers, 1985, 1–20.

81. Hale JE and Morgan MN. Simple renal cysts. Postgraduate Medical Journal 1969, 45, 767–772.

82. Hartnett M and Bennett W. External Manifestations of cystic renal disease. In: Gardner KD Jr, ed., Cystic disease of the kidney. New York: Wiley, 1976, 201–219.

83. Hatfield PM and Pfister RC. Adult polycystic disease of the kidney: A follow-up of 284 patients. Journal of the American Medical Association 1972, 222, 1527–1531.

84. Heggo O. A microdissection study of cystic disease of the kidneys in adults. Journal of Pathology 1966, 91, 311–315.

85. Hellerstedt WL, Johnson WJ, Ascher N, Kjellstrand CM, Knutson R, Shapiro FL and Sterioff S. Survival rates of 2,728 patients with end-stage renal disease. Mayo Clinic Proceedings 1984, 59, 776–783.

86. Higgins CC. Bilateral polycystic kidney disease. American Medical Association Archives of Surgery 1952, 65, 318–329.

87. Hossack KF, Leddy CL, Johnson AM, Schrier RW and Gabow PA. Echocardiographic abnormalities in autosomal dominant polycystic kidney disease. New England Journal of Medicine 1988, 319, 907–912.

88. Hricak H, Crooks L, Sheldon P and Kaufman L. Nuclear magnetic resonance imaging of the kidney. Radiology 1983, 146, 425–432.

89. Huseman R, Grady A, Welling D and Grantham J. Macropuncture study of polycystic disease in adult human kidneys. Kidney International 1980, 18, 375–385.

90. Iglesias CG, Torres VE, Offord KP, Holley KE, Beard CM and Kurland LT. Epidemiology of adult polycystic kidney disease, Olmsted County, Minnesota: 1935–1980. American Journal of Kidney Diseases 1983, 2, 630–639.

91. Ishibashi A. Renal imagings in the diagnosis of polycystic kidney disease. Japan Journal of Nephrology 1981, 23, 1003–1013.

92. Ito Y, Singh S and Pollack VE. General features of autosomal dominant polycystic kidney disease: Efficacy of dialysis treatment. In: Grantham JJ and Gardner KD Jr, eds., Problems in Diagnosis and Management of Polycystic Kidney Disease. Kansas City: PKR Foundation, 1985, 160–168.

93. Kääriänen H. Polycystic kidney disease in children: A genetic and epidemiological study of 82 Finnish patients. Journal of Medical Genetics 1987, 24, 474–481.

94. Kaehny W, Bell P, Earnest M Stears J and Gabow PA. Family clustering of intracranial aneurysms (ICA) in autosomal dominant polycystic kidney disease (ADPKD). The American Society of Nephrology 1986, 19, 47A.

95. Kaehny WD, Tangel DJ, Johnson AM, Schrier and Gabow PA. Uric acid handling in autosomal dominant polycystic kidney disease. Kidney International 1988, Abstr., 33, 211.

96. Kaplan BS, Rabin I, Nogrady MB and Drummond KN. Autosomal dominant polycystic renal disease in children. Journal of Pediatrics 1977, 90, 782–783.

97. Kaye C and Lewis PR. Congenital appearance of adult-type (autosomal dominant) polycystic kidney disease. Journal Pediatrics 1974, 85, 807–810.

98. Kenner CH, Evan AP, Blomgren P, Aronoff GR and Luft FC. Effect of protein intake on renal function and structure in partially nephrectomized rats. Kidney International 1985, 27, 739–750.

99. Kimberling WJ, Fain PR, Kenyon JB, Goldgar D, Sujansky E and Gabow PA. Linkage

heterogeneity of autosomal dominant polycystic kidney disease. New England Journal of Medicine 1988, 319, 913–918.

100. Kleinman HK, Klebe RJ and Martin GR. Role of collagenous matrices in the adhesion and growth of cells. Journal of Cell Biology 1981, 88, 473–485.

101. Kolibash AJ, Kilman JW, Bush CA, Ryan JM, Fontana ME and Wooley CF. Evidence for progression from mild to severe mitral regurgitation in mitral valve prolapse. American Journal of Cardiology 1986, 58, 762–767.

102. Kramer P, Broyer M, Brunner FP, Brynger H, Donckerwolcke RA, Jacobs C, Selwood NH and Wong AJ. Combined report on regular dialysis and transplantation in Europe. In: Davison A and Guillou PJ. Proceedings of the European Dialysis and Transplant Association. London: Pitman Press, 1982, 4–59.

103. Kramer SA, Hoffman AD, Aydin G and Kelalis P. Simple renal cysts in children. Journal of Urology 1982, 128, 1259–1261.

104. Kupin W, Norris C, Levin NW, Johnson C and Joseph C. Incidence of diverticular disease in patients with polycystic kidney disease (PCKD). The International Society of Nephrology 1987, 43.

105. Kutcher R, Schneider M and Gordon DH. Calcification in polycystic disease. Radiology 1977 122, 77–80.

106. Lalli AE and Poirer VC. Urographic analysis of the development of polycystic kidney disease. American Journal of Roentgenology 1973, 119, 705–709.

107. Lambert PP. Polycystic disease of the kidney: A review. Archives of Pathology 1947, 44, 34–58.

108. Lawson TL, McClennan BL and Shirkhoda A. Adult polycystic kidney disease: Ultrasonagraphic and computed tomographic appearance. JCU 1978, 6, 297–302.

109. Leung AWL, Bydder GM, Steiner RE, Bryant DJ and Young IR. Magnetic resonance imaging of the kidneys. AGR 1984, 143, 1215–1227.

110. Levey AS, Pauker SG and Kassirer JP. Occult intracranial aneurysms in polycystic kidney disease: When is cerebral arteriography indicated? New England Journal of Medicine 1983, 308, 986–994.

111. Levine E. Diagnosis of autosomal dominant polycystic kidney disease: Complications and radiologic recognition. In: Grantham JJ and Gardner KD Jr, eds., Problems in Diagnosis and Management of Polycystic Kidney Disease. Kansas City: PKR Foundation, 1985, 34–39.

112. Levine E and Grantham JJ. The role of computed tomography in the evaluation of adult polycystic kidney disease. American Journal of Kidney Diseases 1981, 1, 99–105.

113. Lieberman E, Salinas-Madrigal L, Gwinn JL, Brennan LP, Fine RN and Landing BH. Infantile polycystic disease of the kidneys and liver: Clinical, pathological and radiological correlations and comparison with congenital hepatic fibrosis. Medicine 1971, 50, 277–318.

114. Lipshutz DE and Easterling RE. Spontaneous perforation of the colon in chronic renal failure. Archives of Internal Medicine 1973, 132, 758–759.

115. Loh JP, Haller JO, Kassner EG, Aloni A and Glassberg K. Dominantly- inherited polycystic kidneys in infants. Association with hypertrophic pyloric stenosis. Pediatric Radiology 1977, 6, 27–31.

116. London RD, Malik AA and Train JS. Infection in a patient with polycystic kidney and liver disease: Noninvasive localization and treatment. American Journal of Medicine 1988, 84, 1082–1085.

117. Lundin PM and Oglow I. Polycystic kidneys in newborns, infants and children. A clinical and pathological study. Acta Paediatrica 1961, 50, 185–200.

118. Main D, Mennuti MT, Cornfield D and Coleman B. Prenatal diagnosis of adult polycystic kidney disease. Lancet 1983, 2, 337–338.

119. Martin DC and Goodwin WE. Renal trasplantation in polycystic renal disease. Journal of the American Medical Association 1967, 202, 654–657.

120. Martinez-Maldonado M, Yium JJ, Eknoyan G and Suki WN. Adult polycystic kidney disease. Studies of the defect in urine concentration. Kidney International 1972, 2, 109–113.

121. Matsumura M, Wada H, Nojiri K, Ohwada A and Shinoda T. Unruptured intracranial aneurysms in polycystic kidney disease. Acta Neurochir 1986, 79, 94–99.
122. Mehrizi A, Rosenstein J, Pusch A., Askin JA and Taussig HB. Myocardial infarction and endocardial fibroelastosis in children with polycystic kidneys. Bulletin of the Johns Hopkins Hospital 1964, 115, 92–98.
123. Mendez R, Mendez RG, Payne JE and Berne TV. Renal transplantation: In adults with end stage polycystic kidney disease. Urology 1975, 5, 26–28.
124. Milutinovic J and Agodoa L. Potential causes and pathogenesis in autosomal dominant polycystic kidney disease. Nephron 1983, 33, 139–144.
125. Milutinovic J, Fialkow LJ, Agodoa LY, Phillips LA, Rudd TG and Bryant JI. Autosomal dominant polycystic kidney disease: symptoms and clinical findings. Quarterly Journal of Medicine 1984, 53, 511–522.
126. Milutinovic J, Fialkow PJ, Agodoa LY, Phillips LA and Bryant JI. Fertility and pregnancy complications in women with autosomal dominant polycystic kidney disease. Obstetrics and Gynecology 1983, 61, 566–570.
127. Milutinovic J, Fialkow PJ, Rudd TG, Agodoa LY, Phillips LA and Bryant JI. Liver cysts in patients with autosomal dominant polycystic kidney disease. American Journal of Medicine 1980, 68, 741–744.
128. Mir S, Rapola J and Koskinies O. Renal cysts in pediatric autopsy material. Nephron 1983, 33, 189–195.
129. Mohr JP, Kistler JP, Zabramski JM, Spetzler RF and Barnett HJM. Intracranial aneurysms. In: Barnett HJM, Stein BM, Mohr JP and Yatsu FM, eds., Stroke. New York: Churchill Livingstone, 1986, 643–677.
130. Muther RS and Bennett WM. Cyst fluid antibiotic concentrations in polycystic kidney disease: Differences between proximal and distal cysts. Kidney International 1981, 20, 519–522.
131. Nash DA. Hypertension in polycystic kidney disease without renal failure. Archives of Internal Medicine 1977, 137, 1571–1575.
132. Ng RCK and Suki WN. Renal cell carcinoma occirring in a polycystic kidney of a transplant recipient. Journal of Urology 1980, 124, 710–712.
133. Novick AC. General features of autosomal dominant kidney disease: Renal transplantation. In: Grantham JJ and Gardner KD Jr, eds., Problems in Diagnosis and Management of Polycystic Kidney Disease. Kansas City: PKR Foundation, 1985, 172–179.
134. Oken DE. Chronic renal diseases and pregnancy: A review. American Journal Obstetrics and Gynecology 1966, 94, 1023–1043.
135. Oldrizzi L, Rugiu C, Valvo E, Lupo A, Loschiavo C, Gammaro L, Tessitore N, Fabris A, Panzetta G and Maschio G. Progression of renal failure in patients with renal disease of diverse etiology on protein-restricted diet. Kidney International 1985, 27, 553–557.
136. Oppenheimer GD. Polycystic disease of the kidney. Annals of Surgery 1984, 100, 1136–1158.
137. Oreopoulos DG, Bell TK and McGeown MG. Liver function and the liver scan in patients with polycystic kidney disease. British Journal of Urology 1971, 43, 273–276.
138. Osathanondh V and Potter EL. Pathogenesis of polycystic kidneys: Type 3 due to multiple abnormalities of development. Archives of Pathology 1964, 77, 485–501.
139. Pechan W, Novick AC, Braun WE, Nakamoto S, Popowniak K and Steinmuller D. Management of end stage polycystic kidney disease with renal transplantation. Journal of Urology 1981, 125, 622–624.
140. Perey DYE, Herdman RC and Good RA. Polycystic renal disease: A new experimental model. Science 1967, 158, 494–496.
141. Potter EL. Normal and Abnormal Development of the Kidney. Chicago: Year Book Publishers, 1972.
142. Poutasse EF, Gardner WJ and McCormack LJ. Polycystic kidney disease and intracranial aneurysm. Journal of the American Medical Association 1954, 154, 741–743.
143. Pretorius DH, Lee ME, Manco-Johnson ML, Weingast GR, Sedman AB and Gabow PA.

Diagnosis of autosomal dominant polycystic kidney disease in utero and in the young infant. Journal of Ultrasound Medicine 1987, 6, 249–255.

144. Preuss H, Geoly K, Johnson M, Chester A, Kliger A and Schreiner G. Tubular function in adult polycystic kidney disease. Nephron 1979, 24, 198–204.

145. Proesmans W, Van Damme B, Casaer P and Marchal G. Autosomal dominant polycystic kidney disease in the neonatal period: Association with cerebral arteriovenous malformation. Pediatrics 1982, 70, 971–975.

146. Reeders ST, Breuning MH, Davies KE, Nicholls RD, Jarman AP, Higgs DR, Pearson PL and Weatherall DJ. A highly polymorphic DNA marker linked to adult polycystic disease on chromosome 16. Nature 1985, 317, 542–544.

147. Reeders ST, Zeeres K, Gal A, Propping P, Waldherr R, Davies KE, Zerres K, Hogenkamp T, Schmidt W, Dolata MM and Weatherall DJ. Prenatal diagnosis of autosomal dominant polycystic kidney disease with a DNA probe. Lancet 1986, 2, 6–8.

148. Reubi FC. General features of autosomal dominant polycystic kidney disease: Hypertension. In: Grantham JJ and Gardner KD Jr, eds., Problems in Diagnosis and Management of Polycystic Kidney Disease. Kansas City: PKR Foundation, 1985, 121–128.

149. Ritter R and Siafarikas K. Hemihypertrophy in a boy with renal polycystic disease: Varied patterns of presentation of renal polycystic disease in his family. Pediatric Radiology 1976, 5, 98–102.

150. Ross DG and Travers H. Infantile presentation of adult type polycystic kidney disease in a large kindred. Journal of Pediatrics 1975, 87, 760–763.

151. Rostand SG, Kirk KA, Rutsky EA and Pate BA. Racial differences in the incidence of treatment for end-stage renal disease. New England Journal of Medicine 1982, 306, 1276–1279.

152. Rutkai K and Czeizel A. Obstetric features of mothers giving birth to infants with polycystic disease of the kidneys. Archivse of Gynecology 1982, 231, 235–240.

153. Salvatierra O Jr, Wolfson M, Cochrum K, Amend W and Belzer FO. End stage polycystic kidney disease: Management by renal transplantation and selective use of preliminary nephrectomy. Journal of Urology 1976, 115, 5–7.

154. Sanfilippo FP, Vaughn WK, Peters TG, Bollinger RR and Spees EK. Transplantation for polycystic kidney disease. Transplantation 1983, 36, 54–59.

155. Scheff RT, Zuckerman G, Harter H, Delmez J and Koehler R. Diverticular disease in patients with chronic renal failure due to polycystic kidney disease. Annals of Internal Medicine 1980, 92, 202–204.

156. Schmike RN. Hereditary features of autosomal dominant polycystic kidney disease: A genetic approach. In: Grantham JJ and Gardner KD Jr, eds., Problems in Diagnosis and Management of Polycystic Kidney Disease. Kansas City: PKR Foundation, 1985, 187–193.

157. Schwab SJ. Efficacy of chloramphenicol in refractory cyst infections in autosomal dominant polycystic kidney disease. American Journal of Kidney Diseases 1985, 5, 258–261.

158. Schwab SJ. General features of autosomal dominant polycystic kidney disease: Experience with chloramphenicol in refractory renal infection. In: Grantham JJ and Gardner KD Jr, eds., Problems in Diagnosis and Management of Polycystic Kidney Disease. Kansas City: PKR Foundation, 1985, 106–110.

159. Schwab SJ, Bander SJ and Klahr S. Renal infection in autosomal dominant polycystic kidney disease. American Journal of Medicine 1987, 82, 714–718.

160. Schwab SJ, Hinthorn D, Diederich D, Cuppage F and Grantham JJ. pH- dependent accumulation of clindamycin in a polycystic kidney. American Journal of Kidney Diseases 1983, 3, 63–66.

161. Schwab SJ and Weaver ME. Penetration of trimethoprim and sulfamethoxazole into cyst in patients with autosomal dominant polycystic kidney disease. American Journal of Kidney Diseases 1986, 7, 434–438.

162. Sedman A, Bell P, Manco-Johnson M, Schrier R, Warady BA, Heard EO, Butler-Simon N and Gabow P. Autosomal dominant polycystic kidney disease in childhood: A longitudinal study. Kidney International 1987, 31, 1000–1005.

163. Segal AJ, Spataro RF and Barbaric ZL. Adult polycystic kidney disease: A review of 100 cases. Journal of Urology 1977, 118, 711–713.
164. Shokeir MHK. Expression of "adult" polycystic renal disease in the fetus and newborn. Clinical Genetics 1978, 14, 61–72.
165. Sholder AJ and Grayhack JT. General features of autosomal dominant polycystic kidney disease: Management of pain and hemorrhage. In: Grantham JJ and Gardner KD Jr, eds., Problems in Diagnosis and Management of Polycystic Kidney Disease. Kansas City: PKR Foundation, 1985, 111–120.
166. Siegel MJ and McAlister WH. Simple cysts of the kidney in children. Journal of Urology 1980, 123, 75–78.
167. Simon HB and Thompson GJ. Congenital renal polycystic disease: A clinical and therapeutic study of three hundred sixty-six cases. Journal of the American Medical Association 1955, 159, 657–662.
168. Stickler GB and Kelalis AP. Polycystic kidney disease recognition of the "adult form" (autosomal dominant) in infancy. Mayo Clinic Proceedings 1975, 50, 547–481.
169. Stillwell TJ, Gomez MR and Kelalis PP. Renal lesions in tuberous sclerosis. Journal of Urology 1987, 138, 477–481.
170. Sugimoto T and Rosansky SJ. The incidence of treated end-stage renal disease in the eastern United States: 1973–1979. American Journal of Public Health 1984, 74, 14–17.
171. Sweet R and Keane WF. Perinephric abscess in patients with polycystic kidney disease undergoing chronic hemodialysis. Nephron 1979, 23, 237–240.
172. Thomas JO, Cox AJ Jr and DeEds F. Kidney cysts produced by diphenylamine. Stanford Medical Bulletin 1957, 15, 90–93.
173. Thompson JS and Thompson MW. Patterns of single-gene inheritance. In: Thompson JS and Thompson MW, eds., Genetics in Medicine. Philadelphia: WB Saunders Company, 1986, 44–77.
174. Torres VE, Erickson SB, Smith LH, Wilson DM, Hattery RR and Segura JW. The association of nephrolithiasis and autosomal dominant polycystic kidney disease. American Journal of Kidney Diseases 1988, 11, 318–325.
175. Torres VE, Holley KE and Offord KP. General features of autosomal dominant polycystic kidney disease: Epidemiology. In: Grantham JJ and Gardner KD Jr, eds., Problems in Diagnosis and Management of Polycystic Kidney Disease. Kansas City: PKR Foundation, 1985, 49–69.
176. Valvo E, Gammaro L Tessitore N, Panzetta G, Lupo A, Loschiavo C, Oldrizzi L, Fabris A, Rugiu C, Ortalda V and Maschio G. Hypertension of polycystic kidney disease: Mechanisms and hemodynamic alterations. American Journal of Nephrology 1985, 5, 176–181.
177. Wakabayashi T, Fujita S, Ohbora Y, Suyama T, Tamaki N and Matsumoto S. Polycystic kidney disease and intracranial aneurysms: Early angiographic diagnosis and early operation for the unruptured aneurysms. Journal of Neurosurgery 1983, 58, 488–491.
178. Walker FC Jr, Loney LC, Root ER, Melson GL, McAlister WH and Cole BR. Diagnostic evaluation of adult polycystic kidney disease in childhood. American Journal of Roentgenology 1984, 142, 1273–1277.
179. Ward JN, Draper JW and Lavengood RW Jr. A clinical review of polycystic kidney disease in 53 patients. Journal of Urology 1967, 98, 48–53.
180. Wiebers DO, Whisnant JP and O'Fallon WM. The natural history of unruptured intracranial aneurysms. New England Journal of Medicine 1981, 304 696–698.
181. Williams G, Mitcheson HD and Castro JE. Transplantation for polycystic kidney disease. Urology 1978, 12, 628–630.
182. Wilson PD, Schrier RW, Breckon RD and Gabow PA. A new method for studying human polycystic kidney disease epithelia in culture. Kidney International 1986, 30, 371–378.
183. Wolf GB, Rosenfield AT, Taylor KJW, Rosenfield N, Gottlieb S and Hsia YE. Presymptomatic diagnosis of adult onset polycystic kidney disease by ultrasonography. Clinical Genetics 1978, 14, 1–7.

184. Wolfson M, Amend WJC, Cochrum KC, Belzer FO and Salvatierra O Jr. Transplantation in end-stage renal kidney disease. Dialysis and Transplantation 1976, 5, 66,102.
185. Zerres K, Weiss H, Bulla M and Roth B. Prenatal diagnosis of an early manifestation of autosomal dominant adult-type polycystic kidney disease (letter). Lancet 1982, 2, 988.

13
Autosomal Recessive Polycystic Kidney Disease

B. R. Cole

Abstract

Autosomal recessive polycystic kidney disease (ARPKD) is a specific disease of the kidneys and liver, characterized by renal collecting tubule ectasia and invariably accompanied by biliary dysgenesis and portal fibrosis. In the past the disease has been called "infantile" polycystic kidney disease because of the predominant presentation in infancy. In recent years, however, presentation at later ages and survival into adulthood have become obvious. This chapter will describe the evolution of our knowledge of ARPKD, the diagnosis and management of the condition, and a summary of what is known about pathogenetic mechanisms.

Key words   Autosomal recessive polycystic kidney disease;
                 Congenital hepatic fibrosis;
                 Recessive polycystic kidney disease

1. Historical perspective

Publications four decades ago[41,53] reviewed a century of observations about polycystic disease. As early as 1855, renal cystic disease was described and hypothesized to originate from tubular obstruction. A half-century later, in 1902, a report of the age distribution of 239 patients with presumed polycystic kidney disease showed two peaks of presentation. Twenty-five percent were stillborn babies, and an additional 9% were under the age of 20 years. A second large peak was between 30 and 60 years[41].

Much later, histopathologic studies verified morphologic differences between these two populations[37,47]. Potter[47] described one form of polycystic disease in which there were dilated and elongated tubular structures accompanied by a normal amount of connective tissue. A second form had globular tubular cysts and greater than normal connective tissue. Staemmler (cited by Lundin and Olow[41]) described three cystic kidney diseases: first, a very large kidney occupied by large cystic structures; second, a moderately enlarged kidney that appeared "spongy" on the cut surface; and third, a small kidney with a few cysts. In a monumental study of renal cystic disease in Denmark, Dalgaard[18] surveyed available parents of affected neonates. No parent studied had any evidence of cystic disease, providing the first evidence that this condition, now known as autosomal recessive polycystic kidney disease

(ARPKD), was inherited differently from the disease presenting in adults, now known as autosomal dominant polycystic kidney (ADPKD). Osathanondh and Potter in 1964[45,46,48] characterized, by microdissection, four conditions associated with cysts. Type I was consistent with ARPKD and type III with ADPKD. The other two types had the features of renal dysplasia and of hydronephrosis. Early reports then described a multiplicity of renal cystic diseases. Classifications in the 1960's were based on morphologic and radiographic features[8,9,19,25,28,29,36].

It was recognized in early studies that the renal abnormality of ARPKD was almost always accompanied by hepatic involvement. Kissane[36] wrote that the livers of such patients contained "either multiple epithelial cysts ... or bizarre proliferations of portal bile ducts". Kerr and colleagues[35] noted the occurrence of polycystic kidneys in patients with congenital hepatic fibrosis, a condition morphologically similar to hepatic involvement in ARPKD. Blyth and Ockenden[11] described four groups of patients with infantile PKD and congenital hepatic fibrosis. In the perinatal form, the major feature was bilateral renal enlargement, with dilatation of 90% of the renal tubules. At the other end of the spectrum, children classified as having the juvenile form presented, usually at an older age, with hepatomegaly and frequent portal hypertension. In these children, fewer than 10% of the renal tubules were dilated. The other two groups were intermediate. Although every child in the study had some degree of involvement of both liver and kidneys, other studies of congenital hepatic fibrosis have shown radiologic evidence of renal cystic disease in 50–60% of patients[35,36,53,60].

If kidney biopsies had been performed in all patients with congenital hepatic fibrosis, the correlation might have been better. Alvarez et al.[1] suggest that a combination of clinical, radiologic and anatomic diagnostic tools yields a diagnosis of some form of renal involvement in "virtually all patients with congenital hepatic fibrosis". Although congenital hepatic fibrosis may be associated with other types of renal disease, ARPKD with congenital hepatic fibrosis constitutes an entity.

2. Comparison of ARPKD with other renal cystic diseases

Three other major cystic renal conditions must be considered in the differential diagnosis of cystic disease in children (Table 13.1).

An increasing number of reports attest to the occurrence of ADPKD in infancy[17,32], even in utero[50]. The enlarged kidneys contain globular dilatations that may occur in any or several segment(s) of the nephron or collecting ducts, including glomeruli. Many patients have cysts in other organs[23], including the liver. In general, children with this disease are asymptomatic, although some develop hypertension and chronic renal insufficiency during childhood[17,58,64].

Table 13.1 Differentiation of ARPKD, ADPKD, glomerulocystic kidney disease and cystic dysplasia

	ARPKD	ADPKD	Glomerulocystic kidney disease	Cystic dysplasia
Age of presentation	Childhood *most frequently*	All ages, *most frequently* in 3rd–4th decade	Infancy	Frequently in infancy, may be found incidentally at any age
Inheritance	Autosomal recessive	Autosomal dominant	Sporadic, occasionally dominant	Usually sporadic, may accompany syndromes and is occasionally familial
Incidence	1:10,000– 1:40,000	1:500– 1:1000	Rare	Most common unilateral abdominal mass in newborn; bilateral, rare
Gross anatomic features	Enlarged reniform masses; smooth contours; "sponge-like" on cut surface	Enlarged kidneys with bosselated surfaces; huge globular cysts on cut surface	Enlarged reniform kidneys	Small non-reniform masses with occasional cysts to huge, irregularly shaped masses
Tubular abnormality	Ectasia of collecting ducts	Globular dilatations of any portion or collecting duct; occasional glomerular cysts	Marked dilatation of Bowman's spaces	Primitive tubules in undifferentiated mesenchyme; often islands of cartilage
Accompanying features	Congenital hepatic fibrosis	Hepatic cysts in 20–40%, pancreatic cysts, cerebral artery aneurysms	Usually normal livers; may be associated with multiple malformation syndromes	Ureteric abnormality; contralateral kidney may be hydronephrotic if unilateral; common association with cardiovascular, gastrointestinal and CNS malformations

Glomerulocystic disease is a term that was coined by Taxy and Filmer in 1976[63], although Baxter[7] had described the phenomenon earlier. The kidney cysts are predominantly glomerular. Many patients succumb early in life, and others survive into late childhood[56]. The condition is usually sporadic, but has been reported in families[57]. It may also accompany multiple malformation syndromes, such as tuberous sclerosis, oral-facial-digital syndrome, and brachy-mesomelia–renal syndrome[21]. Glomerular cysts, along with cysts in other nephron segments, are frequently seen in ADPKD.

Multicystic dysplasia usually occurs unilaterally, occasionally bilaterally.

The unilateral condition is the most common abdominal mass in the new-born[36]. When bilateral, the condition is incompatible with life, and, even in the apparently unilateral condition, the contralateral kidney may be hydroneph-rotic because of obstruction at the ureteropelvic junction[36]. The ureter of the multicystic kidney is absent, atretic or severely stenotic. The child with the bilateral condition is usually born with huge flank masses and the features of Potter association (oligohydramnios, abnormal face, low-set ears, pulmonary hypoplasia). The early literature describing polycystic kidney disease in chil-dren often included what is now known to be cystic dysplasia. Multicystic kidneys contain primitive tubules and islands of cartilage[36].

It is obvious, then, that certain features of these conditions have con-siderable overlap[4]. Thus, it behooves the physician to seek all clinical, radio-logical and histologic data to assure accurate diagnosis and appropriate genetic counselling.

3. Clinical manifestations

3.1 Epidemiology

The exact incidence of ARPKD is unknown. Many reports have come only from autopsied patients, and the numbers of survivors are not known. Other reports speak only of the survivors, with no data on the numbers of deaths or the population of the referral area. Occasionally a number is quoted, such as that by Bosniak and Ambos[14], but without identification of source (Table 13.2).

Table 13.2 Epidemiology of ARPKD

	Incidence	Sex preponderance
Kääriäinen[33]	1:10,000	none
Bosniak and Ambos[14a]	1: 6,000 to 1:14,000	F:M::2:1
Potter[48]	1:55,000	—
Zerres et al.[66]	1:40,000 "rough estimate"	—
Gwinn and Landing[29]	—	none

[a]Calculated from data, assuming that the "sporadic" cases are ARPKD.

Zerres et al.[66] make a "rough estimate" that the true incidence is 1:40,000. Kääriäinen[32], in a survey of Finnish children, categorized 32, because of affected siblings, as having ARPKD and judged an additional 41, because of negative family histories, to have recessive disease (called "sporadic"). Given that the number of births in Finland over the time period observed was 650,827, the incidence of ARPKD in Finland was approximately 1:10,000. Whether the

Finnish incidence is replicated in other parts of the world is uncertain. Potter[48] had found only two cases of what appeared to be ARPKD in 110,000 births in Chicago.

In Finland[33], as in California[30], there was no sex preponderance (Table 13.2). Bosniak and Ambos[14] are the only authors to suggest a female preponderance.

13.2 Clinical presentation (Table 13.3)

Table 13.3 Clinical presentation of ARPKD

Presentation in infancy
  History of oligohydramnios
  Difficult delivery because of enlarged abdomen
  Potter facies
  Respiratory distress
    pulmonary hypoplasia
    pneumomediastinum, pneumothorax
    atelectasis
    pneumonia
  Hypertension
    left ventricular hypertrophy
    congestive heart failure
  Renal insufficiency

Presentation in childhood
  Renal insufficiency
  Hepatosplenomegaly
  Gastrointestinal bleeding

Most patients with ARPKD present in infancy. Some cases will have been suspected or diagnosed by fetal ultrasonography; others present at birth with huge flank masses that complicate delivery[11,14,17,24,41]. Oligohydramnios results from poor renal output[14,41]. Potter[47] described the physiognomy now known as "Potter facies" in which there are deep eye creases, a flat, snubbed nose, micrognathia and large, floppy, low-set ears. Contractures of the extremities may also be seen. The Potter association has been thought to result from restriction imposed by the paucity of amniotic fluid; it may accompany any type of kidney disease with poor intrauterine function.

The principal early neonatal complication is pulmonary distress[17,34]. Most of the infants now succumbing in early infancy have pulmonary insufficiency, and renal insufficiency is an uncommon cause of death[11,34,41].

Hypertension is very common[17,24,40,52], and congestive heart failure may develop[29]. Blood pressure elevation is common in both affected infants and older children[24,40].

Children who present with ARPKD later in childhood do so most often with one of two problems. Perhaps more common is congenital hepatic fibrosis[11,40], with either gastrointestinal bleeding from varices or hepatospleno-megaly. The less common presentation comprises the secondary effects of chronic renal insufficiency[11,28,34], such as anemia, growth failure and renal osteodystrophy. Some cases may be detected because of hypertension found on routine physical examination[52] or during evaluation of hematuria precipitated by trauma.

3.3 Complications

Of the three complications of ARPKD, the first to be considered is hypertension. Hypertension begins in the first few months of life, affecting approximately 90% of children with ARPKD[17,24,34]. It may be present in children with normal renal function, requiring treatment with antihypertensive agents.

Urinary tract infections are frequent[34], often accompanied by pyuria[11,53]. Because communicating cysts in early ARPKD become pinched off and more rounded as the disease progresses[12,40,62], just as in ADPKD[26], stasis developing within the cysts may predispose to bacterial infection[27]. Pyuria in ARPKD, even without demonstrable bacteriuria, strongly suggests renal infection and indicates the need for vigorous antibacterial therapy.

Bacterial cholangitis is the third serious complication. It is not common, but may be fatal[34]. It may be suggested by clinical and laboratory evidence of hepatocellular injury, but it should also be considered in the differential diagnosis of any intercurrent fever.

4. Radiologic assessment

4.1 Renal findings

In the past, certain features were said to be "typical" of ARPKD. Current experience indicates that none of them occurs exclusively in patients with ARPKD. Patients with ADPKD occasionally have identical abnormalities.

Ultrasonography is frequently employed as a non-invasive initial diagnostic tool. The kidneys in the affected neonate or infant are enlarged, usually symmetrical, commonly with obscure margins. Diffusely increased echogenicity obscures demarcations among the renal cortex, medulla and sinus.

Macroscopic cysts may be present[12,15,43,44] (Figs. 13.1A, B). Melson and colleagues[43] classified cases on the basis of sonographic findings: Group I, patients with 8–14 mm rims of normal cortex; Group II, patients with 2–3 mm rims of normal cortex; Group III, patients with diffuse hyperechogenicity and no recognizable rim of normal cortex. The patients in Group I remain well at 3–16 years, although one has reduced renal function and controlled hypertension. One survivor of infancy in Group II developed endstage renal failure at

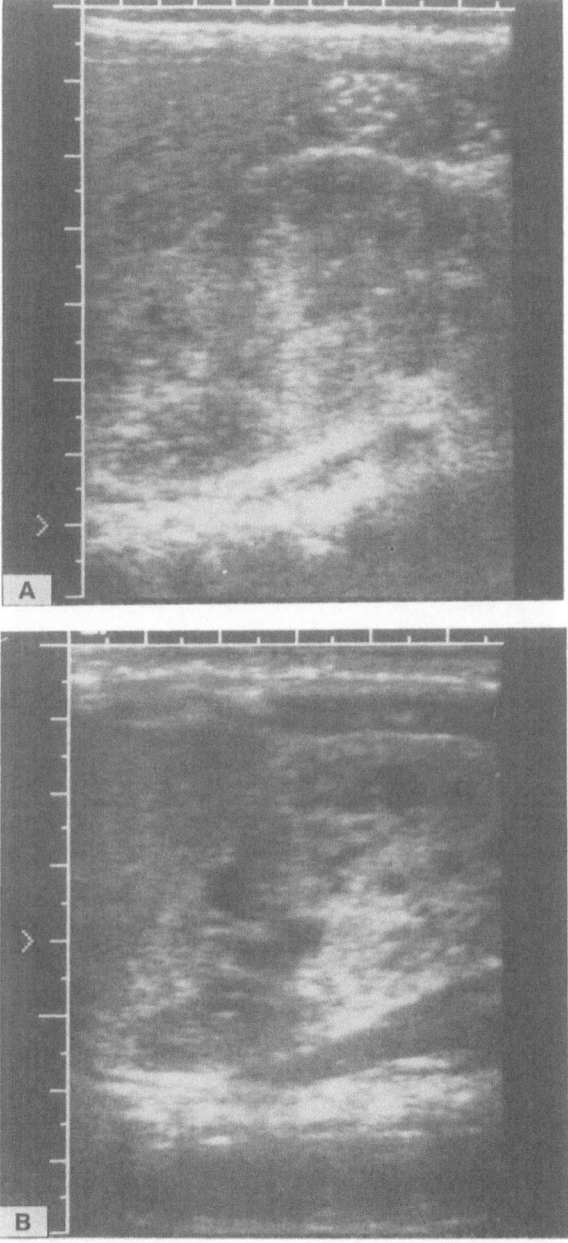

Figure 13.1 A. Sonogram of right kidney of a 6-week-old infant with ARPKD whose cystic kidneys had been detected by fetal ultrasound. The echogenicity of the kidney is greater than that of the liver (upper left corner), and several 0.5–0.8 mm cysts are present in the cortex. This patient had a sibling who had post-mortem renal and hepatic findings consistent with ARPKD. B Left kidney of patient in 13.1A. Sonographically resolvable cysts are more distinct. Blood urea nitrogen and serum creatinine levels are normal.

334

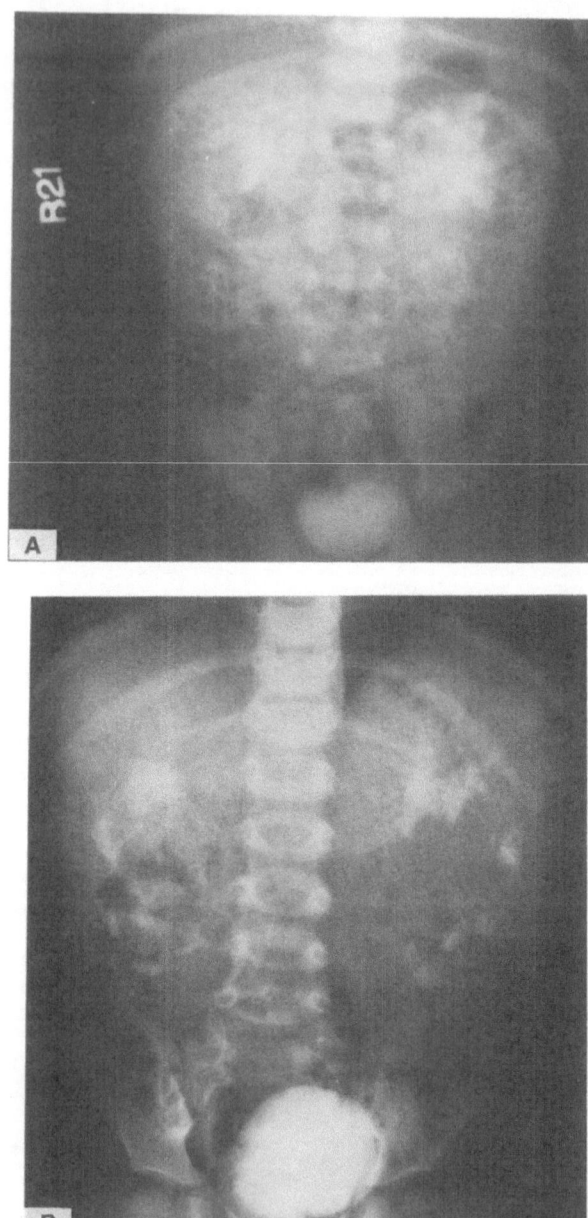

Figure 13.2 A Excretory urogram of infant with ARPKD. Large reniform kidneys are outlined. Contrast medium is concentrated in collecting tubules, producing a mottled appearance. B. Urogram of the same patient at age 2 years. The kidneys remain very large and the contrast medium is concentrated in a striated fashion.

9 years. Three of four patients in Group III have survived, one with normal renal function and no hypertension. Thus, the conjecture[43] that those patients with the greatest amount of sonographically normal cortex would have the best prognosis has not been substantiated, although none of the patients in Group I died during infancy.

Excretory urography, until recently the most commonly used radiographic tool, typically shows enlarged kidneys with a mottled or striated appearance due to accumulation of contrast material in dilated collecting tubules[15,19,25] (Figs. 13.2A, B). In severe cases of neonatal ARPKD, visualization by excretory urography may be slight and very prolonged, with persistence of the nephrogram for days[15]. Computed tomography with enhancement also shows linear or radial opacification in enlarged kidneys[33,62].

The radiographic differential diagnosis includes nephroblastomatosis and bilateral Wilms tumor. The visualization of striations in a dilated collecting system by excretory urography argues against these tumors, but biopsy may be necessary in some cases. Other conditions may mimic the radiographic or sonographic findings of ARPKD, e.g. glomerulocystic disease[42], pyelonephritis[6], transient nephromegaly[61], radiocontrast nephropathy[5] and glomerulonephritis[20]. ADPKD can also present as renal enlargement in the newborn period. Macroscopic cysts can be detected in infants with ADPKD[33], but they are also present in infants with ARPKD[12,65].

The radiographic picture of ARPKD may change in the older child and resemble more strongly the findings in ADPKD[40,49]. The kidneys may become smaller, and striations may disappear and be replaced by rounded cysts[40,49].

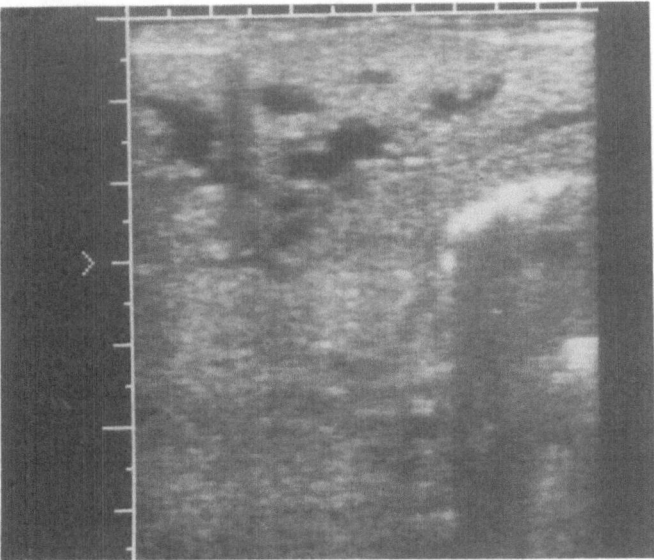

Figure 13.3 Hepatic sonogram of a 3-week-old male with ARPKD, showing extremely dilated biliary ducts. The child died of pulmonary insufficiency at 25 days.

4.2 Liver findings

The liver in ARPKD is usually normal in size and less echogenic than the kidneys. Dilated intrahepatic biliary ducts may be demonstrated sonographically, even in the neonate[49] (Fig. 13.3).

Older children have massive hepatomegaly and splenomegaly, and the liver is hyperechoic. Hepatic venous catheterization may confirm portal hypertension in the older child, and esophageal varices may be demonstrated by barium swallow[40,49].

5. Gross and microscopic pathology

5.1 Kidney

The morphological appearance of ARPKD is reasonably uniform in severely affected newborns and young infants, but changes somewhat as survivors age. Perhaps the best way to approach the disease is to recognize the morphologic appearance in the infant, to identify the variations and to understand the evolution.

The neonate with ARPKD has enlarged kidneys, sometimes huge and distending the abdominal cavity. Individual kidneys have been reported to be

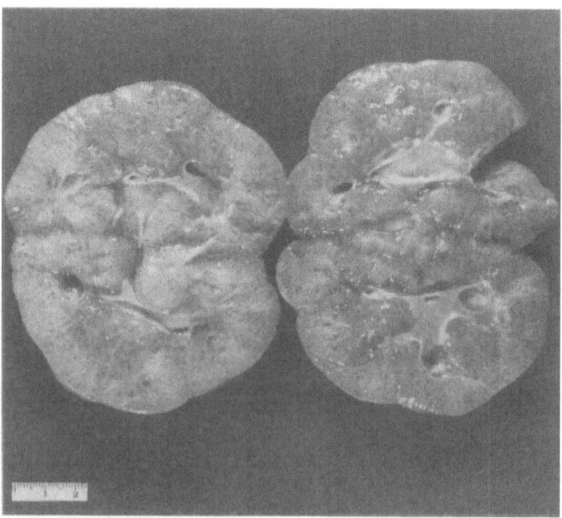

Figure 13.4 Gross specimens of kidneys of patient from Fig. 13.3. The right kidney weighed 177 g, the left 122 (normal 24 g). The cut surfaces reveal a normal lobar configuration, with elongated cortical and rounded medullary cysts.

300–400 g, 10–12 times the normal weight[19]. The kidneys retain their reniform contours, and the external surfaces are smooth with fetal lobulations (Fig. 13.4).

Pinpoint cysts corresponding to the ends of dilated cortical collecting tubules may dot the capsular surface[36]. The cut surface (Fig. 13.5) displays elongated cysts in radial arrangement.

This appearance is frequently described as "spongy"[40], but must not be confused with medullary sponge kidney, a completely different entity seldom seen in childhood[36].

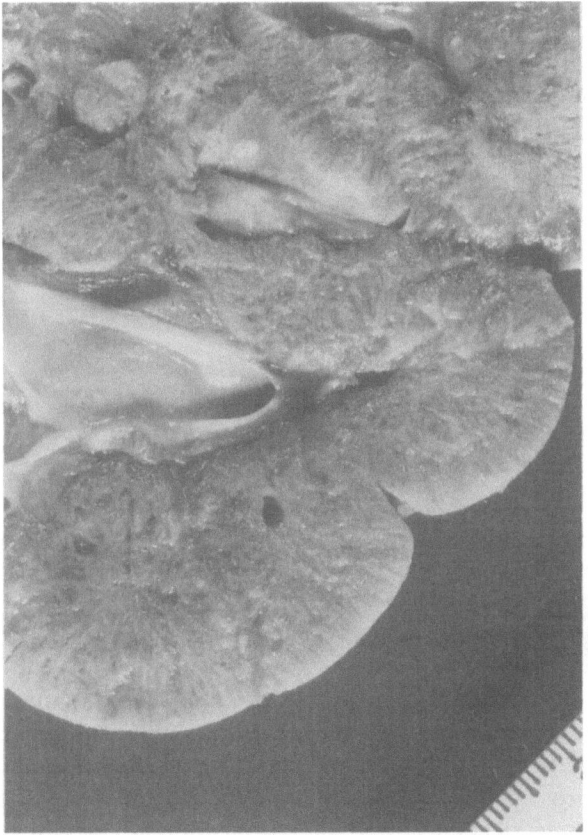

Figure 13.5 Closer inspection of the cut surface of the kidney from the patient from Fig. 13.3. The cortex is traversed by radially oriented fusiform cysts arising in collecting ducts. Cortico-medullary markings are obscured.

The cysts, confirmed by microdissection to be dilated collecting tubules and ducts[46], may be limited to the medullary area and may make differentiation from uremic medullary cystic kidney difficult[14], or may extend throughout the medulla and cortex. These differences probably explain the sonographic spec-

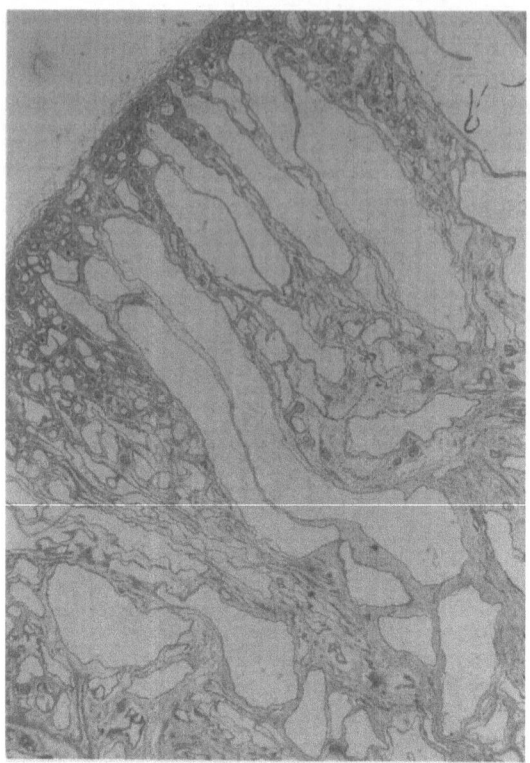

Figure 13.6 Light microscopic section of the kidney of the patient from Fig. 13.3. The cystic spaces, extending throughout the cortex, were lined by simple cuboidal or low columnar epithelium. The glomeruli appeared few in number.

trum described by Melson and colleagues[43], in which a normally echoic rim of cortex may be visible.

The cysts usually are dilated structures lined by low columnar or cuboidal epithelium (Fig. 13.6). The cyst walls are not extremely attenuated, indicating that the cysts are formed by cell proliferation[8,46]. The glomeruli and other tubular structures appear to be few in number, probably the visual result of the striking collecting duct ectasia and interstitial edema. The glomeruli are rarely dilated[36]. The collecting system and renal vessels appear normal.

Blyth and Ockenden[11] noted that the degree of tubular ectasia varied. The proportion of kidney occupied by dilated tubules ranged from 80% or more in newborns who died of the disease to as little as 10% in older children who survived to develop hepatic fibrosis and portal hypertension.

Some histologic studies testify to the evolution of cyst morphology. Lieberman and colleagues[40] described a transition from radially disposed, ectatic collecting ducts to irregular, spherical cysts without orientation during a period of several years. Gang and Herrin[24] described increased fibrosis and chronic inflammation in later specimens from patients who had typical collecting duct dilation during infancy. The evolution of the abnormality leads, in older patients, to an appearance resembling that of ADPKD, and to potential confusion if the earlier findings are not taken into consideration[33].

5.2 Liver

The liver in the newborn is also abnormal. Its size may be somewhat increased, but hepatomegaly is usually a later phenomenon. The abnormality may vary from a slightly increased number of biliary ducts, usually accompanied by portal fibrosis, to an intricate mesh of dilated and communicating biliary ducts, surrounded by increased fibrous tissue[36] (Fig. 13.7).

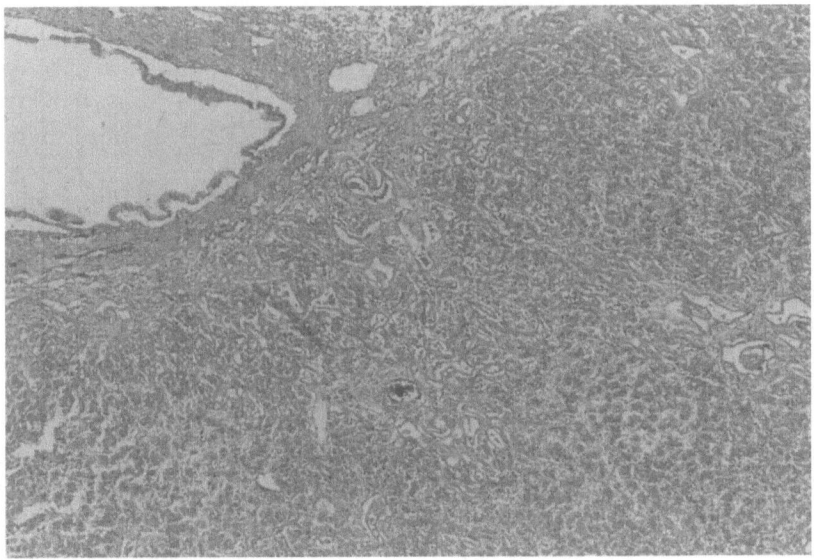

Figure 13.7 Light microscopic section of the liver of patient from Fig. 13.3. Bile duct proliferation appeared in both the protal areas and hepatic lobules. One duct is dilated to almost gross proportions, and small ducts contain inspissated bile. There is minimal fibrosis.

The hepatic cells are usually histologically normal. Although the liver in neonatal ADPKD is sometimes abnormal, with a similar histopathologic appearance, it is seldom as severely affected as in ARPKD.

In later years the hepatic abnormalities progress to hepatomegaly and portal hypertension, which dominate the clinical picture. Portal fibrosis may become more severe, and intrahepatic biliary ectasia may result in Caroli disease (intrahepatic communicating biliary ectasia). The ectatic ducts are visible as intrahepatic cysts[10]. Lieberman and colleagues[40] found, by microdissection and serial-section reconstructions, that the hepatic abnormality consistently involved the Hering ducts and adjacent interlobular ducts. Splenomegaly results from the portal hypertension, but other organs are seldom affected. Small pancreatic cysts occur rarely. Previous reports have suggested pulmonary cysts, but Bernstein[8] believes these to be misdiagnoses.

6. Genetics

Dalgaard[18] addressed the question of whether "congenital polycystic kidneys" could be due to chance occurrence. The frequency of affected sibs and the lack of affected parents led him to conclude that chance occurrence was highly unlikely and that the likely mode of transmission was "recessive heredity", but he could not prove his assumption.

Zerres and colleagues[66] discussed heredity at some length, indicating that recessive inheritance had been proved statistically. Studies of histopathologically homogeneous specimens have supported that conclusion[19,36]. There has been no reported case of the occurrence of ARPKD in more than one generation.

Two matters remain unclear, however. One is whether the neonatally lethal form of the disease is a separate genetic entity from those forms appearing in childhood survivors. Blyth and Ockenden[11] saw no overlap in individual sibships and proposed that each of their four clinical groups was due to a separate genetic abnormality. Others have been unable to substantiate the claim of intrafamilial homogeneity, finding discordance among affected sibs[24,32,66].

One of the difficulties with many of these studies is that they rely on retrospective review. Complications from severe hypertension undoubtedly caused death in a number of infants reported in the past. Speedy diagnosis and effective therapeutic measures applied today may lessen the infant mortality rate, and prospective studies may provide an answer to this question.

The other genetic question is whether congenital hepatic fibrosis and ARPKD are the same disease. Blyth and Ockenden[11] believed that "infantile" and "juvenile" patients, those who presented with primarily hepatic complaints, were each separate genetic entities. Landing and colleagues[31,39] also separated congenital hepatic fibrosis from polycystic kidney disease and found differences in renal abnormalities of the two groups. The deep collecting ducts were affected in congenital hepatic fibrosis, whereas the peripheral ducts were also affected in ARPKD.

The issue is complicated by the occasional appearance of Caroli disease in ARPKD livers, with similar histopathologic biliary abnormalities[8], and by the occurrence of an abnormality similar to that of congenital hepatic fibrosis in diseases other than ARPKD, e.g. hereditary tubulointerstitial nephritis (juvenile nephronophthisis)[13,30] and renal dysplasia[51].

Bernstein et al.[10] described an evolution with age of the hepatic abnormality in ARPKD, just as the renal abnormality changes with age. Increasing fibrosis may be enhanced by intercurrent cholangitis or intrahepatic cholestasis, and the separate groups defined by others[11,38,39] on histopathologic grounds may be resolved into the spectrum of a single entity.

7. Patient survival

Table 13.4 Survival of patients with ARPKD

Reference	Number of patients surviving/ Number of patients reported	Age of presentation	Age at report	Complications in group
10	1/6 ("neonatal")	1 month	8 months	Chronic renal failure
	2/4 ("infantile")	3, 6 month	1½ ,4 yrs	Chronic renal failure and portal hypertension
	1/1("infantile")	7 y	10 y	Polydipsia, polyuria
	3/5 ("juvenile")	1–5 y	> 12 y (pt 4 died at age 20)	Portal hypertension
3	8/14 (called "infantile PKD")	newborn and early infancy	3–18 y	Systemic and portal hypertension, chronic renal insufficiency[a], growth failure
	5/5 (called "congenital hepatic fibrosis")	newborn to 11 y	2–12.5 y	Systemic and portal hypertension; hepatomegaly alone
26	5/11	?(biopsies obtained at 4 d to 21 y)	27 months– 21 y	Systemic hypertension; chronic renal insufficiency[b]
16	15/17	1–12 month	6.1± 4.3 (SD) y	5/17:endstage renal disease 8–197 month; systemic hypertension, portal hypertension, (6/15)
35	14/73[c]	neonatal period	3–18 y	Systemic and portal hypertension, chronic renal insufficiency, hepatosplenomegaly, urinary tract infections

[a]one renal transplant at 7 1/2 y.
[b]one renal transplant at 21 y.
[c]includes patients with known affected sibling and those with no family history.

Just as the true incidence of ARPKD remains obscure, the prognosis of affected patients is also difficult to assess. In general, the accounting of neo-natally lethal cases has been provided by pathologists and the clinical descriptions of survivors provided by clinicians. Kääriäinen's data[32–34] constitute perhaps the most extensive population study, separating ARPKD from other cystic diseases and providing a comparison of the numbers of children dying and surviving (Table 13.4).

The Finnish data suggest that a minority of children, 19% in this series, survive, but this study, like most others, is retrospective. The patients had been cared for by several doctors, and their awareness of the severity of hypertension and its complications is not known. On the other hand, the data suggest that pulmonary complications were the primary causes of death, and that the degree of pulmonary insufficiency may be the discriminating feature for longterm survival. Only four of the 18 who survived the first month of age succumbed.

Cole et al.[17] found that only two of 17 patients surviving the first month died during the first year of life. Mean survival of the remainder was 6.1±4.3 (SD) years. Renal replacement therapy (dialysis and transplantation) will now prevent the deaths of those who would have otherwise succumbed from renal insufficiency.

8. Diagnosis and management

8.1 Recommendations for diagnostic evaluation in a child with suspected cystic kidney disease (Table 13.5)

Table 13.5 Diagnostic evaluation of suspected polycystic kidney disease in a child

Clinical presentation	Genetic studies
History and physical examination	Extended family history
Histologic studies	Radiographic assessment of family members
Radiographic assessment	Evaluation of genetic markers when appropriate

First, it is important that any potentially treatable disease, such as Wilms tumor, be discovered. Second, a specific diagnosis will help the clinician in subsequent clinical evaluation and early intervention for secondary complications. Third, most young parents are eager for genetic counselling.

Initial ultrasound examination of the kidneys and liver is helpful. In infancy or early childhood, the echogenicity of the kidneys usually exceeds that of the liver. The hyperechoic large kidneys may contain sonographically resolvable small cysts. The ultrasound examination will usually rule out multicystic renal dysplasia and hydronephrosis. Liver ultrasonography may detect dilated biliary ducts or more often be normal. As the child increases in age, increased hepatic echogenicity may be somewhat patchy, indicating areas of portal fibrosis.

Excretory urography is helpful in demonstrating that both kidneys function and excluding the diagnosis of multicystic renal dysplasia. The typical striations of contrast material in ectatic collecting tubules are typical of ARPKD, but this picture has also been recorded in ADPKD[17].

Neither ultrasonography nor excretory urography can differentiate glomerulocystic disease from ARPKD or ADPKD[65]. Other considerations, such as renal enlargement due to leukemia or lymphoma, will depend on associated clinical findings. Bilateral Wilms tumor and congenital nephrotic syndrome may be associated with large, hyperechoic kidneys in the neonate and may require tissue diagnosis.

Evaluation should include a history of any renal disease in the extended family, especially grandparents. Parents of children with renal cystic disease may be young enough that signs or symptoms of ADPKD have not yet developed. After careful consideration of the ethical implications of investigating asymptomatic individuals, renal and hepatic ultrasound examinations may be undertaken in available family members, including siblings, parents and grandparents. The presence of one or more cysts in both kidneys or three cysts in a single kidney is thought to be suggestive, and five or more in both kidneys diagnostic of polycystic kidney disease[23]. The absence of any cystic disease in all of the family members makes the diagnosis of ARPKD more probable. In the event that family members do have cystic disease, confirmation by gene linkage markers[54] may be helpful in identifying dominant disease. Thorough counselling of the family members should always precede performance of the tests.

Ultimately, the diagnosis of ARPKD may require tissue examination. Since hepatic involvement is virtually invariable in ARPKD, examination of both liver and renal tissue is optimum. It can be argued that renal tissue should also be examined for complete exclusion of tumors and other rare entities that clinically mimic ARPKD.

The diagnosis of renal cystic disease may also be suspected during prenatal ultrasound examination. The differentiation among types of cystic disease may not be made reliably, however. ADPKD may present as increased echogenicity alone or with definable cysts[50]. ARPKD may also have both of these features[22,55]. It should be noted that *in utero* diagnosis may not be possible until the third trimester[3]. Oligohydramnios and renal masses are sometimes demonstrable in some fetuses during the second trimester, but normal-looking kidneys at that time do not insure absence of disease[3,59]. Oligohydramnios may not be apparent until 20–21 weeks. Finally, most of the reports of *in utero* diagnosis are of severe disease with oligohydramnios; mild involvement with relatively normal renal function may not be detected until after birth.

8.2 Pulmonary complications

Respiratory distress with inadequate ventilation is the first and most formidable complication with which the clinician has to deal. Pulmonary insufficiency is the most frequent cause of death in neonatal ARPKD. Artificial ventilatory measures may be successful in treating newborns with pneumonia, pneumothorax, or pneumomediastinum, whereas babies with pulmonary hypoplasia rarely survive. Those few with hypoplastic lungs who eventually are weaned from ventilatory support may succumb to later pulmonary complications. The degree of pulmonary hypoplasia is difficult to assess at birth, becoming clear only when respiratory insufficiency develops.

8.3 Hypertension

The frequency of hypertension, even in the young infant, has been emphasized earlier in this chapter. The hypertension may be severe and difficult to control. Several agents are available, and multiple drugs must often be employed[16]. This author has had considerable success with captopril, even in patients with relatively normal peripheral renin activity. It is important, however, to utilize the principle of making the regimen as simple as possible, starting with a converting enzyme inhibitor or a primary vasodilator and adding diuretics and βadrenergic blocking agents as necessary to control sodium retention and reflex tachycardia.

Hypertension appears to persist in many patients, necessitating longterm treatment. Nevertheless, some patients do appear to have diminution or even cessation of the high blood pressure[43]. Thus, clinicians should not take the condition for granted. There is little information on the effects of longterm antihypertensive treatment on linear growth, but it stands to reason that agents such as diuretics, which lead to losses of electrolytes, might interfere with normal growth.

8.4 Kidney and liver function

Although some infants are born with poor renal function that results in oligohydramnios and Potter facies, many children have normal glomerular function for their age. The major early and continuing abnormality is tubular, one of abnormal urinary concentrating ability[2,34]. The maximum urinary osmolality is commonly under 500 mOsm/kg. Acid–base balance and serum electrolytes are often normal[34], but others have asymptomatic metabolic acidosis due to impaired secretion of acid.

Proximal tubule functions appear to be normal. Aminoaciduria does not occur[2,34], and phosphaturia occurs only with progressive renal failure[2].

The glomerular filtration rate is variable. Many have normal values for many years[2,17,24,34], but others may develop renal insufficiency within months[17,34,38]. Cole *et al.*[17] noted that calculated creatinine clearances rose throughout the first six months of life in those children surviving beyond one month of age. A few children had values within the normal range at twelve months of age, and some did not develop renal insufficiency until later childhood.

Proteinuria and hematuria have also been reported[17,34]. Hematuria can be gross, sometimes arising from blood-filled cysts, as in ADPKD[27]. Pyuria occurs[40,53], often without significant bacteriuria. With the likelihood that only one or a few cysts are infected, one must maintain a strong index of suspicion that the pyuria is, in fact, a sign of infection.

Progressive portal hypertension occurs in many of these patients. Esophageal varices become symptomatic. Hypersplenism causes leukopenia and thrombocytopenia. On the other hand, hepatocellular function is rarely deranged[40]. Occasionally, isolated enzyme values are mildly elevated[34], but hepatic failure has not been recorded in the literature. Hyperbilirubinemia and elevated serum enzyme values should prompt consideration of concomitant cholangitis.

8.5 Renal insufficiency

The rate at which renal function fails is highly variable. When oligohydramnios occurs, renal function in the infant is likely to be severely compromised. These infants, however, usually succumb to pulmonary insufficiency. Some infants may develop endstage renal failure during the first year of life, but the majority of those children surviving the first month of life do not develop severe renal insufficiency until later childhood or adolescence. Therefore, the clinician is well-advised to observe the children closely and to measure renal function often. Secondary hyperparathyroidism may begin when glomerular filtration rate falls under 50% of normal, resulting in renal osteodystrophy. Reduction in phosphorus intake may prevent or reverse the secondary hyperparathyroidism, particularly in the older child. On the other hand, dietary intake of phosphorus in the young child must be maintained at a level sufficient for growth of new cells. Calcium and Vitamin D supplementation and phosphorous binders, such as calcium carbonate or citrate, may also be necessary, particularly as renal insufficiency progresses.

Growth failure occurs, usually when glomerular function is 20–40% of normal. The factors leading to growth failure are presumably the same as in other kinds of childhood renal diseases, although rarely would proteinuria be a contributing factor. The factors, which are poorly understood, include inadequate caloric intake secondary to anorexia or a rigid dietary regimen, uncontrolled hypertension and acidemia. Close attention to these possibilities can lead to early intervention.

Even when hypertension has not been an early phenomenon, it may occur late and become severe before symptoms develop. Glomerular function is then commonly below 20% of normal, and sodium and water retention cause the hypertension. Dietary sodium and fluid restriction are indicated, and diuretic therapy may be needed. Below this level of renal function, these therapies may be inadequate, necessitating initiation of dialysis.

Anemia also occurs at this level of renal function and, until recombinant erythropoietin is approved for use in children, packed red cell transfusions are the only treatment. Most children have few symptoms as long as the hemoglobin does not fall below 7 g/dl.

Treatment for endstage renal failure by dialysis or renal transplantation is usually required when glomerular filtration rate reaches 10–15% of normal. Both hemodialysis and continuous ambulatory peritoneal dialysis may be utilized; even in the child with considerable renomegaly and hepatosplenomegaly there may be sufficient peritoneal space to dialyse adequately. On the other hand, neither method of dialysis provides an optimum lifestyle or maximizing of growth potential. Renal transplantation is an effective treatment, providing a more normal lifestyle for children. Bilateral nephrectomies or splenectomy may be necessary prior to transplantation. Massively enlarged kidneys, renin-mediated hypertension, or evidence of urinary tract infection would prompt nephrectomy; hypersplenism with leukopenia or thrombocytopenia makes appropriate post-transplantation immunosuppressive medication difficult and thus prompts splenectomy. The patients with ARPKD who receive renal transplants do well, depending on the complications of their congenital hepatic fibrosis.

8.6 Congenital hepatic fibrosis

Complications arise from progressive portal hypertension. Abdominal girth may be exceptional, particularly if liver, spleen and the kidneys are greatly enlarged. Esophageal varices are common; hemorrhoids may develop later. Hypersplenism causes attendant leukopenia and thrombocytopenia. Splenectomy may be necessary, leading to increased susceptibility to overwhelming bacterial infections. Pneumococcal vaccine and penicillin prophylaxis are warranted in post-splenectomy patients.

Hypersplenism may hinder post-transplantation immunosuppressive medication. One other complication of portal hypertension is the production of many intra-abdominal collateral vessels, which interfere with pretransplantation nephrectomy.

8.7 Infections

Urinary tract infections are relatively common[17,34], and many necropsy specimens have shown evidence of pyelonephritis[11]. Since the cysts change in shape and configuration and become more globular, urinary tract infections may be as common as in ADPKD[27]. One infected cyst may provide insufficient bacteria to provide bacteriuria, and the clinical index of suspicion must remain high. Pyuria, even in the absence of significant bacteriuria, should prompt treatment with agents known to penetrate cyst walls effectively[27]. Lethal cholangitis has also been reported[10] and should be considered in the febrile patient.

References

1. Alvarez F, Bernard O, Brunelle F, Hadchouel M, Leblanc A, Odièvre M and Alagille D. Congenital hepatic fibrosis in children. J Pediatrics 1981, 8, 370–375.
2. Anand SK, Chan JC and Lieberman E. Polycystic disease and hepatic fibrosis in children. American Journal of Diseases of Children 1975, 129, 810–813.
3. Argubright KF and Wicks JD. Third trimester ultrasonic presentation of infantile polycystic kidney disease. American Journal of Perinatology 1987, 4, 1–4.
4. Avner ED. Renal cystic disease. Insights from recent experimental investigations. Nephron 1988, 48, 89–93.
5. Avner ED, Ellis D, Jaffe R and Bowen A. Neonatal radiocontrast nephropathy simulating infantile polycystic kidney disease. Journal of Pediatrics 1982, 100, 85–87.
6. Bacopoulos C, Karpathios T, Nicolaidou P, Thomaidis T and Matsaniotis N. Acute infantile pyelonephritis simulating polycystic kidney disease. Journal of Pediatrics 1979, 94, 437–438.
7. Baxter TJ. Cysts arising in the renal corpuscle: a microdissection study. Archives of Diseases of Childhood 1965, 40, 455–463.
8. Bernstein J. Polycystic disease. In: Edlemann CM, ed., Pediatric Kidney Disease. Boston: Little, Brown and Co 1978, 562–565.
9. Bernstein J. and Meyer R. Parenchymal maldevelopment of the kidney. In: Brennerman-Kelley, ed., Practice of Pediatrics. Vol. 3, Hagerstown: Harper and Row, 1967.
10. Bernstein, J, Stickler, GB and Neel IV. Congenital hepatic fibrosis: evolving morphology. APMIS 1988, 4 (Suppl), 17–26.
11. Blyth H and Ockenden BG. Polycystic disease of kidneys and liver presenting in childhood. Journal Medical Genetics 1971, 8, 257–284.
12. Boal DK and Teel RL. Sonography of infantile polycystic kidney disease. American Journal of Roentgenology 1980, 135, 575–580
13. Bodaghi E, Honarmand MT and Ahmadi M. Infantile nephronophthisis. International Journal of Pediatrics and Nephrology 1987, 8, 207–210.
14. Bosniak MA and Ambos MA. Polycystic kidney disease. Seminars in Roentgenology 1975, 10, 133–143.
15. Chilton SJ and Cremin BJ. The spectum of polycystic disease in children. Pediatric Radiology 1981, 11, 9–15.
16. Cole BR. Renal cystic disease. In: Nelson NM, ed., Current Therapy in Neonatal–Perinatal Medicine. Philadelphia: BC Decker, 1985, 289–294.
17. Cole BR, Conley SB and Stapleton FB. Polycystic kidney disease in the first year of life. Journal of Pediatrics 1987, 111, 693–699.
18. Dalgaard OZ. Bilateral polycystic disease of the kidneys. A follow-up of two hundred and eighty-four patients and their families. Acta Medica Scandinavica 1957, Suppl 328, 1–251.

19. Elkin M and Bernstein J. Cystic diseases of the kidney: radiological and pathological considerations. Clinical Radiology 1969, 20, 65–82.
20. Evans JB, Shapeero LG and Roscelli JD. Infantile glomerulonephritis mimicking polycystic kidney disease. Journal of Ultrasound in Medicine 1988, 7, 29–32.
21. Fitch SJ and Stapleton FB. Ultrasonic features of glomerulocystic disease in infancy: similarity to infantile polycystic kidney disease. Pediatric Radiology 1976, 16, 400–402.
22. Fong KW, Rahmani MR, Rose TH, Skidmore MB and Connor TP. Fetal renal cystic disease: sonographic–pathologic correlation. American Journal of Roentgenology 1986, 146, 767–773.
23. Gabow PA, Ikle DW and Holmes JH. Polycystic kidney disease, prospective analysis of nonazotemic patients and family members. Annals of Internal Medicine 1984, 101, 238–247.
24. Gang GL and Herrin JT. Infantile polycystic disease of the liver and kidneys. Clinical Nephrology 1986, 25, 28–36.
25. Gleason DC, McAlister WH and Kissane J. Cystic disease of the kidneys in children. Radiology 1967, 100, 135–145.
26. Grantham J, Geiser JL and Evan AP. Cyst formation and growth in autosomal dominant polycystic kidney disease. Kidney International 1987, 31, 1135–1152.
27. Grantham J and Slusher SL. Management of renal cystic disorders. In: Suki WN and Massry SG, ed., Therapy of Renal Diseases and Related Disorders. Boston: Martinus Nijhoff, 1985: 383–404.
28. Grossman H, Winchester PH and Chisar FV. Roentgenographic classification of renal cystic disease. American Journal of Roentgenology 1968, 319–331.
29. Gwinn JL and Landing BH. Cystic diseases of the kidneys in infants and children. Radiol Clin North America 1968, 6, 191–204.
30. Harris HWJr, Carpenter TO, Shanley P, Rosen S, Levey RH and Harmon WE. Progressive tubulointerstitial renal disease in infancy with associated hepatic abnormalities. American Journal of Medicine 1986, 81, 169–176.
31. Helczynski L, Wells TR, Landing B and Lipsey AI. The renal lesion of congenital hepatic fibrosis–pathologic and morphometric analysis with comparison to renal lesions of infantile polycystic disease. Pediatric Pathology 1984, 2, 441–455.
32. Kääriäinen H. Polycystic kidney disease in children: a genetic and epidemiologic study of 82 Finnish patients. Journal of Medical Genetics 1987, 24, 474–481.
33. Kääriäinen H, Jääskeläinen J, Kirirsaari L, Koskimies O and Norio R. Dominant and recessive polycystic kidney disease in children: classification by intravenous pyelography, ultrasound and computed tomography. Pediatric Radiology 1988, 18, 45–50.
34. Kääriäinen H, Koskimies O and Norio R. Dominant and recessive polycystic kidney disease in children: evaluation of clinical features and laboratory data. Pediatric Nephrology 1988, 2, 296–302.
35. Kerr DNS, Harrison CV, Sherlock S and Walker RM. Congenital hepatic fibrosis. Quarterly Journal of Medicine 1961, 30, 91–118.
36. Kissane JM. Congenital malformations. In: Heptinstall RH, ed., Pathology of the Kidney. Boston: Little, Brown & Co. 1966, 1974: 69–119.
37. Lambert PP. Polycystic disease of kidney. Archives of Pathology 1947, 44, 34–58.
38. Landing BH, Wells TR and Claireaux AE. Morphometric analysis of liver lesions in cystic diseases of childhood. Human Patholoyg 1980, 11 (Suppl): 549–560.
39. Landing BH, Wells TR, Reed GB and Narayan MS. Diseases of the Bile Ducts in Children. Baltimore: Williams and Wilkins, 1973, 480.
40. Lieberman E, Salinas-Madrigal L, Gwinn JL, Brennan LP and Fine RN. Infantile polycystic disease of the kidneys and liver. Medicine 1971, 50, 277–318.
41. Lundin PM and Olow I. Polycystic kidneys in newborns, infants and children, a clinical and pathological study. Acta Paediatrica 1961, 50, 185–200.
42. McAlister WH, Seigel MJ, Shackelford G, Askin F and Kissane JM. Glomerulocystic Kidney. American Journal of Roentgenology 1979, 133, 536–538.

43. Melson GL, Shackelford GD, Cole BR and McClennan BL. The spectrum of sonographic findings in infantile polycystic kidney disease with urographic and clinical correlations. Journal Clinical Ultrasound 1985, 13, 113–119.

44. Metreweli C and Garel C. The echogenic diagnosis of infantile polycystic disease. Annals of Radiology 1980, 23, 103–107.

45. Osathanondh V and Potter EL. Pathogenesis of polycystic kidneys: historical survey. Archives of Pathology 1964, 77, 459–465.

46. Osathanondh V and Potter EL. Pathogenesis of polycystic kidneys. Type I due to hyperplasia of interstitial portions of collecting tubules. Archives of Pathology 1964, 77, 466–473.

47. Potter E. Pathology of the Fetus and the Newborn. Chicago: Year Book Medical, 1952.

48. Potter EL. Normal and Abnormal Development of the Kidney. Chicago: Year Book Medical, 1972.

49. Premkumar A, Berdon WE, Levy J, Amodio J, Abramson SJ and Newhouse JH. The emergence of hepatic fibrosis and portal hypertension in infants and children with autosomal recessive polycystic kidney disease: initial and follow-up sonographic and radiographic findings. Pediatric Radiology 1988, 18, 123–129.

50. Pretorius DH, Lee ME, Manco-Johnson ML, Weingast GR, Sedman AB and Gabow PA. Diagnosis of autosomal dominant polycystic kidney disease in utero and in the young infant. Journal of Ultrasound in Medicine 1987, 6, 249–255.

51. Proesmans W, Moerman Ph, Depraetere M and vanDamme B. Association of bilateral renal dysplasia and congenital hepatic fibrosis. International Journal of Pediatrics and Nephrology 1986, 7, 113–116.

52. Rahill WJ and Rubin MI. Hypertension in infantile polycystic renal disease. Clinical Pediatrics 1972, 11, 232–235.

53. Rall JE and Odel HM. Congenital polycystic disease of the kidney: review of the literature, and data on 207 cases. American Journal of Medical Science 1949, 218, 399–407.

54. Reeders ST, Bruening MH, Corney G, Jeremiah SJ, Khan PM, Davies KE, Hopkinson DA, Pearson PL and Weatherall DJ. Two genetic markers closely linked to adult polycystic kidney disease on chromosome 16. British Medical Journal 1986, 292, 851–853.

55. Reilly KB, Rubin SP, Blanke BG and Yeh M-N. Infantile polycystic kidney disease: a difficult antenatal diagnosis. American Journal Obstetrics and Gynecology 1979, 133, 580–582.

56. Reznik VM, Griswold WT and Mendoza SA. Glomerulocystic disease: a case report with 10 year follow-up. International Journal of Pediatrics and Nephrology 1982, 3, 321–323.

57. Rizzoni G, Loirat C, Levy M, Milanesi C, Zachello G and Mathieu H. Familial hypoplastic glomerulocystic kidney. A new entity? Clinical Nephrology 1982, 18, 263–268.

58. Sedman A, Bell P, Manco-Johnson M, Schrier R, Warady BA, Heard EO, Butler-Simon N and Gabow P. Autosomal dominant polycystic kidney disease in childhood: a longtitudinal study. Kidney International 1987, 31, 1000–1005.

59. Simpson JL, Sabbagha RE, Elias S, Talbot C and Tamura RK. Failure to detect polycystic kidneys in utero by second trimester ulltasonography. Human Genetics 1982, 60, 295.

60. Sommerschild HC, Langmark F and Mauraseth K. Congenital hepatic fibrosis: Report of two new cases in review of the literature. Surgery 1973, 73, 53–58.

61. Stapleton FB, Hilton S, Wilcox J and Leopold GR. Transient nephromegaly simulating infantile polycystic disease of the kidneys. Pediatrics 1981, 67, 554–557.

62. Stapleton FB, Magill HL and Kelly RR. Infantile polycystic kidney disease: an imaging dilemma. Urological Radiology 1983, 5, 89–94.

63. Taxy JB and Filmer RB. Glomerulocystic kidney: report of a case. Archives in Pathology and Laboratory Medicine 1976, 100, 186–188.

64. Walker FC Jr, Loney LC, Root ER, Melson GL, McAlister WH and Cole BR. Diagnostic evaluation of adult polycystic kidney disease in childhood. American Journal of Roentgenology 1984, 142, 1273–1277.

65. Worthington JL, Shackelford GD, Cole BR, Tack ED and Kissane JM. Sonographically

detectable cysts in polycystic kidney disease in newborn and young infants. Pediatric Radiology 1988, 18, 287–293.

66. Zerres K, Volpel M-C and Weiss H. Cystic kidneys: genetics, pathological anatomy, clinical picture and prenatal diagnosis. Human Genetics 1984, 68, 104–135.

14
Acquired Renal Cystic Disease

I. Ishikawa

Abstract

Acquired renal cystic disease (ARCD) is a recently described disorder. It was appreciated only after the survival of patients with endstage renal disease was prolonged by dialysis. ARCD is a bilateral multiple cystic disorder occurring in patients whose original renal illness was unrelated to cystic disease. The most important influence on its development is the duration of uremia. Moderate impairment of renal function (e.g. serum creatinine levels of 3 mg/dl) is necessary before cyst growth begins. Subsequent dialysis treatment, regardless of whether it is hemodialysis or peritoneal dialysis, accelerates cyst development. The overall incidence of acquired cysts among dialysis patients is 40–50%. Males generally show more extensive cystic changes than females. Successful renal transplantation results in cyst regression.

Key words   Acquired renal cystic disease;
Endstage renal disease;
Hemodialysis;
Epithelial hyperplasia;
Renal cell carcinoma;
Renal neoplasm.

1. Introduction

In 1977, Dunnill *et al.*[22] described a new disorder, bilateral multiple renal cystic disease. It occurred among hemodialysis patients whose original illness had not been cyst related. Fourteen of 30 hemodialysis patients had developed renal cysts. Six of these went on to display renal tumors and one subject died of metastatic cancer. A survey of the classical German literature has revealed that cystic changes in endstage renal disease were described by Frerichs in 1851[29] and by Peipers in 1894[84]. In the English literature, Bell (1935)[6] and Tuttle *et al.* (1971)[99] reported the presence of multiple small cysts in diseased kidneys. However, Dunnill *et al.*[22] are the first to present results from systematic autopsies of kidneys of dialysis patients and to place emphasis on tumor formation in acquired renal cystic disease (ARCD).

    Long-term hemodialysis is complicated by, and has been associated with, many diseases: dialysis amyloidosis, dialysis dementia and aluminium osteo-arthropathy. ARCD now joins the list. Understanding its process of development and the, as yet, undetermined true biological activity of tumors in ARCD is very important because the incidence of tumor formation is so high. ARCD has more epithelial hyperplasia and tumor formation than does autosomal dominant polycystic kidney disease (ADPKD)[39].

One recommended title for this disease is "acquired cystic disease in hemodialysis patients"[35], but cysts also develop in patients treated with continuous ambulatory peritoneal dialysis (CAPD)[46].

2. Definition of acquired renal cystic disease

ARCD is a bilateral cystic disorder that develops in kidneys with endstage renal disease. The degree of cystic transformation required to allow diagnosis of ARCD is somewhat arbitrary. In a series of autopsy studies, Dunnill et al.[22] did not define this condition precisely and described it simply as "extensive bilateral cystic disease". Other studies were more specific; Feiner et al.[28] stipulated that at least 40% of renal parenchyma should be replaced by multiple cysts, while Gehrig et al.[33] suggested that at least 25% of parenchyma need be changed.

On the other hand, in clinical investigations using computed tomography or sonographic examination, Ishikawa et al.[48], Bommer et al.[11] and Mickisch et al.[76] all proposed that ARCD is present if at least one cyst is present in either kidney. Jabour et al.[62] suggested that 3, Narasimhan et al.[80] that 4, and Levine et al.[69] that 5 cysts need to be detected in one kidney for the diagnosis of ARCD. Unfortunately, sometimes even computed tomography (CT) scan or ultrasonic study does not reveal small, multiple cysts. A kidney larger than expected, taking into account the duration of dialysis and presence of one or more cysts on renal imaging, may be sufficient.

3. Frequency of acquired renal cystic disease

The incidence of ARCD in patients undergoing hemodialysis is 40–50% in reports[4, 11,17,22,24,27,28,32,36,37,43,66,76,78,79,98] of autopsy and surgical specimens and of clinical studies. Ishikawa[47] collected findings from 1,103 patients examined in various reports and ascertained that 47.1% of them had acquired cystic disease, a further 4.8% had renal tumors, and 1.5% had renal cell carcinomas (Table 14.1). Similarly, in 601 subjects (some of whom were represented in Ishikawa's study), Grantham and Levine[37] found that 43.6% had acquired cystic disease and 7.1% had renal tumors. The occurrence of acquired cystic disease depends on the duration of hemodialysis[48,69], whether the patient has had a successful renal transplantation[49], and whether the subject is male or female[50]. However, the incidence does not depend on the patient's age[48], treatment modality (i.e. hemodialysis or CAPD), or the nature of the original

Kidney Volume after Induction of Chronic Hemodialysis

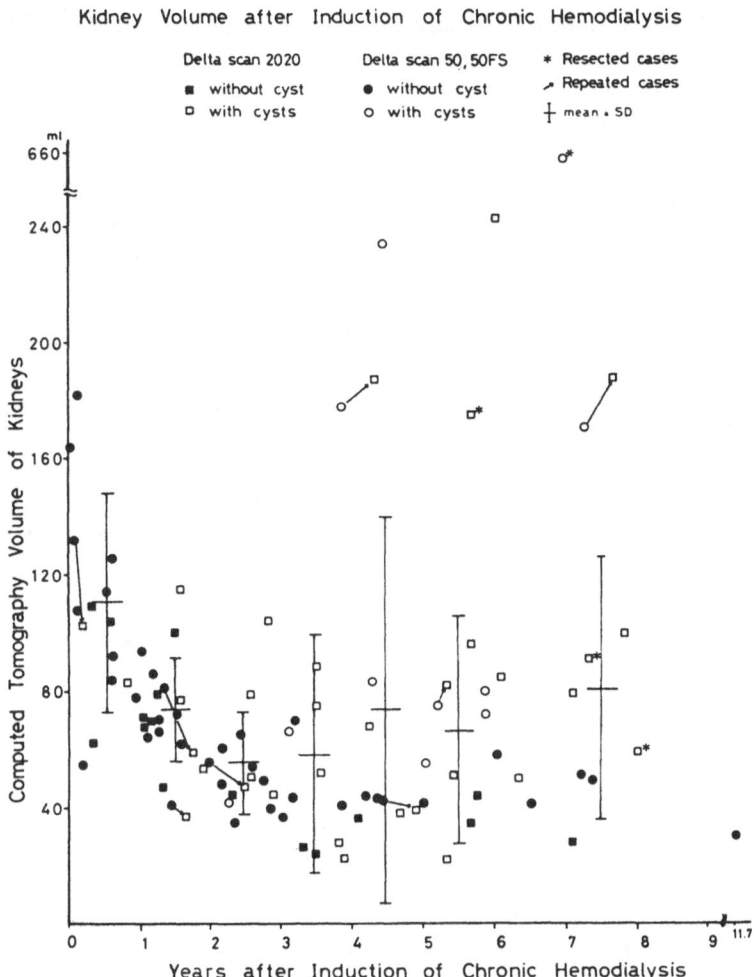

Figure 14.1 Kidney volume and development of acquired cysts after the start of chronic hemodialysis. Volume decreases gradually up to 3 years of dialysis. Thereafter volume may increase, in some cases due to cyst development. Almost all enlarged kidneys have multiple cysts. Three out of four resected specimens revealed renal cell carcinoma. (Reprinted from Ishikawa I, Saito Y, Onouchi A, *et al*. Development of acquired cystic disease and adenocarcinoma of the kidney in glomerulonephritic chronic hemodialysis patients. Clin Nephrol 1980; 14:1–6. With permission).

disease[22]. ARCD develops prior to dialysis in 7–22% of patients[76,80] whose serum creatinines exceed 3 mg/dl[11,76].

Ishikawa *et al.*[48] found that the volume of the kidney, determined by computed tomography (CT), decreases in the first 3 years of dialysis and then increases as the rate of cyst formation increases (Fig. 14.1). Specifically, the incidence of cyst formation in patients with less than 3 years of hemodialysis is 43.5%, after more than 3 years, 79.3% (Fig.14.1).

From 8 Japanese reports, 109 (90.0%) of 121 hemodialysis patients who had been treated for more than 10 years had ARCD. A further 6 (5%) exhibited renal cell carcinoma. Clearly, patients undergoing hemodialysis for more than 10 years have a higher incidence of acquired cysts and adenocarcinomas of the kidney.

Recently, ARCD was described with a 33% incidence in children on dialysis[68]. In general, there are no differences in occurrence of acquired cysts among patients with different renal diseases[22]. Some authors[76] have described a low incidence of ARCD in association with diabetic nephropathy and reflux nephropathy and a high incidence with analgesic nephropathy. However, diabetic and perhaps reflux patients tend to receive shorter courses of dialysis. Others[51] have suggested that autosomal dominant polycystic kidney disease (ADPKD) treated with dialysis may be complicated by ARCD because enlargement of polycystic kidneys is seen occasionally. Whether such a possibility exists, however, is uncertain. ADPKD usually is excluded when ARCD is studied.

Geographic differences have been pointed out by Gardner and Evan[30] and Hughson et al.[44]. Frequencies of ARCD and renal tumors are said to be higher in Japan than in the United States, probably because of differences in the definition of ARCD and the higher number of screening tests carried out for renal malignancy in Japan.

4. Pathologic findings

4.1 Gross findings

Kidneys with acquired cysts are usually smaller than normal kidneys[22]. Occasionally they are normal in size, rarely enlarged to the size of polycystic kidneys[33,48]. The mean weight of a kidney with acquired cysts is around 70 g, range 51–250 g[22,27,28,33], whereas ADPKD kidneys are typically more than 800 g[28]. Gehrig et al.[33] investigated cases of ARCD in large kidneys (340–1,250 g/kidney), and found frequent renal cell carcinomas and hematomas.

Multiple small cysts are visible on the external and cut kidney surfaces (Figs. 14.2, 3).

They are present mainly in the cortex, but occur in the corticomedullary region or occasionally in the medulla. Sixty percent of the cysts are smaller than 0.2 cm[52], but may vary from microscopic to 2–3 cm in diameter[22,43]. There are two extreme variations in pattern: uniformly small cysts less than 2–4 mm in diameter and, at the other extreme, relatively large cysts reaching diameters of 2–3 cm. Cysts commonly contain clear fluid; occasionally they are hemorrhagic.

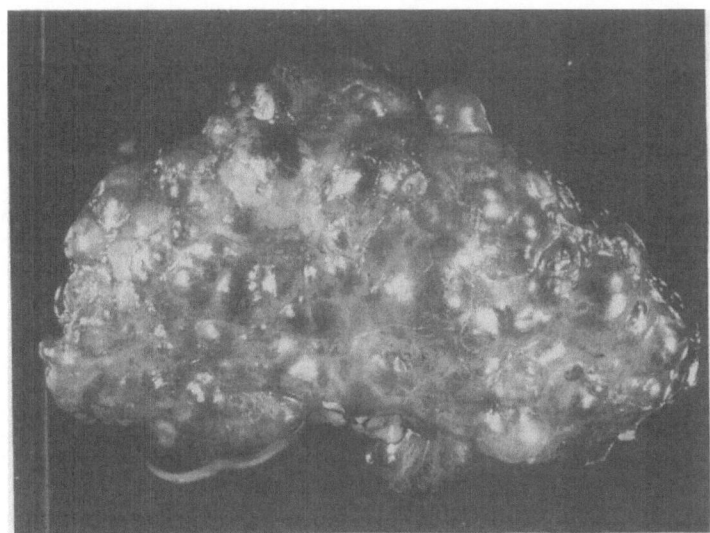

Figure 14.2 Outer surface of acquired renal cystic disease in a 31-year-old male on hemodialysis for 7 years and 8 months. Small cysts up to 2 cm appear as a bunch of grapes. The kidney size is larger than expected given the duration of hemodialysis. A renal cell carcinoma 2.5 cm in diameter was present inside this kidney. No protrusion of tumor is observed in this case. (Scale indicates 0.5 .cm intervals).

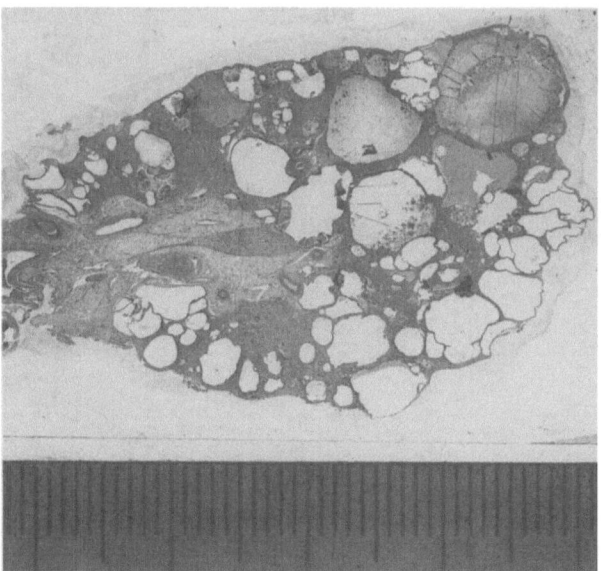

Figure 14.3 Axial cut section of acquired renal cystic disease in a 47-year-old male on hemodialysis for 10 years and 7 months (Hematoxylin–eosin stain). (Scale indicates 1 mm intervals). The renal parenchyma is replaced by multiple cysts. Almost all cysts are less than 5 mm in diameter. Cysts are present in the cortex and medulla. Some contain protein-rich fluid.

Proteinaceous stones of a brown-black color are sometimes found in the renal pelvic region.

4.2 Microscopic findings

Many cysts are multilocular and most are lined with flat or cuboidal epithelial

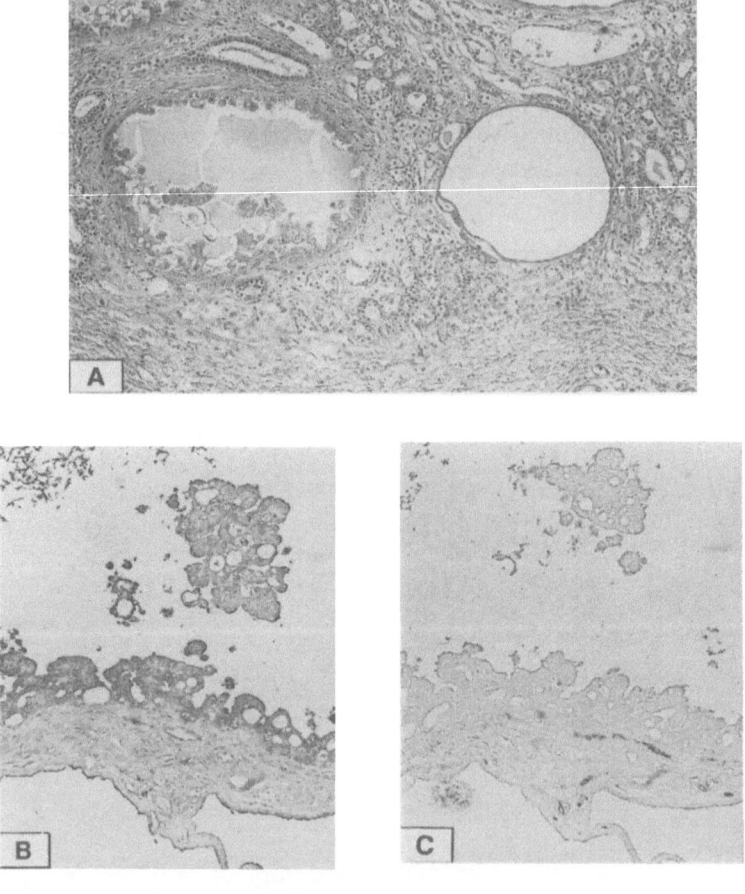

Figure 14.4 Acquired renal cystic disease. A. The right cyst was lined by single layered flat epithelium. The left cyst contained multilayered hyperplastic epithelium, a so-called atypical cyst (x 68). Lectin conjugate reactivity is positive for *Tetragonolobus lotus*, an indicator of proximal tubule origin, (14.4B), but is negative for peanut lectin, an indicator of distal tubule origin, (4C) in one cyst with multilayered hyperplastic epithelia (above) and in two cysts with single layered flat epithelia (below) (x 170). (4B and 4C: Reprinted from Ishikawa I, Horiguchi T, Shikura N. Lectin peroxidase conjugated reactivity in acquired cystic disease of the kidney. Nephron 1989; **51**: 211–214. With permission).

cells in a single layer[22]. However, in 60% of ARCD cases, at least some of the cysts are lined with hyperplastic multilayered epithelium with clear or granular cytoplasm. Hughson *et al.*[43] have labelled these "atypical cysts" and have found them in up to one-third of patients undergoing hemodialysis (Figure 14.4).

Renal tumors are observed in 5–10% of dialysis patients[16,31,33,37,47]. Tumors occur in three basic forms[22,23]: papillary, tubular and solid. Papillary

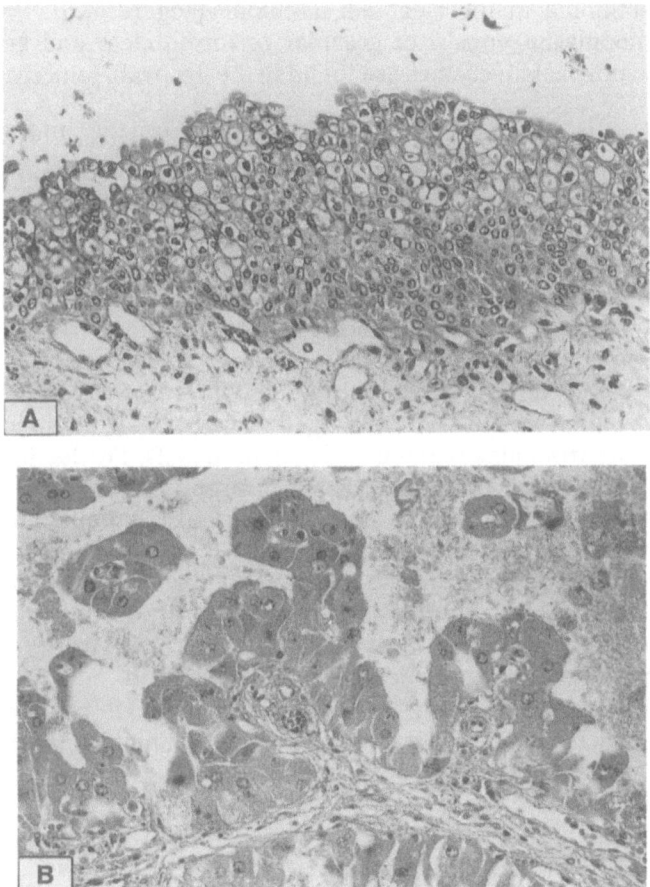

Figure 14.5 Acquired renal cystic disease. A. Hyperplastic epithelia with clear cytoplasm in an atypical cyst in a 47-year-old male on hemodialysis for 10 years and 7 months (× 70). B. Hyperplastic epithelium with granular cytoplasm in an atypical cyst seen in the same patient (×170).

tumors with small, hyperchromatic nuclei and scanty basophilic cytoplasm are characterized by projections into the cyst cavity. Some cells have a rather foamy or eosinophilic granular appearance. Tubular tumors have cells with granular eosinophilic or foamy cytoplasm (Figure 14.5).

Solid tumors are composed of cells with foamy or acidophilic cytoplasm.

Most tumors are small and are considered to be adenomas. More than one type may be present in a single kidney[22]. Some 1.5% of dialysis patients exhibit renal cell carcinoma, mainly clear cell carcinoma (Figure 14.6).

These neoplasms consist of granular or mixed clear and granular cell types[22]. Calcium oxalate crystals are found in the cyst wall, lumen and interstitium.

Electron microscopic study of cyst linings by Mickisch et al.[76] revealed two types of cells, one with an apical brush border configuration and the other with a cobblestone appearance. These correspond to the proximal and the distal or collecting tubules, respectively. However, the authors did not indicate which was the main component of the most frequently seen cysts.

Using microdissection, Feiner et al.[28] reported that cysts begin as fusiform tubular dilatations or saccular outpouchings and communicate with tubules. Glomeruli remained attached to tubules in some nephrons.

Recently a histochemical study examined the reactivity of lectin–peroxidase conjugate in ARCD[53]. The investigation was carried out on paraffin-embedded samples from nine patients with acquired cysts. The lectins used were *Tetragonolobus lotus* (winged pea), with a high affinity for proximal tubules, and *Arachis hypogaea* (peanut), with a high affinity for distal tubules and collecting ducts. Ninety-two percent of the cysts with single layered epithelia and 88% of those with multilayered epithelia were tetragonolobus-positive and peanut-negative (Fig. 14.4). Similar results were obtained for most solid adenomas and renal cell carcinomas. These results indicate that most acquired cysts have characteristics suggesting a proximal tubular origin.

In conclusion, the data suggest that the epithelium affected in ARCD has a high tendency toward proliferation and that cells lining cysts derive mainly from the proximal tubular cells of the kidney.

5. Natural history of acquired renal cystic disease

The most important factor in cyst development is the duration of uremia/dialysis[48]. This observation has been confirmed by Levine et al.[69], Turani et al.[98] and Gehrig et al.[33]. Kidneys and cysts enlarge with time (Fig. 14.7).

Kidney size and cysts regress after successful renal transplantation (Figure 14.8).

Vaziri et al.[101], Levine et al.[69], Minar et al.[78] and Thompson et al.[93] have presented similar findings. The phenomenon of regression suggests that uremia or hemodialysis plays an important role in the pathogenesis of cysts and tumors in ARCD. After transplantation, some native kidneys retain cysts, either because of mild elevations of serum creatinine levels or because they are unrelated simple cysts, cystadenomas or non-communicating acquired cysts[49]. If uremia is present, even the transplanted kidney may develop acquired cysts[19].

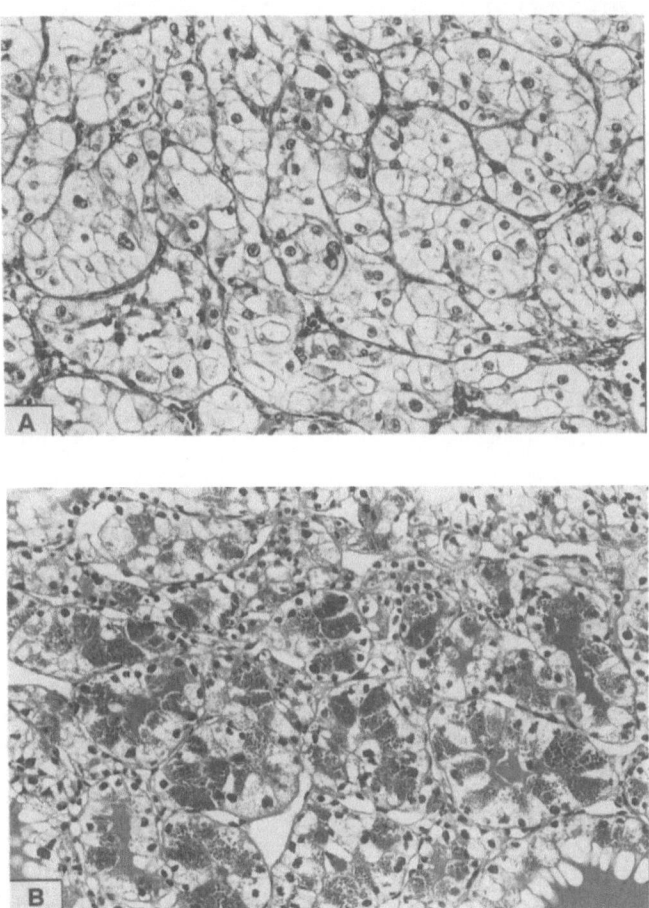

Figure 14.6 Renal cell carcinoma complicated by acquired renal cystic disease. A. Clear cell carcinoma in a 28-year-old male on hemodialysis for 5 years and 8 months (x 170). B. Granular and clear cell carcinoma in a 31-year-old male on hemodialysis for 7 years and 8 months (x 170).

ARCD has gender-related differences in its occurrence and manifestation[50]. Males tend to have more acquired cysts and thus greater kidney enlargement (Fig. 14.9A), whereas young females tend not to develop cysts even after several years of dialysis (Fig. 14.9B). Post-menopausal females also seem to be disposed towards exhibiting cystic changes. A relationship between gender and

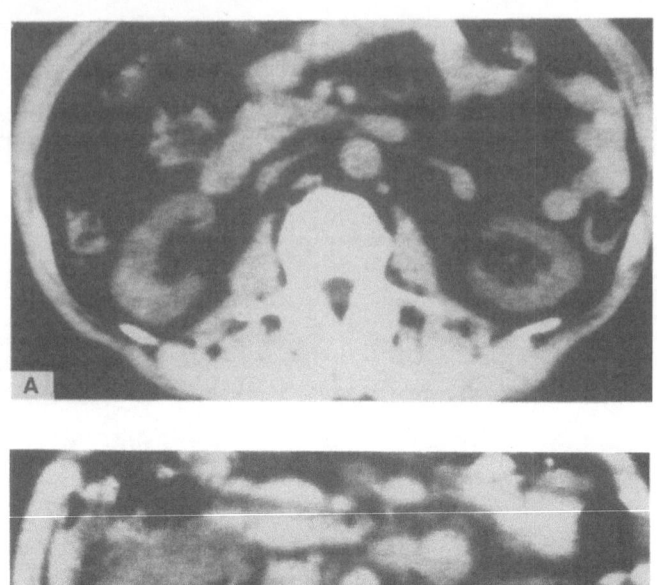

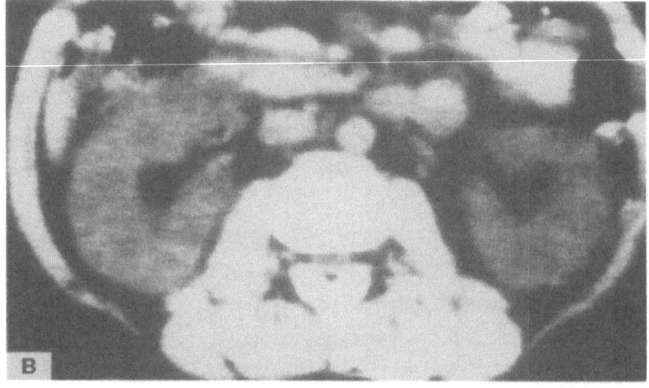

Figure 14.7 Effect of hemodialysis and uremia on acquired cysts. A. Computed tomography reveals small kidneys in a 49-year-old male. B. Four years and 4 months later, both kidneys have enlarged 3.6 times due to progressive development of acquired cysts. The cysts are too small (less than 5 mm in diameter) to be visible. The low density of the kidney is attributable to the presence of multiple small cysts. (Reprinted from Ishikawa I. Uremic acquired cystic disease of kidney. Urology 1985; 26: 101–108. With permission).

ARCD has been confirmed by Narasimhan *et al.*[80] and Smith *et al.*[90], but has been found not significant by Mickisch *et al.*[76], Thomson *et al.*[94] and Bellinghieri *et al.*[7]. No correlation has been found between age and ARCD.

6. Etiology and pathogenesis

The etiology of cyst formation in kidneys with ARCD is unknown, but various theories have been advanced. In 1977, Dunnill *et al.*[22] suggested, from pathological findings, that obstruction of tubules by interstitial fibrosis or calcium oxalate crystals might cause cysts to form. Recently, Ono *et al.*[83] reported that

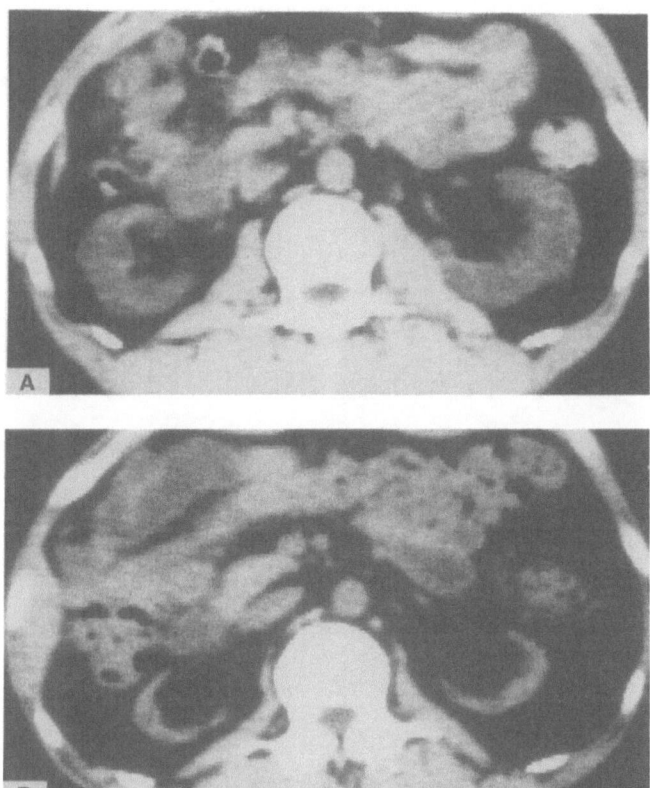

Figure 14.8 Successful renal transplantation in acquired renal cystic disease. A. A 35-year-old male on hemodialysis for 8 years, one month before transplantation, the kidneys are slightly enlarged because of acquired cysts. B. Three months after transplantation, both kidneys are smaller, one-sixth of previous size, because of cyst regression. (Reprinted from Ishikawa I. Uremic acquired cystic disease of kidney. Urology 1985; 26: 101–108. With permission).

the oxalate levels in plasma from patients with acquired cysts are higher than in patients without cysts. They found no relation between the levels of oxalate and the duration of hemodialysis, although the incidence of ARCD correlated with the length of hemodialysis treatment. The role of oxalate in the patho-genesis of ARCD is unclear.

Fayemi *et al.*[27] have proposed that cysts result from ischemia in diseased kidneys. Linke *et al.*[71] suggested nephron obstruction by $beta_2$-microglobulin fragments. However, only two out of eight dialysis patients developed $beta_2$-microglobulin-derived amyloid in tubules[54]. Electron microscopic examin-ation of cyst walls has suggested that partial obstruction is caused by the micropolyps that result from focal hyperplasia in tubular epithelia[30]. It also has

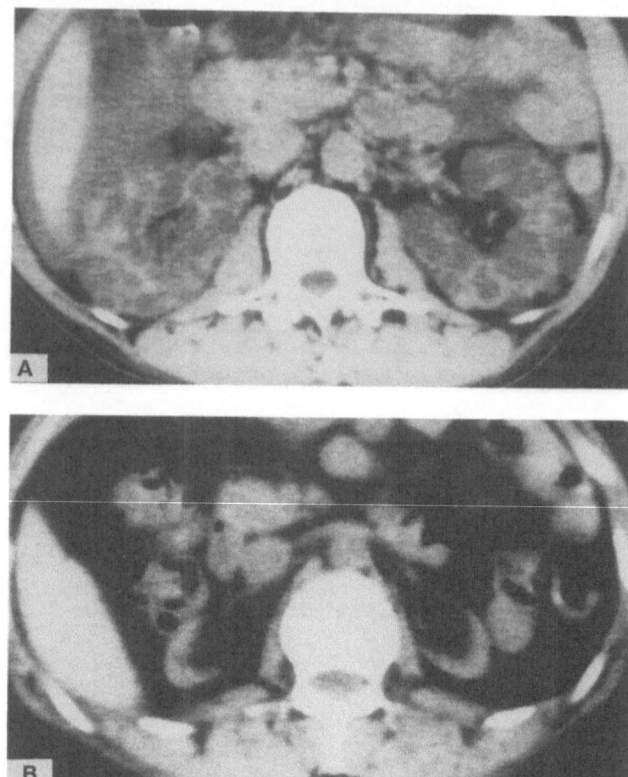

Figure 14.9. Sex differences in acquired renal cystic disease. A. A 42-year-old male on hemo-dialysis for 10 years exhibits extensive multiple cystic transformation of both kidneys (enhanced CT scan). B. A 36-year-old female on hemodialysis for 11 years has severe contracted kidneys without acquired cysts.

been suggested that the accumulation of uremic metabolites contributes to the development of ARCD[1].

The incidence and degree of cystic transformation appear closely related to the duration of dialysis and uremia[48,50]. Successful renal transplantation leads to regression of ARCD and to reduction in the size of affected native kidneys[49]. CAPD patients develop ARCD[20,46,62,64,80,90,94] as do hemodialysis patients. These results suggest that neither hemodialysis *per se* nor the equipment and chemicals associated with hemodialysis (such as plasticizers, formaldehyde and dimethylnitrosamine) are the sole causes of cyst formation.

Epithelial hyperplasia and development of renal tumors and renal cell carcinomas characterize ARCD[9,22]. Decrease in nephron mass due to the original renal disease stimulates hyperfiltration in the remnant nephrons[33,37]. Thus, the increased delivery of some kind of potentially cystogenic, renotrophic growth factor may stimulate epithelial hyperplasia causing abnormal outward cell growth, and sometimes micropolyps that lead to cyst formation[30,33,37,47]. This compound could be a uremic metabolite such as polyamine or nitrogenous waste[1]. Progressive hyperplasia also has a greater likelihood of causing renal cell carcinoma.

Another hypothesis states that cysts represent an extreme example of dilatation, and that the disorder is the result of the normal aging process[32]. Gardner[32] has suggested that neutrophil infiltrates and interstitial reactions – an injury-response mechanism – should be investigated in the future with reference to ARCD.

7. Cyst fluid analysis

Grantham and Levine[37] have found that the pH values of cyst fluid in patients with ARCD are lower than corresponding values in their blood. In a 1985 study, Ishikawa et al.[55,56] demonstrated that acquired cysts have a unique chemical composition. Fluid from 26 acquired cysts in three patients who had received hemodialysis for more than 10 years showed a mean composition as follows: sodium 144.7 mEq/l, potassium 6.5 mEq/l, urea nitrogen 52.4 mg/100 ml, creatinine 63 mg/100 ml, beta$_2$-microglobulin 1.22 mg/l and protein 0.45 g/100 ml. Creatinine levels were higher than those found in either ADPKD or simple cysts, while beta$_2$-microglobulin was lower than in simple cysts.

Table 14.1 Cyst fluid/serum ratio of sodium, creatinine and β_2-microglobulin

| | | Cyst fluid/serum ratio | | |
	Case	Sodium	Creatinine	β_2-microglobulin
ARCD	1	1.096± 0.036[a] (7)[b]	7.058± 1.311 (7)	0.053± 0.057 (7)
	2	1.087± 0.027 (10)	5.363± 1.396 (10)	0.060± 0.022 (8)
	3	1.038± 0.012 (9)	6.855± 1.465 (9)	0.004± 0.008 (7)
	mean	1.072± 0.036 (26)	6.332± 1.581 (26)	0.040± 0.008 (22)
Simple	4	1.075	0.867	1.864
cysts	5	1.077	1.000	0.846
	6	1.109	1.375	
	mean	1.087± 0.019 (3)	1.081± 0.263	1.355 (2)
ADPKD	7	1.007	0.843	–

[a], mean±SD
[b], numbers of cyst examined.

The cyst fluid-to-serum ratio of sodium was 1.07 in acquired cysts (Table 14.1), which is equivalent to ratios determined for simple cysts and for some cysts from patients with ADPKD. A fluid-to-serum ratio of 1.0 suggests that acquired cysts should be classified as proximal cysts, as defined by Huseman *et al.*[45].

On the other hand, the cyst fluid-to-serum ratio of creatinine was 6.3 in the case of acquired cystic disease, 1.1 in studies on simple cysts and 0.8 in patients with ADPKD (Table 14.1). This high creatinine ratio in the presence of a sodium ratio near unity is characteristic of acquired cystic disease and may reflect creatinine secretion.

Levels of beta$_2$-microglobulin were very low in acquired cysts in comparison to respective serum levels, and the fluid-to-serum ratio varied from 0 to 0.06[56] (Table 14.1). In contrast, the ratio ranged between 0.8 and 1.9 for simple cysts, with beta$_2$-microglobulin levels being almost the same in cysts as in serum. In ADPKD, beta$_2$-microglobulin levels in proximal cysts equalled those levels found in serum. On the basis of these chemical analyses, we propose that an acquired cyst is a local dilatation of a functioning proximal tubule. Altered hyperplastic epithelium allows reabsorption of beta$_2$-microglobulin into the serum, and creatinine is either secreted or trapped. Another possibility is that creatinine in the cyst fluid is derived from glomerular filtration, and is concentrated by isosmotic sodium chloride reabsorption in proximal cysts. The continuity of acquired cysts with tubules has been established by nephron dissection[28]. On the other hand, the absence of connection with tubules in 8 out of 11 cysts (72.7%) in subjects with ADPKD[38] indicates that the cyst fluid here probably derives from net transepithelial secretion.

8. Clinical manifestations and differential diagnosis

The incidence of ARCD is high[22,48]; about one-half of all dialysis patients have the disease[31,37,47]. Usually, there are no symptoms. The most common, when present, are gross hematuria, flank pain, renal colic[11,12,28,86], palpable renal enlargement[36,86], fever and rising hematocrit[36,88]. The exact incidence of gross hematuria in ARCD is unknown. A small proportion of dialysis patients (8 of 134 cases in one series) complained of this symptom[57]. Gross hematuria is usually painless, occasionally accompanied by flank or back pain. Although it usually disappears spontaneously within a few days, hematuria may be continuous and cause anemia. Severe renal bleeding, especially when accompanied by retroperitoneal bleeding, causes anemia, hypotension and shock[63,86]. Some patients with gross hematuria have the additional complication of proteinaceous matrix[12] or calcium oxalate ureteral stone formation. Both cyst rupture and ureteral stone formation cause flank pain or renal colic. Kidneys may become palpable, especially if there is a large hematoma or renal cell carcinoma. Work-up of an unknown fever sometimes reveals ARCD complicated by renal cell carcinoma. Rapid increase in hematocrit suggests the presence of ARCD[33,36,86,88]. In addition, there has been one report of hypoglycemia in a patient with acquired cysts and renal cell carcinoma[5]. Rarely, metastatic cancer is the initial symptom with subsequent discovery of ARCD and renal cell carcinoma[73]. Hypercalcemia is rare[95].

Because intrarenal calcification correlates with the duration of hemodialysis and the severity of cyst formation, plain abdominal roentgenograms showing multiple calcifications in the kidney area should suggest ARCD. The diagnosis of ARCD is usually made by computed tomography (CT) scan[48,69] or ultrasonography[67]. Both CT scan and sonography are valuable methods for detecting cysts greater than 5 mm in diameter[48] and cysts greater than 3 mm in diameter in the outer periphery of the kidney. Of the two, sonographic examination is less expensive and is easier to conduct. However, small diseased kidneys are difficult to image because they register as hyperechoic and are deeply embedded in fat tissue[69]. Furthermore, sonography is not useful for the detection of small tumors less than 1 cm in diameter[69]. CT scan is usually necessary for the diagnosis of ARCD and its complications[17,62,69,80]. Narasimhan et al.[80] reported that ARCD can be ruled out if both CT scan and sonography are negative for cysts. It can be further assumed that if a CT scan indicates the existence of a kidney cyst in a patient undergoing dialysis and if the kidney is slightly enlarged, ten or more cysts of less than 0.5 cm in diameter may also be present[52]. Furthermore, fulfilling classic CT and ultrasonic criteria of cysts is not a diagnostic requirement, since this is often impossible when cysts are less than 5 mm in diameter[62,90].

An important consideration is the diagnosis of the complications of ARCD. In practice, the differentiation of renal tumors from cysts containing hemorrhagic or high protein fluids is of paramount importance. A combination of CT scan and sonography, or dynamic CT scan and magnetic resonance imaging (MRI) is recommended. Dynamic or enhanced CT increases the detectability of ARCD and tumors. Angiography is less often used, but is still important, especially for preoperative examinations.

Differentiation of ARCD from other cystic kidney disorders, such as ADPKD, is sometimes necessary. Kidneys with ADPKD are usually larger than those affected by ARCD. Cyst size also is larger and can reach a diameter of 7 cm; those associated with ARCD have an upper limit of 2–3 cm. Because of overlap in the appearances of the two conditions, it may also be necessary to search for cysts in the liver and to examine the family history. Knowledge of the patient's own history is, of course, of paramount importance. Liver cysts do not develop in association with ARCD, but isolated liver cysts, unassociated with the original kidney disease, may cause great diagnostic confusion. Simple cysts in elderly people usually are larger than those encountered in ARCD. Thus, if a patient receiving hemodialysis has multiple cysts, including some 5–7 cm in diameter and projecting from the outer contour of the kidney, the large projecting cysts are likely to be simple cysts. Additional evidence that favors ARCD over ADPKD or simple renal cyst is the demonstration of high creatinine and low beta$_2$-microglobulin levels in cyst fluid[55,56].

Other cystic kidney diseases such as nephronophthisis–medullary cystic disease complex, unilateral multicystic kidney and hereditary syndromes should be distinguishable from ARCD on the basis of their symptoms and radiographic appearances.

9. Cyst hemorrhage as a complication of ARCD

Renal hemorrhage is a major complication of ARCD[22]. It occurs in two forms: the first is bleeding into the kidney or urinary tract. As it is common to see bloody cysts in excised or autopsied kidneys with ARCD, the incidence of intracystic bleeding without gross hematuria is probably high[47]. The second form is retroperitoneal or perirenal bleeding due to rupture of cysts. In the past, extrarenal hemorrhage in dialysis patients has been described as idiopathic retroperitoneal bleeding[75,99]. Patients present with symptoms of back or flank pain, sometimes hypotension and shock. Physical examination may reveal guarding or muscular spasm after retroperitoneal bleeding. CT scans are used for evaluation[70]. Heparin therapy and platelet dysfunction aggravate gross hematuria.

Different complications of cyst rupture have been described[22,86]. Recurrent bleeding in the retroperitoneal space and recurrence of bleeding after vascular embolization have been reported[63]. Soffer et al.[91] described a patient with one kidney affected by renal cell carcinoma and the other by bleeding due to cyst rupture. In our own experience, we have seen a case of intrarenal and perirenal bleeding precipitated by severe coughing.

Levine et al.[70] managed four out of seven bleeding episodes conservatively, with bed rest and analgesia. Conservative treatment of renal bleeding is initially preferred. If blood transfusion cannot maintain blood pressure, therapeutic renal embolization or nephrectomy can be attempted. Nephrectomy is recommended if renal cell carcinoma has not been specifically excluded, because the risk of undetected renal cell carcinoma is high in patients with retroperitoneal bleeding. Gehrig et al.[33] found that 8 of 24 patients with ARCD and symptomatic renal bleeding had renal cell carcinoma on pathologic examination.

10. Renal cell carcinoma as a complication of ARCD

This is the most important complication of ARCD[22]. Renal cell carcinomas usually represent the full histological spectrum of cyst to tumor development, with papillary, tubular and solid adenomas. Distinction between adenoma and highly differentiated renal cell carcinoma is very difficult, and has sometimes been made arbitrarily on the basis of tumor size, i.e. tumors more than 3 cm in diameter are considered to be renal cell carcinomas. However, Bennington[8] and Dunnill *et al.*[23] have argued that basing the diagnosis of malignancy on the size of the tumor may be fallacious. Feiner *et al.*[28] have described renal cell carcinomas only 1.0 cm in diameter. Almost all investigators[8,16,23,44,47] acknowledge that small tumors may be incipient malignancies. In this sense, ARCD, arising as a consequence of epithelial hyperplasia, is a premalignant condition.

Surveys of the literature reveal a variable incidence of histopathologically identified renal cell carcinomas. Ishikawa found them in 17 of 1,103 hemodialysis patients (1.5%) (Table 14.2)[47].

Table 14.2 Incidence of acquired renal cystic disease and renal cell carcinoma in patients with hemodialysis

Duration of dialysis	Cases	Acquired renal cystic disease	Renal cell carcinoma	Source
Less and more than 10 years	1,103	520 (47.1%)	17 (1.5%)	25 reports in world literature
More than 10 years only	121	109 (90.0%)	6 (5.0%)	8 Japanese reports

His subjects were from Japan and abroad, and there were no differences in incidence ascribable to geographic location[47]. Grantham and Levine[37] found 43 renal neoplasms, not clearly identified as to malignancy, in 601 hemodialysis patients (7.1%) and Bretan *et al.*[16] noted 39 renal neoplasms among 429 dialysis patients (9%) in overlapping surveys of the literature. Gehrig *et al.*[33] found seven renal cell carcinomas among 490 hemodialysis patients (1.4%). Some difficulties arise in determining the incidence of malignancy because of uncertain characterization of tumors.

As of December 1984, 78 cases of renal cell carcinoma in patients undergoing hemodialysis and in endstage patients who had not been treated by dialysis were reported from outside Japan[47]. Among them, five showed metastasis. Only 18 cases were reported as complications of ARCD, perhaps because the relationship had been recognized only relatively recently. Subsequently, as of April 1988, 44 cases of renal cell carcinoma were reported in hemodialysis patients outside Japan[3,10,16,33,34,41,42,62,70,73,74,77,81,82,86,87,89,90,91,100], with 12 of them metastasizing and 33 of 37 complicating ARCD.

We conducted a nationwide survey in Japan on the incidence of renal cell carcinoma in hemodialysis patients[58–60].

As shown in Table 14.3, 34 renal cell carcinomas were reported in 1982[58], 37 in 1984[59], 48 in 1986[60] and 115 in 1988 (unpublished data). The mean age of these 234 Japanese patients was 50.5 ± 11.9 years, which is less than that of the general population. Fifty (21.4%) were in the third and fourth decades of life. Mean duration of hemodialysis treatment was 82.5 ± 51.0 months. Males accounted for 79.9% (Table 14.3). ARCD was found in 174 of 226 patients (77.0%) harboring renal cell carcinoma.

Table 14.3 Renal cell carcinoma in hemodialysis patients (Questionnaire studies performed in Japan)

	1982[a]	1984	1986	1988	Total
Number of renal cell carcinoma (cases)	34	37	48	115	234
male	25	31	40	91	187
female	9	6	8	24	47
Mean age (years)	47.9	49.6	50.5	51.4	50.5 ± 11.9[b]
Mean duration of hemodialysis (months)	49.4	73.6	83.9	94.6	82.5 ± 51.0
Presence of ARCD (%)	23/32 (71.9)	20/31 (64.5)	39/48 (81.3)	92/115 (80.0)	174/226 (77.0)
Number of patients with metastases (%)	7/33 (21.2)	8/33 (24.2)	10/48 (20.8)	17/106 (16.0)	42/220 (19.1)
Number of hemodialysis patients	42,223 (Dec. '81)	53,017 (Dec. '83)	66,310 (Dec. '85)	80,553 (Dec. '87)	

[a] year of study
[b] mean$\pm$SD

The incidence of renal cell carcinoma in dialysis patients has been compared with that found in the general population. Gardner[31] estimated that the rate of occurrence is seven times higher in dialysis patients with ARCD. In another study, MacDougall *et al.*[73], in the United States, found that the annual incidence rate of renal cell carcinoma is 0.27% in dialysis patients, compared to 0.005% in the general population. Thus, in the dialysis setting, the risk of developing this cancer is increased by 50 times.

In Japan, the incidence of renal cell carcinoma in the general population is thought to be three cases per 100,000 per year. However, a survey, which was conducted between 1986 and 1988 and which monitored the progress of 51,469 dialysis patients (total number = 73,537; 70% replied), showed that 61 patients developed renal cell carcinoma in 1987 (unpublished data). This corresponds to a frequency of 119 in 100,000 per year or 40 times the expected rate. Furthermore, all 51,469 cases surveyed had not been screened for cancer, so it is possible that many renal cell carcinomas were undiagnosed, perhaps making the actual frequency even higher.

As of April 1988, 356 cases of renal cell carcinoma (122 outside Japan and 234 from Japan) have been reported in patients undergoing hemodialysis; some of the reports from outside Japan included those with endstage kidney not treated by dialysis. Among them, 59 cancers, 17 outside Japan[10,17,22,27,33,41,47,73,82,86,87,89,90,95,100] and 42 from Japan, had metastasized. Based on these findings, clinical malignancy of renal cell tumors in dialysis patients can hardly be regarded as rare.

Deaths due to metastasis were reported by Dunnill et al.[22] in one patient, Fayemi et al[27] in one, Ratcliffe et al.[86] in one, Olsson et al.[82] in two, Vandenbroucke et al.[100] in one, Cho et al.[17] in one, MacDougall et al.[73] in one, Thomson et al.[95] in one, Boileau et al.[10] in one, Smith et al.[90] in one, Hamilton et al.[41] in one, and Ishikawa in 24 – a total of 36 patients.

Case reports have detailed instances of both rapidly and slowly growing tumors. Tumors 6 cm in size have been identified only a year after negative screening, tumors have grown four-fold within months, and tumors smaller than 2 cm have metastasized. In contrast, other studies have found that renal tumors grew little during 6 months of follow-up, and that tumor size did not change significantly over a 2-year period[69]. Thus, both slowly and rapidly growing tumors may be present in patients with ARCD.

It is extremely difficult to assess the potential for malignancy of any given tumor. Electron microscopic examination, ^{31}P magnetic resonance spectrometry, DNA cytometry and transplantability to nude mice may be useful for such evaluation in the future[16]. The frequency of aneuploidy in ARC-associated tumors is less than the frequency of aneuploidy in the general population of renal cell carcinomas. Perhaps ARCD-associated tumors do have a lower malignant potential[21]. However, matched control studies, comparing tumors at the same stage of development, are required before this conclusion can be confirmed.

Torrence et al.[96] have suggested that cyst fluid in ARCD contains a growth factor.

While renal cell carcinoma is asymptomatic in most dialysis patients, gross hematuria, flank and back pain, fever, anemia and erythrocytosis may be observed. These signs and symptoms occurred in 35 of 234 cases of renal cell carcinomas identified in our questionnaires. Several respondents to our questionnaire reported deformation of the stomach, as revealed radiographically. In advanced stages, emaciation and flank deformation, and in rare cases, metastases may be the initial symptoms or signs of malignancy in the kidney. At present, the best non-invasive diagnostic tool to demonstrate small carcinomas is the CT scan[69], either enhanced or dynamic. Contrast-enhancement of a renal mass during the vascular phase of dynamic CT scan may show it to be a hypervascular renal cell carcinoma. Fine needle aspiration biopsy offers a second approach to diagnosis[81].

Two hypotheses have been advanced to account for renal cell carcinoma in dialysis patients[16,33,37,44,47]. One cites impairment of immune surveillance as a consequence of breakdown of cell-mediated immunity during uremia. The other cites oncogenic stimulation by a carcinogen, possible candidates for which include retained uremic metabolites, aliphatic amines, polyamines and renotrophic factors. Possible exogenous influences, which have yet to be implicated, include plasticizers, formaldehyde, nitrates, nitrites, chloramines, synthetic androgens and smoking. Local, intrarenal features, such as cystic degenerative changes, scarring, repeated infection and trauma of the urinary tract, may also play a role[33].

There appear to be two trends in the occurrence of renal cell carcinomas in hemodialysis patients[58]. One is cancer development in young patients in whom malignancy is associated with cyst formation and long periods of hemodialysis. The other is cancer development in a group of older patients in whom there was little relation between renal cell carcinoma and cyst formation, and in whom the duration of hemodialysis was short.

Twenty to thirty percent of the reported renal cell carcinomas in dialysis patients are not associated with acquired cysts (Table 14.3). In such cases, hyperplastic epithelia or microscopic atypical cysts found in non-cystic segments of tubules are likely sources of renal cell carcinoma[9,44]. Renal cell carcinoma has been reported in patients with endstage kidney disease not treated by dialysis[10] and in patients receiving continuous ambulatory peritoneal dialysis. Cotterell et al.[20], Viner et al.[102], and Smith et al.[90] present one example each, Trabucco et al.[97] present two, and Fallon et al.[26] present three, while three cases have been reported from Japan.

ARCD may regress after successful transplantation[49]. It is suggested that the post-transplantation incidence of renal cell carcinoma in the native kidneys may be low. Evidence to the contrary exists. Renal cell carcinomas in native kidneys following transplantation have been detected by Penn[85] in 58 cases; by Isiadinso et al.[61], Vaziri et al.[101], Struve et al.[92], Griffin et al.[40], Arias et al.[2] and Faber et al.[25] in one case each; and in three cases from Japan. Three examples of metastatic renal cell carcinomas developing after renal transplantation have been supplied by Griffin et al.[40], Faber et al.[25] and Ludmerer and Kissane[72].

Urothelial tumors have also been noted in dialysis patients. Chung-Park et al.[18], Boon and Michael[14], Banerjee et al.[3] and the present author in the 1988 survey, each discovered one or two transitional cell carcinomas. An apparent association between renal cell carcinomas and urothelial tumors cannot be entirely discounted. A common tumorigenic factor may play a role in the pathogenesis of both.

In summary, male patients and relatively young patients of both sexes who undergo longterm dialysis treatment and develop extensive cystic disease have a high risk of developing renal cell carcinoma.

11. Other complications

11.1 Infection of acquired cysts

Ishikawa et al.(1980)[57] reported renal abcesses in 1.7% of patients with ARCD. In 1987, Bonal et al.[13] described cyst infection and renal abscess in two dialysis patients. These patients exhibited long-standing fever and septicemia.

11.2 Ureteral stone

The level of beta$_2$-microglobulin in ARCD cyst fluid is very low compared to that present in serum[56]. However, stones with a matrix derived from beta$_2$-microglobulin are often seen in collecting ducts of the kidney or in the renal pelvis in dialysis patients. These stones are typically fragile, brown-black in color, and 2–3 mm in diameter. Bommer *et al.*[12] and Koga *et al.*[65] have reported that the incidence of matrix stones in dialysis patients is approximately 10%, but whether these tubular obstructions are the cause of ARCD[71] is unknown. Stones may cause ureteral obstruction and transient hydronephrosis. When either of these events occurs, the patient may complain of flank pain and experience gross hematuria[12,65].

11.3 Increase in hematocrit

It has been thought that cystic kidneys cause anemia to remit in some patients receiving dialysis. Erythrocytosis may be the first clue to renal cell carcinoma. There have been many reports of a rapid increase in hematocrit, and subsequent discovery of extensive cystic transformation[36,86,88]. Conversely, dialysis patients with few renal cysts have also been found to have high hematocrits. Therefore, some investigators[69,76,79,80,101] believe that raised hematocrit and cyst development are not always observed together and, when they are, they result from coincidence. Long-term dialysis may itself be associated with improvement of anemia. To prove a relationship between these two phenomena, secretion of erythropoietin by cyst epithelial cells must be demonstrated.

12. Screening

The incidence of renal cell carcinoma in dialysis patients is high, and the cancers may be asymptomatic. Therefore, screening is essential if carcinomas are to be detected early. There is, however, no consensus on the effectiveness of screening programmes, because there has been little agreement concerning the frequency and level of metastatic activity of renal cell carcinoma in dialysis patients[15,44,64,76,94,102].

We[47,48] have recommended yearly CT scans for all dialysis patients. We found that many patients, especially older ones, developed renal cell carcinomas within 3 years of hemodialysis. Based on the high incidence (79.3%) of ARCD after 3 years of hemodialysis[48], Levine *et al.*[69] have suggested that a baseline examination by CT scan or sonography be carried out after 3 years of hemodialysis treatment. Generally, once ARCD is diagnosed, repeated CT scans or sonograms are recommended on a yearly basis[16,33,37,47,69].

A patient with a renal mass less than 2–3 cm in diameter or with symptoms such as gross hematuria or flank pain should be examined every 3–6 months. Screening is expensive. According to Gardner et al.[30], in 1984 it cost $20,800 to detect one case of renal cell carcinoma. In practice, as Gardner[32] mentioned, usually only those patients who display symptoms are screened in the United States. This may also be true in the majority of dialysis centers in Japan, so it is probable that many renal cell carcinomas are missed. In any case, all kidney transplant candidates should be screened for the presence of renal masses prior to transplantation.

13. Nephrectomy

Not all patients in whom screening reveals acquired cysts need be nephrectomized. The procedure is necessary only when there are complications such as hemorrhage and tumor[47]. Urinary tract bleeding usually subsides spontaneously, but if a patient develops uncontrollable bleeding, therapeutic embolization or nephrectomy should be considered.

Nephrectomy should be carried out if a tumor exceeds 2–3 cm in diameter[16,33,47,69]. Malignant tumors are hypervascular, sometimes have calcification and are seen in CT scans to have irregular contours and patches with irregular density. Renal masses less than 3 cm in diameter rarely metastasize. Our questionnaire results, however, indicated that no hard and fast rule applies. We found examples of metastases from a tumor 1.2 cm in diameter and several tumors of 3 cm in diameter. Therefore, we take the presence of a tumor more than 2 cm in diameter to be an indication for nephrectomy. Tumors of this size can be diagnosed readily by CT scan. If it is not certain that a mass is malignant, but if it grows during the follow-up period or if the patient exhibits relevant symptoms, nephrectomy is recommended irrespective of the tumor size. If a patient with tumor or suspected tumor is a renal transplant candidate, nephrectomy should be performed regardless of the tumor size.

Nephrectomy is performed only on the side with a renal mass unless the patient is a transplant candidate. Bilateral nephrectomy complicates subsequent dialysis therapy due to hypotension and severe anemia.

References

1. Annotation; Acquired cystic disease of the kidney. Lancet 1977, 2, 1063.
2. Arias M, de Francisco ALM, Ruiz L, Val F, Gonzalez M and Zubimendi A. Acquired renal cystic disease and renal adenocarcinoma in a long term renal transplant patient. International Journal of Artificial Organs 1986, 9, 271–272.
3. Banerjee SS, Harris M, Lupton EW and Ackrill P. Acquired cystic disease of kidney with multiple renal and urothelial neoplasms. Journal of Clinical Pathology 1985, 38, 864–867.
4. Bansal VK, Ing TS, Daugirdas JT, Chejfec G, Gandhi VC, Geis WP and Hano JE. Cystic change in the kidneys of maintenance hemodialysis patients. ASAIO Journal 1980, 3, 65–68.

5. Bansal VK, Brooks MH, York JC and Hano JE. Intractable hypoglycemia in a patient with renal failure. Archives of Internal Medicine 1979, 139, 100–102.
6. Bell ET. Cystic disease of the kidneys. American Journal of Pathology 1935, 11, 373–423.
7. Bellinghieri G, Savica V, Mallamace A and Consolo F. Evidence for acquired cystic disease during hemodialytic treatment. Clinical Nephrology 1986, 26, 216.
8. Bennington JL. Renal adenoma. World Journal of Urology 1987, 5, 66–70.
9. Bernstein J, Evan AP and Gardner KD Jr. Epithelial hyperplasia in human polycystic kidney diseases: Its role in pathogenesis and risk of neoplasia. American Journal of Pathology 1987, 129, 92–101.
10. Boileau M, Foley R, Flechner S and Weinman E. Renal adenocarcinoma and end stage kidney disease. Journal of Urology 1987, 138, 603–606.
11 Bommer J, Waldherr R, van Kaick G, Strauss L and Ritz E. Acquired renal cysts in uremic patients – in vivo demonstration by computed tomography. Clinical Nephrology 1980, 14, 299–303.
12. Bommer J, Ritz E and van Kaick G. Acute flank pain in dialysed patients. Demonstration of hydronephrosis by computer tomography. Journal of Dialysis 1980, 4, 109–114.
13. Bonal J, Garalps A, Lauzurica R, Serra A, Romero K and Inaraja L. Cyst infection in acquired renal cystic disease. British Medical Journal 1987, 295, 25.
14. Boon NA and Michael J. Multiple neoplasia in a patient on dialysis presenting with haematuria. British Journal of Urology 1984, 56, 96–103.
15. Brendler CB, Albertsen PC, Goldman SM, Hill GS, Lowe FC and Millan JC. Acquired renal cystic disease in the end stage kidney: Urological implications. Journal of Urology 1984, 132, 548–552.
16. Bretan PN Jr, Busch MP, Hricak H and Williams RD. Chronic renal failure: A significant risk factor in the development of acquired renal cysts and renal cell carcinoma. Case reports and review of the literature. Cancer 1986, 57, 1871–1879.
17. Cho C, Friedland GW and Swenson RS. Acquired renal cystic disease and renal neoplasms in hemodialysis patients. Urological Radiology 1984, 6, 153–157.
18. Chung-Park M, Ricanati E, Lankerani M and Kedia K. Acquired renal cysts and multiple renal cell and urothelial tumors. American Journal of Clinical Pathology 1983, 79, 238–242.
19. Cohen AH. Renal pathology forum; Patient 3. American Journal of Nephrology 1985, 5, 309–311.
20. Cotterell L, Egan JD, Wells IC, Hammeke MD, Berman MH, Saigh J and Lynch HT. Significant incidence of ACDK in CAPD patients. Peritoneal Dialysis Bulletin (Suppl) 1986, 6, S5.
21. Deguchi N, Tachibana M, Hata M and Tazaki H. Flow cytometric DNA analysis of neoplastic factors in the kidney of patients on hemodialysis. Abstracts in 10th International Congress of Nephrology, 1987, 498.
22. Dunnill MS, Millard PR and Oliver D. Acquired cystic disease of the kidneys: a hazard of long-term intermittent maintenance hemodialysis. Journal of Clinical Pathology 1977, 30, 868–877.
23. Dunnill MS. Acquired cystic disease. In: Grantham JJ and Gardner KD, eds., Problems in the Diagnosis and Management of Polycystic Kidney Disease. Kansas City, Mo: Polycystic Kidney Research Foundation, 1985, 211–223.
24. Elliott HL, MacDougall AI and Buchanan WM. Acquired cystic disease of kidney. Lancet 1977, 2, 1359.
25. Faber M and Kupin W. Renal cell carcinoma and acquired cystic kidney disease after renal transplantation. Lancet 1987, 2, 1030–1031.
26. Fallon B, Yousef MA and Williams RD. Acquired cystic disease of the kidneys in chronic ambulatory peritoneal dialysis patients. Journal of Urology 1988, 139, 294A.
27. Fayemi AO and Ali M. Acquired renal cysts and tumors superimposed on chronic primary kidney diseases. An autopsy study of 24 patients. Pathology Research Practice 1980, 168, 73–83.

28. Feiner HD, Katz LA and Gallo GR. Acquired cystic disease of kidney in chronic dialysis patients. Urology 1981, 17, 260–264.
29. Frerichs FT. Die Bright'sche Nierenkrankheit und deren Behandlung. Braunschweig: F. Vieweg und Sohn, 1851, 38–40.
30. Gardner KD Jr and Evan AP. Cystic kidneys: An enigma evolves. American Journal of Kidney Diseases 1984, 3, 403–413.
31. Gardner KD Jr. Acquired renal cystic disease and renal adenocarcinoma in patients on long-term hemodialysis. New England Journal of Medicine 1984, 310, 390.
32. Gardner KD Jr. Cystic kidneys. Kidney International 1988, 33, 610–621.
33. Gehrig JJ, Gottheiner TI and Swenson RS. Acquired cystic disease of the end-stage kidney. American Journal of Medicine 1985, 79, 609–620.
34. Gorey T, Spees EK, Sapir D and Mostofi FK. Renal malignancies are increased in transplant candidates. Journal of Urology 1984, 131, 230A.
35. Glassberg KI, Stephens FD, Lebowitz RL, Braren V, Duckett JW, Jacobs EC, King LR and Perlmutter AD. Renal dysgenesis and cystic disease of the kidney: A report of the Committee on Terminology, Nomenclature and Classification, Section on Urology, American Academy of Pediatrics. Journal of Urology 1987, 138, 1085–1092.
36. Goldsmith HJ, Ahmad R, Raichura N, Lal SM, McConnell CA, Gould DA, Gyde OHB and Green J. Association between rising hemoglobin concentration and renal cyst formation in patients on long term regular hemodialysis treatment. Proceedings of the European Dialysis and Transplant Association 1982, 19, 313–318.
37. Grantham JJ and Levine E. Acquired cystic disease: Replacing one kidney disease with another. Kidney International 1985, 28, 99–105.
38. Grantham JJ, Geiser JL and Evan AP. Cyst formation and growth in autosomal dominant polycystic kidney disease. Kidney International 1987, 31, 1145–1152.
39. Gregoire JR, Torres VE, Holley KE and Farrow GM. Renal epithelial hyperplastic and neoplastic proliferation in autosomal dominant polycystic kidney disease. American Journal of Kidney Diseases 1987, 9, 27–38.
40. Griffin SC and Williams G. Metastatic hypernephroma from a native kidney after cadaver renal transplantation. Postgraduate Medical Journal 1985, 61, 471–472.
41. Hamilton Dutoit SJ and Baillod RA. Systemic amyloidosis of β_2-microglobulin type and acquired renal cystic disease with disseminated carcinoma arising in a patient on long term hemodialysis. Journal of Pathology 1988, 154, 46A.
42. Henson JHL, Al-Hilli S, Penry JB and Mackenzie JC. The development of acquired renal cystic disease and neoplasia in a chronic hemodialysis patient. British Journal of Radiology 1985, 58, 1215–1217.
43. Hughson MD, Hennigar GR and McManus JFA. Atypical cysts, acquired renal cystic disease, and renal cell tumors in end stage dialysis kidneys. Laboratory Investigation 1980, 42, 475–480.
44. Hughson MD, Buchwald D and Fox M. Renal neoplasia and acquired cystic kidney disease in patients receiving long-term dialysis. Archives of Pathology and Laboratory Medicine 1986, 110, 592–601.
45. Huseman R, Grady A, Welling D and Grantham J. Macropuncture study of polycystic disease in adult human kidneys. Kidney International 1980, 18, 375–385.
46. Ishikawa I, Moncrief JW, Aguirre F, Brindley BW and Mott CL. Acquired cystic kidney disease in continuous ambulatory peritoneal dialysis patients. In: Maekawa M, Nolph KD, Kishimoto T and Moncrief JW, eds., Machine-Free Dialysis for Patient Convenience: The Fourth ISAO Official Satellite Symposium on CAPD. Cleveland: ISAO Press, 1984, 131–133.
47. Ishikawa I. Uremic acquired cystic disease of kidney. Urology 1985, 26, 101–108.
48. Ishikawa I, Saito Y, Onouchi Z, Kitada H, Suzuki S, Kurihara S, Yuri T and Shinoda A. Development of acquired cystic disease and adenocarcinoma of the kidney in glomerulonephritic chronic hemodialysis patients. Clinical Nephrology 1980, 14, 1–6.
49. Ishikawa I, Yuri T, Kitada H and Shinoda A. Regression of acquired cystic disease of the

kidney after successful renal transplantation. American Journal of Nephrology 1983, 3, 310–314.

50. Ishikawa I, Onouchi Z, Saito Y, Tateishi K, Shinoda A, Suzuki S, Kitada H, Sugishita N and Fukuda Y. Sex differences in acquired cystic disease of the kidney on long-term dialysis. Nephron 1985, 39, 336–340.

51. Ishikawa I, Tateishi K, Kitada H and Shinoda A. Regression of adult type polycystic kidney during chronic intermittent hemodialysis. Is it a universal phenomenon? Nephron 1984, 36, 147.

52. Ishikawa I, Shikura N, Horiguchi T, Morimoto S, Tamai Y, Masuzaki S and Shinoda A. Size distribution of acquired cysts in chronic hemodialysis patients. Journal of Kanazawa Medical University 1988, 13, 171–175.

53. Ishikawa I, Horiguchi T and Shikura N. Lectin peroxidase conjugate reactivity in acquired cystic disease of the kidney. Nephron 1989, 51, 211–214.

54. Ishikawa I, Horiguchi T, Kitada H, Matsuno H, Shinoda A, Saito Y and Onouchi Z. β_2-microglobulin-derived amyloid deposition in acquired cystic disease of the kidney with renal cell carcinoma. Nephron 1987, 46, 101–102.

55. Ishikawa I. Unusual composition of cyst fluid in acquired cystic disease of the end stage kidney. Nephron 1985, 41, 373–374.

56. Ishikawa I. β_2-microglobulin level of cyst fluid in uremic acquired cystic disease of the kidney. Nephron 1986, 44, 381.

57. Ishikawa I, Saito Y, Kitada H, Onouchi Z and Shinoda A. Comoputed tomography of kidneys with hemodialysis. Journal of Kanazawa Medical University 1980, 5, 146–154.

58. Ishikawa I and Shinoda A. Renal adenocarcinoma with or without acquired cysts in chronic hemodialysis patients. Clinical Nephrology 1983, 20, 321–322.

59. Ishikawa I. Adenocarcinoma of the kidney in chronic hemodialysis patients in Japan. In Man N-K, Mion C, Henderson LW, eds., Blood Purification in Perspective: New Insights and Future Trends. Cleveland: ISAO Press, 1987, 86–88.

60. Ishikawa I. Adenocarcinoma of the kidney in chronic hemodialysis patients. International Journal of Artificial Organs 1988, 11, 61–62.

61. Isiadinso OA, Stubenbord WT and Rubin AL. Renal cell carcinoma postrenal transplant. Discovered accidentally. New York State Journal of Medicine 1976, 76, 2024–2025.

62. Jabour BA, Ralls PW, Tang WW, Bowell WD Jr, Colletti PM, Feinstein EI and Massry SG. Acquired cystic disease of the kidneys: Computed tomography and ultrasonography appraisal in patients on peritoneal and hemodialysis. Investigative Radiology 1987, 22, 728–732.

63. Kassirer JP and Gang DL. Weekly clinicopathological exercises, Case records of the Massachusetts General Hospital, Case 16–1982. New England Journal of Medicine 1982, 306, 975–984.

64. Katz A, Sombolos K and Oreopoulos DG. Acquired cystic disease of the kidney in association with chronic ambulatory peritoneal dialysis. American Journal of Kidney Diseases 1987, 9, 426–429.

65. Koga N, Nomura G, Yamagata Y and Koga T. Ureteric pain in patients with chronic renal failure on hemodialysis. Nephron 1982, 31, 55–58.

66. Krempien B and Ritz E. Acquired cystic transformation of the kidneys of hemodialysed patients. Virchows Archiv A. Pathology, Anatomy and Histology 1980, 386, 189–200.

67. Kutcher R, Amodio JB and Rosenblatt R. Uremic renal cystic disease: Value of sonographic screening. Radiology 1983, 147, 833–835.

68. Leichter HE, Dietrich R, Salusky IB, Foley J, Cohen AH, Kangarloo H and Fine RN. Acquired cystic kidney disease in children undergoing long-term dialysis. Pediatric Nephrology 1988, 2, 8–11.

69. Levine E, Grantham JJ, Slusher SL, Greathouse JL and Krohn BP. CT of acquired cystic kidney disease and renal tumors in long-term dialysis patients. American Journal of Roentgenology 1984, 142, 125–131.

70. Levine E, Grantham JJ and MacDougall ML. Spontaneous subcapsular and perinephric

hemorrhage in end stage kidney disease: Clinical and CT findings. American Journal of Roentgenology 1987, 148, 755–758.

71. Linke RP, Bommer J, Ritz E, Waldherr R and Eulitz M. Amyloid kidney stones of uremic patients consist of beta₂-microglobulin fragments. Biochemestry and Biophysics Research Communications 1986, 136, 665–671.

72. Ludmerer KM and Kissane JM. Clinicopathologic conference. A new chest mass in a 49-year-old man with a transplanted kidney. American Journal of Medicine 1988, 84, 121–128.

73. MacDougall ML, Welling LW and Wiegmann TB. Renal adenocarcinoma and acquired cystic disease in chronic hemodialysis patients. American Journal of Kidney Diseases 1987, 9, 166–171.

74. Meares EM Jr, Sant GR, Mitcheson HD and Ucci AA Jr. Acquired renal cystic disease and adenocarcinoma in endstage kidneys – Urologic implications. Journal of Urology 1988, 139, 431A.

75. Meyrier A, Verger C, Ang KS, Sraer JD, Kourilsky O and Jablonsky JP. Acute internal hemorrhage due to spontaneous visceral ruptures in hemodialysis patients. Kidney International 1979, 16, 97.

76. Mickisch O, Bommer J, Bachmann S, Waldherr R, Mann JFE and Ritz E. Multicystic transformation of kidneys in chronic renal failure. Nephron 1984, 38, 93–99.

77. Miller L, Soffer O and Nassar VH. Tumorous degeneration of acquired renal cystic disease in ESRD: An autopsy of 155 cases. Kidney International 1987, 31, 210.

78. Minar E, Tscholakoff D, Zazgornik J, Schmidt P, Marosi R and Czembirek H. Acquired cystic disease of the kidneys in chronic hemodialysed and renal transplant patients. European Urology 1984, 10, 245–248.

79. Mirahmadi MK and Vaziri ND. Cystic transformation of end stage kidneys in patients undergoing hemodialysis. International Journal of Artificial Organs 1980, 3, 267–270.

80. Narasimhan N, Golper TA, Wolfson M, Rahatzad M and Bennett WM. Clinical characteristics and diagnostic considerations in acquired renal cystic disease. Kidney International 1986, 30, 748–752.

81. Nunez D Jr, Yrizarry JM, Nadji M, Beerman R and Morillo G. Renal cell carcinoma complicating long-term dialysis: Computed tomography-guided aspiration cytology. Journal of Computed Tomography 1986, 10, 61–66.

82. Olsson PJ, Fierer JA, Kelly CE, Wright RW, Blaise D, Anderson KB, Peterson JC and Alexander RW. Renal carcinoma and dialysis in end stage renal disease. Southern Medical Journal 1985, 78, 507–512.

83. Ono K, Yasukohchi A and Kikawa K. Pathogenesis of acquired renal cysts in hemodialysis patients. Transctions of the Association for Artificial Internal Organs 1987, 33, 245–249.

84. Peipers A. Ueber eine besondere Form von Nierensteinen. Munchen Med Wochenschrift 1894, 41, 531–532.

85. Penn I, Brunson ME. Cancers after cyclosporine therapy. Transplantation Proceedings 1988, 20 (Suppl. 3), 885–892.

86. Ratcliffe PJ, Dunnill MS and Oliver DO. Clinical importance of acquired cystic disease of the kidney in patients undergoing dialysis. British Medical Journal 1983, 287, 1855–1858.

87. Schillinger F, Montagnac R, Milcent T, Nollez F and Hopfner C. Acquired cystic disease and adenocarcinoma of the kidney in chronic hemodialysis patients. Kidney International 1988, 33, 1040.

88. Shalhoub RJ, Rajan U, Kim VV, Goldwasser E, Kark JA and Antoniou LD. Erythrocytosis in patients on long-term hemodialysis. Annals Internal Medicine 1982, 97, 686–690.

89. Siegel SC, Sandler MA, Alpern MB and Pearlberg JL. CT of renal cell carcinoma in patients on chronic hemodialysis. American Journal of Roentgenology 1988, 150, 583–585.

90. Smith JW, Sallman AL, Williamson MR and Lott CG. Acquired renal cystic disease: Two cases of associated adenocarcinoma and a renal ultrasound survey of a peritoneal dialysis population. American Journal of Kidney Diseases 1987, 10, 41–46.

91. Soffer O, Miller LR and Lichtman JB. CT findings in complications of acquired renal cystic disease. Journal of Computer Assisted Tomography 1987, 11, 905–908.
92. Struve C, Zabel P and Roggensack H-O. Hypernephroides Nierenkarzinom einer glomerulonephritischen Schrumpfniere nach Nierentransplantation. RÖFO 1984, 141, 587–588.
93. Thompson BJ, Jenkins DAS, Allan PL, Winney RJ, Dick JCB, Wild SR, Anderton JL and Chisholm GD. Acquired cystic disease of the kidney: indication for renal transplantation? British Medical Journal 1986, 293, 1209–1210.
94. Thomson BJ, Jenkins DAS, Allan PL, Elton RA and Winney RJ. Acquired cystic disease of the kidney in patients with end stage chronic renal failure: A study of prevalence and aetiology. Nephrology Dialysis Transplantation 1986, 1, 38–43.
95. Thomson BJ, Allan PL and Winney RJ. Acquired cystic disease of kidney: Metastatic renal adenocarcinoma and hypercalcaemia. Lancet 1985, 2, 502–503.
96. Torrence RJ, Elbers JD, Seline P and Clayman RV. The effect of renal cyst fluid from patients with acquired cystic disease of the kidneys (ACDK) upon the growth of benign and malignant human renal cells. Journal of Urology 1988, 139, 211A.
97. Trabucco AF, Bozek SA, Johansson SL, Egan JD and Taylor RJ. Acquired renal cystic disease and neoplasia in patient on chronic peritoneal dialysis. Journal of Urology 1987, 137, 233A.
98. Turani H, Levi J, Zevin D and Kessler E. Acquired cystic disease and tumors in kidneys of hemodialysis patients. Israel Journal of Medical Science 1983, 19, 614–618.
99. Tuttle RJ, Minielly JA and Fay WP. Spontaneous renal hemorrhage in chronic glomerular nephritis and dialysis. Radiology 1971, 98, 137–138.
100. Vandenbroucke JM, Huaux JP, Guillaume Th, Nöel H, Maldague B and van Ypersele de Strihou C. Capsular synovial and bone amyloidosis: Complications of long-term hemodialysis. Proceedings of the European Dialysis and Transplant Association-ERA 1985, 22, 136–138.
101. Vaziri ND, Darwish R, Martin DC and Hostetler J. Acquired renal cystic disease in renal transplant recipients. Nephron 1984, 37, 203–205.
102. Viner NJ, MacIver AG and Mackenzie JC. Acquired cystic disease of the kidney. Lancet 1987, 1, 121–122.

15
Medullary Sponge Kidney

E. R. Yendt

Abstract

Medullary sponge kidney is a relatively common developmental abnormality in which intrapapillary dilated collecting ducts give the renal medulla a typically spongy appearance. It is found among 20% of stone formers, is accompanied by hypercalciuria in 50% of affected subjects, and may be complicated by hematuria, infection and stone formation. Criteria for its diagnosis are primarily radiologic and are insufficiently sensitive to detect all cases. Its overall prognosis is excellent.

Key Words   Sponge kidney;
Hypercalciuria;
Nephrolithiasis;
Urolithiasis;
Hematuria.

1. Introduction

Medullary sponge kidney (MSK) is a disorder characterized by the presence of dilated collecting ducts and tubules in one or more renal pyramids. The condition was first described in 1939[23], but the clinical, radiographic and morphologic features of the disease were not established until 1949[3].

The true prevalence of MSK is unknown, because it is asymptomatic unless complicated by nephrolithiasis, hematuria, or urinary infection. A systematic examination of the kidneys at autopsy to determine the prevalence of this disorder has not been reported. In unselected patients undergoing excretory urography, the prevalence is approximately 0.5%[30,33]. The reported prevalence of MSK in patients with nephrolithiasis varies widely. Earlier reports suggested a fairly low prevalence of 2.6–3.6%[22,32,47]. In 1981, however, we pointed out that milder degrees of the condition were frequently missed by routine excretory urography, and that 21% of 400 consecutive patients with nephrolithiasis had MSK when milder degrees of the condition were detected[49]. Sage *et al.*[40] subsequently reported that 17% of 200 randomly selected patients with nephrolithiasis had MSK, and Parks *et al.*[35] found the disorder in 12% of 624 male patients and 19% of 175 female patients with nephrolithiasis. Vagelli *et al.*[44] diagnosed MSK in 11.6% of 138 consecutive patients with calcium stones.

2. Pathology and pathogenesis

The pathologic changes of MSK are confined to the renal medulla, especially to the inner portions of the renal pyramids[6,26]. One or more pyramids contain dilated collected ducts and tubules associated with multiple small cysts measuring 1–7.5 mm in diameter. The cysts may communicate with each other, with the dilating collecting ducts, or directly with corresponding minor calyces. The cysts frequently contain densely radiopaque spherical concretions that are shown by X-ray crystallography to be composed wholly or predominantly of apatite[6]. The affected pyramids and associated calyces are often enlarged[26], and there may be generalized renal enlargement when numerous pyramids are involved.

The renal cortex, columns of Bertin, calyces and pelvis appear normal, unless affected by complications of the disease such as pyelonephritis or urinary obstruction.

MSK is probably a developmental anomaly. Supporting evidence includes the histologic appearance of the lesions, the lack of progression in the absence of complications[21], and the occasional presence of embryonal tissue[6]. Co-existent anomalies of the urinary tract are frequent, and there are numerous reports of associations with other developmental abnormalities, especially congenital hemihypertrophy, which has been reported in as many as 25% of patients[12]. Although congenital hemihypertrophy occurs without MSK, the degree of hemihypertrophy occurring in association with MSK is usually not seen in other conditions. Other associated congenital abnormalities include Ehlers–Danlos syndrome[24,29], congenital pyloric stenosis[29], Caroli disease[27], Marfan syndrome[41] and polycystic disease[1,31,38]. Some putative associations have resulted from the misinterpretation of medullary ductal ectasia in autosomal recessive polycystic kidney disease and in Caroli disease, because medullary ductal ectasia and MSK are radiographically indistinguishable. Morris et al.[29] suggested that the urographic pattern generally considered to be diagnostic of MSK actually reflects several different disease processes.

Familial cases of MSK have occasionally had pedigrees consistent with autosomal dominant inheritance[20,21]. Although it has been suggested that a hereditary basis is unlikely in most families[29], this suggestion must be interpreted with caution because the disorder is frequently asymptomatic and because of difficulty in the diagnosis of mild cases by excretory urography.

Two other theories for the pathogenesis of MSK have been proposed. In 1951, Vermooten[45] proposed that the dilatation of the collecting tubules resulted from their occlusion by uric acid crystals during fetal life, but the theory has not received further support. It has also been suggested that MSK might be a consequence of idiopathic hypercalciuria[28] but the evidence cited is unimpressive and the recognition of MSK following the appearance of nephrolithiasis may result from either cyst enlargement or better urographic visualization.

3. Pathogenesis of urolithiasis in medullary sponge kidney

The intrarenal concretions were composed of pure apatite in seven of ten patients and a mixture of apatite and calcium oxalate in the remaining three[6]. Several factors possibly contribute to the formation of the concretions. Urinary supersaturation with apatite, a prerequisite for the nucleation of apatite crystals, could result from impaired acidification and increased pH of the tubular fluid (see section 5). The frequent occurrence of hypercalciuria in MSK also favors supersaturation with apatite, although stone formation occurs in normocalciuric patients. Perhaps the fluid in ectatic ducts has higher pH values and calcium concentrations than the fluid in unaffected collecting ducts, even though the pH value and calcium concentration of the final urine are normalized by a preponderance of unaffected collecting ducts.

   Other factors are urinary stasis within the ectatic lesions and the intracavitary accumulation of hyaline material and cellular debris[6], which act as matrices for stone formation.

   Although the intrarenal concretions were all found to contain apatite and some to contain only apatite, the passage of pure apatite stones is uncommon. Approximately 50% of the stones passed in the absence of infection consist of an admixture of calcium oxalate and apatite, and the remainder are composed entirely of calcium oxalate. It is likely that some of the papillary concretions find their way into the calyces, probably by erosion through cyst walls, but they almost always acquire a coating of calcium oxalate crystals. The initial site of formation of pure calcium oxalate stones and their pathogenesis is uncertain. However, hypercalciuria favors urinary supersaturation with calcium oxalate. We have also found that urine oxalate excretion in MSK patients is higher than in normal subjects or in patients with idiopathic calcium oxalate stones[52]. This is undoubtedly of major importance in oxalate stone formation, because oxalate concentration is of greater importance than calcium concentration in supersaturating the urine with calcium oxalate[39,46]. In our experience, urinary citrate excretion in MSK patients does not differ significantly from normal[52].

   Stone formation in the majority of patients occurs in the absence of urinary infection. However, infection with urease-producing organisms may occasionally result in the explosive production of struvite stones.

4. Clinical features

MSK is asymptomatic unless complicated by nephrolithiasis, hematuria, or infection, and MSK should always be considered in patients presenting with these problems. The onset of symptoms often occurs during childhood or the second decade of life, occasionally as late as the sixth decade. We have found the prevalence of MSK in stone patients younger than 20 years to be at least twice as high as the prevalence in our entire group of stone patients[52]. The prevalence is higher in female than in male stone patients[35,52]. The prevalence is even higher in hypercalciuric female stone patients; 25% of 100 consecutive hypercalciuric female stone patients presenting to our clinic had this disorder[52].

Hematuria is the second most common initial symptom. Hematuria is unrelated to stones or infection, and it may be recurrent. The bleeding is usually painless, but colic is occasionally caused by the passage of clots.

Urinary tract infection is another common complication, regardless of nephrocalcinosis and nephrolithiasis, and it may be the sole clinical manifestation of the disorder. Ekström et al.[6] estimated that 11% of their patients had developed chronic pyelonephritis, but the frequency of pyelonephritis is reduced by modern antibacterial therapy. Urinary infection occurs more frequently in MSK stone patients than in idiopathic stone patients[35]. Infections are much more apt to occur in female than in male patients with stone and MSK; Parks et al.[35] found that more than two infections occurred in approximately 35% of their female patients but in only 5% of their male patients[35].

The prevalence of hypertension is not increased in MSK patients who do not have pyelonephritis[6,13].

5. Renal function

Urinalysis, glomerular filtration rate and renal plasma flow are normal in the absence of complications[5,10,15]. However, we have found that 24-hour endogenous creatinine clearance is significantly lower in male patients with MSK and stones than in male patients with idiopathic calcium oxalate stones[52]. Urinary concentration is often diminished[6,10,15,21]. The concentrating defect is not due to impaired active chloride reabsorption across the thick descending limb of Henle, and it is vasopressin-resistant[15]. Urinary dilution is not impaired[10,15].

Impaired urinary acidification after acute ammonium chloride loading occurs in some patients[5] because the terminal portion of the collecting duct, the site of the abnormality, loses its ability to generate steep pH gradients between tubular fluid and interstitial fluid in acidosis[9]. Higashihara et al.[15] found that four of eleven MSK patients were unable to lower their urine pH below 5.3 after acute ammonium chloride loading and Houillier et al.[17] found a similar abnormality in two of nine MSK patients. In the first of these studies, the impaired ability to lower urine pH was associated with reduced excretion of titratable acid despite normal ammonium excretion[15]. In the second study, however, maximal response in titratable acidity, ammonium excretion and net acid excretion in the patients did not differ significantly from these responses in controls[17]. All of these patients had extensive bilateral disease. Information concerning renal function in MSK patients with less than extensive involvement is limited; urinary concentration was impaired and acidification was normal in one patient with segmental disease and one with unilateral disease[16]. The acidification defect in most MSK patients is not accompanied by systemic acidosis and is not of clinical consequence. However, a few cases of systemic acidosis have been described[4,13,19,24,29], and one of them presented with hypokalemic paralysis due to renal potassium-wasting[19]. We have not encountered a single example of systemic acidosis or hypokalemia in our series of 159 MSK patients; mean urinary citrate excretion in the MSK patients did not differ significantly from normal[52].

High fractional excretion of sodium is an almost universal feature of the disease, even in patients with only slight changes affecting a few renal pyramids[10]. An impaired kaliuretic response to short-term potassium infusions has also been reported in three patients having impaired urinary concentration and acidification; these patients were able to preserve potassium balance during long-term potassium loading or depletion[11].

Proximal tubular function appears to be normal in MSK. Glucosuria and hypouricemia are not features of the disease[5,35], and urinary amino acid excretion is normal[43].

6. Hypercalciuria and medullary sponge kidney

The reported prevalence of hypercalciuria in MSK patients varies from 40 to 50%[6,13,35]. Thirty percent of our first 140 MSK patients had hypercalciuria: 45% of 74 males and 26% of 66 females.

The cause of hypercalciuria is uncertain. Net calcium reabsorption has been demonstrated to occur along the medullary collecting duct of the rat[2], and it is a possibility that hypercalciuria may be yet another functional manifestation of a primary abnormality in the terminal collecting duct. A primary renal calcium leak could produce parathyroid stimulation that in turn could lead to hypophosphatemia. There is disagreement in the literature concerning the nature of hypercalciuria in MSK patients. Maschio et al.[28] reported the hypercalciuria to be due to a renal calcium leak in eight and to intestinal calcium absorption in two MSK patients, whereas O'Neill et al.[32] classified the hypercalciuria as absorptive in ten renal in three and unclassified in two patients. In the latter study, serum PTH levels were elevated in the three patients with renal hypercalciuria. O'Neill et al. concluded that MSK patients had the same spectrum of metabolic abnormalities as did the overall population of stone patients. Jaeger et al.[18] found that 6 of 20 patients with renal hypercalciuria had MSK.

A major problem in assessing the nature of hypercalciuria in MSK is caused by difficulty in measuring parathyroid function. The unreliability of many of the early radioimmunoassays for parathyroid hormone (PTH) is well known. Measurement of total urinary cyclic AMP (expressed as a function of glomerular filtrate) in our experience also lacks the sensitivity required to detect slight to modest degrees of PTH hypersecretion; we have found that urinary cyclic AMP excretion is normal in most patients with a surgically proven parathyroid tumor when the degree of hypercalcemia is slight and when the parathyroid adenoma weighs less than 1 g[51]. In recent years we have used an improved radioimmunoassay, commercially available in a kit, based on the method of Lindall et al.[25]. The sensitivity of this assay in patients with parathyroid adenomas weighing more than 300 mg is on the order of 85%, but only on the order of 30% in patients with adenomas weighing less than 300 mg[51]. Using this assay, we have found elevated plasma PTH levels in two of eleven patients with MSK, whereas plasma PTH levels were normal in all of 41 patients with idiopathic calcium oxalate stones[52]. Thus, hypercalciuria associated with secondary hyperparathyroidism appears to be an important association of MSK, and we have been unable to demonstrate secondary hyperparathyroidism in idiopathic calcium oxalate stone disease. Because of the low sensitivity of the radioimmunoassay, the data may underestimate the prevalence of secondary hyperparathyroidism in MSK patients. We have also found that serum inorganic phosphate levels are significantly lower in patients with MSK than in patients with idiopathic calcium oxalate stones, and the prevalence of frank hypophosphatemia is higher in the MSK patients[52]. These data are also consistent with the occurrence of secondary hyperparathyroidism in MSK.

We[52] have found other major differences between hypercalciuric patients with MSK and hypercalciuric patients with idiopathic calcium oxalate stones. Urinary magnesium, phosphate, uric acid, sodium and zinc are all higher than normal in male patients with idiopathic calcium oxalate stones. These abnormalities, which we believe to be related to increased dietary protein intake, are much less prominent in male MSK patients. Furthermore, serum uric acid levels are significantly lower in male MSK patients. Thus, hypercalciuria appears less likely to be related to dietary abnormalities in patients with MSK than in those with idiopathic calcium oxalate stones.

The occurrence of secondary hyperparathyroidism in MSK, albeit in a minority of patients, suggests that chronic parathyroid stimulation may sometimes result in tertiary hyperparathyroidism. Six of our patients have had overt hyperparathyroidism corrected by surgical removal of parathyroid adenomas. There are reports of more than 20 other such patients in the literature[20,28]. The only report of an abnormally high prevalence of hyperparathyroidism in MSK is that of Maschio et al.[28], who found seven patients (single adenomas in six, hyperplasia in one) during investigation of 28 patients with MSK. There is still insufficient evidence, however, to prove a direct association between the two disorders.

8. Diagnosis

The diagnosis of MSK is made by excretory urography[6,21,26]. When opacified

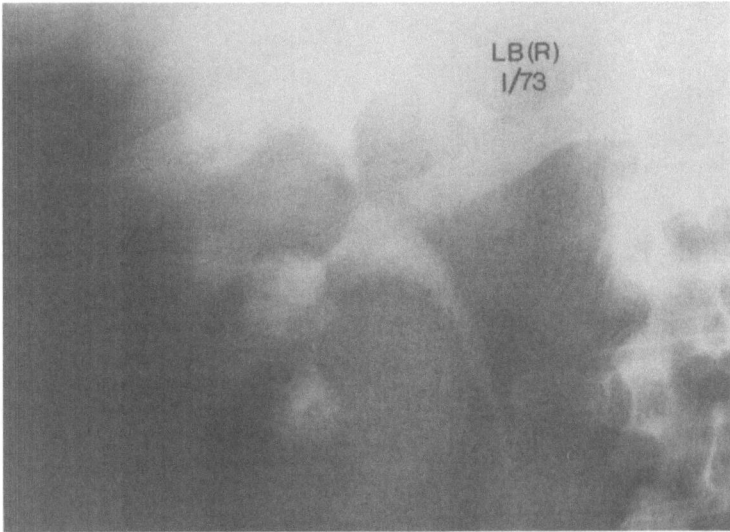

Figure 15.1. Excretory urogram of a patient with medullary sponge kidney showing diffuse linear streaking of the papillae of the right kidney due to contrast medium in dilated collecting ducts and tubules.

by contrast medium, dilated collecting ducts appear either as linear striations that impart a characteristic blush-like pattern to the renal medulla (Figure 15.1) or as spherical cysts (Fig. 15.2). The latter appearance has been described as "bouquets of flowers" or "bunches of grapes". The dilated ducts and cysts fill poorly with contrast medium during retrograde pyelography. The cysts may be the first structures to opacify and the last to empty during excretory urography, but the linear streaking of the pyramids indicative of dilated collecting ducts may be evanescent. Affected renal pyramids and their corresponding calyces may be enlarged. Enlarged pyramids have been described in parts of the kidney lacking ectatic ducts during excretory urography, and histologic examination of these pyramids has shown the typical changes of MSK[6,26]. Dense spherical concretions, occurring in clusters, are frequently seen in plain films (Fig. 15.3), and radiopaque stones may be present within the renal calyces and pelvis. After the injection of the contrast medium, additional concretions may be demonstrated by negative images with the contrast medium. Unilateral enlargement of the pelvic innominate bone indicates an association with hemihypertrophy. Ultrasonography, arteriography and computer tomography have little, if any, role in diagnosis.

There are major difficulties in the radiographic diagnosis of MSK. Although the diagnosis is relatively easy in florid cases, when virtually all pyramids of both kidneys are involved, milder involvement may not be easily apparent. A satisfactory excretory urogram must clearly opacify the pyelocalyceal sys-

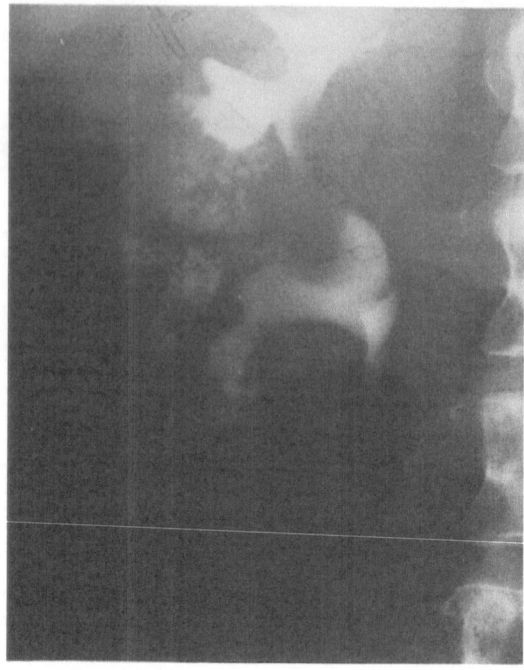

Figure 15.2. Excretory urogram of a patient with medullary sponge kidney showing widespread cystic dilatations of medullary ducts and tubules in right kidney.

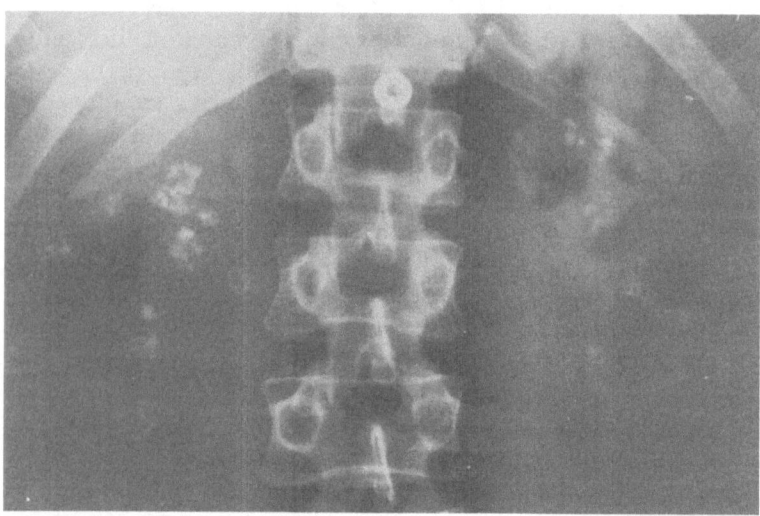

Figure 15.3. Preliminary film of a patient with medullary sponge kidney showing clusters of papillary concretions in both kidneys. (Reproduced from Yendt ER. Medullary Sponge Kidney in Urolithiasis. In: Rous SN, ed: Stone Disease: Diagnosis and Management. Orlando. Grune and Stratton, Inc. Chapter 13. With permission)[50].

tems, including each calyx and its infundibulum, detail must not be obscured by overlying bowel contents, and urinary tract obstruction must not be present. Most excretory urograms in stone patients are performed during episodes of renal colic and tend to be of extremely poor quality[49]. Another problem is that milder degrees of MSK are frequently not recognized or commented on by radiologists, nephrologists and urologists[52]. Even with a satisfactory urogram, there may be difficulty in recognizing MSK. In our clinic we make the diagnosis when discrete dye-filled ectatic ducts are demonstrated in at least three renal papillae. The diagnosis is not made when papillary blushing is the sole radiographic abnormality. These criteria are arbitrary and may exclude patients who have the disorder. It is established that the disorder may be confined to only one or two renal pyramids, and the diagnosis is justified if numerous characteristic lesions are identified in the same pyramids.

Another problem in the radiographic diagnosis of MSK is the significance of diffuse opacification or "blushing" of the renal pyramids during excretory urography. On reviewing 2,465 excretory urograms, Palubinskas[34] noted papillary blushing without other evidence of MSK in 21 cases, an incidence of less than 1%. In individual cases of MSK he found that the radiographic changes in different papillae ranged from papillary blushing, through a few distinguishable dilated tubules combined with papillary blushing, to the classic appearance of multiple cystic lesions. He also found that the characteristic dilated collecting ducts were found histopathologically in pyramids that demonstrated only a blush or enlargement on excretory urography. Moreover, the technique of magnification excretory urography has demonstrated individually dilated tubules in renal pyramids that otherwise showed only a blush[14]. Therefore, many instances of papillary blush probably represent minor degrees of MSK. Kuiper[21] stated that pyramidal blushing is diagnostic of MSK when it is diffuse, persistent in successive examinations, and present on both early and delayed films without the use of compression, especially if accompanied by pyramidal enlargement, intraductular papillary concretions, or linear or cystic dilatations. Although we do not make the diagnosis of MSK when papillary blushing is the sole radiographic abnormality, we do entertain a strong suspicion of MSK.

In summary, excretory urography as routinely performed may be a fairly insensitive diagnostic test for MSK because of the unsatisfactory quality of many of the examinations. The recognition of minor forms of the disease and the assessment of papillary blushing when it is the sole radiographic abnormality are additional problems. Furthermore, the characteristic lesions of MSK have been demonstrated histopathologically in a papilla that urographically appeared completely normal[18]. A more sensitive test is clearly needed.

9. Differential diagnosis

The diagnosis of florid MSK with diffuse pyramidal involvement in typical clinical circumstances is a relatively easy matter. The single, most frequently confused condition is autosomal recessive polycystic kidney disease, which has an almost identical radiographic appearance in older children and adults. This similarity has confounded radiologists and cluttered the literature. The pitfall can be avoided through careful evaluation of the clinical circumstances and family history. When the changes are minimal, involving a single pyramid or only a few pyramids, the disorder must be differentiated from calyceal diverticula, renal tuberculosis, renal papillary necrosis and other causes of nephrocalcinosis. MSK must also be distinguished from pyelotubular stasis, a fine brush-like opacification of the renal pyramids resulting from the application of excessive abdominal pressure during excretory urography. No cystic lesions are present, however, and repeat examination without ureteral compression does not reproduce the findings. Pyelovenous backflow, another abnormality that must be distinguished from MSK, is a lacy dye pattern produced by raised intrapelvic pressure and the disruption of the calyceal fornices. This may result from excessive injection pressure in the renal pelvis during retrograde pyelography, in which case the changes are not reproducible during excretory urography. Pyelovenous backflow may also occur during excretory urography when stones produce acute ureteric occlusion. Microcalyces may also produce peculiar opacifications around papillae, simulating the lesions of MSK[36].

10. Course, prognosis and treatment

The management of patients with asymptomatic and uncomplicated MSK is relatively straightforward. The patient should be informed of the benign nature of the disorder when uncomplicated, but should also be alerted to the potential complications of stone formation, urinary infection and hematuria. Periodic urinalyses and urine cultures are advisable, even in asymptomatic patients.

The management of nephrocalcinosis and nephrolithiasis is the same as when these complications occur in the absence of MSK. In our experience, active and progressive stone formation can nearly always be arrested by thiazides[48,50], which have now been proven efficacious in preventing calcium stones[8]. Thiazides are effective in both normocalciuric and hypercalciuric patients. In hypercalciuric patients, there is no need to classify the hypercalciuria as absorptive or renal before initiating thiazide treatment.

Inorganic phosphates have also been used to arrest the progression of stone disease in MSK patients[42]. We use thiazides as the agent of first choice because of their proven efficacy, convenience and low cost. However, if thiazides are contraindicated or poorly tolerated, inorganic phosphate therapy is well worth a try. Inorganic phosphates should not be used, however, in patients with a urinary tract infection due to a urease-producing organism because of the danger of producing struvite stone.

Urinary tract infection in MSK patients should be treated with antibacterial agents in the usual manner. There is a tendency for the infections to recur after discontinuation of antibacterial therapy, and long-term therapy may be necessary in some patients. Infection with a urease-producing organism may lead to an explosive progression of the stone disease in MSK patients. The offending organism is frequently a coagulase-negative staphylococcus that should not be ignored, even when colony counts seem insignificant. Treatment is indicated if the same organism is grown on repeated culture, and the careful monitoring of these patients with frequent cultures is essential.

Hematuria occurring in the absence of stones or infection requires no specific treatment. Unfortunately, however, MSK is frequently not considered in the differential diagnosis of hematuria, or the diagnosis of MSK may have been dismissed on the basis of poor quality excretory urograms. These patients may undergo repeated and unnecessary urologic procedures before the correct diagnosis is established.

With the proper management of complications, the long-term prognosis of MSK patients is excellent and the development of serious renal damage is uncommon, although it was fairly frequent in the earlier Swedish experience[6]. In the past, nephrectomy and partial nephrectomy were occasionally necessary to alleviate symptoms[6,37], but these procedures should now rarely be necessary.

References

1. Abreo K and Steele FH. Simultaneous medullary sponge kidney and adult polycystic kidney disease: the need for accurate diagnosis. Archives of Internal Medicine 1982, 142, 163–165.
2. Bengele HH, Alexander EA and Lechene CP. Calcium and magnesium transport along the inner medullary collecting duct of the rat. American Journal of Physiology 1980, 239, F24–F29.
3. Cacci R and Ricci V. Sur une rare maladie kystique multiple des pyramides renales, le "rein en eponge". Journal of Urology Nephrol (Paris) 1948, 55, 497–519.
4. Deck MDF. Medullary sponge kidney with renal tubular acidosis. A report of 3 cases. Journal of Urology 1965, 94, 330–335.
5. Defronzo RA and Thier SO. Functional abnormalities in renal cystic diseases. In: Gardner KD, ed, Cystic Diseases of the Kidney. New York: Wiley, 1976, 65–81.
6. Ekström T, Engfeldt B and Lagergren C. Medullary Sponge Kidney. Stockholm: Almqvist and Wiksell, 1959.
7. Ettinger B, Citron J and Tang A. Controlled studies in stone prophylaxis: Comparison of placebo versus allopurinol/chlorthalidone/magnesium hydroxide. Urology Research 1984, 12, 491 (abstract).
8. Ettinger B, Citron JT, Livermore B and Dolman LI. Chlorthalidone reduces calcium oxalate calculous recurrence but magnesium hydroxide does not. Journal of Urology 1988, 139, 179–684.
9. Graber ML, Bengele HH and Schwartz JH. pH and pCO_2 profiles of the rat inner medulla. American Journal of Physiology 1981, 241, F659–f668.
10. Granberg PO, Lagergren C and Theve NO. Renal function studies in medullary sponge kidney. Scandinavian Journal of Urology Nephrol 1971, 5, 177–180.
11. Green J, Szylman P, Sznajder I, Winaver J and Better OS. Renal tubulr handling of

potassium in patients with medullary sponge kidney. A model of renal papillectomy in humans. Archives of Internal Medicine 1984, 144, 2201–2204.

12. Harris RE, Fuchs EF and Kaempf MJ. Medullary sponge kidney and congenital hemihypertrophy: Case report and literature review. Journal of Urology 1981, 126, 676–678.

13. Harrison, AR and Rose GA. Medullary sponge kidney. Urology Research 1979, 7, 197–207.

14. Hayt DB, Perez LA and Blatt CJ. Direct magnification intravenous pyelography in the evaluation of medullary sponge kidney. Roengenol Radium Ther Nucl Medicine 1973, 119, 701–704.

15. Higashihara E, Nutahara K and Tago K. Medullary sponge kidney and renal acidification defect. Kidney International 1984, 25, 453–459.

16. Higashihara E, Nutahara K and Tago K. Unilateral and segmental medullary sponge kidney: Renal function and calcium excretion. Journal of Urology 1984, 132, 743–745.

17. Houillier P, Leviel F, Daudon M, Paillard M and Jungers P. Response to acute acid load in patients with medullary sponge kidney and calcium nephrolithiasis. Urology Research 1988, 16, 209 (abstract).

18. Jaeger P, Portmann L, Ginalski JM, Campiche M and Burckhardt P. Dietary factors and medullary sponge kidneys as causes of the so-called idiopathic renal leak of calcium. American Journal of Nephrology 1987, 7, 257–263.

19. Jayasinghe KSA, Mendis BLJ and Mohideen R. Medullary sponge kidney presenting with hypokalemic paralysis. Postgraduate Medical Journal 1984, 60, 303–304.

20. Kuiper JJ. Medullary sponge kidney in three generations. New York State Journal of Medicine 1971, 71, 2665–2669.

21. Kuiper JJ. Medullary sponge kidney. In: Gardner KD, ed., Cystic Diseases of the Kidney. New York: Wiley, 1976, 151–171.

22. Lavan JN, Neale FC and Posen S. Urinary calculi: Clinical, biochemical and radiological studies in 619 patients. Medical Journal of Australia 1971, 2, 1049–1061.

23. Lenarduzzi G. Reperto pielograficco poco commune (dilatazione delle vie urinarie intrarenali). Radiol Med (Torino) 1030, 26, 346–347.

24. Levine AS and Michael AF. Ehlers–Danlos syndrome with renal tubular acidosis and medullary sponge kidney. Journal of Pediatrics 1967, 71, 107–113.

25. Lindall W, Elting J, Ells J and Roos BA. Estimation of biologically active intact parathyroid hormone in normal and hyperparathyroid sera by sequential N-terminal immunoextraction and midregion radioimmunoassay. Journal of Clinical Endocrinology and Metabolism 1983, 57, 1007–1014.

26. Lindvall N. Roentgenologic diagnosis of medullary sponge kidney. Acta Radiologica 1959, 51, 193–206.

27. Mall JC, Ghahremani GG and Boyer JL. Caroli's disease associated with congenital hepatic fibrosis and renal tubular ectasia. Gastroenterology 1974, 66, 1029–1035.

28. Maschio G, Tessitore N and D'Angelo A. Medullary sponge kidney and hyperparathyroidism...a puzzling association. American Journal of Nephrology 1982, 2, 77–84.

29. Morris RC, Yamauchi H, Palubinskas AJ and Howenstine J. Medullary sponge kidney. American Journal of Medicine 1965, 38, 883–892.

30. Myall GF. The incidence of medullary sponge kidney. Clinical Radiology 1970, 21, 171–174.

31. Nemoy, NJ and Forsberg L. Polycystic renal disease presenting as medullary sponge kidney. Journal of Urology 1968, 100, 407–411.

32. O'Neill M, Breslau NA and Pak CYC. Metabolic evaluation of nephrolithiasis in patients with medullary sponge kidney. Journal of the American Medical Association 1981, 245, 1233–1236.

33. Palubinskas AJ. Medullary sponge kidney. Radiology 1961, 76, 911–918.

34. Palubinskas AJ. Renal pyramidal structure opacification in excretory urography and its relation to medullary sponge kidney. Radiology 1963, 81, 963–970.

35. Parks JH, Coe FL and Strauss AL. Calcium nephrolithiasis and medullary sponge kidney in women. New England Journal of Medicine 1982, 306, 1088–1091.
36. Pollack HM. Some limitations and pitfalls of excretory urography. Journal of Urology 1976, 116, 537–543.
37. Pyrah LN. Medullary sponge kidney. Journal of Urology 1966, 95, 274–283.
38. Reilly BJ and Neuhauser EBD. Renal tubular ectasia in cystic disease of the kidneys and liver. American Journal of Roentgenology 1960, 84, 546–554.
39. Robertson WG, Peacock M and Nordin BEC. Measurement of activity products in urine from stone-formers and normal subjects. In: Hench LL, Smith LH and Finlayson B, eds., Urolithiasis: Physical Aspects. Washington: National Academy of Sciences, 1972, 79.
40. Sage MR, Lawson AD, Marshall VR and Ryall RL. Medullary sponge kidney and urolithiasis. Clinical Radiology 1982, 33, 435–438.
41. Schoeneman MJ, Plewinska M, Mucha M and Mieza M. Marfan syndrome and medullary sponge kidney: case report and speculation on pathogenesis. International Journal of Pediatric Nephrology 1984, 5, 103–104.
42. Thomas WC Jr. Use of phosphates in patients with calcareous renal calculi. Kidney International 1978, 13, 390–396.
43. Thomas WC Jr, Malagodi MH and Rennert OM. Amino acids in urine and blood of calculous patients. Investigative Urology 1981, 19, 115–118.
44. Vagelli G, Ferraris V, Calabrese G, Mazotta A, Pratesi G and Gonella M. Medullary sponge kidney and calcium nephrolithiasis. Urology Research 1988, 16, 201 (Abstract).
45. Vermooten V. Congenital cystic dilatation of the renal collecting tubules. Yale Journal of Biolical Medicine 1951, 23, 450–453.
46. Werness PG, Brown CM, Smith LH and Finlayson B. Equil 2: A basic computer program for the calculation of urinary saturation. Journal of Urology 1985, 134, 1242–1244.
47. Wikstrom B, Backman U and Danielson BG. Ambulatory diagnostic evaluation of 389 recurrent renal stone formers. A proposal for clinical classification and investigation. Klin Wochenschrift 1983, 61, 85–90.
48. Yendt ER and Cohanim M. Prevention of calcium stones with thiazides. Kidney International 1978, 13, 397–409.
49. Yendt ER, Jarzylo S and Finnis W. Medullary sponge kidney (tubular ectasia) in calcium urolithiasis. In: Smith LH, Robertson WG and Finlayson B, eds., Urolithiasis: Clinical and Basic Research. New York: Plenum Press, 1981, 105–112.
50. Yendt ER. Medullary sponge kidney and urolithiasis. In: Rous SN ed., Stone Disease: Diagnosis and Management. Orlando: Grune and Stratton, Inc, 1987, 135–146.
51. Yendt ER and Cohanim M. Clinical and laboratory approaches for evaluation of nephrolithiasis. Journal of Urology. 1989, 14, 764–769.
52. Yendt ER, Jarzylo S and Cohanim M. Medullary sponge kidney. In: Proceedings of the Seventh International Symposium on Urolithiasis. New York: Plenum Press. (In press).

16
Congenital Multicystic Kidney

C. F. Piel

Abstract

The congenital multicystic kidney is composed of cysts of varying size and number supported by mesenchymal stroma. It is dysplastic, always containing primitive ducts considered evidence of faulted organogenesis. The ureter is usually atretic. A normal reniform contour is not present, and function cannot be demonstrated. The majority of abdominal masses in the neonate are of renal origin, and multicystic dysplastic kidney and hydronephrosis account for approximately 90% of them. Multicystic kidney is generally considered to be non-hereditary. It occurs more frequently on the left side than on the right and in males more often than in females. Bilateral involvement rarely occurs, although abnormalities (primarily hydronephrosis or dysplasia) exist relatively frequently in the contralateral kidney. Other systems may be involved, particularly the gastrointestinal tract (esophageal atresia). Ultrasonography readily reveals the diagnosis anti- and post-natally. Radionuclide study or computed tomography confirms it. Removal of the mass in infancy is not necessary unless size is a problem. Whether surgical removal is indicated at any time remains controversial.

1. Introduction

The congenital multicystic kidney is a grossly cystic, dysplastic kidney associated with an atretic ureter. It is frequently described as resembling a "bunch of grapes", even though it does not look like one. Normal gross architecture is not seen, but small lobes of renal tissue are occasionally present. No function can be demonstrated by intravenous pyelography or isotopic techniques, although high doses of contrast medium ("total body opacification") may visualize the kidney. The contralateral kidney may be normal, but not uncommonly multicystic, dysplastic or hydronephrotic. In addition, other systems are often involved.

The dysplastic multicystic kidney characteristically presents in infancy as an abdominal mass, but may be found in later life, sometimes with symptoms, sometimes as an incidental finding. In the majority of affected individuals there is no hereditary pattern.

The following discussion includes those reports which, in the view of this author, contribute to the current understanding of congenital multicystic kidney.

2. History

The term "unilateral multicystic kidney" was first proposed by Schwartz[70] in 1936, when he described a large abdominal mass removed from a well seven-month-old infant. The mass proved to be a kidney totally replaced by varying sized cysts; normal tissue was not present. Many authors have since described similar cases, usually as single case reports using varying terminology. In 1955, Spence[72] established multicystic kidney as an entity distinct from polycystic kidney disease. He reviewed 15 cases from the literature and added four. Most patients were well infants who presented with palpable flank masses in the first weeks or months of life, but there were also a four-year-old with rickets and renal failure and a 70-year-old with recurrent urinary tract infections. Plain films of the abdomen revealed calcific rings in the renal fossae in the two oldest patients. There was no predilection for sex or side of involvement. Nephrograms performed preoperatively revealed no function on the affected side. The ipsilateral ureteral orifice was lacking in half of the patients who underwent cystoscopy, and the other half had ureteral obstruction. The resected kidneys were replaced by cysts of varying size and were without normal renal architecture. Solid tissue components consisted of embryonal elements, ducts, ductules, tubules and glomeruli that had failed to differentiate normally.

Spence concluded that the multicystic kidney presented as a palpable, non-tender, freely movable flank mass, usually in a newborn or infant and unassociated with symptoms unless the mass was large enough to impinge on other abdominal organs. He stated that the lesion could occur in adults. He further noted that the lesion was unilateral and the prognosis good, provided the opposite kidney was normal.

Spence's observations and conclusions fit with current concepts of the abnormality. In 1959, Friedman and Abeshouse[27] found 76 cases in the literature, usually single case reports. They added three and found that 36 were under the age of one year; 23, however, were older than 30 years. Calcification was present in 25 of the 79 kidneys, 15 of these in patients over the age of 30 years. Both Spence and Freidman and Abeshouse recognized the need to ascertain function of the contralateral kidney. Both of these papers, as well as many others published in the 1950s, recommended nephrectomy as the treatment of choice.

3. Incidence

The true incidence of multicystic dysplastic kidney is difficult to assess (Table 16.1).

Table 16.1 Incidence of multicystic dysplasia of the kidney in children

Authors	Date	Place	Years of observation	Hospital admissions	Autopsy reviews	Uni-lateral	Bi-lateral
Fine and Burns[26]	1959	Tulane	20	829,292[a], 349,414		0 6	0 0
Parkkulainen et al.[59]	1959	Scandinavia	12	32,000	2,900	6 12	1
Gummess et al.[32]	1960	Los Angeles		> 1,000,000		9	
Rubenstein et al.[67]	1961	Detroit	10		2,153 (180 renal abnormalities)	7	
Vellios and Garrett[79]	1961	Indiana	8			7	
Pathak and Williams[60]	1963	London	12	107,000		20	1
Staubitz et al.[75]	1963	Buffalo	20	20 cystic renal cases		7	
Greene et al.[30]	1971	Mayo Clinic	>30	Records		19 11[b]	8
Risdon[65]	1971	London	15	150 cases for nephrectomy	121 with GU anomalies	14 6	0 3
Daniel et al.[19]	1972	Mayo Clinic	10	2,709[c]		10	0
Griscom et al.[31]	1975	St Louis	> 30	Records		44	2
Felson and Cussen[24]	1975	Cincinnati	10		Records	18	2
Lebowitz & Griscom[46]	1977	Boston	30	146 infants with hydro-nephrosi		6	
Mir et al.[53d]	1983	Finland	30		6,521	23	28

[a]Adult admissions.
[b]Over the age of 16 years.
[c]Review of renal masses demonstrated by IVP or abdominal film.
[d]Not clear in this paper if these children truly had multicystic dysplastic kidney disease as defined in the beginning of this chapter.
[e]Three of these cases were from the Pathology Museum – not admissions during the period.

The reported occurrence rate is based primarily on surveys of hospital admissions or on reviews of autopsies. The frequently published statement that the multicystic kidney is "the most common cause of abdominal mass in the newborn"[24,44] is based on the 1958 review of admissions to the surgical service at Boston Children's Hospital[49]. During a 20-year period, 32 infants were admitted to the surgical service of that hospital for abdominal masses discovered in the first day of life. Sixteen of the masses were renal, 15 multicystic kidneys, two of them bilateral and one mass was a hydronephrotic kidney.

In 1959, Melicow and Uson[52] reviewed the records of 653 infants and children who were hospitalized between 1934 and 1956 at Columbia Presbyterian Center in New York City because of palpable abdominal masses. The majority of these children, 372, had "medical" conditions. Nine of 31 children with renal cystic diseases were classified as having unilateral multicystic kidney. Fifty-six infants had hydronephrosis, with obstruction of the ureteropelvic junction in 34.

A third paper a decade later described the incidence of abdominal masses in children under one year of age seen in the pediatric surgical services at Cook County Children's Hospital and the Cook County Hospital[64]. In a 13-year period, seven of 31 infants had unilateral multicystic kidney disease. One of them had a small Wilms tumor in the wall of one cyst. Six infants had hydronephrosis resulting from ureteropelvic obstruction.

The last two papers illustrate the comparable occurrence of unilateral multicystic kidney disease and hydronephrosis in infancy, confirmed by additional reports (Table 16.1). Multicystic kidney occurs infrequently and quite rarely may be bilateral. Multicystic kidney disease occurs in 0.02–0.05 per 100,000 hospital admissions. The frequency increases in series of patients studied by radiographic techniques to demonstrate and evaluate abdominal masses and in studies of autopsy material. The periods of observation included in these papers vary from 8 to 30 years.

4. Clinical presentation

By far, the most frequent presentation of multicystic kidney disease is the incidental finding of a non-tender, freely movable mass in the left or right flank of an asymptomatic newborn or infant. The mass may occasionally be transilluminated. The mass is sometimes large enough to crowd the abdominal space and induce symptoms of distention and vomiting. Urinary tract findings, such as proteinuria, hematuria and infection, may infrequently initiate studies that lead to the discovery of the multicystic kidney. These signs relate to the contralateral kidney. There is occasional occurrence of or presentation with hypertension[17,39]. In older individuals, abdominal pain may lead to the discovery of the mass, characterized radiographically by concentric rings of calcium that outline the walls of the cysts. Identical calcific rings may also be an incidental finding during evaluation for an unrelated problem[1].

In 1955, when Spence identified the multicystic kidney as a distinct entity, he stressed its unilaterality, but by 1957, it was recognized to be occasionally bilateral[49] (Table 16.1). Affected infants presenting with bilateral flank masses succumb shortly after birth. In their review of the lesion, Mir et al.[53] did not clearly define multicystic kidney. Many of their patients, identified as having cystic dysplasia, with or without obstruction, survived for extended periods of time. The multicystic kidney as defined in this chapter essentially does not function. Bilateral occurrence is not compatible with survival beyond a few weeks. One patient is reported to have lived for 64 days[41].

It is commonly stated that there is no sex predilection. However, a review of papers reporting the largest numbers of cases indicates that there is not only a preponderance of males, but also a more frequent occurrence of the lesion on the left than on the right[24,26,30-32,53,55,59,60,65,75,79]. Although Spence realized that function of the contralateral kidney required evaluation and management, it has since become apparent that the opposite kidney is frequently compromised (Table 16.2).

Table 16.2 Unilateral multicystic kidney: The contralateral kidney

References	Number involved/ total number of patients	Hydronephrosis ureteropelvic junction obstruction	Hydronephrosis ureteral stenosis or dilatation	Kidney agenesis	Foci of cysts or dysplasia
Parkkulainen et al.[59]	5/19	2		1	2
Pathak and Williams[60]	16/20	5	6		5
Greene et al.[30]	7/38	3	3	1	
Risden[65]	2/14	2			
	4/6	1	1	1	1
Griscom et al.[31]	7/44	7			
Mir et al.[53]	15/23	3			12
Curry et al.[18]	31/80			6	
DeKlerk et al.[20]	7/29	2	1		4
Kleiner et al.[42]	11/27	2		3	6

Sixteen of the 20 children with multicystic kidney disease reported by Pathak et al.[60] had lesions of the contralateral kidney. The contralateral kidney may be hydronephrotic due to obstruction at the ureteropelvic or ureterovesical junction, stenosis along the course of the ureter, megaureter, or vesicoureteric reflux. The kidney may also contain areas of dysplasia. Small multicystic kidneys, sometimes little more than a nubbin of tissue, constitute a spectrum with the large, more typical forms and have been categorized as "aplastic".

Anomalies of systems other than the urologic tract may seriously compromise many children with multicystic dysplasia. Only five of 19 patients described by Parkkulainen et al.[59] and one-third of 38 cases at the Mayo Clinic[30]

had no associated anomalies. One of the more frequent abnormalities is esophageal atresia, often with tracheo–esophageal fistula (Table 16.3).

Table 16.3 Multicystic kidney dysplasia: other organ involvement

Reference	26	59	60	30	65	55	31	24	53	18	20	42
No. of cases	6	19	21	38[b]	20	27	46	20	23	31	29	27
Cardiovascular								4[a]	3[a]			
Tetralogy of Fallot						2						
Truncus arteriosus		1										
Right-sided aortic arch			1									
Left superior vena cava			1									
Abnormal rt subclavian artery			1									
Overriding aorta			1									
Coarctation of aorta			2		1							
Pulmonary stenosis		1			1							
Ventricular septal defect	1	1	3	1	1	1					2	1
Atrial septal defect					2							
Hypoplastic left ventricle	1									3		
Patent ductus arteriosus		1	3	1	3					5	1	
Gastrointestinal												
Esophageal atresia				1			1		10[c]			
Tracheo-esophageal fistula		5		1	2							
Duodenal atresia					1						2	
Exomphalos	1											
Universal mesentery								1				
Rectal atresia		2	2	1	5			1		3	1	1
Hirschsprung disease								1				
Annular pancreas			1		1							
Agenesis of gall bladder					1							
Nervous system												
Arnold–Chiari deformity					1							
Meningomyelocele			1	1	1							
Hydrocephalus			1	1				1				
Anencephalia			1									
Musculoskeletal												
Absent abdominal muscle			1									
Talipes	1		2	1							1	
Absent radii		1										
Harelip and cleft palate	1		1				1	3			1	
Spina bifida				1								
Micrognathia								2				
Sagittal synostosis							1					
Pterygium colli							1					
Genital										5[b]		
Gonadal dysgenesis		1									2	
Absent bladder		1										
Bicornate uterus		1										
Inguinal hernia					3							
Hypospadias										2		

[a]Precise lesion not stated.
[b]Type of abnormality, number of cases not stated.
[c]10 of 28 children with bilateral cystic dysplasia. An additional 14 of 23 with unilateral renal cystic dysplasia with and without obstruction also had alimentary tract abnormalities. Not stated in the article if these are cases of multicystic renal dysplasia.

It has been suggested, therefore, that all babies with esophageal atresia have sonography of the kidneys prior to surgical intervention[53]. Compensatory hypertrophy of a normal contralateral kidney is not present at birth, but does occur later in life[31,55].

The multicystic dysplastic kidney is considered to be non-hereditary. There are no published reports of involvement of siblings or of inheritance from one generation to the next. However, there are documented cases of multicystic dysplasia occurring in families with other urologic abnormalities, primarily agenesis[18,66,73]. Additionally, there is a recent paper describing a syndrome in two sibs and one first cousin composed of cystic dysplasia of the kidney and digital and cerebral abnormalities[23]. Cystic dysplasia of the kidney has been recognized for a long time to be an integral part of a variety of rare syndromes.

5. Pathology

5.1 Gross appearance

A reniform shape is not present. The cystic mass, which varies in size from smaller than normal to very much larger, replaces the normal kidney (Fig 16.1). The abnormal kidney is composed of cysts of varying size and number held together by connective tissue. It usually lies in the renal fossa, but ectopic kidneys may also be dysplastic[54]. The pelvis is usually not identified. The calyces and pelvis were entirely absent in 20 of the 21 cases reported by Pathak et al.[60]. The ureter may be dilated proximally, but is usually stenotic somewhere along its course; it may be completely atretic and fibrous. Total atresia of the ureter is associated with absence of the ipsilateral ureterovesical orifice and hemitrigone.

Osathanondh and Potter[58] described two types of gross appearance: one is a cluster of cysts with no identifiable pelvis; the other a cluster of cysts with a dilated cavity in the renal pelvic area, which may include a few centimetres of the dilated ureter above a stenosed segment. Griscom and his associates[31] excluded this "hydropelvic" type and consider pelvo-infundibular atresia essential for the definition of multicystic dysplastic kidney. Felson and Cussen[24] describe cases of what they call multicystic dysplastic kidneys with both alterations, some with pelvic atresia, which is the most common variety, and some with a dilated pelvis. However, the hydronephrotic type of multicystic dysplasia is probably a form of dysplasia associated with almost any kind of urinary tract obstruction, with distinct morphologic differences from multicystic dysplasia.

Cysts are generally considered not to communicate with one another. However, in a few instances communications have been demonstrated both in the late phase of intravenous urography and by the injection of contrast medium above the stenosed ureter in the surgically removed specimen[24]. Using percu-

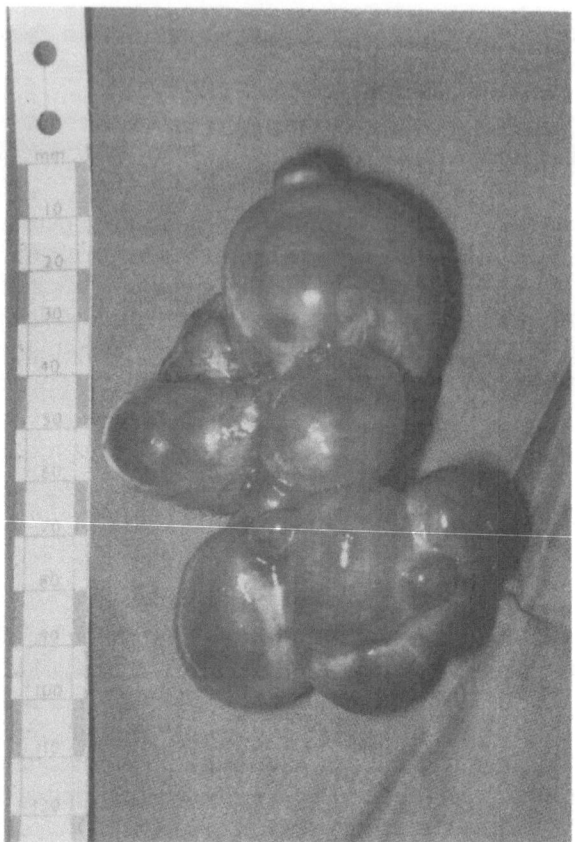

Figure 16.1 Left unilateral multicystic kidney removed at operation. The ureter was identified, but could not be cannulated. Note variably sized cysts. (Courtesy of Barry A. Kogan MD).

taneous pyelography, Saxton *et al.*[69] demonstrated communication between cysts through tortuous tubules. They advocated this procedure to distinguish between multicystic dysplastic kidney and severe neonatal hydronephrosis. Perhaps communication between cysts would be found more frequently if this procedure were in general use. The vasculature is miniaturized, in an abnormal position, or impossible to identify[24,31,59]. Bladder and urethra are normal, except the ipsilateral hemitrigone is lacking in cases of total ureteral atresia.

5.2 Microscopic appearance

The criteria necessary to make the diagnosis of renal dysplasia were established in 1958 by Ericsson and Ivemark[21,22]. For them, the presence of primitive ducts and cartilage was acceptable evidence of malformation during renal differentiation. In multicystic disease, the prominent feature is the presence of numerous cysts (Fig. 16.2), which are lined with cuboidal epithelium and contain clear fluid usually comparable in composition to extracellular fluid[30,31].

Fluid has been found to contain taurine, considered evidence of nephron activity[59].

Cuboidal or columnar epithelium, often ciliated, lines the primitive ducts. The ducts occur singly and in clusters, surrounded by varying amounts of usually dense connective tissue and smooth muscle fibres (Fig. 16.3).

These primitive ducts may be restricted to the hilar area, but also extend out to the subcapsular region. They are considered to be altered derivatives of the metanephric duct. The foci of cartilage are primarily located in the cortical areas and appear to be derived from metanephric blastema[9]. By microdissection, Osathanondh and Potter[58] demonstrated fewer generations of tubules derived from the ureteric buds, only 4–12 instead of 12–20. Some primitive ducts radiate out from the pelvic area and terminate in cysts; some of the last generations terminate in normal nephrons without dilatation. The septa among the cysts contain primitive ductules, some dilated, others more normal and lined with cuboidal or flat epithelium, islets of cartilage, small areas of lymphoid-like tissue, vessels, nerve trunks and clusters of nephrons. Glomeruli are

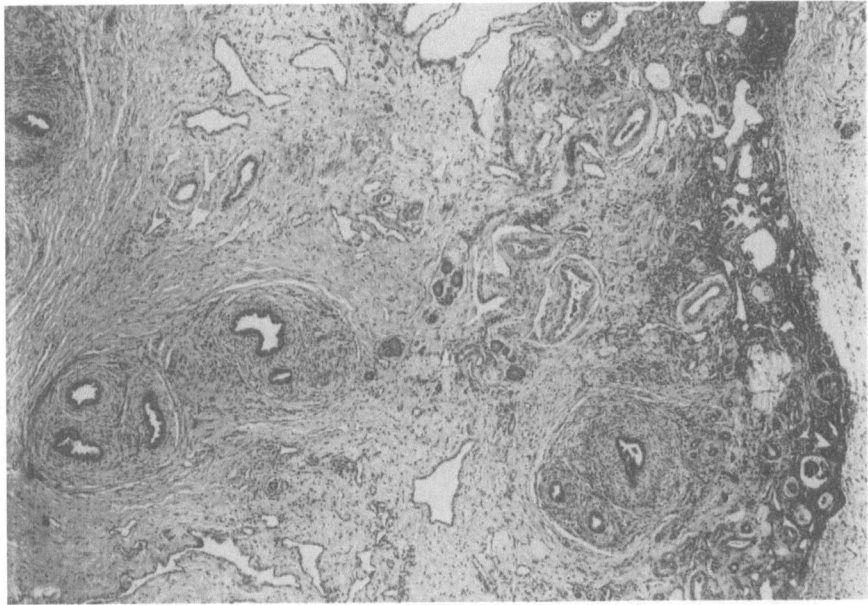

Figure 16.2 Histologic examination of multicystic dysplastic kidney. On the lower left side are two clusters of primitive ducts, each surrounded by a collar of dense fibrous tissue. Several small cysts lined with flat epithelium are seen at the top and bottom of this section. On the right is an area of primitive glomeruli, tubules bordered by fibrous mesenchyma and several thick-walled vessels. The tissue in the centre consists of embryonic stroma. (Courtesy of Barry A. Kogan MD) × 27.

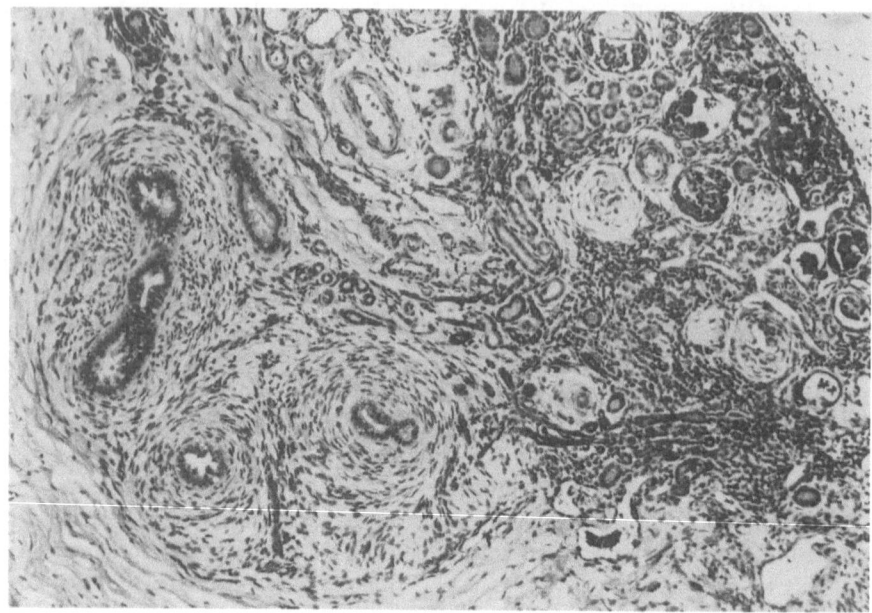

Figure 16.3 Photomicrograph of dysplastic kidney. On the lower left is a cluster of primitive ducts lined with high columnar epithelium and surrounded by a concentric arrangement of primitive connective tissue and smooth muscle. On the right is a focus of primitive glomeruli, some of which are sclerosed. The surrounding lymphocytes are considered to be associated with hematopoiesis. (Courtesy of Barry A. Kogan MD) × 68.

primitive – poorly vascularized and small, with segmental hyalinization. The primitive ductules may be traced through the pelvic area to the cortex where they lie close to, but not connected with, the immature glomerular and tubular structures[12].

Ljungqvist[48] showed, by microangiography of specimens, that large hilar vessels branch repeatedly and fan out into the subcapsular region. Such large subcapsular vessels do not exist in normal or other abnormal kidneys. Ljungqvist described the vasculature of the cyst walls as being similar to that of the normal renal pelvis, and the vasculature around the primitive ducts as having a medullary pattern. He judged the vessels between the primitive ducts and the cortex to be arcuate arteries, and considered the arteriole–glomerular units to be similar to normal fetal ones that involute shortly after infancy.

There is general agreement that the presence of primitive ducts is essential for the diagnosis of renal dysplasia[10,22]. Whether islets of cartilage can occur in normal kidneys[63] or in association with chronic inflammation[78] without foci of dysplasia is controversial. Primitive glomeruli, tubules and ductules may appear in reparative states such as those occurring in neonatal renal necrosis[11], renal trauma in the experimental animal[10], and post-biopsy scarring.

6. Pathogenesis

Normal renal structure depends on the orderly penetration of the ureteric bud into the normally positioned and constituted metanephric blastema. Osatha-nondh and Potter[58] concluded that inadequate ampullary activity caused failure of induction of normal nephrons and resulted in the cystic abnormality. It is recognized that fetal urine is discharged into the bladder at approximately the 10th to the 11th week of gestation, and that nephron induction is complete at 32–36 weeks of gestation. The earlier in organogenesis that maldevelopment occurs, the more dysplastic the kidney.

Ultrasonography has provided some interesting insights into the natural history of the multicystic kidney and has raised provocative questions about its pathogenesis. Avni et al.[3] found that the multicystic kidney changed dramati-cally both in utero and after delivery. Sonography at a mean gestational age of 28.8 weeks (range 21–35 weeks) showed cysts, whereas previous studies at a mean gestational age of 18.8 weeks (range 14–25 weeks) had not. Perhaps cysts were present but were too small to be identified by sonography. Subsequent fetal sonography showed some kidneys to remain unchanged, cysts in some to increase and cysts in others to decrease. Similarly, post-natal follow-up showed cysts in some kidneys to decrease in size and some cysts to disappear completely after several years. Cyst walls also calcified after a period of time.

Similar observations have been made by others. Arger et al.[2] found cystic disease in nine fetuses, seven with unilateral and two with bilateral in-volvement, in obstetrical ultrasonographic examination of 3,530 patients. The abnormality was first seen at a mean age of 28 weeks of gestation (range 18–34 weeks), and three of the seven with unilateral disease had an earlier ex-amination that did not show the abnormality. Pedicelli et al.[61] observed post-natal disappearance of cystic masses demonstrated antenatally. Hashimoto et al.[36] also found an increase and occasional decrease in size of the cysts with progression of pregnancy. These sonographic observations define the earliest periods in gestation when the diagnosis of multicystic dysplastic kidney can be made, and illustrate the changes in structure that can occur during gestation and after birth. Both total disappearance of the mass and involution of the cysts to form a small, echogenic, aplastic kidney have been described. The apparently involutional changes in the cystic kidneys and the association of small renal arteries with multicystic dysplasia support older theories that faulted vascular development plays a role in the production of this anomaly.

Attempts to produce multicystic dysplasia experimentally have generally been disappointing. Tanagho[77] and Beck[7] produced hydronephrosis, but no dysplasia, by ligating one or both ureters in lambs during mid or late gestation. Fetterman et al.[25] induced dilatation of the loop of Henle when they performed ureteral ligation in the last half of gestation in rabbits. They also found dilata-tion of the peripheral, immature nephrons. Glick et al.[28] produced hydrone-phrosis with histologic lesions of dysplasia by ligating one ureter in 58–66 day-old lamb fetuses. Berman and Maizels[8] were unable, however, to induce dysplasia in chick embryos by ligating the ureters before or after the appearance of nephrons. Only hydronephrosis occurred in this model.

7. Evaluation

The majority of abdominal masses in the infant are of renal origin. The majority of renal masses are either multicystic dysplastic or hydronephrotic kidneys[46]. Originally, the multicystic kidney was differentiated from hydronephrosis, Wilms tumor, and fetal renal hamartoma by routine radiographic procedures if (1) intravenous urography failed to demonstrate function, (2) retrograde pyelography revealed a hypoplastic or atretic ureter, and (3) angiography revealed hypoplastic or absent renal arteries[43,44].

In 1963, O'Connor and Neuhauser[56] observed early total body opacification of the vascular compartment by large doses of contrast medium, and kidney cysts appeared after contrast as non-opacified or radiolucent areas. Leonidas et al.[47] used the high-dose technique, including immediate films after the injection and again at three and five minutes, to demonstrate radiopaque rims surrounding radiolucent areas during the early phase of opacification. The authors interpreted these findings as reflecting visualization of the vascular stroma in the cyst walls. They considered this pattern to be specific to multicystic dysplastic kidneys, clearly differentiating it from other non-visualizing abdominal masses.

Newer contrast agents subsequently became available. Warshawsky et al.[81] found visualization of cystic abdominal masses to occur later in the course of intravenous urography, several minutes after initial total body opacification. Histology of the cystic masses removed at surgery confirmed the presence of glomeruli and tubules in the foci that corresponded to the areas of radiographic visualization. Felson and Cussen[24] also observed calyceal crescents in some patients with multicystic renal dysplasia, but the parenchymal tissue found histologically did not correlate with the location of the crescents. However, contrast medium injection into the surgically removed specimens revealed opacification of many of the cysts, indicating the presence of communication among the cysts and suggesting the presence of pelvic dilatation.

Young et al.[83] observed late puddling of contrast material in cysts after earlier visualization of crescents in one patient. Felson and Cussen[24] interpreted that finding to support their contention that hydropelvis is an acceptable finding in multicystic renal dysplasia, although less common than the more usual occurrence of pelvic atresia.

Although not all investigators agree with this, the idea seems reasonable, since the dysplasia is almost identical in both.

Most recently, ultrasonography has become the initial diagnostic procedure of choice, particularly in children[4,5,6,29,71]. It is non-invasive, harmless,

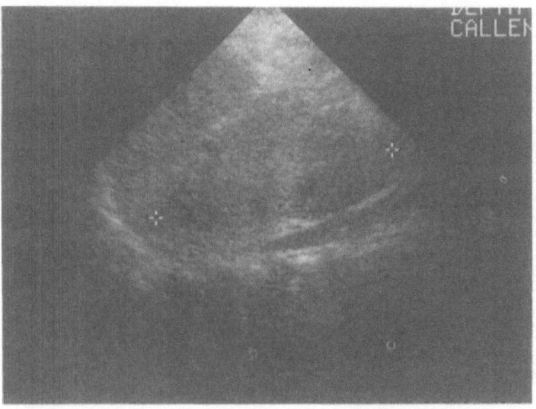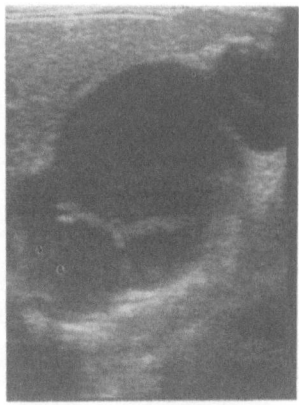

Figure 16.4 Case 1. A male prematurely born after 33 weeks gestation. Normal pregnancy and female twin. Cystic right kidney identified antenatally. On the right is a sonogram of the right kidney performed at 4 months of age. Several large cysts are revealed. On the left is a sonogram of the left kidney which shows homogeneous echotexture without corticomedullary distinction. The serum creatinine at 3 weeks of age was 2.2 mg/dl; at four months, 0.9 mg/dl.

readily accepted by patients and relatively inexpensive[84]. Experienced operators can readily differentiate fluid-filled structures from solid tissues with 90–95% accuracy[62].

Early descriptions[6] of the distinct ultrasonographic features seen in multicystic kidney disease have been expanded by Stuck *et al.*[76] to include: (1) the presence of interfaces between the cysts (Figure 16.4), (2) lateral location of the larger cysts, and (3) no identifiable renal sinus.

The presence of septa (cyst walls) and lateral displacement of the largest cysts establishes the correct diagnosis.

Sonography of the hydronephrotic kidney demonstrates a dilated pelvis with ovoid, hypoechoic areas representing dilated calyces radiating outward from the hilum[29]. The importance of differentiating the hydronephrotic from multicystic dysplastic kidney is self-evident, since prompt relief of obstruction is required in order to salvage renal tissue. However, sonographic findings may be misleading[68], sometimes strongly suggestive of ureteropelvic obstruction[82]. Findings such as these have led many investigators to question the existence of the "hydropelvic" variety of multicystic dysplastic kidney.

Currently, the initial diagnostic procedure for evaluation of an abdominal mass is sonography. In those cases with inconclusive sonographic findings, the next diagnostic step is usually a radionuclide study, which also is less invasive and carries less exposure to radiation than conventional radiographic techniques. In multicystic renal dysplasia, there is no uptake of photons (Fig. 16.5).

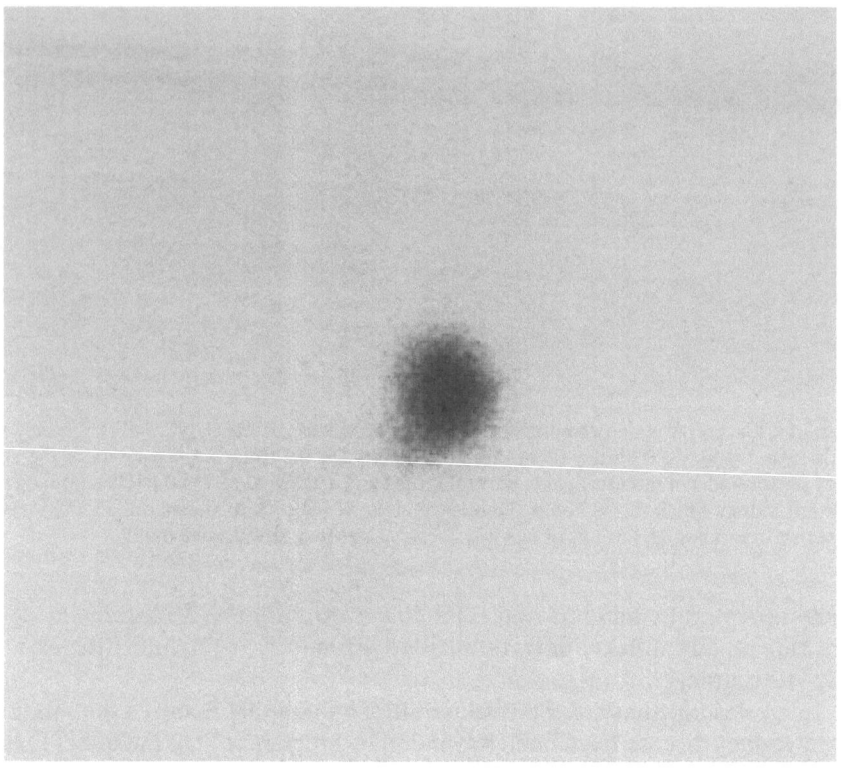

Figure 16.5 DMSA study in Case 1 (Fig. 16.4) demonstrates function on the left, no uptake of photons on the right. DMSA study was identical at birth and at 4 months of age.

An alternative is computed tomography, with or without contrast enhancement[15,51]. The most recently developed modality, magnetic resonance imaging, has not yet proved to offer additional diagnostic accuracy[38,50].

Cystic lesions of the urinary tract in fetuses are easily detected by sonography[34]. Normal fetal kidneys are identified by the 15th post-menstrual week, but normal renal architecture cannot be differentiated until the 20th week. Multicystic kidney dysplasia has been repeatedly recognized *in utero*[57], although cystic lesions may be confused with fluid-filled bowel loops[37]. Since patients with unilateral multicystic disease and a normal contralateral kidney may live a long time, antenatal sonography guides both obstetrical and postnatal management. Whether intrauterine surgical intervention should be undertaken to relieve obstruction of a hydronephrotic contralateral kidney remains debatable. The risks of such surgery must be weighed against the recognized increase in damage that occurs over time in an obstructed kidney.

It is very questionable whether any current modality can detect abnormalities early in gestation when dysplasia begins.

8. Management

Originally, all multicystic kidneys presenting as abdominal masses in the neonatal period were removed surgically, primarily for diagnostic purposes. Many detected at an older age were symptomatic, usually with abdominal pain, and some were found incidentally to other evaluations. Since the diagnosis can be made more accurately with current procedures (sonography and computed tomography) than with the older, conventional modalities (excretory urography, retrograde pyelography and cyst puncture), the need for nephrectomy to confirm the diagnosis has been seriously questioned. In a survey of 136 pediatric urologists published more than 10 years ago[14], 75% were confident of the diagnosis. Forty-four percent believed that exploration was not necessary in asymptomatic patients. Sonographers are demonstrating that the cysts may become smaller or even disappear with time[3,36,61]. However, information about the natural history is scarce. Those who caution against non-intervention express concern about associated malignancy, hypertension, infection and pain. To date, reports of these problems are few. Of the 31 cases identified beyond infancy[1,5,13,35,39], five have been found to contain tumors, three renal cell carcinomas, one mesothelial tumor and one Wilms tumor[35]. Raffensberger and Abousleiman[64] had previously reported a Wilms tumor in the multicystic kidney of a 10-month-old infant.

Hypertension that resolved post-nephrectomy has been reported in three patients, ages 3 weeks[17], 6 years[39] and 21 years[16]. Hypertension was not altered by removal of the cystic mass in four of 27 patients reviewed by Ambrose[1]. Pain in 14 of these 27 patients was relieved by nephrectomy. There is total agreement that surgical exploration is indicated if the diagnosis is questionable. Twenty-five percent of the urologists surveyed by Bloom and Brosman[14] reported misdiagnoses when their patients were explored for presumed multicystic kidneys. It should be noted that, in this report, the preferred procedure used for evaluation of the abdominal masses was intravenous pyelography. The current use of sonography and renal scan has led to increased accuracy and permits non-invasive follow-up. Whether surgical removal is indicated in all cases is greatly debated at this time[40,74,80]. However, if the decision is to leave the cystic mass *in situ*, diligent follow-up is indicated.

References

1. Ambrose S, Gould R, Trulock T and Parrott T. Unilateral multicystic renal disease in adults. Journal of Urology 1982, 128, 366–369.

2. Arger P, Coleman B, Mintz M, Snyder H, Camardese T, Arenson R, Gabbe S and Aquino L. Routine fetal genitourinary tract screening. Radiology 1985, 156, 485–489.
3. Avni E, Thoua Y, Lalmand B, Didier F, Droulle P and Schulman C. Multicystic dysplastic kidney: Natural history from in utero diagnosis and postnatal followup. Journal of Urology 1987, 138, 1420–1424.
4. Baltarowich O and Kurtz A. Sonographic evaluation of renal masses. Urological Radiology 1987, 9, 79–87.
5. Barrett D and Wineland R. Renal cell carcinoma in multicystic dysplastic kidney. Urology 1980, 15, 152–154.
6. Bearman S, Hine P and Sanders R. Multicystic kidney: A sonographic pattern. Radiology 1976, 118, 685–688.
7. Beck A. The effect of intra-uterine urinary obstruction upon the development of the fetal kidney. Journal of Urology 1971, 105, 784–89.
8. Berman D and Maizels M. The role of urinary obstruction in the genesis of renal dysplasia. A model in the chick embryo. Journal of Urology 1982, 128, 1091–1096.
9. Bernstein J. Developmental abnormalities of the renal parenchymal – renal hypoplasia and dysplasia. In: Sommers SC, ed., Pathology Annual. New York: Appleton-Century-Crofts, 1968; 213–247.
10. Bernstein J. The morphogenesis of renal parenchymal maldevelopment (renal dysplasia). Pediatric Clinics of North America 1971, 18, 395–407.
11. Bernstein J and Meyer R. Congenital abnormalities of the urinary system. II. Renal cortical and medullary necrosis. Journal of Pediatrics 1961, 59, 657–668.
12. Bialestock D. Morphogenesis of unilateral multicystic kidney in childhood. Australasian Annals of Medicine 1960, 9, 53–56.
13. Birken G, King D, Vane D and Lloyd T. Renal cell carcinoma arising in a multicystic dysplastic kidney. Journal of Pediatric Surg 1985, 20, 619–621.
14. Bloom D and Brosman S. The multicystic kidney. Journal of Urology 1978, 120, 211–215.
15. Bosniak M. The current radiological approach to renal cysts. Radiology 1986, 158, 1–10.
16. Burgler W and Hauri D. Vitale komplikationen bei multizystischer nierendegeneration (multizystischer dysplasie). Urology International 1983, 38, 251–256.
17. Chen Y, Stapleton F, Roy S III and Noe H. Neonatal hypertension from a unilateral multicystic dysplastic kidney. Journal of Urology 1985, 133, 664–665.
18. Curry C, Jensen K, Holland J, Miller L and Hall B. The Potter sequence: A clinical analysis of 80 cases. American Journal of Medical Genetics 1984, 19, 679–702.
19. Daniel W Jr, Hartman G, Witten D, Farrow G and Kelalis P. Calcified renal masses. Radiology 1972, 103, 503–508.
20. DeKlerk D, Marshall F and Jeffs R. Multicystic dysplastic kidney. Journal of Urology 1977, 118, 306–308.
21. Ericsson N and Ivemark B. Renal dysplasia and pyelonephritis in infants and children. Archives of Pathology and Laboratory Medicine 1958, 66, 255–269.
22. Ericsson N and Ivemark B. Renal dysplasia and urinary-tract infection. Acta Chirurgica Scandandinavica 1958, 115, 58–65.
23. Eronen M, Somer M, Gustafsson B and Holmberg C. New syndrome: A digito–renal–cerebral syndrome. American Journal of Medical Genetics 1985, 22, 281–285.
24. Felson B and Cussen L. The hydronephrotic type of unilateral congenital multicystic disease of the kidney. Seminars in Roentgenology 1975, 10, 113–123.
25. Fetterman G, Ravitch M and Sherman F. Cystic changes in fetal kidneys following ureteral ligation: Studies by microdissection. Kidney International 1974, 5, 111–121.
26. Fine M and Burns E. Unilateral multicystic kidney: Report of six cases and discussion of the literature. Journal of Urology 1959, 81, 42–48.
27. Friedman H and Abeshouse B. Congenital unilateral multicystic kidney; a review of the literature and a report of three cases. Journal of the Mount Sinai Hospital New York 1957, 6, 51–68.

28. Glick P, Harrison M, Noall R and Villa R. Correction of congenital hydronephrosis *in utero* III. Early mid-trimester ureteral obstruction produces renal dysplasia. Journal of Pediatrics Surg 1983, 18, 681–687.

29. Green W and King D. Diagnostic ultrasound of the urinary tract. Journal of Clinical Ultrasound 1975, 4, 55–64.

30. Greene L, Feinzaig W and Dahlin D. Multicystic dysplasia of the kidney: With special reference to the contralateral kidney. Journal of Urology 1971, 105, 482–487.

31. Griscom N, Vawter G and Fellers F. Pelvoinfundibular atresia: The usual form of multicystic kidney: 44 unilateral and two bilateral masses. Seminars in Roentgenology 1975, 10, 125–131.

32. Gummess G, Lombardo L and Lester D. The unilateral multicystic kidney. Report of nine cases. Western Journal of Surgery 1960, 68, 373–377.

33. Gutter W and Hermanek P. Maligner tumor der nierengegend unter dem bilde der knollenniere (nierenblastemcysten). Urology International 1957, 4, 164–182.

34. Hadlock F, Deter R, Carpenter R, Gonzalez E and Park S. Sonography of fetal urinary tract anomalies. American Journal of Roentgenology 1981, 137, 261–267.

35. Hartmann G, Smolik L and Shochat S. the dilemma of the multicystic dysplastic kidney. American Journal of Diseases in Children 1986, 140, 925–627.

36. Hashimoto B, Filly R and Callen P. Multicystic dysplastic kidney *in utero*: Changing appearance on US. Radiology 1986, 159, 107–109.

37. Henderson S, Van Kolken R and Rahatzad M. Multicystic kidney with hydramnios. Journal of Clinical Ultrasound 1980, 8, 249–250.

38. Hricak H, Williams R, Moon K Jr., Moss A, Alpers C, Crooks L and Kaufman L. Nuclear magnetic resonance imaging of the kidney: Renal masses. Radiology 1983, 147, 765–772.

39. Javadpour N, Chelouhy E, Moncada L, Rosenthal I and Bush I. Hypertension in a child caused by a multicystic kidney. Journal of Urology 1970, 104, 918–921.

40. King L. The management of multicystic kidney and ureteropelvic junction obstruction. In: King L, ed., Urologic Surgery in Neonates and Young Infants. Philadelphia: W. B. Saunders Company, 1988, 140–154.

41. Kishikawa T, Toda T, Ito H, Yamaguchi S, Kuroda M and Matsuyama K. Bilateral congenital multicystic dysplasia of the kidney. Japanese Journal of Surgery 1981, 11, 198–202.

42. Kleiner B, Filly R, Mack L and Callen P. Multicystic dysplastic kidney: Observations of contralateral disease in the fetal population. Radiology 1986, 161, 27–29.

43. Kyaw M. Roentgenologic triad of congenital multicystic kidney. American Journal of Roentgenology 1973, 119, 710–719.

44. Kyaw M and Koehler P. Congenital multicystic kidney. In: Gardner KD Jr ed., Cystic Diseases of the Kidney. New York: John Wiley and Sons 1976, 115–123.

45. Lange E and Gershanik J. Multicystic dysplastic kidney: Diagnostic considerations and management. Southern Medical Journal 1978, 71, 888–891.

46. Lebowitz R and Griscom N. Neonatal hydronephrosis: 146 cases. Radiological Clinics of North America 1977, 15, 49–59.

47. Leonidas J, Strauss L and Krasna I. Roentgen diagnosis of multicystic renal dysplasia in infancy by high dose urography. Journal of Urology 1972, 108, 963–965.

48. Ljungqvist A. Arterial vasculature of the multicystic dysplastic kidney. A micro-angiographical and histological study. Acta Pathologica Microbiolica Scandinavica 1965, 64 309–317.

49. Longino L and Martin L. Abdominal masses in the newborn infant. Pediatrics 1958, 21, 596–604.

50. Marotti M, Hricak H, Fritzsche P, Crooks L, Hedgcock M and Tanagho E. Complex and simple renal cysts: Comparative evaluation with MR imaging. Radiology 1987, 162, 679–684.

51. McClennan B, Stanley R, Melson G, Levitt R and Sagel S. CT of the renal cyst: Is cyst aspiration necessary? American Journal of Roentgenology 1979, 133, 671–675.

52. Melicow M and Uson A. Palpable abdominal masses in infants and children: A report based on a review of 653 cases. Journal of Urology 1959, 81, 705–710.

53. Mir S, Rapola J and Koskimies O. Renal cysts in pediatric autopsy material. Nephron 1983, 33, 189–195.

54. Moe P and Crofford W. Ectopic unilateral multicystic kidney in infant. Journal of Diseases of Childhood 1960, 99, 51/35–54/38.

55. Newman L, Simms K, Kissane J and McAlister W. Unilateral total renal dysplasia in children. American Journal of Roentgenology 1972, 116, 778–783.

56. O'Connor J and Neuhauser E. Total body opacification in conventional and high dose intravenous urography in infancy. American Journal of Roentgenology 1963, 90, 63–71.

57. Older R, Hinman C, Crane L, Cleeve D and Morgan C. *In utero* diagnosis of multicystic kidney by gray scale ultrasonography. American Journal of Roentgenology 1979, 133, 130–131.

58. Osathanondh V and Potter E. Pathogenesis of polycystic kidneys. Type 2 due to inhibition of ampullary activity. Archives of Pathology and Laboratory Medicine 1964, 77, 474–484.

59. Parkkulainen K, Hjelt L and Sirola K. Congenital multicystic dysplasia of the kidney. Acta Chirurgica Scandinavica (Supplement) 1959, 244, 5–46.

60. Pathak I and Williams D. Multicystic and cystic dysplastic kidneys. British Journal of Urology 1964, 36, 318–331.

61. Pedicelli G, Jequier S, Bowen A and Boisvert J. Multicystic dysplastic kidneys: Sponteneous regression demonstrated with US. Radiology 1986, 160, 23–26.

62. Pollack H, Banner M, Ager P, Peters J, Mulhern C Jr and Coleman B. The accuracy of gray-scale renal ultrasonography in differentiating cystic neoplasms from benign cysts. Radiology 1982, 143, 741–745.

63. Potter E, ed. Normal and Abnormal Development of the Kidney. Chicago: Year Book Medical Publishers, 1972.

64. Raffensberger J and Abousleiman A. Abdominal masses in children under one year of age. Surgery 1968, 63, 514–521.

65. Risdon A. Renal dysplasia. Journal of Clinical Pathology 1971, 24, 57–71.

66. Roodhooft A, Birnholz J and Holmes L. Familial nature of congenital absence and severe dysgenesis of both kidneys. New England Journal of Medicine 1984, 310, 1341–1345.

67. Rubenstein M, Meyer R and Bernstein J. Congenital abnormalities of the urinary system. I. A postmortem survey of developmental anomalies and acquired congenital lesions in a children's hospital. Journal of Pediatrics 1961, 38, 356–366.

68. Sanders R and Hartman D. The sonographic distinction between neonatal multicystic kidney and hydronephrosis. Radiology 1984, 151, 621–625.

69. Saxton H, Golding S, Chantler C and Haycock G. Diagnostic puncture in renal cystic dysplasia (multicystic kidney). Evidence on the etiology of the cysts. British Journal of Radiology 1981, 54, 555–561.

70. Schwartz J. An unusual unilateral multicystic kidney in an infant. Journal of Urology 1936, 35, 259–263.

71. Slovis T and Perlmutter A. Recent advances in pediatric urological ultrasound. Journal of Urology 1980, 123, 613–620.

72. Spence H. Congenital unilateral multicystic kidney: An entity to be distinguished from polycystic kidney disease and other cystic disorders. Journal of Urology 1955, 74, 693–706.

73. Squiers E, Morden R, Bernstein J. Renal multicystic dysplasia: An occasional manifestation of the hereditary renal adysplasia syndrome. American Journal of Medical Genetics Supplement 1987, 3, 279–284.

74. Stanisic T. Review of "The dilemma of the multicystic dysplastic kidney". American Journal of Diseases in Children 1986, 140, 865.

75. Staubitz W, Jewett T Jr and Pletman R. Renal cystic disease in childhood. Journal of Urology 1963, 90, 8–12.

76. Stuck K, Koff W and Silver T. Ultrasonic features of multicystic dysplastic kidney: Expanded diagnostic criteria. Radiology 1982, 143, 217–221.
77. Tanagho E. Surgically induced partial urinary obstruction in the fetal lamb. II. Urethral obstruction. Investigative Urology 1972, 10, 25–34.
78. Taxy J and Filmer R. Metaplastic cartilage in nondysplastic kidneys. Archives of Pathology 1975, 99, 101–104.
79. Vellios F and Garret R. Congenital unilateral multicystic disease of the kidney. A clinical and anatomic study of seven cases. American Journal of Clinical Pathology 1961, 35, 244–254.
80. Walker R, Senior D, Filmer B, Grossman H and Brosman S. Multicystic kidney. Dialogues in Pediatric Urology 1981, 4, 1–8.
81. Warshawsky A, Miller K and Kaplan G. Urographic visualization of multicystic kidneys. Journal of Urology 1977, 117, 94–96.
82. Wood B, Goske M and Rabinowitz R. Multicystic renal dysplasia masquerading as ureteropelvic junction obstruction. Journal of Urology 1984, 132, 972–974.
83. Young L, Wood B, Spohr C and Panner B. Delayed excretory urographic opacification, a puddling effect, in multicystic renal dysplasia. Annals Radiologie (Paris) 1974, 17, 391–396.
84. Zimmer W, Williamson B Jr., Hartman G, Hattery R and O'Brien P. Changing patterns in the evaluation of renal masses: Economic implications. American Journal of Roentgenology 1984, 143, 285–289.

17
Multilocular Cystic Renal Lesions – Malformations, Benign Nephromas, or Differentiated Wilms Tumors?

J. M. Kissane

Abstract

Multilocular cystic lesions are rare, unilateral, solitary, blind, multiloculate, epithelial-lined, septated defects that are found within normal renal tissue. Their prime clinical importance rests in the frequency with which they may be confused with Wilms tumor. The lesions are likely to be detected in increasing numbers as more ultrasonographs, computed tomographic scans and nuclear magnetic images are performed. They are amenable to surgery; nephrectomy is the therapy of choice. Ultimate recognition and distinction from Wilms tumor depend on the surgical pathologist's evaluation of excised tissue.

Key Words   Cystadenoma;
Curvilinear calcification;
Nephroma;
Wilms tumor.

Introduction

First described in 1892 by Edmunds[25] as "cystic adenoma" (Fig. 17.1), multilocular cystic lesions of the kidney were systematically considered by Powell and associates only in 1951.

In their report of two cases, these authors promulgated eight criteria for the diagnosis of what they termed "multilocular cysts of the kidney":

(1)   The lesion is unilateral;
(2)   The lesion is solitary;
(3)   The lesion is multilocular;
(4)   Cysts do not communicate with the renal pelvis;
(5)   Locules do not communicate with each other;
(6)   Locules are lined with epithelium;
(7)   Interlocular septa do not contain renal parenchyma; and
(8)   Surrounding renal tissue is normal except for compression.

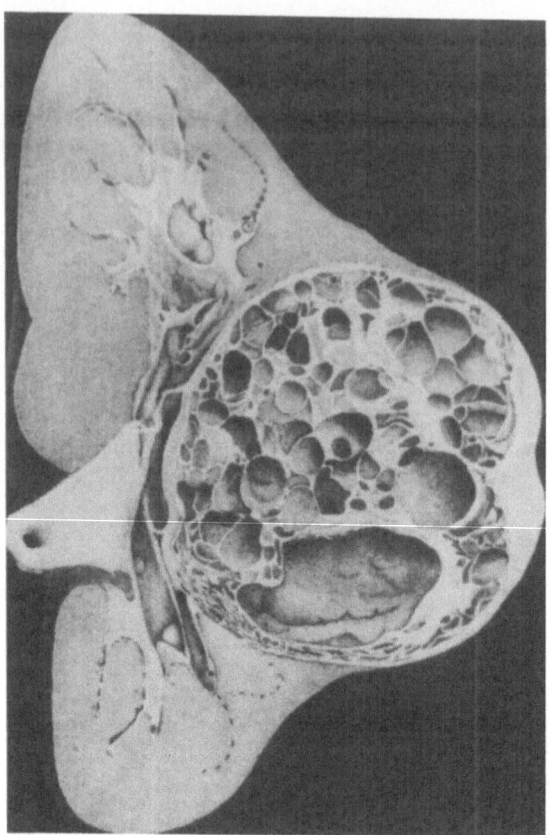

Figure 17.1 Reproduction of Edmunds' case[25] described as a "cystic adenoma of the kidney".

Using these criteria, Powell and associates[62] accepted 13 examples reported previously.

Five years later, Boggs and Kimmelstiel[12] reported two cases, only one of which satisfied the criteria of Powell *et al*. The other had solid cords and tubules within septa between daughter locules. They modified the seventh criterion of Powell *et al*. to exclude fully differentiated renal tissues in septa, and interpreted the epithelial structures in their first case as evidence of neoplastic origin of the lesion. They suggested the name "benign multilocular cystic nephroma".

Aterman and co-workers[5] in 1973 reiterated Boggs and Kimmelstiel's revision of the criteria of Powell *et al*., but reverted to the designation "solitary multilocular cyst of the kidney".

Perlmann's[59] very unusual case (in an adult) was initially considered a lymphangioma. It has since been regarded, in a report of a similar lesion, as a cystic adenoma (Perlmann tumor)[24] and as a multilocular renal cyst[67]. The lesion described by Robinson[67] had smooth muscle in the capsule.

Aterman et al.[5] suggested that several renal lesions reported as "lymphangiomas"[59,75] were actually multilocular cysts, an interpretation accepted by Attwood and Grieve[6]. Exclusively intrarenal lymphangioma (as opposed to renal involvement in a diffuse hemolymphangiomatous hamaromatous process, retroperitoneal hygroma) probably occurs. I agree with Aterman and co-workers that several, perhaps most of the very rare intrarenal "lymphangio-

Table 17.1 Diagnostic designations applied to multilocular cystic renal lesions

Designation	Reference
Multilocular cyst of the kidney	2,5,6,7,9,17,20,65
Multilocular renal cyst	8,14,19,31,53,64,66
Benign multilocular cystic nephroma	12,16
Cystic adenoma or cystadenoma	25,63
Benign adenomatous polycystic kidney tumor	24
Cystic nephroma	1,32
Benign cystic differentiated nephroblastoma	50
Cystic partially differentiated nephroblastoma	14,43,44,46,78
Differentiated nephroblastoma	29
Polycystic nephroblastoma, polycystic Wilms tumor	18,21
Cystic mesoblastic nephromas	69
Cystic nephroblastoma	70
Well-differentiated polycystic Wilms tumor	48,72
Segmental cystic disease	61
Partially polycystic kidney	73
Lymphangioma	42,59,76
Perlmann's tumor	24,67
Multicystic nephroma	13
Mixed tumor of the kidney	75

mas" are multilocular cysts[42]. In the period under discussion and since, a bewildering array of diagnostic designations has been applied (Table 17.1).

Each of these designations appears to have been advocated to express the opinion of the proponents as to the biologic nature of the lesion as:

(1) A congenital abnormality in nephrogenesis
(2) A quasi-neoplastic tumefaction related to the developmental process perhaps phenomenologically best characterized as a "hamartoma";
(3) Partial or complete differentiation of a nephroblastoma (Wilms tumor); and
(4) A neoplasm of the developing kidney related to nephroblastoma (Wilms tumor) in its origin from metanephrogenic tissue (blastema).

What we are left with is a relatively uncommon lesion, but one which is encountered every few years or so on a busy urology or pediatric urology service, and of which retrospective evaluation in a collective experience is often hampered by incomplete documentation of salient features.

2. Clinical characteristics

2.1 Incidence

Multilocular cystic lesions of the kidney are uncommon. In 1951, Powell and associates accepted only 13 previously reported cases as satisfying their criteria. Dainko et al.[20] in 1963 accepted nine cases in patients younger than 18 years of age. In 1973, Aterman et al. accepted 18 cases in children and 22 in adults, noting that many reports lacked sufficient details for classification. Potter[61], referring to the lesion as segmental cystic disease, mentioned encountering eight examples in 12,000 autopsies from 110,000 live births and, with Osathanondh[57], described microdissection of one case in a newborn infant. Probably 80–100 cases had been described in patients of all ages by 1983, when Madewell and co-workers[51] from the Armed Forces Institute of Pathology (AFIP) reported 61 lesions from 58 patients. Except for that unrivalled experience, these lesions are reported as individual cases or as groups of two to several cases from major centers.

There are limited data regarding the incidence of multilocular cystic lesions among abdominal or renal tumefactions. Lattimer[49], in 1961, encountered six solitary multilocular renal cysts among 650 abdominal masses in children. Gallo and Penchansky[32] found four cases among 165 primary renal tumors in children. Gonzalez-Crussi and co-workers[36] found six among 216 primary renal tumors in children. It thus appears that multilocular cystic lesions of the kidney constitute a very small proportion of renal mass lesions in children, placing them probably slightly less common than congenital mesoblastic nephroma. The relative contribution by these lesions to series of renal tumefactions in adults is very much less and undoubtedly underreported because of incomplete separation from other renal cystic lesions, chiefly simple cysts. There have been no familial cases.

There appear to be no ethnic, national or anthropologic concentrations of multilocular cystic renal lesions. The AFIP experience documents cases in whites, blacks, orientals and Native Americans[51]. Isolated reports include Americans of Hispanic background[20,41]. Cases have been reported from Latin America[32], Australia[29,50], India[44] and the Far East[45,75,77]. Joshi[43] illustrated a multilocular cystic renal lesion from an opossium (sic).

2.2 Age

A distinctive feature in the epidemiology of multilocular cystic lesions of the kidney is the distribution of cases with respect to age. At least by 1973, it had emerged that about half of these lesions occurred in children, half in adults. In that year, Aterman et al. noted that there were virtually no reported cases between the ages of 5 and 18 years. This bimodal age distribution has been consistent since then. In the AFIP report of 61 lesions, only four occurred between ages of four and thirty years. Very few cases, however, have been reported in newborn infants[57,61]. The lesion in a newborn infant reported by Randolph[64] was, however, obviously a multicystic dysplastic kidney[61].

2.3 Sex

Pediatric cases of multilocular cystic renal lesions are approximately equally distributed between the two sexes. Parenthetically, it may be pointed out that the sex distribution of Wilms tumor (nephroblastoma) is approximately equal in most large series of cases. In contrast, multilocular cystic renal lesions presenting in adulthood are distinctly and consistently more common in women than men. This is in distinct contrast with the sex distribution of other renal masses in adults.

2.4 Symptoms

The presence of an abdominal or flank mass is the most common and often the only clinical feature of multilocular cystic renal lesions. There is no predominance in one or the other side. Bilateral lesions have been rarely recognized either synchronously[52] or asynchronously[34]. A few patients have had hematuria with or without pain[6]. These features have sometimes been attributable to herniation of locules of the renal mass into the upper collecting system[15,35,71]. Rare patients have had hypertension, which may revert to normal after nephrectomy[38]. Infection is now uncommon, but was encountered formerly[55]. Ravitch's case[65] had tubercles in a multilocular cystic kidney (accepted by Powell et al.[62]).

Multilocular cystic renal lesions are not associated with lesions in other organ systems, unlike the association of multicystic renal dysplasia with ureteral or gastrointestinal atresia, defects of cardiac septation and lumbar meningomyelocele, of autosomal dominant polycystic disease with epithelial-lined cysts of other organs and with aneurysm of cerebral arteries, or of autosomal recessive polycystic disease with biliary proliferations in the liver. One case of a multilocular cystic renal lesion had a contralateral simple renal cyst not sampled histologically[36]. In the large series of multilocular cystic renal lesions

418

from the AFIP, one occurred in a horseshoe kidney, one had ureteropelvic stenosis on the opposite side, and one patient had a cervical meningomyelocele[51]. One of Boggs' and Kimmelsteil's cases[12] had an ileal intussusception. One case had a "bullous lesion" of a lung (not examined pathologically)[1]. Potter's case[61] had multiple congenital anomalies. The 20-year-old patient reported by Hutchins *et al.*[40] had had a testicular embryonal carcinoma. Peterson's[60] (bilateral) case was associated with hypoplasia of ureters and bladder. That case seems to have been an example of bilateral renal dysplasia, a distinctive lesion although undeniably "multilocular" and "cystic". Multilocular cystic renal lesions have been found incidentally at autopsies in adults dead of various causes[55]. The 48-year-old woman reported by Friday *et al.*[31] had diabetes.

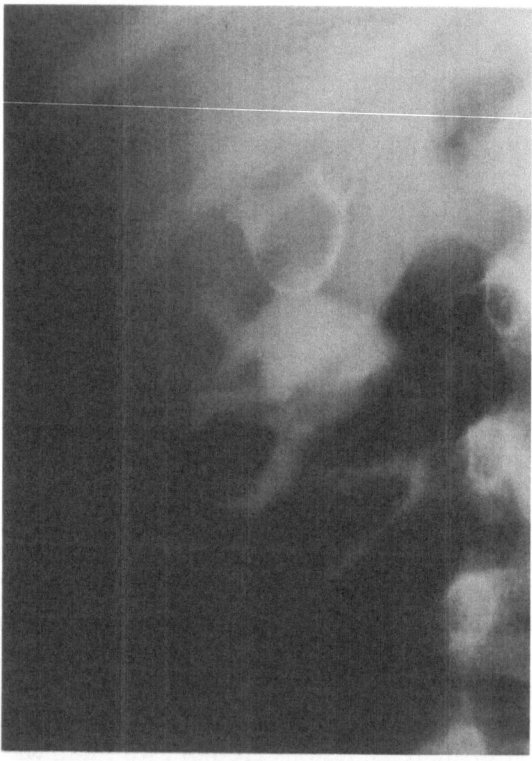

Figure 17.2 Intravenous urogram on an 8-year-old boy who had a history of a swollen penis. The right kidney shows a filling defect in the upper pole. (Figure contributed by W. H. McAlister MD, Chief Pediatric Radiology, St Louis Children's Hospital).

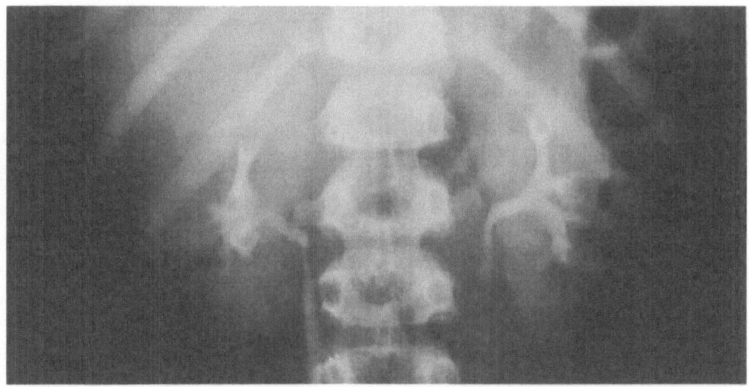

Figure 17.3 An 8-year-old boy entered with microscopic hematuria. An intravenous urogram demonstrates a mass in the midlateral portion of the right kidney with some calyceal distortion. (Figure contributed by W. H. McAlister MD, Chief Pediatric Radiology, St Louis Children's Hospital).

3. Diagnosis

Plain radiographs usually disclose a soft tissue mass either by distortion of contiguous soft tissue structures or displacement of gas-filled loops of intestine[51]. Calcification or ossification may be seen as small, delicate, curvilinear densities[8].

Excretory urography practically always demonstrates an intrarenal mass either by distortion or displacement of contiguous renal tissue or a focally absent nephrogram[52]. The mass is characteristically round and sharply marginated. The pyelocalyceal system is often distorted (Figs. 17.2–5).

Delayed excretion or non-visualization often indicates herniation of components of the cyst into the upper collecting system. In these cases, a smooth filling defect in the renal pelvis may be noted at retrograde urography. McAlister *et al.*[53] described veins in the capsules of two multilocular cystic lesions in early phases of excretory urograms.

Angiograms often demonstrate an avascular or hypovascular mass[22,27], uncommonly a hypervascular mass[7,26,31]. No arteriovenous shunts are demonstrated.

Sonograms characteristically demonstrate a complex intrarenal mass[39], usually with acoustic enhancement. Discrete septation may be seen to divide the mass into multiple sonolucent locules (Fig. 17.6A).

Computed tomography usually demonstrates a discrete intrarenal mass. A definite outer capsule and delicate locular septa are often visualized (Figs. 17.6B,C).

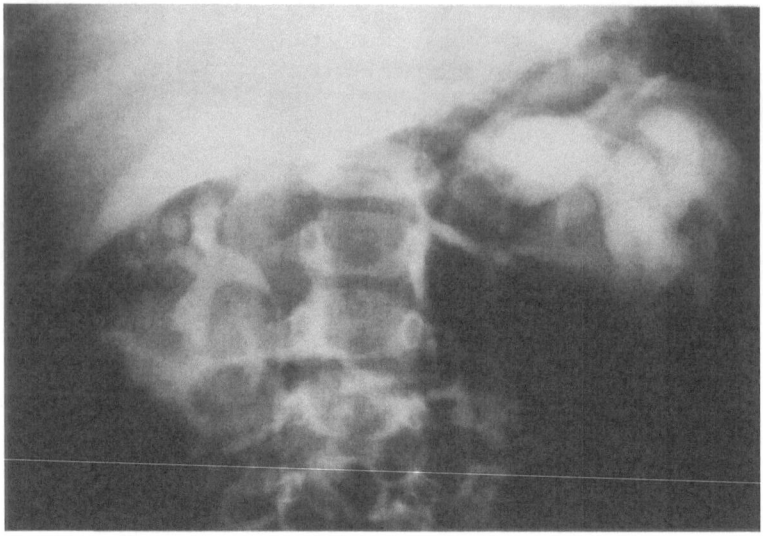

Figure 17.4 A 1-year-old boy entered with a large left-sided abdominal mass. An intravenous urogram demonstrates the mass to be within the left kidney. The calyces of the left kidney are dilated and distorted. (Figure contributed by W. H. McAlister MD, Chief Pediatric Radiology, St Louis Children's Hospital).

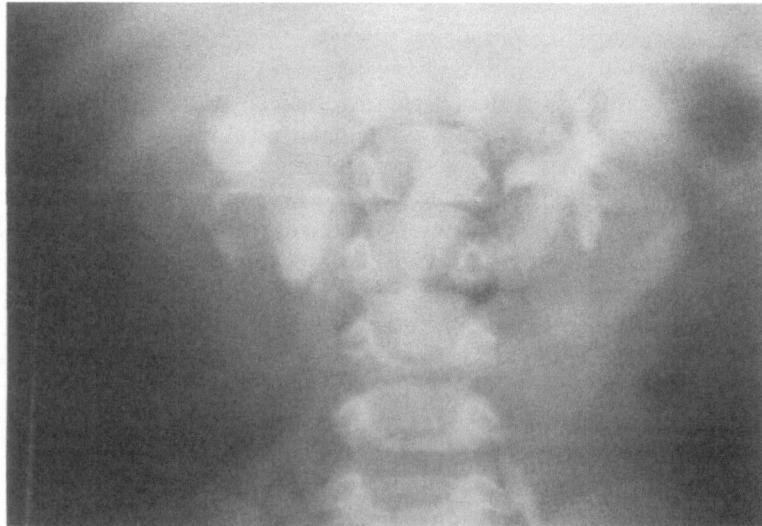

Figure 17.5 A 4-year-old boy had a mass palpated in the right side of the abdomen on a routine physical examination. An intravenous urogram demonstrates a large mass in the lower pole of the right kidney. (Figure contributed by W. H. McAlister MD, Chief Pediatric Radiology, St Louis Children's Hospital).

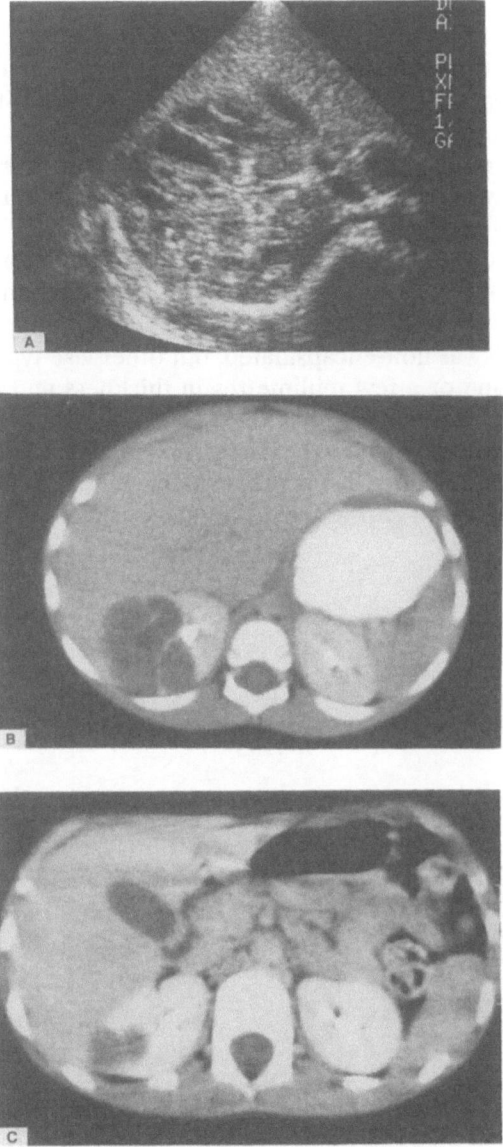

Figure 17.6 A 3-year-old boy entered with a hematuria and diffuse abdominal pain. He was found to be febrile, but the blood and urine cultures were negative. A repeat ultrasound (A) demonstrates a large mass involving the right kidney with multiple sonolucent and echogenic areas within the mass. Computerized tomography after the administration of intravenous contrast material demonstrates a large mass involving the right kidney. (B) The mass has decreased attenuation but contains multiple septa. (C) In the superior portion of the mass two loculated areas can be seen. (Figure contributed by W. H. McAlister MD, Chief Pediatric Radiology, St Louis Children's Hospital).

4. Pathology

Multilocular cystic renal lesions are large and may be very large. The whole renal lesion is usually approximately spherical and ranges from a few to many centimetres in diameter (Fig. 17.7).

A discrete outer capsule (some authors refer to it as a pseudocapsule) characteristically separates the lesion from contiguous renal tissue, which, except for compression by the expansile mass, is normal.

We have seen a lesion from an adult in which the outer capsule was focally discontinuous, and fully-differentiated, histologically benign epithelial-lined cysts had "spilled over" into extracapsular renal parenchyma. The case of Hutchins et al.[40] was non-encapsulated, but otherwise typical. The outer capsule is usually one or a few millimetres in thickness and may contain brittle spicules of calcification or ossification[7,8,16,19,23].

Within this outer capsule, the lesion is divided into a few to several dozen roughly spherical locules. The septa between these daughter locules are, in contrast with the outer capsule, usually thin, parchment-like and semi-trans-

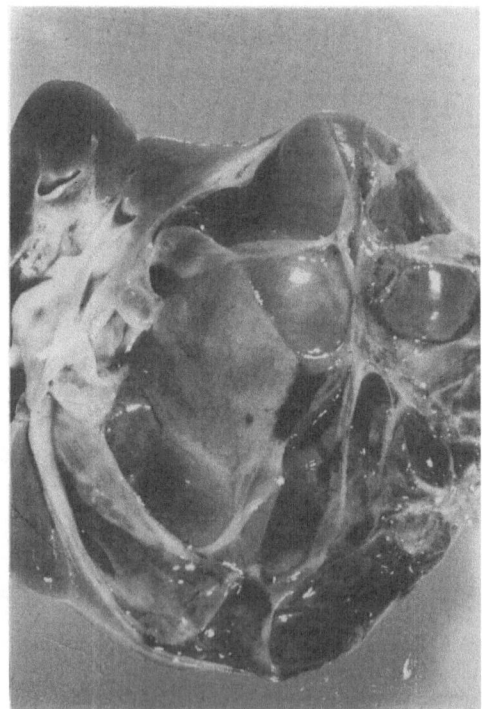

Figure 17.7 Gross photograph of a multilocular renal cyst consisting of roughly spherical locules enclosed in an outer capsule and compressing contiguous normal kidney.

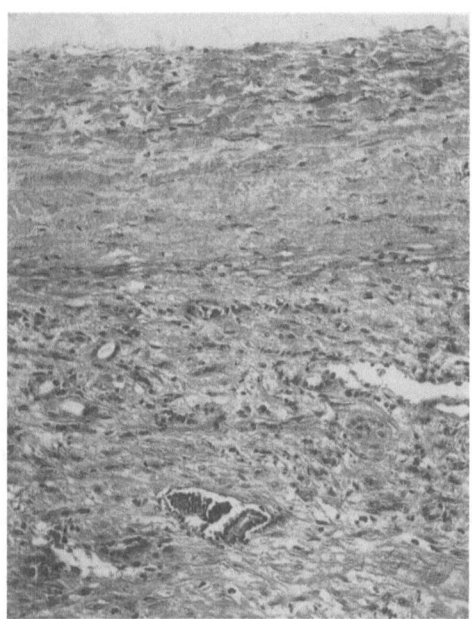

Figure 17.8 Photomicrograph of outer capsule of a multilocular cystic renal lesion which contains fascicles of smooth muscle and a trapped glomerlus.

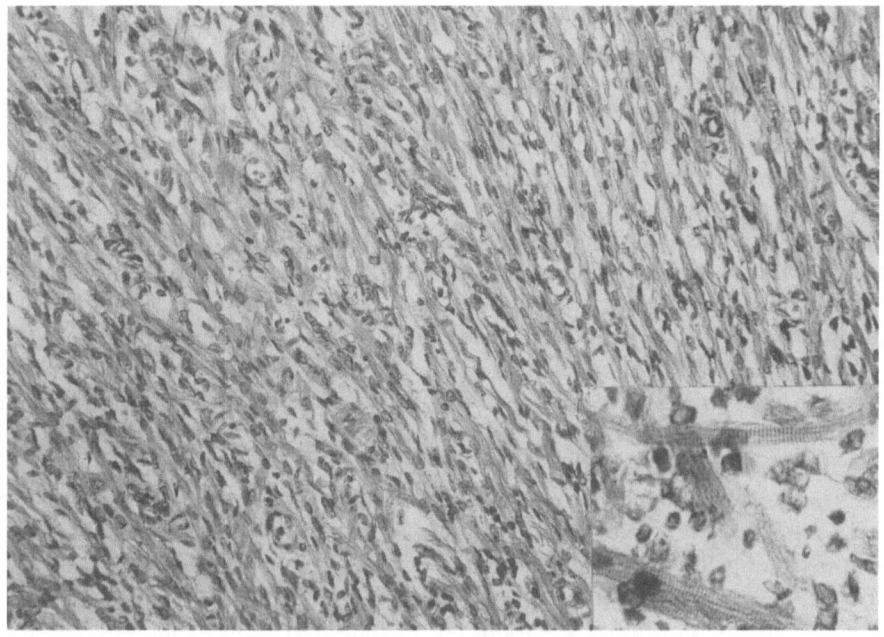

Figure 17.9 Outer capsule of a multilocular cystic renal lesion showing fascicles of differentiated rhabdomyocytes with (inset) recognizable cross striations.

parent. They separate roughly spherical locules from the lower limit of naked eye visibility to one or a few centimetres in diameter. The daughter locules contain clear yellow or faintly bluish fluid. When analyzed, the cyst fluid has a chemical composition similar to that of serum[62] and has been shown to contain prostaglandins[1]. Blood or altered blood is rarely described[66]. The daughter locules communicate neither with each other nor with the upper collecting system[31,62].

In some cases, one or a few daughter locules can be seen to have prolapsed into the pyelocalyceal system, and there may be appreciable hydronephrosis in the kidney surrounding the lesion[15,35,71]. Sometimes, septa between daughter locules may be thick and opaque either diffusely or in a nodular fashion. These areas should be assiduously sought and sampled histologically[13,39].

Microscropically, the outer capsule usually consists of spindle cells (fibroblasts), blood vessels, sparse mononuclear cells and interstitial collagen. Frequently, the capsule includes atrophic tubules and shrunken, partially or completely sclerotic glomeruli (Figure 17.8).

This obvious incorporation of elements of contiguous normal kidney leads some authors to characterize this sheath as a "pseudocapsule". Quite often, there are fascicles of mature smooth muscle[1,6,20,62]. This feature alone is quite in contrast with the lining of the familiar simple renal cyst. Parenthetically, it should be pointed out that Sirola[68] identified smooth muscle in two of nine simple cysts he studied – an observation that would have to be characterized as unusual. I regard the presence of dysontogenic tissue as distinguishing a true capsule from a pseudocapsule.

Besides smooth muscle, other dysontogenic tissues may be identified in the outer capsule. Well-differentiated skeletal muscle cells with cytoplasmic cross striations may be found[14,32,36,44] (Fig. 17.9). Bone or non-osseous foci of calcification may be seen[7,8,16,19,23], and are perhaps better regarded as dystrophic rather than dysontogenic. Differentiated adipose tissue has been described[38,75,78]. I have once seen spicules of cartilage in the outer capsule of a multilocular cystic lesion that was clearly not a multicystic dysplastic kidney in which cartilage is a much more common finding. Young et al.[78] also found cartilage in a multilocular cystic lesion.

The cysts that comprise a multilocular renal lesion are, by definition, lined with epithelium. This is usually a nondescript simple cuboidal or low columnar epithelium, occasionally in a hobnail or picket fence pattern (Fig. 17.10). Papillary epithelial intracystic proliferations occur but are uncommon[30].

The stroma of the septa between daughter locules is variable and constitutes the most important feature upon which biologic interpretations of these lesions are based. Usually, this stroma consists of undistinguished spindle cells and scanty extracellular matrix without epithelial components. In fact, it was the absence of epithelial components in daughter septa that Powell et al. insisted upon in their definition of multilocular renal cysts. Very soon thereafter, exceptions to this criterion came to be recognized specifically by the

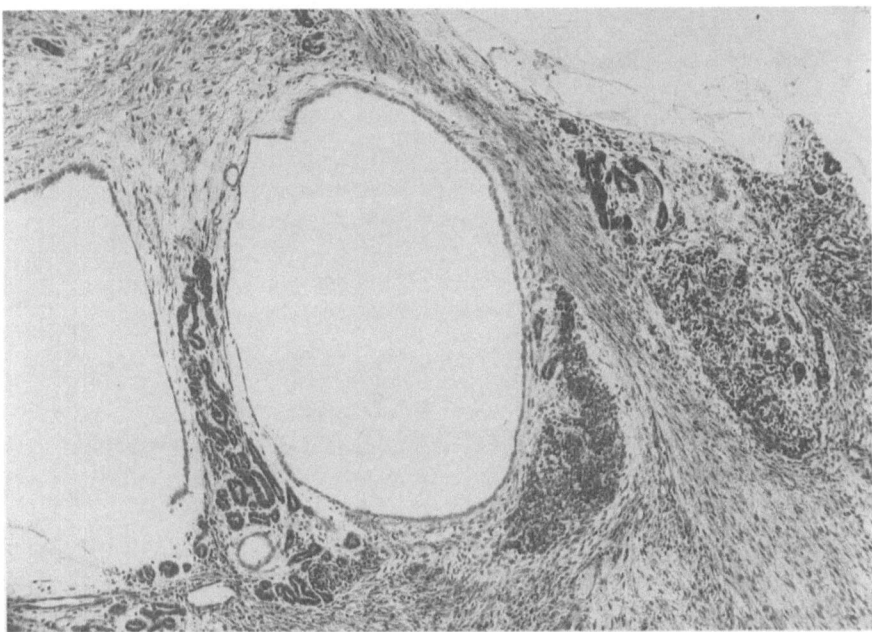

Figure 17.10 Photomicrograph of a multilocular cystic renal lesion showing epithelial-lined cysts (centre and right), undifferentiated blastema (centre) differentiated tubules (right) and partially differentiated blastema and tubules (left).

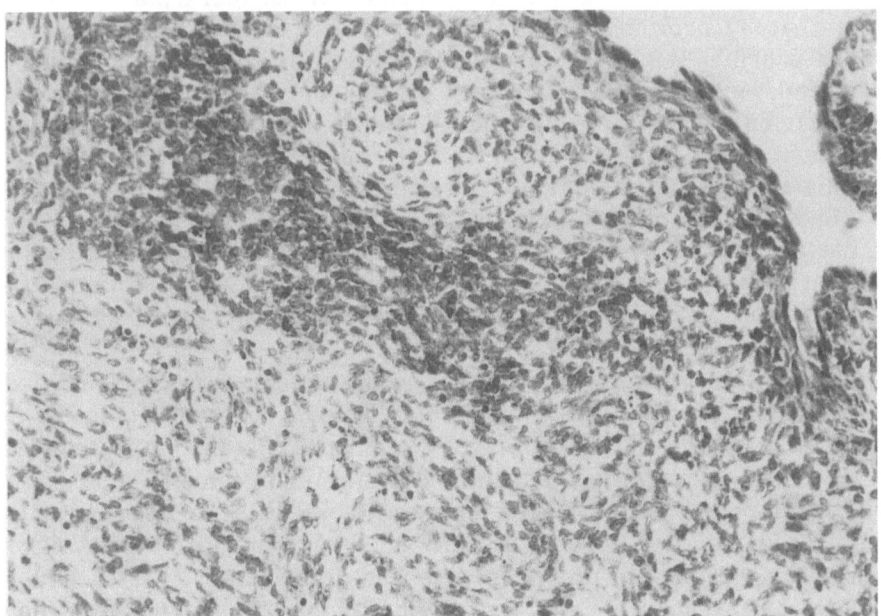

Figure 17.11 Photomicrograph showing undifferentiated blastema in a septum of a multilocular cystic renal lesion.

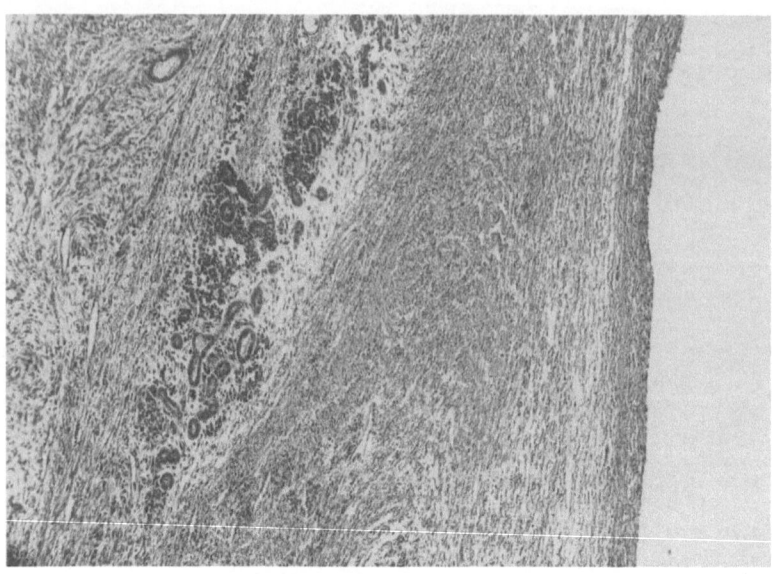

Figure 17.12 Photomicrograph showing partially differentiated blastema in a septum of a multilocular cystic renal lesion which also contains smooth muscle and cords and tubules of epithelium.

presence of solid or tubular epithelial structures in daughter septa[12,19,21,29,30]. Others have recognized abortive glomeruli in these septa[11,14].

In daughter septa, some multilocular cystic renal lesions contain aggregates of renal blastema, pavement-like arrays of small to medium size cells that are reminiscent of those of the metanephrogenic blastema (Fig. 17.11) with or without atypical tubular structures[3,11,14,18,32,42,46] (Fig. 17.12), rarely differentiated to abnormal glomerular structures.

In other cases, differentiation to mature tissue elements, smooth or skeletal muscle, adipose tissue, or bone may be identified. In a few cases, either an isolated septal nodule or more diffuse microscopic involvement recognizable as nephroblastoma (Wilms tumor) may be identified and made the basis of post-operative therapy[2,3,38,46].

One case in the series reported by Gonzalez-Crussi *et al.* had a grossly recognized nodule that proved microscopically to be nephroblastoma (Wilms tumor). The AFIP series had four cases with nephroblastoma in multilocular cystic lesions. In reporting a case of multicystic Wilms tumor, Wood *et al.*[74] state that fourteen cases had been reported previously. Andrews *et al.*[3] added another example. Beckwith and Kiviat[10] state that four cases in the *National Wilms Tumor Study* had prominent cysts and developed metastases. One of Gallo and Penchansky's[32] cases had a Wilms tumor in the kidney contiguous with, but separate from, a multilocular cystic lesion. Merten *et al.*[56] described a case of multicystic Wilms tumor that also had features of a mesoblastic nephroma.

In adults, renal adenocarcinoma has been described in association with multilocular cystic lesions[58]. The large AFIP experience includes four cases of sarcoma in kidneys of adults with multilocular cystic lesions[51]. The histologic features of the sarcomas were not described.

Three of these patients died with metastatic disease histologically similar to the renal lesion.

5. Treatment

Nephrectomy alone has been overwhelmingly the most frequently applied treatment of multilocular cystic renal lesions. In children, the preoperative diagnosis has usually been nephroblastoma (Wilms tumor), and the finding on pathologic study of a multilocular cystic lesion without pathologically alarming features has often militated against multiagent therapy.

When intraoperative examination of preoperative radiographic studies has suggested the diagnosis of a multilocular cystic lesion, partial nephrectomy has occasionally been performed with favorable results[23,28]. Unroofing of cysts has been followed by "recurrence" (clinically overt persistence) in at least one case[34].

In a few cases, chemotherapy (vincristine and actinomycin D) and irradiation were administered preoperatively to shrink large lesions[15,41]. In several other cases, post-operative chemotherapy, with or without irradiation, has been administered because of pathologic findings in multilocular cystic lesions[2,3,32,36,38,46,66].

6. Prognosis

From the reported experience, the prognosis of multilocular cystic renal lesions appears to be excellent. One of the patients reported by Boggs and Kimmelstiel and one reported by Gallo and Penchansky died of post-operative complications. Three adult patients in the AFIP series with sarcoma in a multilocular cyst died with metastases[51]. Those seem to have been the only deaths reported in patients with this general category of lesions. Gallo and Penchansky's case[32] of a nephroblastoma (Wilms tumor) contiguous to a multilocular cystic lesion was alive and free of disease 7.5 years after nephrectomy. One patient in the group reported by Gonzalez-Crussi et al.[36] was alive with a grossly recognizable nodule of typical nephroblastoma. Four cases in the AFIP series who had nephroblastoma in a multilocular cystic renal lesion were alive and well 2.75 to 9 years after nephrectomy[51]. Beckwith and Kiviat[10] have, however, seen four nephroblastomas with prominent cysts that had metastasized. Details were not provided. Merten *et al.*[56] reported a case of a multicystic Wilms tumor (with some features of mesoblastic nephroma) who was alive. In reporting a patient with multicystic Wilms tumor who was alive and well 8 months after nephrectomy, vincristine and actinomycin D, Wood and co-workers[74] state that there had been 14 previous cases of multicystic Wilms tumors, none of whom had died of tumor after periods of follow-up from 2 to 11 years.

7. Discussion

Multilocular cystic renal lesions have been variously interpreted as:

(1) Conventional congenital malformations[62]
(2) Tumefactions related to the developmental process, "hamartomas"[4];
(3) Examples of partial or complete differentiation of a nephroblastoma (Wilms tumor)[3,14,43]; or
(4) Benign variants of nephroblastoma[21,33,48,74].

These interpretations have usually been based upon the histologic features of the stroma of the outer capsule or more frequently, of the septa between daughter locules of the multilocular lesion.

The non-specific blandness of the fibroblastic outer capsule and daughter septa led Powell and associates[62] to regard lesions with these features as congenital malformations that occur during nephrogenesis. Features against this hypothesis, which emerged relatively promptly, are the great rarity of multilocular cystic lesions, as defined, in newborn infants and the few cases (all adults) in whom a multilocular renal cystic lesion had become demonstrable some years after a normal radiographic examination[34,40,51,71].

There are embryologic objections to regarding multilocular cystic lesions of the kidney as conventional anomalies in nephrogenesis. Here, perhaps it is appropriate to distinguish renal multilocular cystic lesions from the much more common lesion, renal dysplasia on situational, clinical and morphologic grounds. In its most familiar form, unilateral multicystic renal dysplasia is present at birth, often associated with ureteral malformations, especially atresia, and it often occurs in infants with other reflections of disturbed ontogeny in the fourth week of gestation, e.g. anomalies of cardiac septation, anomalies of intestinal canalization and anomalies in neural tubularization. These associations have never been described (barring one case with a *cervical* meningomyelocele)[51] in patients with multilocular renal cystic lesions as herein considered. The closest similarity of an undoubted congenital malformation with a segmental multilocular renal abnormality is the frequent occurrence of dysplastic features, including the presence of cartilage, in segments (almost always rostral) of a kidney drained by a supernumerary ureter through an ectopic ureterocele. The association with ureteral anomalies and the fact that segmental renal dysplasia associated with ectopic ureteroceles is not encapsulated, clearly distinguish the two classes of lesions.

Regarding multilocular cystic renal lesions as tumefactions related to disturbed ontogeny, broadly designated as hamartomas, is initially comforting but rarely satisfying. Adami's original designation of "hamartoma" as opposed to "choristoma" (or, their malignant variants, "hamartoblastoma" vs "chorioblastoma") has almost vanished from systematic pathology. the only marginally viable vestige of that largely intellectual conceptualization has been "hamartoma," which has remained useful as designating aggregations of tissue that appear as tumefactions, apparently of developmental origin, and that are composed of tissues normal to the ontogeny of an organ or tissue but abnormal in relative distribution. Clearly, many multilocular renal cystic lesions do not qualify as "hamartomas." Smooth muscle, skeletal muscle, cartilage (rare), adipose tissue and bone (perhaps dysplastic rather than dysontogenic) however distributed, are not components of the normal kidney.

The presence of solid or tubular epithelial components in the intracystic septa of a multilocular renal cystic lesion led Boggs and Kimmelstiel[12] to the designation "multilocular cystic nephroma" entailing the contrasting views of true renal neoplasia vs abnormal renal differentiation. Many authors who express this point of view designate lesions as a "nephroma" if they include epithelial cords or tubules in the capsule or in the septa[12].

That multilocular cystic renal lesions represent partial or total differentiation of a nephroblastoma (Wilms tumor) has since been suggested by several authors[3,14,43]. Dysontogenic, but undoubtedly differentiated tissue, most commonly smooth and skeletal muscle, came relatively promptly to be recognized in what were interpreted as "differentiated nephroblastomas." The presence of smooth muscle has somehow been interpreted as less justification of the designation "nephroblastoma" than has skeletal muscle.

Additionally, cases with incompletely differentiated renal blastema came to be recognized. These are not cases of undoubted nephroblastoma (Wilms tumor). They are cases in which grossly guided or randomly taken microsections of a multilocular cystic lesion disclose areas of "renal blastema" undifferentiated metanephrogenic tissue with or without areas of differentiation along nephric lines (tubules or glomeruli) or stromal lines (smooth or striated muscle or, more rarely, cartilage or adipose tissue). They have been designated, in consideration of the degree of differentiation of the blastema, as partially differentiated or differentiated "nephroblastomas".

Adherents to the theory that multilocular renal cystic lesions result from a previously existing nephroblastoma (Wilms tumor) generally express that concept in such diagnostic designation. The presence of dysontogenic tissue or tissues with or without blastema has often been taken to justify the designation "nephroblastoma", "differentiated", if mature, "partially differentiated", if immature; "multicystic nephroblastoma"if manifested by the presence of metanephrogenic blastema and atypical epithelial elements only. These usages

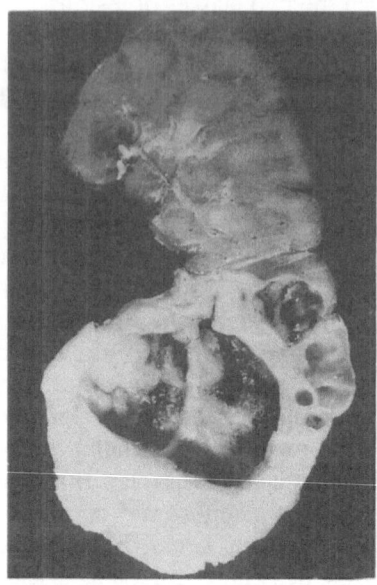

Figure 17.13 Gross photograph of a multilocular cystic renal lesion with thick septa which showed features of a congenital mesoblastic nephroma.

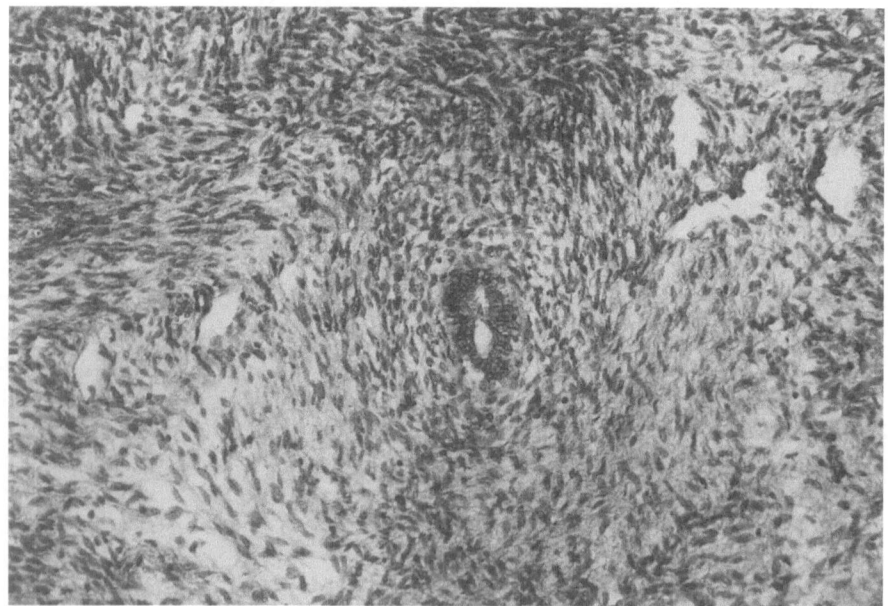

Figure 17.14 Photomicrograph of lesion illustrated in Fig. 17.13 showing spindle cells and epithelial-lined structures.

have become reasonably consistently applied and, by students of the lesions, fairly comprehensively understood. At least consistent with the interpretation of multilocular cystic renal lesions as resulting from maturation of nephroblastoma (Wilms tumor) is the crude preponderance of both lesions in young patients and, *a priori*, the presence in some multilocular cystic lesions of tissue components that are generally considered as precursors of nephroblastoma, e.g. metanephrogenic blastema.

Against this hypothesis is that differentiation of an established nephroblastoma to a benign lesion has not been described. In reported sequential observations, the evolution has been towards less well-differentiated, rather than better differentiated lesions. Additionally, the mean age of children with multilocular cystic renal lesions is less, rather than greater than the mean age of children with acknowledged Wilms tumor, as would be expected had one lesion differentiated from another. Beckwith and Kiviat[10] state that congenital mesoblastic nephromas are grossly cystic in "most" cases. Without arguing the point of "most", I would agree that mesoblastic nephromas certainly may be grossly cystic[33,54]. Often these locules are not lined with epithelium and,

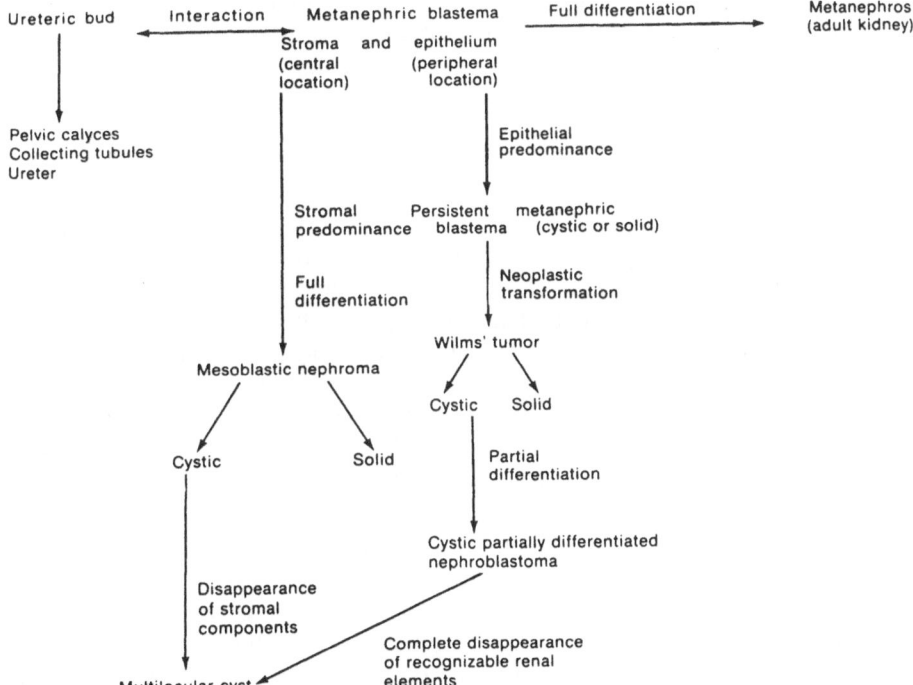

Figure 17.15 Schematic representation of relationships between various derivatives of metanephric blastema. (Reproduced with permission from Granich and co-workers, Human Pathol. 12: 1039, 1981, W B Saunders Co., publishers).

therefore, fail to qualify as multilocular renal cystic lesions[47], but multiple epithelial-lined cysts certainly occur in renal lesions that otherwise present features of mesoblastic nephroma[33]. I have seen such a case (Figs. 17.13, 17.14) and others have been described[54].

Cases of congenital mesoblastic nephroma with some features of multi-locular renal cystic lesions have compelled attractive theories of histogenesis[33] (Fig. 17.15).

Like multilocular cystic renal lesions, mesoblastic nephroma has generally had an excellent prognosis, but metastasis has been reported[37].

Some have come to the conclusion that while multilocular cystic renal lesions do not represent differentiation of a pre-existing nephroblastoma (Wilms tumor) they share with that lesion a common origin in metane-phrogenic blastema, vestiges of which may remain in various stages of differen-tiation when the lesion comes available for microscopic examination, just as nodules of persistent renal blastema may be found in cases of Wilms tumor. These features are more common in lesions from young patients.

Andrews et al.[3], in describing a case of "polycystic Wilms tumor" (their case 2) state that blastema has been reported in multilocular cystic lesions only in children. However, the case of Behr et al.[11], a 77-year-old woman, had blastema with tubular and glomerular differentiation in a multilocular cystic renal lesion interpreted by the authors as a cystic nephroblastoma.

8. Conclusions

Multilocular cystic lesions constitute a relatively circumscribed constellation of renal lesions in both children and adults. The lack of lesions from intervening ages remains unexplained, but raises legitimate questions regarding the unity of lesions that share multilocular morphology. Such lesions at different ages may well differ in pathogenesis, natural history and their very biologic nature. Practically all multilocular cystic renal lesions have an excellent prognosis after nephrectomy only. The commonest expression of lesions in the category of multilocular cystic renal lesions is a lesion in a patient of any age, which, on appropriately thorough microscopic examination, contains neither immature nor dysontogenic tissues. Such a lesion should be diagnosed "multilocular renal cyst" and diagnostic terms that imply theories of pathogenesis specifically avoided. These lesions are appropriately treated by nephrectomy alone in the expectation of an excellent prognosis. The presence of appropriate renal structures, solid or tubular, or abortive glomeruli may be taken to justify the pathologic designation "multilocular cystic nephroma" if one interprets the presence of those features as indicating a neoplastic (hence the suffix "-oma") as opposed to a dysplastic pathogenesis of the lesion.

When, as becomes increasingly likely with advances in imaging tech-niques, the diagnosis of a multilocular cystic renal lesion is suggested preoperatively, partial nephrectomy may be legitimately considered if deemed anatomically feasible. In point of fact, this will rarely become a consideration because uninvolved renal tissue usually exists as a narrow concentric rim about the cystic lesion and is not technically amenable to salvage.

Rare examples of multilocular cystic Wilms tumor are usually readily recognized and generally pose no problem either conceptually or in choosing therapy. They justify the diagnostic designation "nephroblastoma" (almost always clinical stage 1) and are appropriately treated as such, generally anticipating an excellent prognosis.

Between these two classes of lesions – namely on the one hand histologically benign multilocular renal cystic lesions with or without appropriate nephric elements, whatever their pathogenesis, and on the other hand Wilms tumors that happen to contain many epithelial-lined cysts – lies a group of biologically provocative, therapeutically controversial cases. Purely biologically, though not necessarily clinically predictively, metanephrogenic tissue (renal blastema) or dysontogenic results of non-nephric differentiation of those anlagen in a renal mass justify the designation "nephroblastoma". The degree of histologic differentiation of that precursor tissue can be descriptively characterized, and the present clinical prediction is for an excellent prognosis.

References

1. Abt, AB, Demers, LM and Shochat, J. Cystic nephroma: An ultrastructural and biochemical study. Journal of Urology 1979, 122, 539.
2. Akhtar, M and Qadeer, A. Multilocular cyst of kidney with embryonic tissue. Urology 1980, 16, 90.
3. Andrews, MJ Jr, Askin, FB, Fried, FA, McMillan, CW and Mandell, J. Cystic partially differentiated nephroblastoma and polycystic Wilms' tumor: A spectrum of related clinical and pathologic entities. Journal of Urology 1983, 129, 577.
4. Arey, JB. Cystic lesions of the kidney in infants and children. Journal of Pediatrics 1959, 54, 429.
5. Aterman, K, Boustani, P and Gillis, DA. Solitary multilocular cyst of the kidney. Journal of Pediatric Surgery 1973, 8, 505.
6. Attwood, HD and Grieve, J. Solitary multilocular cyst of the kidney. British Journal of Urology 1958, 30, 78.
7. Austin, SR and Castellino, RA. Multilocular cysts of kidney. Urology 1973, 1, 546.
8. Banner, MP, Pollack, HM, Chatten, J and Witzelben, C. Multilocular renal cysts: radiologica-pathologic correlation. Americal Journal of Roentgenology 1981, 136, 239.
9. Baldauf, MC and Schulz, DM. Multilocular cyst of the kidney. Report of three cases with review of the literature. American Journal of Clinical Pathologyol 1976, 65, 93.
10. Beckwith, JB and Kiviat, NB. Editorial. Multilocular renal cysts and cystic renal tumors. Americal Journal of Roentgenology 1981, 136, 435.
11. Behr, G and Duari, M. Cystic nephroblastoma in an adult. British Journal of Urology 1975. 47, 268.
12. Boggs, LK and Kimmelstiel, P. Benign multilocular cystic nephroma: Report of two cases of so-called multilocular cyst of the kidney. Journal of Urology 1956, 76, 530.
13. Bolande, R. Commentary: Multicystic nephroma. What it is and its relationship to Wilms tumor. Pediatric Radiology 1982, 12, 46.

14. Brown, JM. Cystic partially differentiated nephrobalstoma. Journal of Patholgy 1975, 115, 175.
15. Burrell, NL. Multilocular cysts of the kidney. Journal of Urology 1940, 43, 656.
16. Carlson, DH, Carlson, D and Simon, H. Benign multilocular cystic nephroma. Americal Journal of Roentgenology 1978, 131, 621.
17. Chang, SH. Wilms' tumor in a multilocular cyst of the kidney (cystic Wilms' tumor). Southern Medical Journal 1976, 69, 1623.
18. Christ, ML. Polycystic nephroblastoma. Journal of Urology 1968, 98, 570.
19. Coleman, M. Multilocular renal cyst. Case report, ultrastructure and review of the literature. Vichow's Archives (A) 1980, 387, 207.
20. Dainko, EA, Dammers, WR and Economou, SG. Multilocular cysts of the kidney in children. Journal of Pediatrics 1963, 63, 249.
21. Datnow, B and Daniel, WW Jr. Polycystic nephroblastoma 1976, Journal of the American Medical Association 1976, 236, 2528.
22. Davides, KC, King, LM, Siconolfi, E and Paat, F. Multilocular kidney disease; unusual angiographic appearance. Journal of Urology 1976, 116, 246.
23. Dias, R and Fernandes, M. Multilocular cystic disease of the kidney. Urology 1979, 13m 58.
24. Dobben, GD. Benign adenomatous polycystic kidney tumor (Perlmann's tumor). Radiology 1961, 76, 100.
25. Edmunds, W. Cystic adenoma of the kidney. Transations of the Pathological Society of London 1891-92, 43, 89.
26. Epstein, L, Wacksman, J, Daughtry, J and Straffon, RA. Multilocular cysts of kidney: A diagnostic dilemma. Urology 1978, 11, 573.
27. Felman, AH, Hawkins, IF Jr, Hackett, RL and Talbert, JL. Multilocular cyst of the kidney. A case report with angiographic findings. Radiology 1973, 106, 629.
28. Fobi, M, Mahour, GH and Isaacs, H Jr. Multilocular cyst of the kidney. Journal of Pediatric Surgery 1979, 14, 282.
29. Fowler, M. Differentiated nephroblastoma: Solid, cystic or mixed. Journal of Pathology 1971 105, 215.
30. Frazier, TH. Multilocular cysts of the kidney. Journal of Urology 1951, 65, 351.
31. Friday, RD, Crummy, AB and Malck, GH. Multilocular cyst. Angiographic, ultrasonic, and cyst-puncture findings. Urology 1974, 3, 354.
32. Gallo, CE and Penchansky, L. Cystic nephroma. Cancer 1977, 39, 1322.
33. Ganeck, DJ, Gilbert, EF, Beckwith, JD and Kiviat, N. Congenital cystic mesoblastic nephroma. Human Pathology 1981, 12, 1039.
34. Geller, RA, Pataki, KI and Finegold, RA. Bilateral multilocular renal cysts with recurrence. Journal of Urology 1979, 121, 808.
35. Gibson, TE. Multilocular cyst of the kidney: Case report. Transactions of the American Association for Genetourinary Surgery1961, 53, 53.
36. Gonzalez-Crussi, F, Kidd, JM and Hernandez, RJ. Cystic nephroma: Morphologic spectrum and implications. Urology 1982, 20, 88.
37. Gonzalex-Crussi, F, Sotelo-Avila, C and Kidd, JW. Malignant mesenchynal nephroma of infancy: report of a case with pulmonary metastases. American Journal of Surgical Pathology 1980, 4, 185.
38. Havers, W and Stambolis, C. Benign cystic nephroblastoma. European Journal of Pediatrics 1979, 131, 119.
39. Hunt, JB, Rao, RN, Vanderzalm, T, Smith, AM and Witherington, R. Abdominal mass in a young child. Journal of Urology 1979, 121, 482.
40. Hutchins, KR, Mulholland, SG and Edson, M. Segmental polycystic disease. New York State Journal of Medicine 1972, 72, 1850.
41. Johnson, EE, Ayala, AH, Medellin, H and Wilbur, J. Multilocular renal cystic disease in children. Journal of Urology 1973, 109, 101.

42. Joost, J, Schafer, R and Altwein, JE. Renal lymphangioma. Journal of Urology 1977, 118, 22.
43. Joshi, VV. Cystic partially differentiated nephroblastoma: an entity in the spectrum of infantile renal neoplasia. Perspectives in Pediatric Pathology 1979, 5, 217.
44. Joshi, VV, Banejee, AK, Yadev, K and Pathak, JC. Cystic partially differentiated nephroblastoma. Cancer 1977, 40, 789.
45. Kawamura, J and Miyakawa, M. Multilocular cyst of the kidney in a male infant: Report of a case. Acta Urologica Japan 1969, 15, 759.
46. Keegan, GT, Peterson, RF, Stucki, WJ and Street, L. Case report: Cystic partially differentiated nephroblastoma (Wilms' tumor). Journal of Urology 1979, 121, 362.
47. Kelly, DR. Case 2: Cystic cellular mesoblastic nephroma. Pediatric Pathology 1985, 4, 157.
48. Landing, BH. Case 11: Well differentiated and polycystic (benign?) Wilms' tumor. Cancer Seminars 1958, 2, 110.
49. Lattimer, J. In discussion of Gibson, T. Multilocular cyst of the kidney. Case report. Transactions of the American Association for Genitourinary Surgery 1961, 53, 53.
50. Lazner, J and Juriedini, KF. Benign cystic differentiated nephroblastoma in an infant. South Australia Clinics 1971, 5, 279.
51. Madewell, JE, Goldman, SM, Davis, CJ Jr, Hartman, DS, Feigen, DS and Lichtenstein, JE. Multilocular cystic nephroma: A radiologic–pathologic correlation of 58 patients. Radiology 1983, 146, 309.
52. Madewell, JE, Hartman, DS and Lichtenstein, JE. Radiologic pathologic correlations in cystic disease of the kidney. Radiology Clinics of North America 1979, 17, 261.
53. McAlister, WH, Siegel, MJ, Askin, FB, Kissane, JM and Shackelford, GD. Multilocular renal cysts. Urological Radiology 1979, 1, 89.
54. McAlister, WH, Siegel, MJ, Askin, F and Shackelford, GD. Congenital mesoblastic nephroma. Radiology 1979, 132, 356.
55. Meland, EL and Braasch, WF. Multilocular cysts of the kidney. Journal of Urology 1933, 29, 505.
56. Merten, DF, Yang, SS and Bernstein, J. Wilms' tumor in adolescence. Cancer 1976, 37, 532.
57. Osathanondh, V and Potter, EL. Pathogenesis of polycystic kidneys. Type 2 due to inhibition of ampullary activity. Archives of Pathology 1964, 77, 479.
58. Pearlman, C. Coexisting renal carcinoma and cyst. Journal of International Surgery 1964, 41, 620.
59. Perlmann, S. Uber einen Fall von Lymphangioma cysticum der Niere. Virchow's Archives 1928, 268, 524.
60. Peterson, RO. Urologic Pathology. Philadelphia: JB Lippincott Co, 1986, 29-32 and 66-68.
61. Potter, EL. Normal and Abnormal Development of the Kidney. Chicago: Year Book Medical Publishers, 1972.
62. Powell, T, Shackman, R and Johnson, MD. Multilocular cysts of the kidney. British Journal of Urology 1951, 23, 142.
63. Power, S. Cystadenoma of the kidney. British Journal of Urology 1955, 37, 285.
64. Randolph, M. Congenital multilocular renal cyst in a newborn infant. Clinical Proceedings of the Children's Hospital 1947, 3, 248.
65. Ravich, A. Multilocular tuberculous cyst of kidney. Journal of Urology 1931, 25, 223.
66. Redman, JF and Harper, DL. Nephroblastoma occuring in a multilocular cystic kidney. Journal of Urology 1978, 120, 356.
67. Robinson, GL. Perlmann's tumor of the kidney. British Journal of Surgery 1956, 44, 620.
68. Sirola, L. Simple cysts of the kidney. Report of nine cases. Annals Chirurgie Gynecologie Fenn 1957, 46, 267.
69. Slasky, BS, Penkrot, RJ and Bron, KM. Cystic mesoblastic nephroma. Urology 1982, 19, 220.
70. Stambolis, C. Cystic nephroblastoma – a benign variant of Wilms' tumor. Pathological Research Practice 1978, 163, 168.

71. Uson, AC and Melicow, MM. Multilocular cysts of the kidney withintrapelvic herniation of a "daughter" cyst: Report of 4 cases. Journal of Urology 1963, 89, 341.
72. Uson, AC, Rosario, CD and Melicow, MM. Wilms' tumor in association with cystic renal disease: Report of two cases. Journal of Urology 1960, 83, 262.
73. Wakely, CPG. Case of unilateral polycystic kidney in a child age one year and eight months. British Journal of Surgery 1930, 18, 162.
74. Wood, BP, Muurahaiven, N, Anderson, VM and Ettinger, LJ. Multicystic nephroblastoma: Ultrasound diagnosis (with a pathologic–anatomic commentary). Pediatric Radiology 1982, 12, 43.
75. Wu, SD. Mixed tumors of the kidney. Chinese Medical Journal 1938 (Suppl 2) p 193.
76. Wynn-Williams, D and Morgan AD. Lymphangioma of the kidney. British Journal of Surgery 1949, 37, 346.
77. Yanezawa, S, Tokunaga, M, Sato, E, Arima, E, Ohzono, H, Kumagai, N and Tokita N. "Cystic partially differentiated nephroblastoma" and multilocular cyst of the kidney. Report of two cases of so-called multilocular cyst of the kidney. Acta Pathologica Japan 1979, 29, 471.
78. Young, G, L'Heureux, PL and Dehner, LP. Cytstic nephroma (so-called polycystic Wilms' tumor) of childhood. A CT-pathologic study. American Journal of Pediatric Hematology and Oncology 1979, 1, 179.

Index

444